A PRACTICAL REFERENCE

For Transgender and Gender-Nonconforming Adults

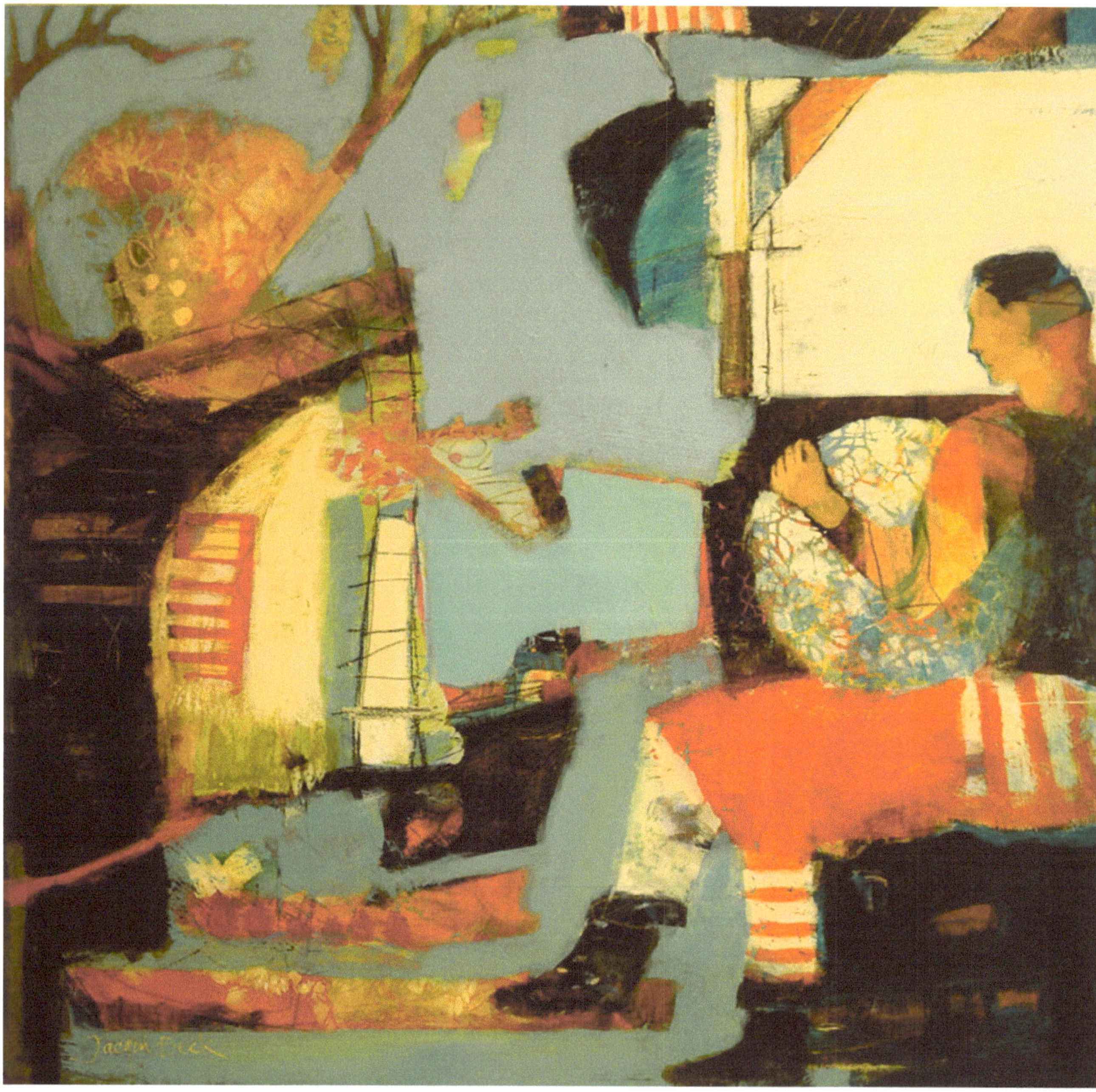

Holding the World

A PRACTICAL REFERENCE

For Transgender and Gender-Nonconforming Adults

Linda Gromko, MD

Foreword by Marsha Botzer

OTHER BOOKS BY LINDA GROMKO, MD

Complications: A Doctor's Love Story

Let Me Go When the Banter Stops:
A Doctor's Fight for the Love of Her Life

Arranging Your Life When Dialysis Comes Home:
The Underwear Factor
by Linda Gromko, MD and Jane C. McClure

Where's MY Book? A Guide for Transgender and Gender Non-Conforming Youth,
Their Parents, & Everyone Else

Bainbridge Books, Seattle, Washington

Cover image by Jacqui Beck

Print edition ISBN: 978-0-9825143-4-4
eBook edition ISBN: 978-0-9825143-5-1
Library of Congress Control Number: 2021915294

MEDICAL DISCLAIMER
This book contains general information about gender dysphoria and related medical and surgical topics. It discusses depression, suicidality, sexuality, sexually transmitted infections, and a range of other health-related topics.

This book should not, however, be relied upon to diagnose or treat any illness, condition, or disease—or to manage any postoperative complications. This is what your healthcare providers are for! Consult your healthcare practitioner before beginning any new diet or exercise program. Certainly, take this book to your healthcare provider with your questions about anything in this book. I heartily encourage you not to purchase medications online without the assistance of your healthcare provider.

The author and contributors disclaim any liability or responsibility for injury or damage to persons or property incurred, directly or indirectly, from application of any of the contents of this book. It is the reader's responsibility to know and follow the recommendations of their healthcare providers who have specific knowledge of the reader's circumstances.

DEDICATION

**This book is gratefully dedicated to my friend, David,
who has taught me important lessons about gender and life.**

David carved out a unique life against steep odds. Surviving an intolerant childhood, David transitioned gender in young adulthood at a time when very few people managed that. He became an accomplished scientist. He married his soulmate Ann, loving her throughout their life together and after her death. David nurtured his golden retriever soul dog Sam and later the rambunctious puppy named "M."

When I met him, David was in his early seventies, deliberately moving through his stealth life with stubbornness and courage. He actively pursued his personal growth, reading extensively and conquering the goblins of childhood. His world expanded with improving health, regular swimming, and new and old friendships alike.

David began attending trans support meetings at Ingersoll Gender Center. He became a champion of the youth book I wrote, *Where's MY Book? A Guide for Transgender and Gender Non-Conforming Youth, Their Parents, & Everyone Else,* donating copies for fundraising raffles and recommending the book to parents of trans youth. I imagine my books would have eased David's way, and David's support made it easier for the next person on the path.

In December of 2019, David suffered an unthinkable accident. At home with M, David fell somehow. Driving his hard head nearly through a plasterboard wall, David landed on his face and knees, forcing his head and neck into unnatural positions. David told me later he couldn't move at all. He couldn't possibly have summoned anyone even if he had had an alert necklace or his phone. Four days after that dreadful accident, a swimming buddy (Judy) thought it was odd that David hadn't shown up at the pool. It was she who initiated the police welfare check that saved David's life. The police found an immobile David and his loudly barking M. The medics transferred David to the hospital.

David had become a high quadriplegic in that split-second horror. With blood clots in his legs and his lungs, he clearly should have died.

But he didn't die.

Suddenly, "stealth" in any fashion was no longer possible and no longer protective of anything. Everything was exposed. Minute to minute, David landed on metaphorical feet, forging on with that stubborn head and sincere heart. I have never seen anyone quite as durable as David, and I've seen durable before.

I've never given a birthday book dedication before. I know he likes the idea of the book. So, to him, and in honor of all who have survived against steep odds, I dedicate this effort.

Happy Birthday, my friend.

— Linda Gromko, MD

Please see page 462 for the epilogue to this dedication.

TABLE OF CONTENTS

SECTION 4 | GENDER-AFFIRMING SURGERIES

SECTION 5 | SURVIVING AND THRIVING

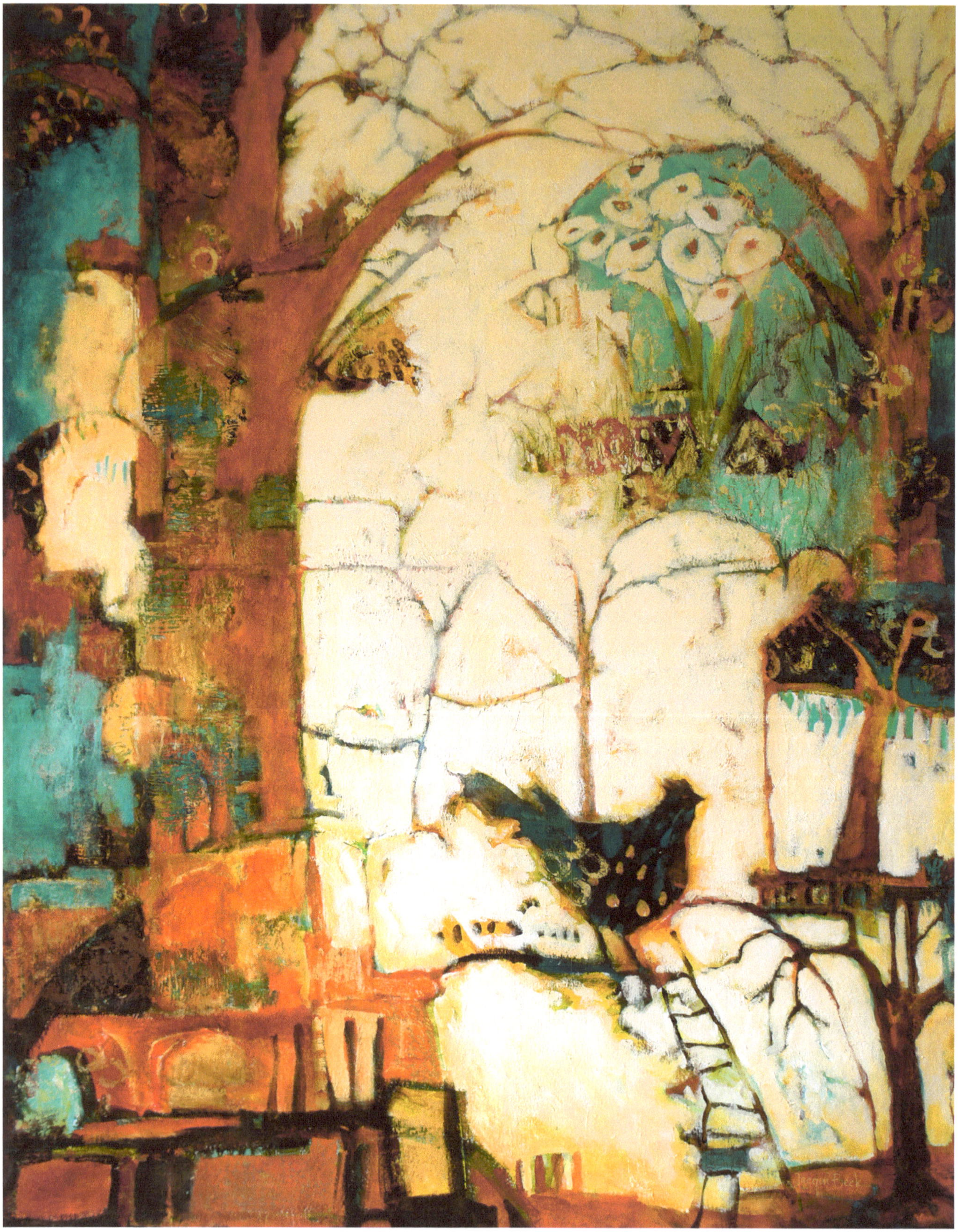

Tree House

FOREWORD

By Marsha Botzer, Founder of the Ingersoll Gender Center Seattle, Washington

Here is Dr. Linda Gromko's second great gift to our transgender and gender-nonconforming community. Her first book graciously gave families, youth, "and everyone else" an honest and dependable resource reference of great clarity. Lives changed for the better.

Now comes a truly rare thing: a companion book equal to the first, and surpassing it in the only way possible with an even wider examination of what it means to be healthy across a lifetime experience of gender and identity expression.

The focus this time is on adults and, as before, on providing assistance in the most practical and useful forms. Written discussion and visual images are offered to you in the welcoming way of a good conversation respectfully engaged. This is a book filled with art, photographs, guidance, and the wisdom that comes from learning through direct service practice over many years.

I founded Ingersoll Gender Center and still serve our organization. We are now in our fourth decade offering support and resources, and very early in our history, we saw how much we had to learn about providing effective service for the people who came to us. In the preface to Dr. Gromko's first book, I told the story of how she visited Ingersoll's weekly support group, how we talked, and how over many months a trusted professional relationship developed. By the time of her visit we had learned, often through hard-won trial-and-error experience, that we needed to take great care in choosing our professional providers. We had learned that we needed partners who could build, grow, and advance with us *together*.

Through her visit all those years ago and her resulting years of commitment to our work, Dr. Gromko has proven herself to our organization.

The world learns and changes, and our access to relevant information must keep up. Today we ask new questions about our bodies, our sexuality, and our total physical and mental health throughout our full lives. We need the latest from the worlds of medicine and research. And where once we might have hoped for only the most basic guides, today we require and rightly expect much more.

At this moment in history, I find that what matters most to me is quality care, clear support, and honest respect for all trans and gender-nonconforming people. These things are just what the new book provides. It is a source for understanding the best currently available care and medical options. Reading this book assures that you are informed as you experience, explore, and express your identity and gender. It is also a most helpful resource for those around you who care for your successful progress.

And let me offer this: Nothing in the way of service to transgender and gender-nonconforming people has come into being on its own. All of it—support, research, service, community safety, and more—is the result of work done by individuals and groups of caring people. Dr. Gromko is a wonderful part—and a superb member—of this expanding community of helpers and makers.

Please consider, if you will, that in some future time you might bring your own voice to this ongoing work. For what we have made we have made *together*, across a long mutual act of care—mind to mind, heart to heart, hand to hand.

I hope you will join the conversation offered here, that you will sit with Dr. Gromko and hear the voice of a skilled caregiver. When kindness is born from skill and love, the world is enlightened. This book is part of our journey.

— Marsha Botzer

PREFACE

A Practical Reference for Transgender Adults from an Elder Cisgender Medical Doctor

I've been involved in healthcare since I was a candy striper some 50 years ago. I graduated with a bachelor's in nursing from the University of Washington in 1973 and completed the University of Washington Family Nurse Practitioner Program in its infancy in 1975. It was during my years as a nurse practitioner and educator at Planned Parenthood that I identified a true calling to go to medical school. Not as an escape. I loved everything I did in nursing, but simply wanted to extend the depth and breadth of what I knew.

With a 2-year-old son in tow, I went back to school for the painful science prerequisites: a couple more years of chemistry, a couple of calculus courses, and a year each of physics and biology. My nursing background bought me no credit in the medical school entrance process. One advisor told me, "the kind of people who become nurses aren't the kind of people who become physicians!"

But when I started as a first-year University of Washington medical student in 1980, I realized instantly that my nursing background brought me solid advantages. For one thing, I was fluent in *speaking and writing medicine*—and its many abbreviations and expressions. Moreover, I knew how medical tasks got done, and I knew how the medical hierarchy operated.

Clinically, I had performed some 3,000 pelvic exams (and examined twice as many breasts) as a nurse practitioner at Planned Parenthood. I could confirm the duration of pregnancies with reasonable accuracy and could manage contraceptive options and treat sexually transmitted infections by rote.

Most of all, however, I recognized that my nursing background gave me the capacity to walk into any patient room at any time with something *to offer—even if that was purely my ability to interpret the language of medicine.*

After finishing medical school in 1984, I selected the University of Washington Family Practice Residency Program because I truly enjoyed all my clinical rotations in medical school. While I was drawn to obstetrics and women's healthcare, I didn't want to exclude men or children from my practice. I sought out additional experiences in psychiatry and surgery, gaining hours of extra experience in these areas.

The decision to go into family medicine wasn't a given, even at the University of Washington, which is widely known as one of the best primary care schools in the nation. When I was in medical school and expressed an interest in primary care, I remember a senior surgeon commenting, "Family practice—you'll be able to do a lot of things—*poorly*."

But I knew then—and have confirmed time and time again—that there is a critical need for first-rate generalists. Our training and experience *do* stress breadth over depth, so we primary care providers are the ones who naturally scan and see the larger picture, much as the emergency room physician does. We may be the ones who save your medical neck because we haven't forgotten to look at all the medications or treatments in your medical scenario. We may be the ones who *interpret* diagnoses and treatments on behalf of some of our specialist colleagues. And when longevity of care is involved, we are the ones who can celebrate your personal victories and ache with you in your losses because we've been right there *with* you over the years.

Besides, when you're on an airplane and a medical crisis unfolds, does the flight attendant ask if there's an ophthalmologist (eye specialist) on the plane? For my money, I hope there's a family medicine or internal medicine provider or an emergency room doctor—someone with the "scanning" skills to size up the total picture quickly and move on to a logical plan.

Good healthcare requires both *general* and *specialty care*. Neither is done in a vacuum, and neither is more important than the other. What is important is knowing what is needed for a particular patient at a particular time.

After completing my family practice residency at the University of Washington, I worked for a couple of years as an emergency room physician, and as a "moonlighter" in a clinic that defended women's reproductive freedoms. These experiences enhanced my knowledge base and procedural skills—and confirmed my gut sense that I was cut out to work for myself (perhaps not unemployable but destined to be my own boss).

I opened my sturdy little family practice in 1989, located on the foot of Seattle's Queen Anne Hill, the neighborhood where I went to high school in the 1960s. We are still located there today, 30 years later.

From experience, I now understand why doctors may *not* wish to open their own independent practices. A small medical practice is a complicated little business: gritty and rugged and fraught with insurance struggles. There's a bit of financial skydiving required with no safety nets or subsidies to protect a small independent clinic. And, as in any small business, the owner is paid last—*after* we make the staff payroll. Intent on "doing the right thing," our practice covered the staff's medical and dental insurance from day one, and the practice payroll most certainly went on my personal Visa card from time to time.

But with several superb nurse practitioners and a seasoned and loyal staff, I can attest that opening an independent family medicine practice was the perfect choice *for me*. This style of practice suited *my* temperament. It satisfied my requirement to respond urgently to patient needs without having to okay reasonable policies with anyone other than myself and my colleagues, and perhaps my malpractice insurance carrier. The "higher power" I answered to was the standard of excellent medical care. My style of practice honored a clear commitment to doing what was right for each patient at a given time. And the small size of our practice made us nimble: able to recognize problems and find practical solutions by the close of the business day.

Over the years, I have learned that family practice is messy. Humans are complicated. Responding to humans' needs and doing our level best to help them through crises takes time. We have found consistently that no single protocol fits all people. *Human time and consideration will always be the currency of exchange in good medicine.*

I have noticed that the patients who seek out care in *our* practice are sincere, contributory individuals who truly aim to make the world a better place. Rather than seeing themselves as victims of circumstance, *our* patients tend to roll up their sleeves and work on their problems. And my staff and I ride right alongside them whether the issue is a problem pregnancy, a learning variance, a career mismatch, a relationship struggle, mental illness, alcohol dependency, aging parents, or the desire to navigate the end of life with as much control as a human can have.

One day in 1998, a caller asked our receptionist, "Does Dr. Gromko treat transgender women?"

When the receptionist asked me the caller's question, I replied, "Not yet."

But I asked the receptionist to explain to the client that I was an absolute beginner in the field, and that I would be learning right along with her, and that I was likely to be learning *from* her. The caller said she was okay with all of that; very few Seattle doctors provided care for transgender clients. While I wouldn't choose to require a patient to become my teacher, it seems valid that we *always* learn from our patients. Truly, we don't stop learning until we stop listening.

As I write this, I recall that there *had* been another transgender woman who had asked if I would take her on as a patient. And I had said "no." After all, I had no training in transgender medicine in either my nursing or my medical education. At the time, it seemed medically appropriate—even responsible—to decline.

But by the time the second woman asked, perhaps only months later, it occurred to me that *my* comfort level was going to have to take second place. Here were real patients who needed care that I could learn to provide, even if it meant structuring my own learning.

Setting out to learn about transgender medicine, I contacted the three physicians I knew who might know something, *anything*, about it. I read the WPATH Standards of Care. (The World Professional Association for Transgender Health, formerly the Harry Benjamin Society, has grown to be *the* international organization that serves as a clearinghouse and educational resource for clinicians.)

Locally, I contacted Marsha Botzer, the founder of Seattle's Ingersoll Gender Center. Marsha started Ingersoll in 1979 as a self-help organization that facilitated support groups and provided participants the limited information available on where to seek therapy and medical care, and even less information on surgical care.

Marsha invited me to attend a Friday night Open Group to learn more about the transgender community. The groups typically start with an around-the-group check-in, followed by a second hour focusing on a specific issue of the group's choosing.

I went to one group and just kept going every Friday evening for several months. This became the true foundation of my transgender education.

In the group, I learned about "gatekeeping." At the time, transgender people were required to work with a therapist for a minimum of 3 months and obtain a letter in support of receiving hormone therapy. While I've always been an advocate of counseling for *everybody*, it seemed that the policy could create an adversarial relationship between therapists and clients and between clients and prescribers. I believe the policy may have sent some folks to the Internet to prescribe their own hormones, something I've seen occur less often as time has passed. Worst of all, gatekeeping seemed to imply that a client couldn't be trusted to know what was best for them.

In the groups, I learned the impact that "coming out as trans" had on relationships, particularly with spouses and children. When I joined the group in 1999, couples seemed to split apart, as if by default. It was agonizing. Over the years, this has seemed far less automatic; many people are realizing that *it's the person, not the gender identity* that counts. And many more people now seem to find that the financial realities and emotional costs of breaking up a long-term relationship are simply too high. Today, I see more couples redefining their partnerships, either expanding their own sexual identities or recharacterizing their relationships as platonic.

I learned about the day-to-day struggles of transitioning. One woman described her three painful facial electrolysis treatments per week. (Having undergone a few upper-lip electrolysis treatments in college myself, this alone would have sealed my understanding that transitioning was not "a phase.") I heard the heartbreak of casual insults and the anguish of poorly concealed slights in the workplace. I witnessed the financial hardships experienced by people even trying to get the required therapist's letter to begin hormone therapy, let alone pay for their hormones or surgeries. Such services were almost never covered back then, although they are increasingly covered now.

The most critical point I discovered in the group was that a person's gender identity is not elective. It is not a discretionary definition that a person chooses. Certainly, an individual may elect to enter into the process of gender transition. But I learned that *that* decision—that is, to transition or not—was often a life-or-death matter.

Armed with my embryonic awareness of the transgender community, I began to see more transgender clients. Word spread that there was a family doctor who had *some* information and was open to treating trans patients.

I remember the first trans male I treated. I called the University of Washington's Medcon service (a telephone consulting service for area providers) to get the little information they had, and I reviewed recommended testosterone dosing with a willing ally.

My client signed the consent form I had written (and reviewed with Ingersoll and my malpractice company). The clinic was so busy on that particular day that I had to meet my client in the clinic's baby room, which had a climbing ladder on the exam table and a floor-to-ceiling giraffe graphic in the corner. I apologized to the client, thinking he might have felt belittled by the ambiance of the infant room. But he just smiled and said,

"Well, it sort of *is* my birthday!"

From that moment on, I knew we'd be fine. Our intentions were evident, and our clientele was grateful.

In 2009, I was approached by Aidan Key, the founder of Gender Odyssey, an internationally known Seattle conference dealing with transgender issues. Aidan is also the founder of Gender Diversity, a support group network for transgender children and their parents.

It had become clear to Aidan that there was a need for providers who were willing and able to treat transgender adolescents with puberty blockers and cross-sex hormones. Aidan facilitated a trip for me and a local naturopathic physician, Christopher Bosted, ND, to travel with Aidan to Vancouver, British Columbia, to meet with Dan Metzger, MD, a Canadian endocrinologist who was an expert in the field. From Dan, I was able to learn important basic information and to confirm my understanding that many children were aware of gender asynchrony from toddlerhood. From my practice, I had witnessed repeatedly the despair of trans women who had ached to forestall the onset of secondary sex characteristics like facial hair, height, stereotypically male facial features, and a deep voice. I could attest to the misery I witnessed in trans men wearing chest binders or having menstrual periods they hated. What a benefit it might be for some of my clients to reach their gender goals at an age where costly surgeries would not become necessary, where living a *lifetime* in their true gender was a possibility.

Since then, I have learned to insert the implantable histrelin puberty blockers into the arms of early-puberty kids, to give them the gift of "pausing" the puberty process. I typically also start cross-sex hormones in young adolescents, provided they and their parents are clear and well-informed.

In 2015, I published a book entitled *Where's MY Book? A Guide for Transgender and Gender Non-Conforming Youth, Their Parents, & Everyone Else.*

My reasons for writing the book were starkly clear to me.

**Maybe it will become common for a teenager to say,
"I've always been male, but I was born with female genitals."**

For one thing, a 17-year-old trans male in our practice died by suicide. He had orchestrated his death using helium suffocation; it was not an impulsive act. In his suicide note, the young man had written that one of his greatest concerns was that he would be misgendered after death! We never saw the suicide coming, and it broke my heart. (We know that nearly half of all transgender individuals have made a suicide attempt.)[1]

The second reason was that the puberty class presented at Seattle's Children's Hospital featured the popular book *Will Puberty Last My Whole Life?* by Julie Metzger, RN, MN, and Robert Lehman, MD. It was

1 Statistics for adolescent suicide attempts from 2015 data: "Nearly 14% of adolescents reported a previous suicide attempt; disparities by gender identity in suicide attempts were found. Female to male adolescents reported the highest rate of attempted suicide (50.8%), followed by adolescents who identified as not exclusively male or female (41.8%), male to female adolescents (29.9%), questioning adolescents (27.9%), female adolescents (17.6%), and male adolescents (9.8%)." Russell B. Toomey, Amy K. Syvertsen, and Maura Shramko, "Transgender Adolescent Suicide Behavior," *Pediatrics* 142, no. 4 (October 2018): 1, https://doi.org/10.1542/peds.2017-4218.

Statistics for adult suicide attempts from 2015 data: "In a national study, 40% of transgender adults reported having made a suicide attempt. 92% of these individuals reported having attempted suicide before the age of 25." Sandy E. James et al., *The Report of the 2015 U.S. Transgender Survey* (Washington, DC: National Center for Transgender Equality, 2016), 24, https://transequality.org/sites/default/files/docs/usts/USTS-Full-Report-Dec17.pdf. Please also see https://www.thetrevorproject.org/resources/guide/preventing-suicide.

An analysis of the National Transgender Discrimination Survey (NTDS) from 2008 cites the following statistics: "Suicide attempts among trans men (46%) and trans women (42%) were slightly higher than the full sample (41%) ... the prevalence of suicide attempts is elevated among those who disclose to everyone that they are transgender or gender-nonconforming (50%)." Jody L. Herman, Ann P. Haas, and Philip L. Rodgers, *Suicide Attempts among Transgender and Gender Non-Conforming Adults* (Los Angeles: The Williams Institute, UCLA, 2014), 2, https://escholarship.org/uc/item/8xg8061f.

written directly from questions that arose from the actual puberty classes, so it was reality-based. But one half of the book was rimmed in blue for boys and the other half in raspberry pink for girls. There was little information on sexual orientation and nothing at all on gender diversity. (In fairness, this has changed some with the latest edition.)

I knew from experience that the kids I treated had been all over the Internet by the time they consulted me about gender dysphoria; they needed something more suited for them. So, *Where's MY Book? A Guide for Transgender and Gender Non-Conforming Youth, Their Parents, & Everyone Else* was born. I rated the book "R" for "Realistic."

I loved the book because it was conversational in tone and resonated with the gentle but realistic information we shared with our own patients. The book was beautifully sprinkled with the whimsical paintings of Seattle artist Jacqui Beck, who created her collection "Gender Personal" when her own child transitioned. I also appreciated the many contributions from staff, colleagues, and patients as they shared stories and practical tips to make the book more useful. Factual information on hormones, presentation, and surgery collided with the "Surviving and Thriving" chapters to create a work that has served families across the country, one Amazon purchase at a time.

The book was recognized with several awards in 2016: the ASSECT (American Association of Sexuality Educators, Counselors, and Therapists) Book of the Year; two Benjamin Franklin Silver Medals from the Independent Book Publishers Association in the categories of LGBT and Teen Nonfiction; a Gold Medal in the Global eBook competition in the category of LGBT Nonfiction; and First Place in the Health Category of the Eric Hoffer Book Award.

Through the years of the practice, we saw more and more trans women and trans men who were having gender-reassignment surgeries, both pre- and postoperatively.

One of the requisites for the surgical creation of a vagina, or vaginoplasty—at least with most surgeons—is the removal of genital hair by electrolysis or laser. The consequence of not having adequate hair removal before surgery is hair in the vagina after vaginoplasty, or medically worse, hair in the urethra after phalloplasty (the surgical creation of a penis).

One day in about 2013, I was prescribing EMLA cream (a topical numbing medicine) and a narcotic pain reliever for one of my patients to address pain during electrolysis.

In a light-bulb moment, I thought, *We could do this. And not only could we do this, we could do electrolysis and laser in-house with better anesthetic options.*

It was then that I personally took electrolysis training, as required by my malpractice insurance carrier. My partner-in-crime was one of our receptionists, Lauren Christophersen, who also trained. Lauren, it turned out, was an electrolysis savant—she was amazingly skilled right from the start.

Our practice bought two electrolysis machines. We also bought a Vectus laser that was designed exclusively for hair removal.

Then we addressed the issue of pain management. I desperately wanted hair removal in my clinic *not* to represent "yet another punishment for being transgender." My cosmetic surgery colleague, Tony Mangubat, MD, gave me the recipe for an effective prescription-strength topical medication called "BLT" (benzocaine, lidocaine, tetracaine) that could be used before painful treatments.

While at a WPATH conference in Bangkok in 2014, I spoke with surgeon Toby Meltzer. Toby showed me how to perform a spermatic cord block on a napkin during a dinner cruise. We've modified our technique over the years to do mostly scrotal field blocks, but it was a tremendous start. We have some clients who sleep through their electrolysis treatments.

Then, in Seattle, I asked the dentist upstairs in my building if he would be willing to do dental blocks for our patients before having facial electrolysis or laser hair removal.

"Linda," responded Dr. Ryan Tennant, "I'll teach you how to do it. It'll just take me a few minutes."

And while I'd never claim to be as skilled as a dentist, I can do a serviceable dental block that takes most of the trauma away from patients undergoing painful upper- and lower-lip hair removal procedures.

As time has gone on and our aesthetic offerings have become more popular, my practice envisioned other ways that we might help the trans community. We developed an approach to what we called "more affordable" aesthetics: nonsurgical procedures that could help an individual masculinize or feminize.

For example, CoolSculpting (spot-reduction of fat) can reshape a person's body contours to make them appear more masculine or feminine. It's not designed to reduce *weight*, but it can reduce the amount of fat tissue in a belly "pooch," the chin, or the flanks. A trans male, for example, might elect to reduce fat in the hips or thigh area; a trans female might choose to contour the midsection, such as the abdomen and flanks, to enhance a more feminine contour.

We learned that neurotoxins and dermal fillers can reshape a face, at least temporarily. We found that injecting neurotoxins in the strong masseter muscles of the jaw can soften the jaw and make a person look more feminine. Likewise, dermal fillers injected into the cheek area can highlight the eyes for a more feminine appearance. In contrast, and also in "off-label use," dermal fillers can create the contour of a more prominent brow bone or jaw angle for a trans man. These are much less expensive than surgical approaches; plus, surgery for masculinizing or feminizing faces is less frequently covered by insurance.

In addition to providing puberty blockers for adolescents, hormone therapy, pre- and postoperative care in gender-confirming surgeries, and trans-friendly aesthetic services, my practice has come to provide primary care for most of our transgender patients. We see cisgender people as well; in fact, I still treat young adults I delivered nearly 30 years ago.

But the point that we provide primary care for transgender patients ranging in age from 5 to 85 years is something that brings me considerable pride and satisfaction.

I have found it equally satisfying to share transgender medical information with professional colleagues. All of our staff members are culturally competent and well-versed in transgender care. Our outstanding nurse practitioners provide full transgender care, including anesthetic blocks for hair removal.

I have been lecturing in the area of transgender medicine since about 2011. Since that time, I've participated in every transgender medicine elective course at the University of Washington School of Medicine. I've spoken at Gender Odyssey in Los Angeles and Seattle, the Trans Wellness Conference in Philadelphia, and at First Event in Boston. I have delivered lectures to the University of Washington School of Nursing, the Harborview Residency Program in Emergency Medicine, Physicians' Insurance (my malpractice carrier), the Washington Association of Osteopathic Medicine, the Washington Physician Assistants Association, and even the Annual Dialysis Conference and the northwest chapter of the American Nephrology Nurses Association. In total, this has amounted to over 70 lectures on transgender medicine delivered to healthcare workers.

In recent years, I've heard folks lament that there aren't enough transgender healthcare providers. I couldn't agree more, and there will be *many* more in short order. As it stands, we *do* have outstanding transgender providers who offer a personal sensitivity I can only imagine.

For now, I am grateful to have been present in the somewhat early days of transgender medicine, appreciating and responding to the needs of an amazing community of people. Having worked with the transgender and gender-nonconforming community for 20 years, I'm hoping for 20 more.

With great personal respect for a most resilient community,

— Linda Gromko, MD

Queen Anne Medical and Transformative Aesthetics
200 West Mercer #104
Seattle, Washington 98119

Linda@LindaGromkoMD.com
LindaGromkoMD.com (Website and blog)
QueenAnneMedicalAssociates.com (Office)

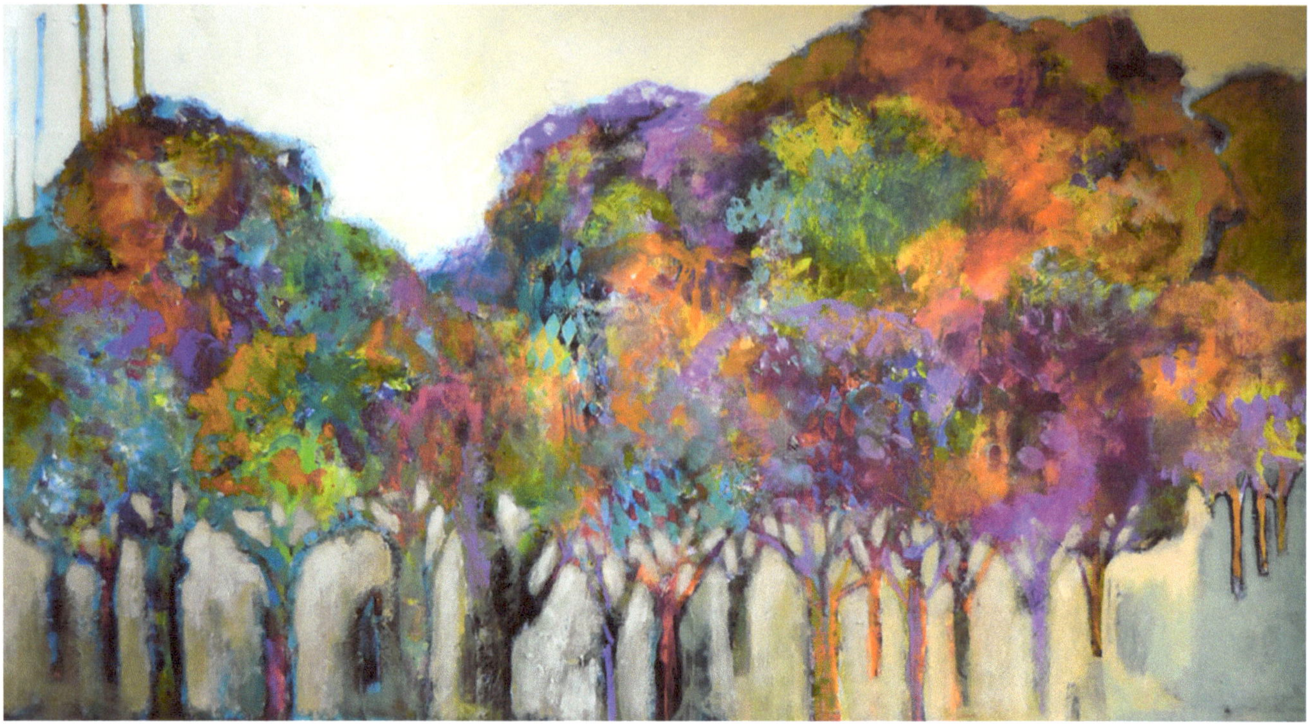

In the Trees

INTRODUCTION

How to Use This Book

If you are reading this book, you are likely examining issues of gender in your life or in the life of someone you care about. Perhaps you have identified as transgender, at least on some level, since you were a small child. Perhaps you were aware of this as simply a feeling that "something was different" for you. Maybe your gender identification has been evolving, becoming clearer as time has passed. Like many people, you may have begun to realize that being transgender is a real thing, and that there are positive steps that can be taken to relieve the gender dysphoria you've experienced. You've known or read about other adults who have transitioned. Or possibly, you have witnessed the transition of teenagers who see the promise of a gender-synchronous life that was only a dream until now.

(For efficiency, I'll be using the term "transgender" throughout this book. Consider this term—for this reading anyway—to represent "transgender and gender-nonconforming." I'll be discussing the dilemmas of language in a later chapter. I apologize for any offense or discomfort this may cause for anyone.)

I am a board-certified family practice doctor with more than 30 years of experience as a physician, plus two nursing degrees before that. I have worked with the transgender community since 1998, and I have come to value and respect the community enormously.

If you have read my earlier book for trans youth (*Where's MY Book? A Guide for Transgender and Gender Non-Conforming Youth, Their Parents, & Everyone Else*), you will recognize that my writing style is blunt. I rated the earlier book as "R" for "Realistic." Because I wrote *this* book for adults, it goes a bit further, maybe an "R-plus." (Genitalia and sexuality will be given more prominent roles.) I believe that if we cannot be clear about information, we cannot possibly be effective in sharing the information that counts.

Please understand that this book is not intended as a substitute for working with your healthcare provider. Your medical situation is unique; your healthcare provider can tailor recommendations specifically to you and your circumstances.

Nor is this book intended to represent a scholarly work. You will find excellent resources cited, of course, and ways to tap into academic works if that's what you need. Rather, this book is intended to serve as a friendly collection of information and practical tips to help you through your journey; things a benevolent big sister might tell you.

Much of the information in this book will likely be a review for you; some of the information may be new territory. Some information may apply to you, and some won't. You may certainly disagree with me; let me know if you'd like to discuss something I've written. And please do tell me if you find something that is incorrect or offensive to you.

If you read my earlier book, you will undoubtedly find repetition and full-on plagiarism of the first book. Scan the content; read the book cover-to-cover; skip around. Take what is useful for you. Use the book as a springboard from which to formulate new questions and gather more information.

You will find that this book is divided into five major subject areas:

1. Basic information about gender identity, sexual orientation, gender dysphoria, and a review of both puberty and the treatment of transgender children and youth.

2. Basic information about hormones.

3. Presentation: the nonsurgical things people can do to feminize or masculinize one's appearance.

4. Surgical treatments: gender-affirmation surgeries, along with preoperative and postoperative considerations.

5. Surviving and thriving: an assembly of information too diverse to characterize. This section deals with sex and relationships, work, fertility preservation, education, name and document changes, and safety—in short, a variety of factors that may help in very practical ways. (If you can find even a couple of tidbits that make your life better, I will have done my job.)

Please understand that this book was not intended to be the "only reference you'll ever need." There are whole segments of information that have not been included, not because they aren't important, but rather because the field is so broad that there is simply far too much to cover. You'll detect the flavor born of a "beige little practice in the heart of high-tech Seattle"—that is, mostly Caucasian with a well-represented computer industry. Please tell me what you notice and how this book might have been more valuable to you.

Know that this book has drawn from a host of contributors: physicians who were kind enough to review the book for accuracy, my years of clinical practice with the transgender and gender-nonconforming community, and the stories and helpful gems of personal advice from willing clients.

I wish you the very best in your journey and hope that this book will help you along the way.

—Linda Gromko, MD

Challenges with Online Links and Internet References

Even though all online links to reference citations and websites were checked and current at the time of the book's printing, some may no be longer available. And if we've linked to a periodical reference, the reference may have changed. What to do?

- Try entering the title or topic in the search bar of your browser.
- If an address of a link is spread out over two lines, you may have to type in the whole link to get it to work.

SECTION I

GENDER, SEXUAL ORIENTATION, PUBERTY, AND GENDER DYSPHORIA

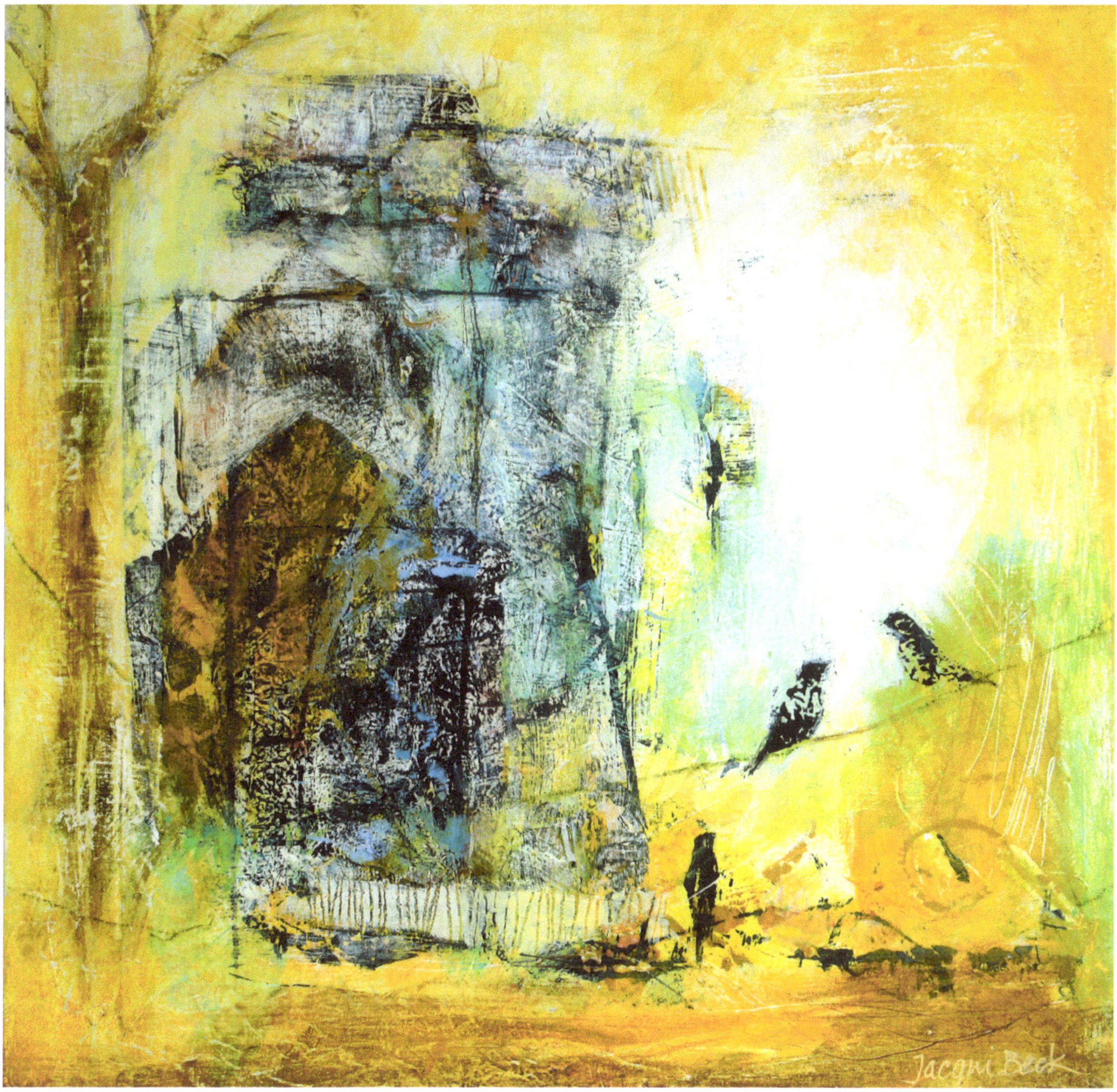

Avian Gossip

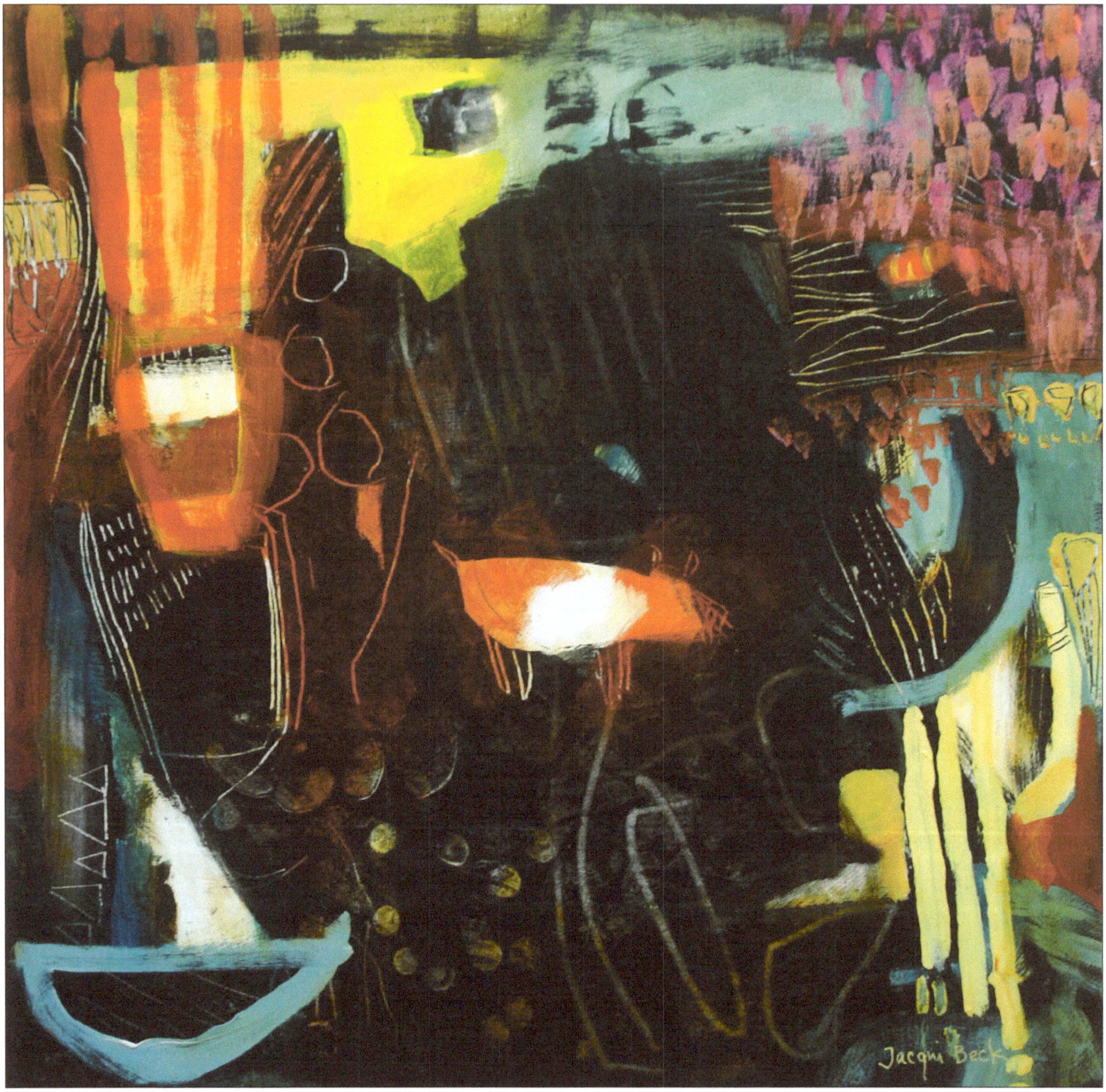

In the Very Middle

CHAPTER 1

The Critical 911 Message

What a way to begin a book for transgender adults! If this startles you, let me remind you that nearly half of all transgender individuals report that they *have* made a suicide attempt. If *you* have attempted suicide, or if you have even thought of taking your own life, *the fact that you are reading this book makes you a* **survivor**.

As an adult experiencing gender dysphoria, you may have experienced a great deal of frustration and distress in your life. Perhaps life has felt impossible, or at least unmanageable. You may be afraid that moving into transition more fully may make your life that much more tenuous. You may worry about your relationships, your children, your parents, your work. Will these parts of your life survive transition?

Then again, will you be able to survive *without* transitioning?

These are enormous questions, but they are questions with answers. Whether you acknowledge it or not, you have enormous impact on how your life will unfold. With care and planning, you will be able to come as close to getting what you want as is humanly possible. And this book is designed to get you the correct information if and when you need it.

I know that things can work out for transgender adults and their families because I've seen it happen time and again. I've seen rejecting partners come to the careful realization that happiness in a relationship means that both partners are happy. Both partners *can* get their needs met, although it requires love and understanding—and perhaps a measure of creativity and compromise. I've seen elderly parents buy their adult children gender-appropriate gifts. I've heard the story of a grandchild exclaiming delightedly, "You're so much more fun since you've been *Grandma* Bob!"

I've seen workplaces welcome and support their transgender employees. Many Seattle-based companies demonstrate that commitment by providing comprehensive insurance for gender-affirming surgeries. I've seen companies terminate cisgender employees for making critical and ignorant comments about their transgender coworkers.

Don't get me wrong; I've witnessed the nightmares also. But the point is that things are getting better and they don't have to end badly by default.

But all this envisioning and problem-solving is for later.

I want you to know what to do if you are having dark thoughts of dying **right now**. *I want you to know what to do so that your life has all the possibilities I know it can have!*

What to Do If You Are Having Thoughts about Wanting to Die

- **Please talk to another human right away. Having these thoughts is, after all, a life-threatening emergency. The life that is threatened is *yours*.**

  If you do not have a sympathetic friend, spouse, or counselor available to you right now, call a suicide hotline like one of these:

> Trans Lifeline: **1-877-565-8860**
>
> Crisis Connections (formerly Crisis Clinic): **1-866-427-4747**
>
> National Suicide Prevention Lifeline: **1-800-273-8255**
> They also have an online chat service at
> suicidepreventionlifeline.org/chat
>
> Your nearest city or town likely has one also, and
> **if you cannot locate the number, call 911.**

- **Talk to your doctor or healthcare provider and ask directly for their help.**

  Tell your healthcare provider what you have been thinking. Saying something like, "I've been having dark thoughts and I'm not sure I can go on" should make a healthcare provider sit up and take notice. This is an emergency.

  But if anyone should *minimize* this in any way, say, "I mean it. I am thinking about dying. I'm not sure I can keep from doing something to harm myself."

  At this point, your healthcare provider should be asking you if you have a specific suicide plan and should be assessing the lethality of that plan. They should be asking about your support resources.

  They may want to speak with you about taking antidepressants if you are not taking them already. They may want to get you to a counselor who deals regularly with people in crisis. And if your situation is immediate, they may facilitate your admission to a hospital to help keep you safe.

  At least in Washington State, a healthcare provider cannot just admit you directly into a psychiatric facility without your consent. As a physician, for example, I would be required to contact the local mental health professional (now called the Designated Crisis Responder or DCR) via the Crisis Clinic. The MHP (now the DCR) by law would determine if a temporary involuntary admission is in order—specifically if an individual is homicidal, suicidal, or gravely psychiatrically disabled. This regulation protects a person from a lengthy involuntary commitment without a patient-centered review.

Important: If your healthcare provider does not seem to take your concerns seriously, go to another provider.

- **Get a transgender-friendly counselor or healthcare provider if you do not have one already.**

  While it may not be critical for every transgender person to have a transgender-sensitive provider, it may help you in the long run. You do not have to leave your current provider. But if they do not have the information you need, you may want to see a transgender-friendly provider also.

  If you do not know of such providers in your area, search something like "transgender services in (your area)." I've seen human resources staff find this information for their employees. In Seattle, look up the Ingersoll Gender Center (ingersollgendercenter.org) for a list of counseling and medical providers. You can do the same thing anywhere in the world by going to wpath.org and looking for WPATH members in your area.

- **Go to a hospital emergency room.**

  In Seattle, you can go to any hospital emergency room and say, "I am thinking about hurting myself." They are required to assess you and get you appropriate care. This is their job!

- **Call 911.**

  The 911 dispatcher can get you in touch with other resources or dispatch on-site assistance if needed. You may have a 211 line in your area that can connect you to appropriate resources on a less urgent basis.

- **Don't let anyone make fun of you or belittle your concerns.**

  Sometimes, a family member or healthcare provider will dismiss your concerns. Perhaps this is their way of soothing *themselves*; suicide is frightening and it's easy to say, "Oh, it can't be all that bad."

  But I know that it *can* be that bad. Your feelings are real and deserve to be taken seriously. You deserve to get care from kind and informed people who recognize your potential to have a whole and satisfying life.

- ***Know that your family will be better off with you alive,* whatever has happened in the past, and whatever you might have ever done.**

  I have heard patients state that their children would be better off with a life insurance payout than with a transgender parent.

  Wrong!

  I remember hearing an expression that goes something like this: "The person who suicides finds peace perhaps, but the rest of the world picks up the pieces!"

  There is little that is more difficult for a child or family to deal with than the death of a parent by suicide. Children tend to blame themselves: "If I had been a better kid, my parent would still be alive." Many family members suffer for the rest of their lives, second-guessing what they might have done to prevent the suicide.

But when it's "game over"—when you end your life out of despair—there's no possibility of resolution as we know it.

- **Take measures to safeguard yourself.**

  If you have lethal weapons in your home, ask a trusted friend to keep them for you. Alcohol, which makes us more depressed anyway, clouds our decision-making. Be cautious of your drinking if you are depressed. The same goes for recreational drugs, particularly opiates. Be mindful also of your driving; can you be reasonably certain that nothing will happen to you "by accident"?

  If you are reading this book in the interest of a family member, you may want to quietly remove or disarm weapons or stockpiled medications and put them in a safe place.

  And if opiates are a concern, buy Narcan (naloxone) to have on hand. In most states, Narcan (nasal spray or injection) can be purchased without a prescription. This drug can abort an opiate overdose, saving your life or that of someone you love.

"Anything Else!"

I have a wonderful transgender adult patient in our practice who thinks about suicide every single day. Finally, rather than asking her *if* she was having thoughts of killing herself, I began to ask her, *"What are you doing* **when** *you think about taking your own life?"* Her perfect answer: *"Anything else!"*

That conversation occurred over 5 years ago. My patient struggles daily, but she is still very much alive. "Anything else" for her might mean taking a walk, playing with her dog, talking to her spouse, or surfing the Internet.

"Anything else" for another person might be making cookies, going to a movie (by yourself even), drinking a glass of ice water, taking a bubble bath, getting a tattoo, painting toenails, going to the mall, looking up trans information on YouTube, going on a nature hike, visiting the library, binge-watching *Orange Is the New Black* again, playing music, or doing anything safe that just keeps you going on to the next minute.

**The point is that life can get better—
but only if you're breathing.**

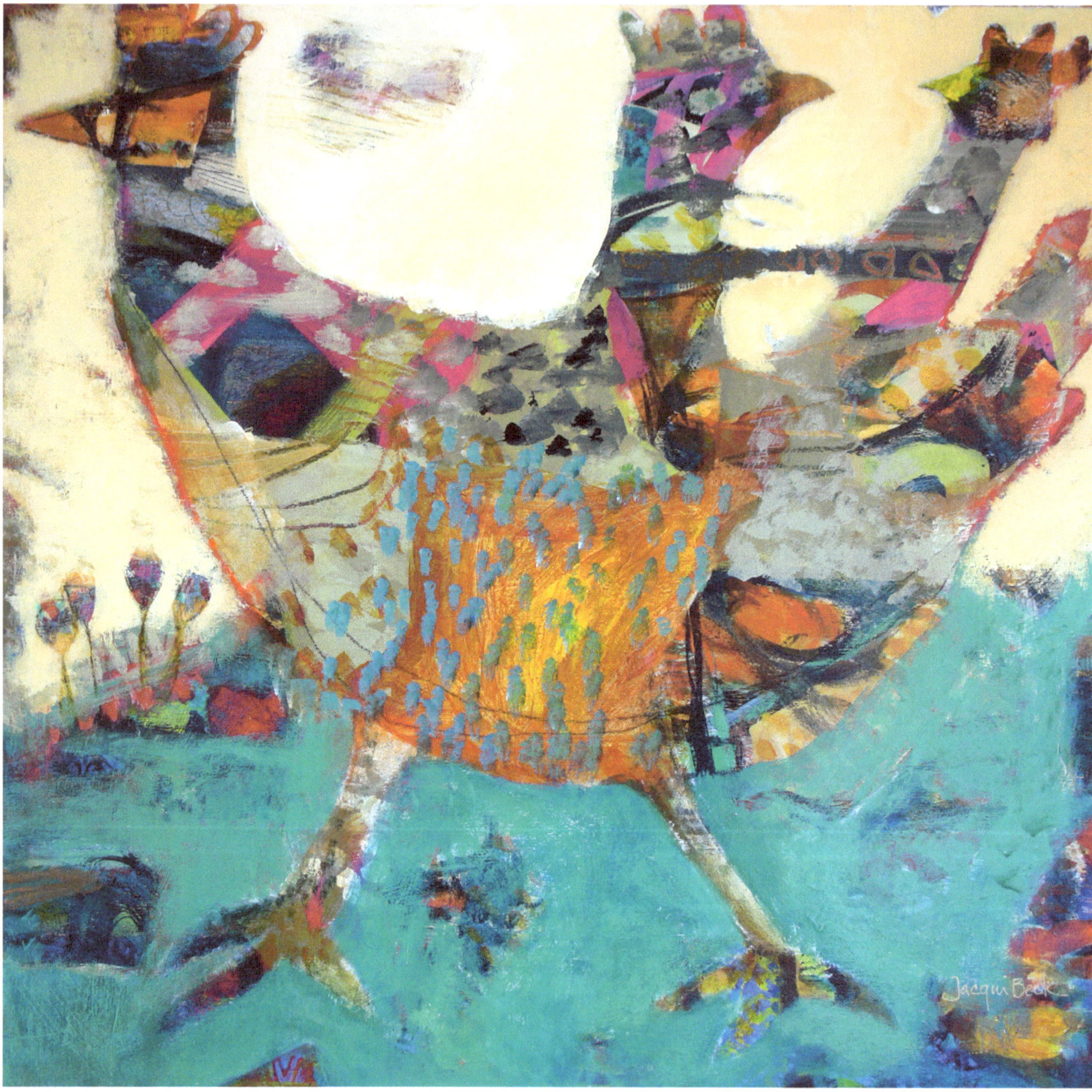

Chicken Connection

CHAPTER 2
Defining Gender

What "Gender" Means

In the most basic terms, gender is whether you were born a boy or a girl. Gender might also be called "sex." This, of course, does not mean that the gender assigned or recorded at your birth is the gender you identify as your own. How *you* identify is what's important. And how you identify is defined by you—and only by you.

The Language Conundrum

Before we go any further, I'd like to comment about the language of gender and the terms we use.

Over the time I've been working with the transgender community, I've seen many evolutions of language. Terms that were acceptable years ago have become "fighting words" today. Terms that were once supportive have become insulting.

So, what's a well-meaning person to do? Here are some thoughts that may help:

- Ask, "What would you like to be called?" or "How would you like to be addressed?" when it comes to addressing *another* person.
- Ask a person what pronouns they use. By pronouns, of course, I mean "he, him," "she, her," "they, them." There are others too, but this is a good start.

Why Using "They" Is Important

It can be confusing when an individual person uses "they" to refer to themself. Using a plural word to describe a singular person would have been a grammar error in school. In the global scheme of things, it may not matter all that much; it just sounds wrong. But it certainly does matter to the individual who requests these pronouns because they are experiencing gender dysphoria with more traditional pronouns.

If you have trouble using the plural "they" to describe a singular person, this would be a good time for you to let it go.

You are feeling awkward; the other person is in pain.

- Think about the pronouns you feel most comfortable with or appreciate most, if we're talking about *you*. To help people remember, kindly remind them—or buy a pronoun lapel pin online (search "pronoun label pin" at etsy.com).

- Ask a transgender community leader or consult a website like ingersollgendercenter.org or transequality.org to see what terminology they use. They are likely to be most current.

- Apologize sincerely and move on if you misgender someone or otherwise insult them without meaning to. This is most important. (And remember, transgender people misgender themselves and one another by mistake also.)

As of this writing, the terminology of the day includes ***transgender, cisgender, gender fluid, gender-nonconforming, and nonbinary.*** But don't hold your breath; this terminology may change soon.

The Trans Language Primer

The language dilemma is at the core of the Trans Language Primer (TLP). Founded by editor-in-chief Greyson Simon in 2016, the TLP grew out of the recognized need for a "resource that could be utilized by the community ... as well as our cohorts and the medical, mental health, and social professionals working with us." From its early beginnings hosted by Outshine NW, the TLP expanded in 2017 to become a dynamic Google document. Further help from the Transgender Justice Funding Project in 2018 allowed the TLP to expand to the robust website seen today (translanguageprimer.com). The TLP is also supported by patrons (patreon.com/TransLanguagePrimer).

According to Simon, "Providing up-to-date working definitions ... has already helped bridge the gap (between the community and supportive professionals) as well as helped questioning fledglings find their way in a vibrant community." (See the Transgender Language Primer at the end of this book.)

The Terms "Transgender" and "Cisgender"

"Cis" comes from the Latin language and means on the side of, or on the *same* side of something. In the context of gender, "cisgender" would refer to a person who was born with male genitals and identifies as male. "Cisgender" would also refer to a person who was born with female genitals and identifies as female. For cisgender people, the assigned gender *and* their identified gender match.

Transgender, on the other hand, would refer to a person who was born with male genitals (assigned male at birth or AMAB) but identifies as female, or a person who was born with female genitals (assigned female at birth or AFAB) but identifies as male. Of course, it isn't as easy as all that. But, again, it's a place to start.

Other Terms People Use to Describe Gender

Although terminology is in flux, look at the following list and my personal comments that follow.

- **Assigned male at birth (AMAB) or assigned female at birth (AFAB)**
  I've never really liked these labels, but they seem to have stuck. AMAB and AFAB are labels that refer ***to how a baby's genitals are identified at birth by the birth attendant***—that is, usually the delivering doctor or midwife.

The terminology further assumes that the doctor or midwife has made an *accurate* identification of the genitals when examining the baby. (We know that some babies may have genitals that are hard to classify, specifically in the cases of ambiguous genitalia—or in babies with "disorders of sex development"—earlier known as intersex.

Rather than announcing in a delivery room, "It's a boy!" we should really announce, "It's a baby human with male genitals!"

- **Recorded male at birth (RMAB) or recorded female at birth (RFAB)**
  This is a variation of the first term, above.

- **Born male or born female (or natal male or natal female)**
  I had liked these terms initially and occasionally still use them. But when I used "natal male" and "natal female" in my youth book, I learned that some people were genuinely offended.

  Today, I believe that when we say that someone is "born male" or "born female," we infer information that is broader in scope than that which is limited to a person's genitals. It implies that all-male or all-female attributes, expectations, and "privilege" (or lack thereof) are extended without buy-in from the person involved.

- **Testicle-bodied or ovary-bodied**
  You really may not know if a baby has testicles or ovaries unless you perform an ultrasound examination to determine this. Testicles do not always descend into the scrotum by the time of birth; ovaries are in the abdomen and are not externally visible. Without these exams, we are making assumptions.

- **Genetic male or genetic female**
  When we refer to *genetics*, it assumes that we know the chromosomal makeup of the individual in question. In truth, we usually do not know the chromosomal makeup of ourselves or anyone else.

  To use the term "genetic male" correctly, we represent that the individual in question has both one X and one Y chromosome. To use the term "genetic female" correctly, we represent that the individual has two X chromosomes. To learn this, you must have access to a person's karyotype, or the number and types of chromosomes a person has. A karyotype can be evaluated from a sample of blood, cells from the cheek (buccal mucosa), amniotic fluid that surrounds a baby before birth, or the chorionic villi (placental precursor cells sampled near the end of the first trimester of pregnancy). So, it's obvious that this information may not be readily available.

  I've had several patients who have asked to have their karyotypes tested from their blood. This is usually not covered by insurance, but it seems to be important information for some people.

  Let's dig a little deeper. (Please skip ahead if your eyes are glazing over.)

  Whenever we talk about "genetic" anything, we are talking about biology—about chromosomes and DNA (deoxyribonucleic acid). As humans, we each have 23 *pairs* of chromosomes (46 chromosomes in all) in the nucleus of almost every cell in our bodies (mature red blood cells do not have nuclei). The very important exceptions to this are the egg (ovum) and sperm (spermatozoon) cells; they have 23 chromosomes each but combine at fertilization to make the total of 46 chromosomes. Thus, 23 chromosomes from the egg and 23 chromosomes from the sperm combine to make up the 46 chromosomes in a fertilized egg that can develop to become a full human.

Each chromosome is packed with DNA that contains the coding information that "tells" our cells what to do and how to make new cells. Your DNA, for example, tells what proteins to make. DNA tells your body what color hair to grow, how tall to grow, or what color eyes you'll have. Very importantly, DNA contains the instructions for a cell to repair itself. This reparative information is critical for cells to live and function normally.

One pair of chromosomes is called the *sex chromosomes*. These are called X and Y chromosomes because of their shape (refer to Figure 2.2 of the human karyotype on page 14). If you were assigned male at birth, you likely have an X and a Y chromosome making up the pair of sex chromosomes. If you were assigned female, you probably have two X chromosomes in this pair.

It is important to know that there are other variations of this, too. These are often referred to as disorders of sex development (DSD) or intersex. Excellent resources include the Intersex Society of North America at **isna.org** and **accordalliance.org**.

So, by looking at a baby's genitalia, you really may not know for *sure* if that particular baby has an X and a Y chromosome (XY), two X chromosomes (XX), one X chromosome only (XO), an X with two Y chromosomes (XYY), or two X chromosomes and a Y chromosome (XXY). You *can* get this information, as stated earlier, through a karyotype evaluation.

But to be medically factual, if you don't have these details, you may not know for certain.

Most of the time, when a parent knows the sex or gender of their baby before birth, it's because they saw a penis or vaginal labia on the baby's ultrasound during pregnancy. Ultrasounds are painless sound wave tests that can tell us a lot of very important information about a baby before birth, like whether the heart and brain look normal, whether the baby has a normal spine, and other things that are critical for a baby's development. Penises and labia (the outer lips of the vagina) are visible also. You've probably heard about "gender reveal parties" where new parents announce the visible gender of their babies during mid-pregnancy. Wouldn't it be great to see a "healthy vital organs" party instead?

Again, the fact that a baby has a penis does not necessarily confirm that their sex chromosomes are XY. Babies with the intersex variations of XXY or XYY will also have penises visible on ultrasound. And a baby may have both labia and the sex chromosomes XO.

For this book, we *assume* that a penis equals the karyotype XY and a vagina equals the karyotype XX. But we must fully acknowledge that an assumption isn't always correct.

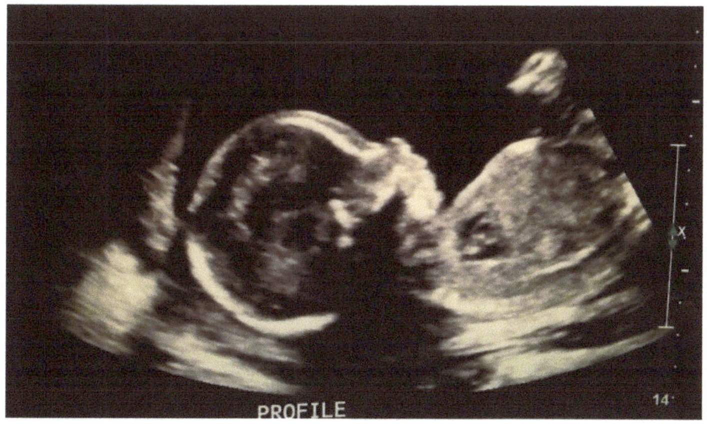

Ultrasound fetal head

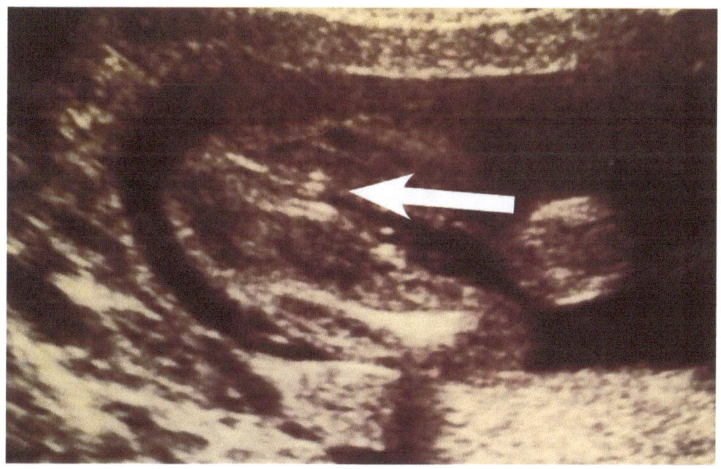

Ultrasound labia (left of the arrow)

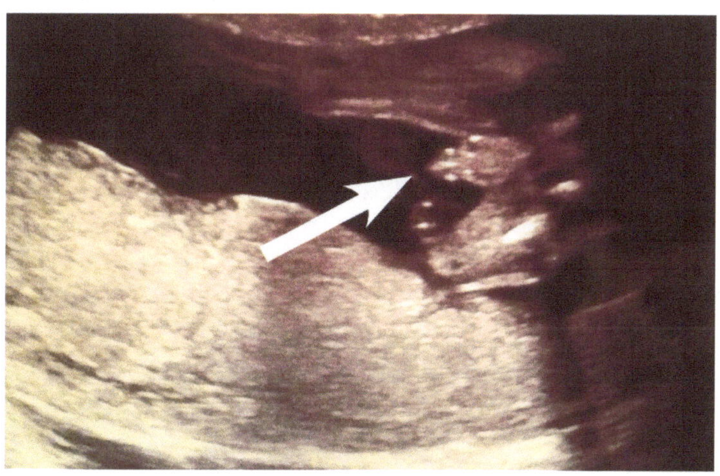

Ultrasound penis (right of the arrow)

Figure 2.1. Gender anatomical characteristics in the fetus.

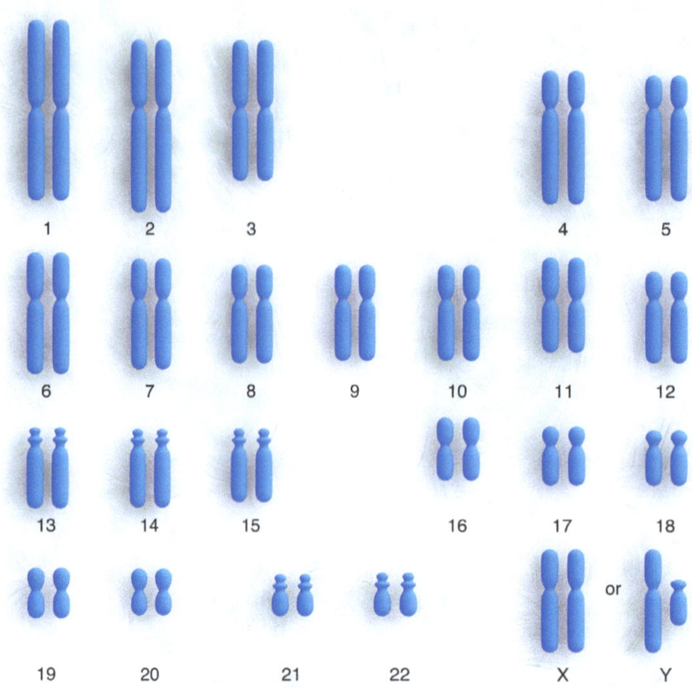

Figure 2.2. Human karyotype, 46 XY.

Defining Gender Identity

Gender identity is whether you see *yourself* as a boy or man, as a girl or woman, as neither, or somewhere in between.

Because gender identity isn't always that clear-cut, many people see gender identity as a continuum. You might think of the gender continuum as a line with "male-identified" on one end and "female-identified" on the other. Many people see themselves definitively on one end or the other. "Gender binary" refers to people who identify strictly as male or strictly as female.

The Gender Continuum

Let's examine this gender continuum diagram:

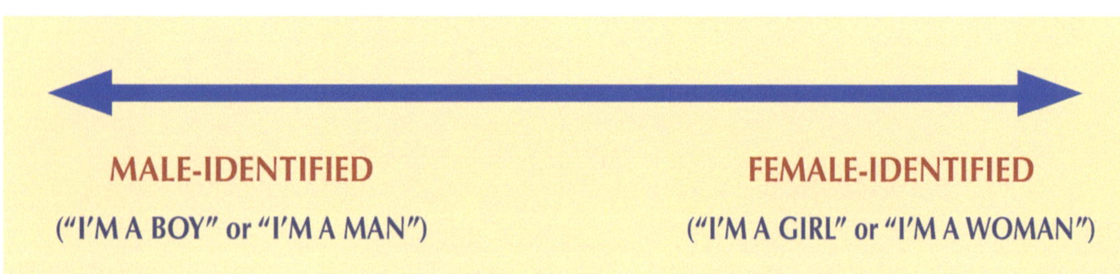

Figure 2.3. The gender continuum.

Some people find themselves somewhere along the continuum, but not strictly at either end. And many people feel that they move along the line of the gender continuum, identifying as more male at certain times and more female at other times. This may vary according to what you're doing, who you're with, your mood, and so on. This is often termed being "gender-fluid." You might hear terms like "male of center" or "female of center."

There are many terms people use to describe themselves. Facebook, for example, has over 50 ways to denote gender identity. While that's probably too many for practical use, it demonstrates how important it is for people to be able to define their own gender identity and the words they select to describe it.

What If You Don't Identify with Either Gender?

Many people do not identify with *either* gender. They may refer to themselves as "nonbinary" and use the pronouns "they" or "them."

Most people—including most trans people—do identify as being either male or female. But, according to the National Center for Transgender Equality, "... some people don't neatly fit into the categories of 'man' or 'woman,' or 'male' or 'female.' For example, some people have a gender that blends elements of being a man or a woman, or a gender that is different than either male or female. Some people don't identify with any gender. Some people's gender changes over time.

"People whose gender is not male or female use many different terms to describe themselves, with nonbinary being one of the most common. Other terms include genderqueer, agender, bigender, and more. None of these terms mean exactly the same thing—but all speak to an experience of gender that is not simply male or female."[2]

What Does Gender-Nonconforming Mean?

Gender-nonconforming (GNC) is a blurry umbrella term. While gender identity describes how we identify or how we define our gender, GNC relates more to how we express our gender. Referring to the Transgender Language Primer (**translanguageprimer.org**), a person who is gender-nonconforming is "someone who does not fully conform to the expectations around their gender that their society enforces.

This may be, but is not limited to, expression, roles, or some other aspect of gender. Being GNC is distinct from being transgender, though some trans people may consider themselves gender-nonconforming." (See the TLP at the end of this book.)

The concept of gender conformity as opposed to nonconformity relies heavily on stereotypes and is constantly changing.

2 National Center for Transgender Equality, "Understanding Non-Binary People: How to Be Respectful and Supportive," *Issues and Resources*, October 5, 2018, https://transequality.org/issues/resources/understanding-non-binary-people-how-to-be-respectful-and-supportive.

Listing Yourself as Nonbinary in an Official Capacity

Jamie Shupe of Oregon applied to the Oregon Department of Motor Vehicles to be listed as nonbinary in 2016. When the DMV refused, Shupe asked a Multnomah County judge for a new gender designation: nonbinary. Shupe won and was probably the first person in the United States to be legally nonbinary, at least for state identification and the driver's license. (Shupe subsequently transitioned back to a gender identity of male.[3])

You can now be listed as "nonbinary" or "Gender X" in other states as well: Washington, Oregon, California, and Washington, DC.

Gender X is a term used to encompass "a gender that is not exclusively male or female, including, but not limited to, intersex, agender, amalgagender, androgynous, bigender, demigender, female-to-male, genderfluid, genderqueer, male-to-female, neutrois, nonbinary, pangender, third sex, transgender, transsexual, two-spirit, and unspecified."[4]

Can a person identify as gender nonbinary for purposes of their birth certificate, social security number, or passport? A nonbinary passport designation is coming soon.[5] For the most current information on changing your official documents, go to **transequality.org** and refer to the "Documents" section.

A third gender option is legally available in India, Pakistan, Australia, and Germany.

Defining Oneself as Agender

A person calls themself "agender" when they don't identify with or conform to a stereotypical gender at all.

Eunuchs

A eunuch is someone who was assigned male at birth and is presumably a genetic male (XY). A eunuch is medically or surgically castrated to remove testicles and sometimes the penis (medical castration means that antitestosterone medication was used to essentially eliminate testosterone in a person's bloodstream).

Historically, eunuchs were castrated males who served harems of women who were the property of kings. Without testicles, eunuchs posed no genetic threat to the lineage of the king. Eunuchs could not reproduce and they presumably had less sex drive. This made them less threatening and they occupied positions of trust with royalty. Some eunuchs were reported to have been castrated before puberty, eliminating the development of the secondary sex characteristics, such as a low voice, facial hair, and adult-sized genitalia.

In modern times, eunuchs are AMAB individuals who are voluntarily castrated by medical or surgical means. Sometimes treated with testosterone and estradiol, eunuchs do not identify as female but rather are gender-neutral or male individuals who wish to eliminate the effects of testosterone.[6]

---

3 Jamie Shupe, "I Was America's First 'Nonbinary' Person. It Was All a Sham," *The Daily Signal*, March 10, 2019, https://www.dailysignal.com/2019/03/10/I-was-Americas-first-non-binary-person-it-was-all-a-sham.

4 Linley Sanders, "What Is Gender X? New Identity Is Accepted in These States, and Washington and Vermont Could Be Next," *Newsweek*, January 19, 2018, https://www.newsweek.com/gender-x-new-identity-states-washington-vermont-775221.

5 Kate Sosin, "U.S. to Add 'X' Gender Marker on Passports," *The 19th*, June 30, 2021, https://19thnews.org/2021/06/u-s-to-add-x-gender-marker-on-passports/.

6 Richard J. Wassersug and Thomas W. Johnson, "Modern-Day Eunuchs: Motivations for and Consequences of Contemporary Castration," *Perspectives in Biology and Medicine* 50, no. 4 (Autumn 2007): 544–56, http://doi.org/10.1353/pbm.2007.0058.

As with any gender-related medical treatment, readers are strongly advised not consider do-it-yourself treatments and to remember that adequate hormone levels are necessary to maintain good bone health.[7]

Gender nullification surgery (informally called "the Smoothie") is available through some surgeons who specialize in gender-affirmation surgeries (see page 250 in Chapter 11).

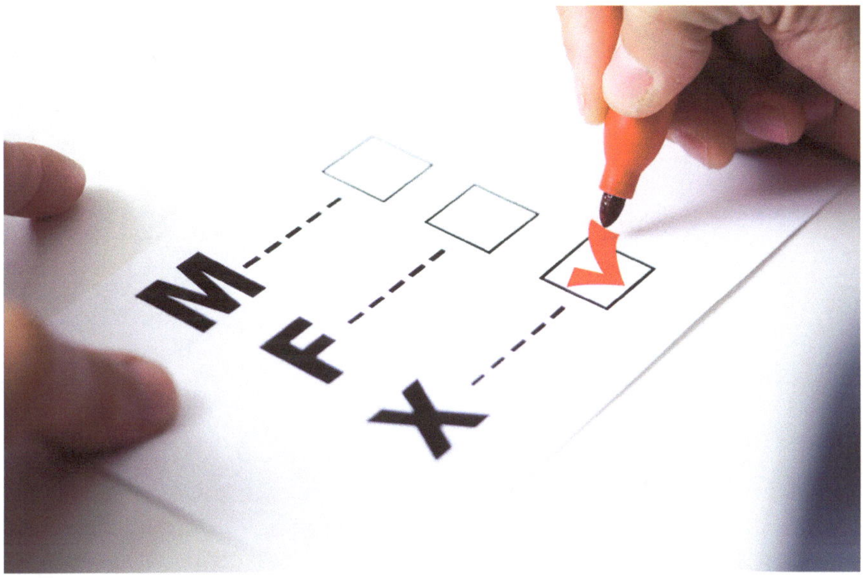

7 Robyn A. Jackowich et al., "Voluntary Genital Ablations: Contrasting the Cutters and Their Clients," *Sexual Medicine* 2, no. 3 (August 2014): 121–32, https://doi.org/10.1002/sm2.33.

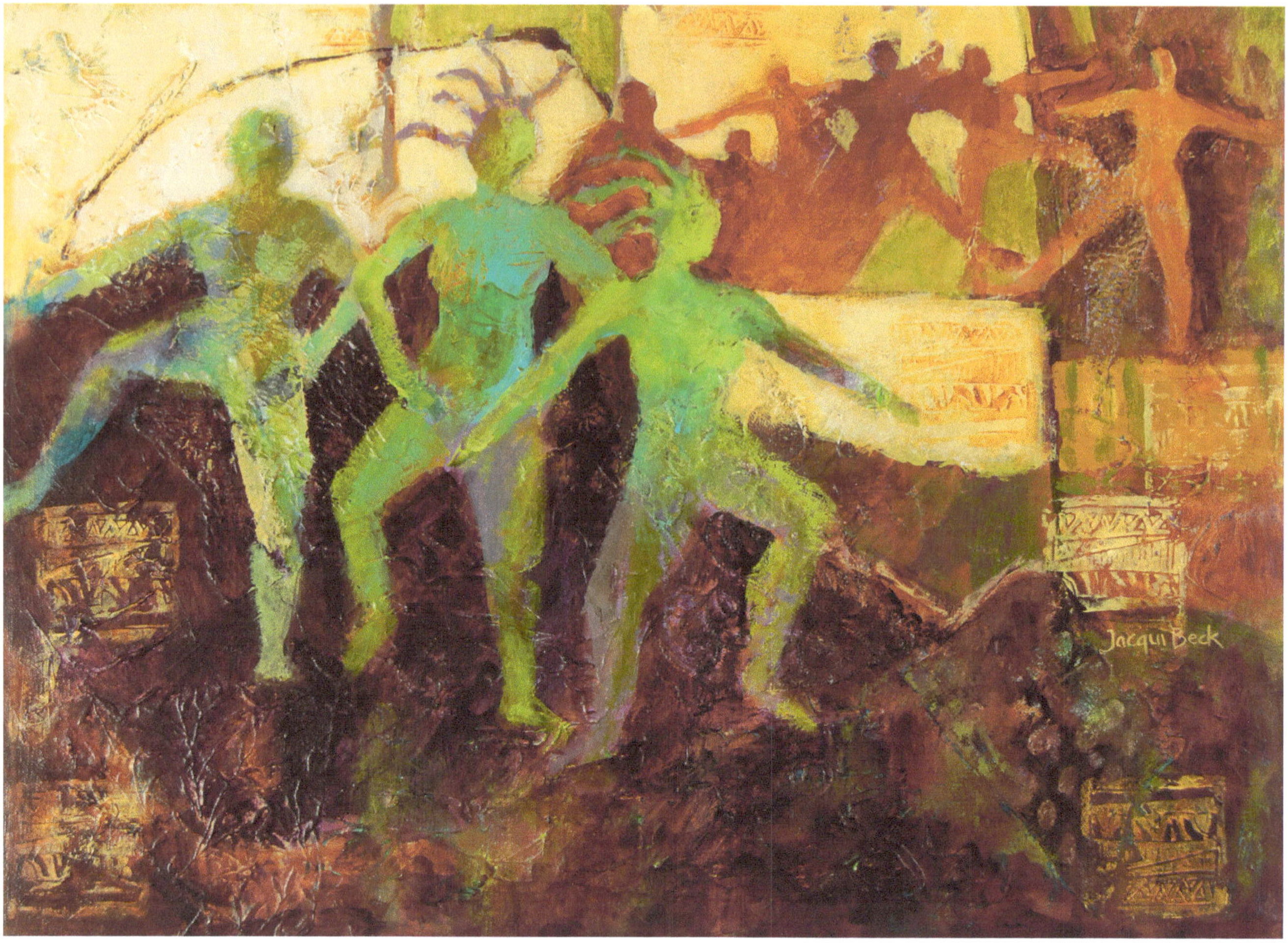

Sister Dance

CHAPTER 3

Sexual Orientation

Sexual orientation is all about who we are attracted to, as well as who we want to love or be with sexually. And just like gender identity, this can get complicated.

As children, we may have been taught to think that men were supposed to fall in love with women and that women were supposed to fall in love with men. Now, of course, we know there's much more to love than that.

Men *can* be attracted to other men. Men can fall in love with other men and they can marry men also. When a man is attracted to other men, this is often called being homosexual or "gay."

> **Gender orientation is who you go to bed as and sexual orientation refers to who you go to bed with.**
>
> — *Jen Hastings, MD*

The US Supreme Court upheld marriage equality legislation in June 2015. This action gave the legal right for all same-sex couples to marry in every state of the Union, at least as of this writing.

In the same way, women can be attracted to and fall in love with other women. Women who are attracted to women or women with female partners, girlfriends, or wives are known as lesbians. Like gay men, lesbians have same-sex relationships. Some people call gay men "men who have sex with men"; you may hear the abbreviation MSM. Some call lesbians "women who have sex with women." (For whatever reason, men tend to be called gay or homosexual, even though these terms apply to women in same-sex relationships, too.)

You may have noticed my wording, "fall in love with," above. As Tina Turner so memorably sang, "What's love got to do with it?" Sometimes nothing, and sometimes everything. Again, the point is that you get to choose.

Many same-sex couples have children. To have a baby, you must have sperm from a partner who was assigned male at birth and an egg from a partner who was assigned female. If two men want a baby who is biologically related to one of them, they work with someone assigned female who provides the necessary egg and carries a pregnancy for them, often using sperm from one of the male partners. This is often referred to as a "surrogate pregnancy." If two women want to have a baby who is biologically related to one of them, they must find a sperm donor whose sperm will combine with one of the women's eggs and produce a baby that way.

It is possible for a trans man to become pregnant, carry, and deliver a baby after he transitions. It does require that the man stops testosterone to allow him to ovulate and remain off testosterone throughout pregnancy and chest-feeding. Also, a trans man would require sperm from a donor (see Chapter 21).

It's not uncommon for people to be attracted sexually or romantically to *both* sexes. So, you might have a man (cis or trans) who is attracted to both men and women. And you might have a woman (cis or trans) who is attracted to both cis or trans women and men. People who are attracted to both sexes are often referred to as "bisexual."

Just as with gender identity, you may want to think about sexual orientation as a continuum. Again, think of a line with "Attracted to the Same Sex" on one end and "Attracted to the Opposite Sex" on the other. Like this:

The Sexual Orientation Continuum

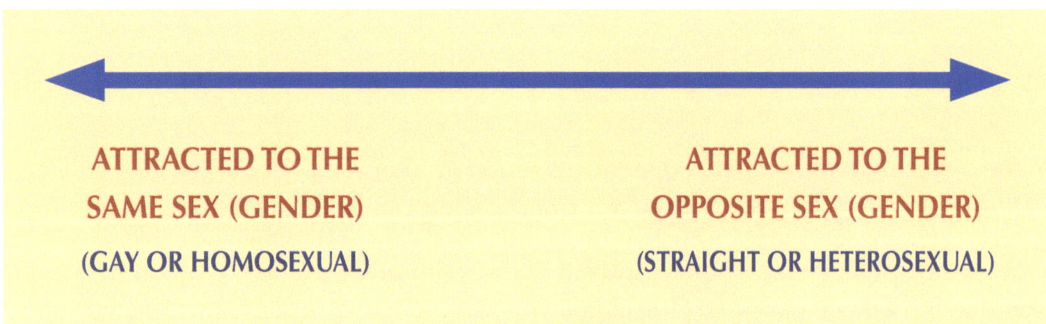

Figure 3.1. The sexual orientation continuum.

Your sexual orientation means who you are attracted to sexually. Again, this does not involve "right" or "wrong." It's something that just *is*.

I appreciate that this may be a bit cumbersome, particularly when the person we are talking about may be transgender or cisgender—and the person they are attracted to may be trans or cis also. So, to clarify:

- If a trans male is attracted to a trans male, they would be in a same-sex relationship—that is, gay or homosexual.
- If a trans male is attracted to a cis male, they are in a same-sex relationship.
- If a trans male is attracted to a trans female, they would be in a straight or heterosexual relationship.
- If a trans male is attracted to a cis female, they are in a straight relationship.

Nonbinary individuals may not fit into these neat categories, if that is even important. A nonbinary couple may refer to themselves as a "queer" couple. Just communicate the information that's important to you to the people whom you want to have the information!

And just as with gender identity, your sexual orientation can be fluid. You may be attracted to men at some point in your life and to women at another time in your life, or both, or neither. When they are attracted to all expressions of gender, a person may call themselves "pansexual." And people who have no sexual desire and are attracted to neither males or females are "asexual."

Q **If you are transgender, does that mean you are gay?**

A **Maybe yes, maybe no. Gender identity and sexual orientation are separate things.**

You have undoubtedly seen the acronym "LGBTQ." This acronym usually stands for "lesbian, gay, bisexual, transgender, queer." Sometimes people use the "Q" to represent "questioning." It can also be sort of an umbrella term that refers to people who are gender-fluid or nonbinary. Note that in the past, "queer" was most definitely considered a derogatory term. That doesn't seem to be the case now, *but be sure about this before you label anyone—other than yourself, of course.*

Then there is the acronym "LGBTQIA+," which can refer to "lesbian, gay, bisexual, transgender, queer, intersex, and allies" (the "A" can also mean "asexual"). Adding the "+" acknowledges the noncisgender and nonstraight identities not included in the acronym. More acronyms will follow, no doubt.

As all this information can be confusing, I think the best way to think about this can be summed up in four important points in the box below:

The Most Important Points

- **Gender** is a biological definition and refers to whether you were assigned male or assigned female at birth. (Or more specifically, gender refers to whether you were born with male genitals or born with female genitals.)
- **Gender identity** is how we see ourselves. It's who we are—that is, male or female, somewhere in between, or "without" gender. Gender identity goes far beyond our genitals.
- **Sexual orientation** refers to who we are attracted to *sexually*.
- Most importantly, your **gender identity** and your **sexual orientation** are defined by you, and only by you.

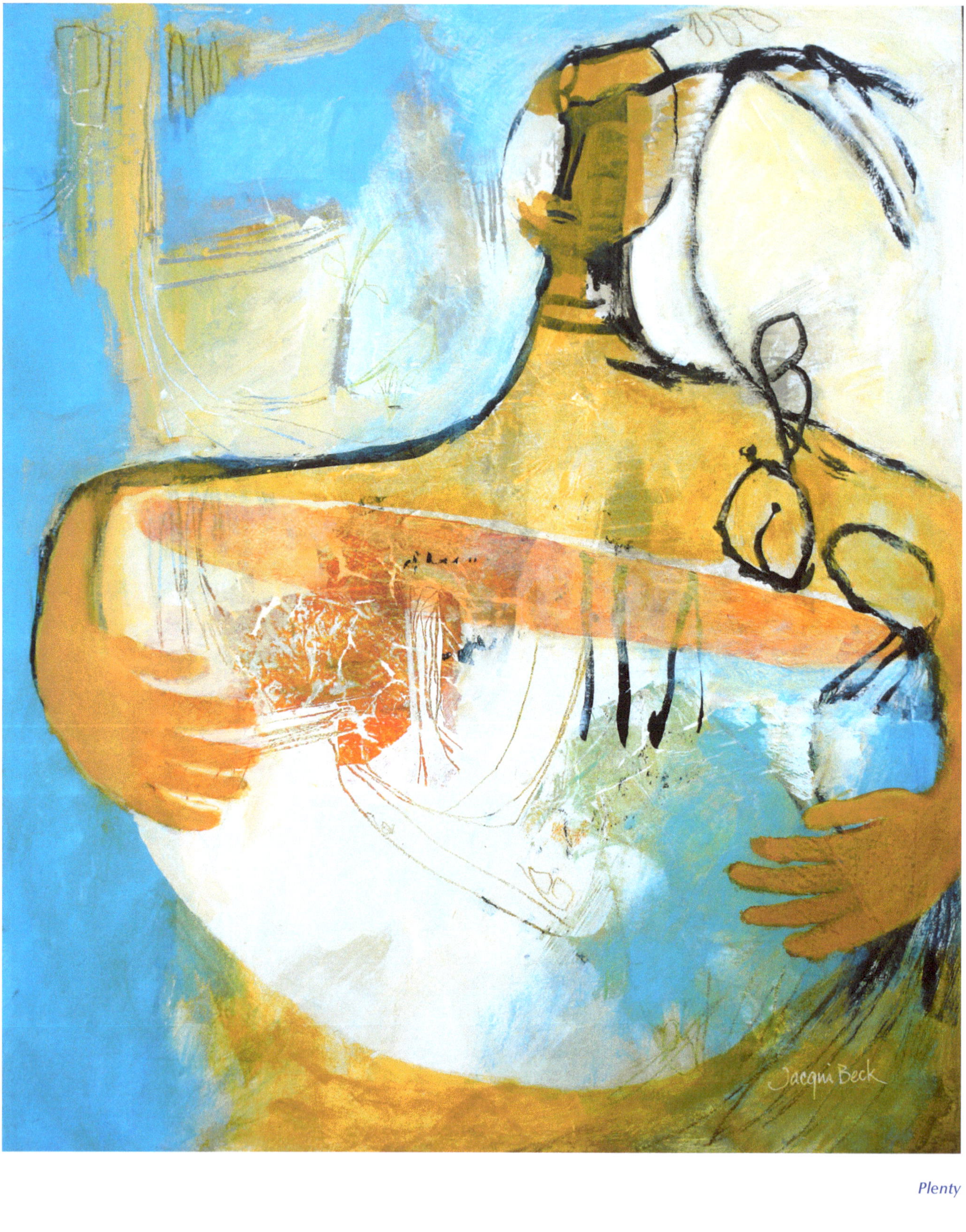

Plenty

CHAPTER 4

Deciding What You Want and Need

When I meet a new transgender or nonbinary patient for the first time, I ask them what they want and need to do to transform their gender. (This is in my role as a physician, of course. Otherwise, this could feel very invasive to ask something so personal after you've just met.)

I ask, "What would you like to see happen if you could do anything you liked concerning your gender?"

Sometimes, I'll ask, "If you won the lottery tomorrow and didn't have to think about anything or anybody else (which, of course, you must do in real life), what would you like to see happen concerning your gender?"

I appreciate that's a broad question, and I know that not everything *is* possible. Medical science cannot change your sex chromosomes, and we cannot send you back to the womb for a do-over (although I've been asked that).

Over the last two decades of working with the transgender community, I've learned that you are far more likely to get exactly what you want—or as close to it as possible—*if you know what you want.*

Let me share some of the remarkable things I've seen:

- I've seen little kids grow up in their identified gender with the benefits of puberty blockers and cross hormones; they are truly as well-adjusted and as happy as any kid can be. (The research of University of Washington psychology professor Kristina Olson, PhD, backs this up: When trans kids receive support from their families and are allowed to express their gender as they define it themselves, they do as well as their cisgender counterparts. They are no more likely to be depressed and they suffer only slightly more anxiety than their cisgender classmates. Dr. Olson was honored with a 2018 MacArthur "Genius" Grant—a fellowship worth $625,000—as well as the National Science Foundation's Alan T. Waterman Award—and its accompanying $1 million grant. Olson is using her winnings to support her TransYouth Project, a 20-year study launched in 2013 and the nation's first large-scale, long-term study of transgender children.[8])

- I listened as one extremely high-risk teenager looked me squarely in the eye and said, "I think I'd be dead now if I hadn't gotten testosterone." In my heart, I know he was probably right.

- I watched as a college woman transformed herself into a veritable lumberjack with a full beard and a twinkle in his eye in only a year. He exuded happiness!

- I dabbed the tears from the cheeks of a sophisticated, professional woman who had emerged from a craggy, bearded face with the benefit of laser hair removal and the precise placement of neurotoxin and dermal filler (no surgery). Appreciating her elegant face as she had only envisioned it, she said, "I never thought this was even remotely possible."

8 Sandi Doughton, "UW Psychologist Kristina Olson Thought the MacArthur Foundation Had the Wrong 'Genius'," *Pacific NW Magazine, Seattle Times*, September 1, 2019, https://www.seattletimes.com/pacific-nw-magazine/uw-psychologist-kristina-olson-thought-the-macarthur-foundation-had-the-wrong-genius/.

- I recall a trans woman who took every tenuous step from hormones and laser facial hair removal to genital hair removal and finally to a gender-affirming genital surgery—all the while knowing that her beloved wife was planning to leave her. She *had* to transition to be herself and to follow her truth. Imagine her joy when her wife reevaluated and did not leave!
- I know an 18-year-old who orchestrated getting testosterone and having top surgery by age 16. He has *already* had his phalloplasty.
- I knew a lovely woman in her 60s who traveled halfway around the world to have the vaginoplasty she'd dreamed of for decades. While far away, she learned by email that her wife had died. I ached just thinking of my patient making cremation arrangements for her spouse via the Internet and coming back to an empty house.
- I remember one of the first patients I assisted with hormones now claiming her place as a trans community matriarch. Two of her children embrace her; two have cast her aside. Yet she radiates the contentment of a life lived with great purpose and dignity.

I witness these stories every day. And while I acknowledge that there exists tremendous pain within the trans community, I see the victories as well. Overall, I have seen many more victories than sadness.

So, what would you like to see happen concerning your gender and gender expression?

Most of my patients say "hormones." And, of course, that's an excellent place to start. Taking hormones will probably give you the most significant changes possible on a day-to-day basis and for the least cost.

Some trans women will identify facial feminization surgery (FFS), although it is less frequently covered by health insurance. (Some of the tech companies *do* cover FFS, so check your benefits.)

Most trans men I treat identify top surgery (gender-affirming chest reconstruction surgery, a reduction mammoplasty done to create a fully male-appearing chest) as a priority, after testosterone.

Many, but not nearly all, trans women seek vaginoplasty (a surgically created vagina). And more and more trans men are seeking genital surgeries, including phalloplasty (a surgically created penis).

We'll discuss all of these in much more detail.

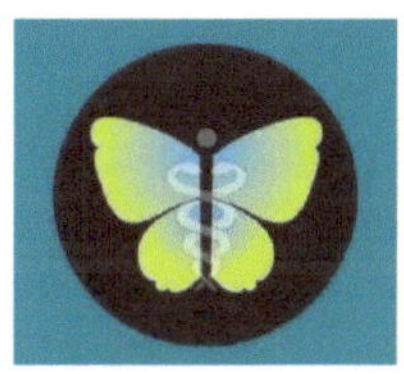

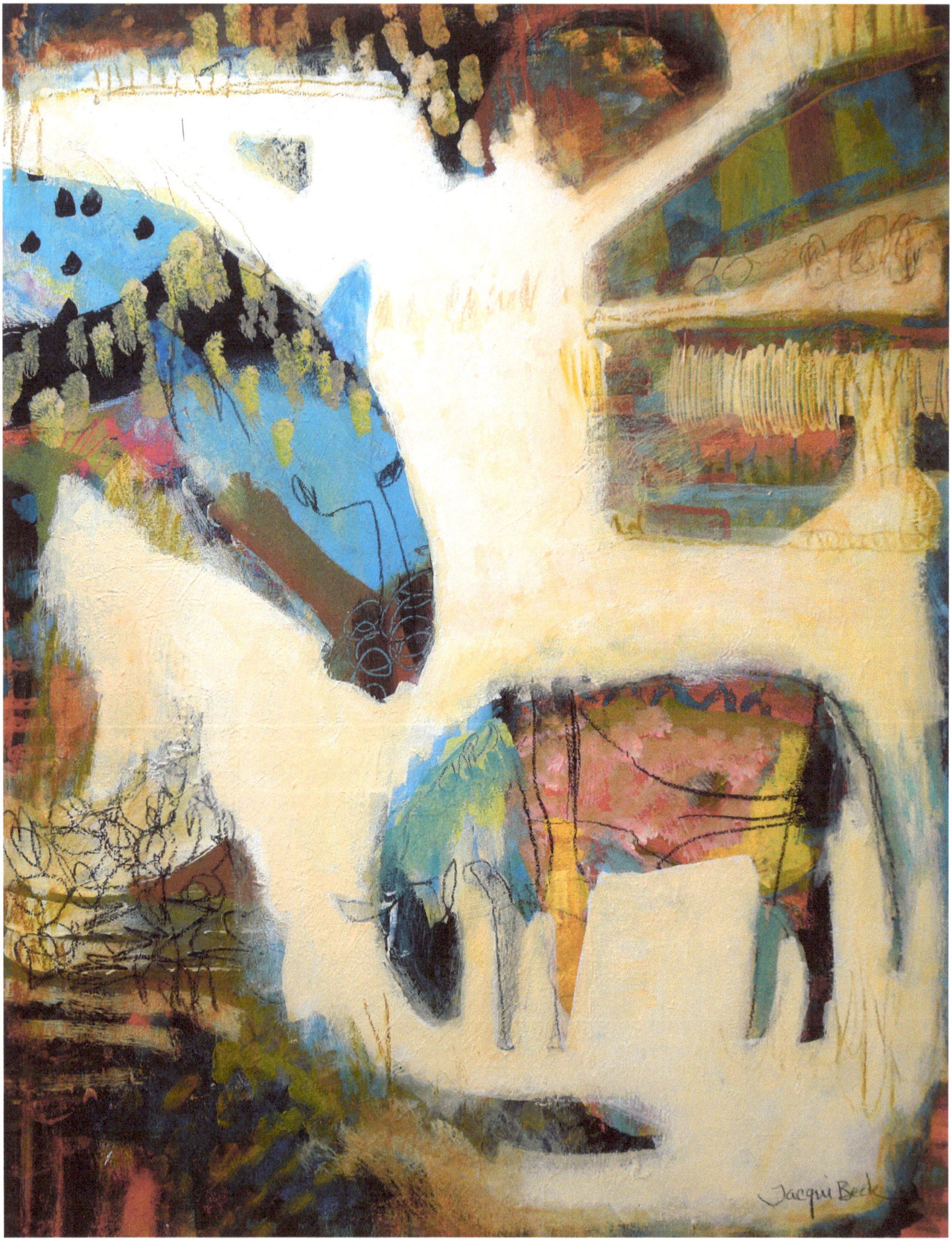

Watching Over

CHAPTER 5
A Review of Puberty and Reproduction

Note: These next portions (including "Medical Treatment for Children and Adolescents with Gender Dysphoria") are modified from the Puberty and Reproduction section of my youth book. Please feel free to skip ahead if the information isn't of use to you.

— *Linda Gromko, MD*

Why Are We Reviewing Puberty?

Who would *want* to revisit puberty? Puberty is tough for most people, but it can be especially hard if you know you're going through the wrong puberty.

I think this is a useful review, however, for these reasons:

- First, many of us never got this information in any real way when we were going through puberty. We'll fix this now.
- Secondly, this will give you an opportunity to see what can be done *today* for young transgender and nonbinary adolescents who want to "pause" their puberty with puberty blockers. Puberty blockers can give kids (and families) time to figure out what they truly want to see happen. Or, the puberty blockers can be followed directly—or supplemented by—cross-sex hormones that feel like the *correct* hormones to a transgender adolescent. Today, you can essentially *transition* as an adolescent before the seemingly indelible secondary sex changes occur (developed breasts and menstrual periods for someone assigned female, or broad shoulders, facial hair, a deep voice, and an Adam's apple for someone assigned male).
- Thirdly, reviewing the puberty process, as well as the earlier process of embryologic development, helps us to understand how gender-affirming genital surgeries work. While puberty blockers may be too late for you as an adult, gender-affirming surgeries are likely still possible if your overall health allows you to undergo a surgery safely. (I had a woman in my practice just come back from vaginoplasty at age 67; she did great.)

Way before Puberty

Before we were born, we all looked pretty much the same. Think of it: All little fetuses in their mothers' uteruses look almost identical to one another!

Then, at about 10 weeks into the pregnancy, we start to have changes that make us look like baby boys or baby girls. This happens because of the influence of the hormone testosterone (the male hormone). Boy fetuses are programmed by the DNA in their Y chromosomes to make testosterone, while girl fetuses are not. As you remember, girl fetuses do not have a Y chromosome at all, but rather, two X chromosomes. People born boys are usually XY in the chromosome department, and people born girls are generally XX.

Testosterone makes the boy-programmed fetus develop a penis, scrotum, prostate, and testicles (male genital and reproductive organs). Girl-programmed fetuses develop a vagina, uterus, fallopian tubes, and ovaries.

Look at Figure 5.1 on page 29 drawn by the late Dr. Frank Netter. You will see how our external genitalia are virtually identical in our early beginnings until they're changed by the programmed influence of the hormone testosterone. It's useful to recognize how similar the male and female genitalia look as they develop, particularly when it comes to understanding gender-reassignment surgery.

I remember surgeon Dr. Toby Meltzer referring to this diagram in a lecture on sexual reassignment surgery. Dr. Meltzer said, "Look, it's *color-coded*!"

The structures *are* color-coded in Dr. Netter's illustrations (not in real life, of course). But you can easily see that the yellow glans penis in the male in Dr. Netter's drawing is analogous to the yellow clitoris in the female. Study this drawing: All the color-coded "matches" are analogous to each other.

Just as there are external genital organs, we have internal reproductive organs as well. The gonads (the glands that produce our gametes—that is, sperm in males and eggs or ova in females) form in the lower abdomen or pelvis. In males, the testicles descend into the scrotum, while in females, the ovaries remain deep within the pelvis. Testicles and ovaries are not the same, of course. But in addition to producing sex hormones, they have the same essential function: producing either sperm in males or eggs in females with the possibility of combining to create a new human.

Even when they are young children, it's hard to tell males and females apart. We all look pretty much the same, except for the genital organs.

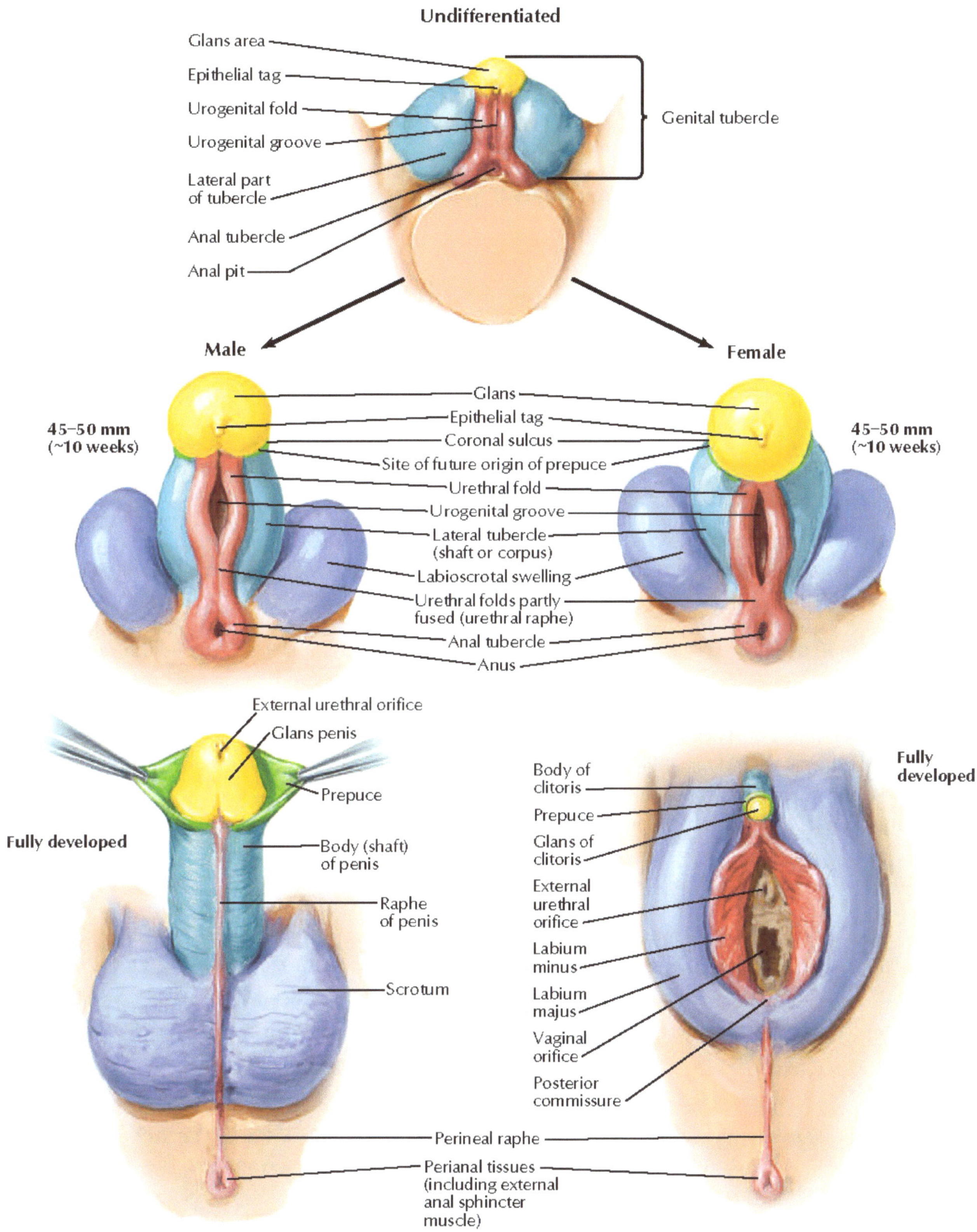

Figure 5.1. Embryologic equivalents in male and female external genitals.

Moving into Puberty

Puberty is the time when kids grow into adults. The process begins a little earlier in kids who are assigned female, starting at around age 9 to 11 years. In kids who are assigned male, puberty begins at around 11 to 13 years of age. The whole process of puberty generally takes several years from start to finish.

It might be convenient if everyone went through puberty at the same predictable time. But it doesn't work that way at all. That's why you may see kids who are the same age, but one looks like a little kid and the other looks like a fully grown adult.

Few of us would want to go back to puberty, even for a visit, unless perhaps to get the puberty blockers that are now available.

Before puberty starts, kids go through a stage called "adrenarche." Adrenarche is when the adrenal glands that sit on top of our kidneys start producing androgen hormones that make us develop underarm hair and body odor. These two changes tell us that puberty is generally well on its way.

Here's What Happens to People Who Are Assigned Female at Birth

As a girl grows into a woman, a girl's body matures to the point where she can become pregnant and have a baby. That does not mean that a girl or woman *must* have a baby, but it means she may be able to have a baby if she wants to.

The breasts begin to develop early in puberty in what is referred to as Tanner Stage 2. (See the Tanner Stages in Figure 5.6 on page 39.) The first change that happens is the development of the breast "bud." The breast bud grows beneath the areola (the colored part of the nipple). It feels sort of like a lentil or a little pinto bean. It sometimes hurts to touch it or even when a T-shirt rubs against it. (You probably know that breast bud formation is an early change that transgender women experience when they first begin estrogen as part of their hormonal transition. Trans women's breasts can get very tender when they start hormones, much like a person assigned female would notice in early puberty.)

> **There are five Tanner Stages. We are prepubertal in Tanner Stage 1; puberty begins in Tanner Stage 2 and ends with Tanner Stage 5. The onset of Tanner Stage 2 is the development of the breast bud in a person assigned female, or the growth of a testicle to 1 inch in length in a person assigned male.**

The breasts continue to grow, first with the areola pointing out like a little cone and later with glandular breast tissue growing around and under the nipple. All these changes allow a woman to breastfeed or "nurse" a baby after she has one. Usually at the time the breasts are starting to develop, a girl is talking to her parents or friends about buying bras. It's no wonder that trans *boys* struggle horribly in puberty when they begin to develop full breasts. They know that the developing breasts are not at all what they want, and they may start using chest binders or dressing in ways that camouflage their chests (see Chapter 9).

Q **Can a transgender woman nurse a baby?**

A **It is possible, but a specific hormonal environment must be created by using supplemental hormones.**

(A trans male may be able to chest-feed a baby also; see Chapter 21.)

Another part of puberty for kids who were assigned female is the start of menstrual periods. Look at the drawings later in this chapter to familiarize yourself with the internal reproductive organs and the hormone fluctuations of the menstrual cycle.

A child who is born a girl will (likely) have a uterus, with fallopian tubes and ovaries on each side of the uterus. *When a girl is born, her ovaries already have all the eggs she will ever have in her whole life.*

(I have always felt that this fact represents a major stroke of gender inequity. Why? If a 40-year-old woman gets pregnant, *her* eggs are 40 years old and are more likely to have chromosomal abnormalities associated with what's called "advanced maternal age." Men make new sperm all the time. So, if a 40-year-old woman mates with an 80-year-old man, her eggs are 40 years old, and his sperm are brand-spanking new!)

At puberty, the ovaries start to release about one egg per month in a process called "ovulation." Ovulation occurs 2 weeks before each menstrual period begins. The tiny egg (ovum) travels to the uterus by way of one of the fallopian tubes. If, along the way the egg meets a sperm (either in the abdominal cavity or in the fallopian tube) from someone assigned male at birth, the two can combine in what is called "fertilization." A fertilized egg can then implant itself into the inner wall of the uterus and grow for the next 9 months until a fully grown baby human is ready to be born. (The baby is then born by moving through the cervix—the "neck" of the uterus—and the vagina in a vaginal birth. Or, the baby can be delivered by cesarean section when a doctor makes an incision in the lower part of the abdomen and uterus and removes the baby through the abdomen.)

Not all pregnancies go to full term. According to the March of Dimes, "as many as half of all pregnancies may end in miscarriage. We don't know the exact number because a miscarriage may happen before a woman knows she's pregnant."[9]

Miscarriages often occur very early in a pregnancy, even before the pregnancy is diagnosed. While it may not be comforting to know this, miscarriage frequently occurs when there's a chromosomal abnormality that prevents the pregnancy from continuing. People also have the option to end a pregnancy, as in an abortion. Thankfully, abortions are now generally safe and available for women who elect not to carry the pregnancy (at least as of this writing).

How the Egg and Sperm Get Together

In years past, puberty books *never* clarified how such chance meetings occurred. Oh, we'd hear about a married man and his wife "holding each other very close in a special way" and then, voilà—a baby would be

9 March of Dimes, "Miscarriage," last reviewed November 2017, https://www.marchofdimes.org/complications/miscarriage.aspx.

born—from somewhere, anyway. Wouldn't you think that how the sperm gets together with the egg would be interesting, even critical, information? Me too! So here goes:

A person assigned female has a vagina, a passageway which leads from the *outside* of the body directly to the opening of the uterus deep *inside* the body. You cannot see the uterus from the outside, although I can see the lower part of the uterus (the cervix) by using a vaginal speculum to separate the vaginal walls when taking a Pap test or a culture for sexually transmitted infections.

When a person assigned female has intimate sexual contact (we'll get to that in a minute) with someone assigned male, sperm can enter the vagina, swim up to the uterus and fallopian tubes, and combine with (or fertilize) an egg to create a pregnancy.

A person who is assigned male at birth produces sperm in the testicles. During sexual activity, sperm come out of the opening at the end of the penis in a milky, off-white liquid called "semen." Semen is different from urine, but it comes out of the same hole you urinate through when you pee. (You don't pass urine during sexual activity, just semen. We'll discuss later that trans women on estradiol may not produce semen at all or may produce a clear ejaculate, on page 413 in Chapter 22.)

Intimate sexual contact often means that the penis enters the vagina, although there are many, many other ways to have sexual intimacy. The penis becomes erect or hard when a person assigned male is sexually excited or aroused. Traditional sexual intercourse between a person assigned male and a person assigned female is the process where the erect penis enters the vagina, moves in and out until the person assigned male is sexually aroused *enough* to have an ejaculation or orgasm (also called a climax). That's when the semen (containing the sperm) comes out of the penis and into the vagina. From there, the sperm can travel up through the uterus and fallopian tubes to join with an egg in the process of fertilization. And, of course, when a fertilized egg nestles into the uterine lining tissue, it can implant and create a pregnancy.

> For your safety, I want you to know that I have taken care of patients who have gotten pregnant when a guy's semen got onto a girl's thigh or when sperm traveled through a girl's underpants. So be aware that if sperm are in the vicinity of the vagina, a pregnancy could result.
>
> You may be wondering if these girls did have sexual intercourse. I examined the young women in these two situations, and they were both anatomically virgins.
>
> — *Linda Gromko, MD*

Of course, you know that a penis can become erect or hard spontaneously, perhaps first thing in the morning, or when its owner is having sexual thoughts. The erection occurs when blood fills the corpora cavernosa, two hollow pontoons within the penis. If the penis is stimulated, perhaps by a person alone in masturbation or with another person during sexual intimacy, the penis becomes hard and ejaculation or orgasm can occur. Or, sometimes a person will ignore the erection and it will go away on its own.

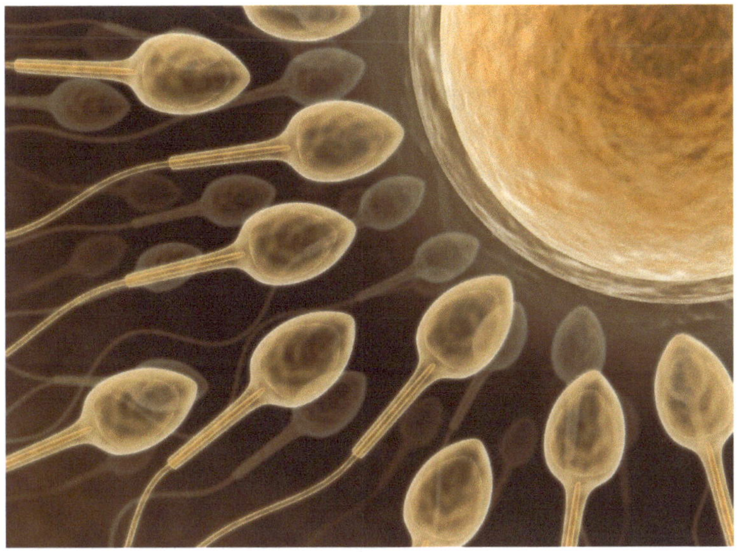

Figure 5.2. Fertilization.

It's interesting to talk to children and adolescents about sexual intercourse, *because so many young people find it, well, inconceivable that their parents might have had this kind of sexual intimacy.*

But of course, their parents did have sexual intimacy, or at least found some way for sperm and egg to get together to create *them*! And the great likelihood is they had sex more than once—probably, many times. Most people, but not all, like to be sexually intimate with someone special because it can feel amazing! (Maybe not right at first when it can feel pretty awkward, but practice makes perfect. And people seem to keep doing it.)

Here's an important warning for people of all ages: Sexual contact that is wanted can be wonderful. Sexual contact that is *unwanted*—or happens against your will—is called sexual assault or rape. Unwanted sexual contact is a serious form of harm that one person can do to another. If you have been a victim of unwanted sexual contact, talk to someone helpful like a therapist or your healthcare provider. A sexual assault can impact many areas of your life experiences going forward. I encourage you to work through this (perhaps in therapy) so that the sexual assault does not become a lasting source of stress or pain throughout your life.

Remember, when you say "No," it means "NO!" (We'll discuss more about consent in a sexual context in Chapter 22.)

From about fifth grade on, kids now learn that sexual contact can have profound consequences like sexually transmitted infections and pregnancy (if sperm and egg are involved). We will talk more about how to prevent undesired sexual consequences later.

Menstruation: From an Early Signal of Sexual Maturation to Making Babies

Every month after a person assigned female starts having periods (usually around age 12 to 13, but sometimes as early as nine), the uterus prepares itself to sustain a pregnancy, even when a person is really much too young to have a baby. The uterus does this by making its lining thicker with an enriched blood supply, thus preparing it to accept a fertilized egg that then nestles into its fluffy lining and grows into a new human.

If there is no sexual contact to allow sperm to fertilize the egg (or if a couple is using birth control), the person assigned female has what is called a "period" or "menstrual period." During a period, the lining tissue that wasn't used for the growth of a pregnancy leaves the uterus through the vagina. It looks like blood, although it may be darker in color than the blood you see when you cut your finger (menstrual blood may be a dark red, maroon, or even brown). The period "flow" is caught by a sanitary napkin, a menstrual cup, a liner worn in the underpants, or a tampon—an expanding cylinder of absorbent material that is inserted deep into the vagina. (Companies that manufacture tampons and pads often have informative websites about menstruation.)

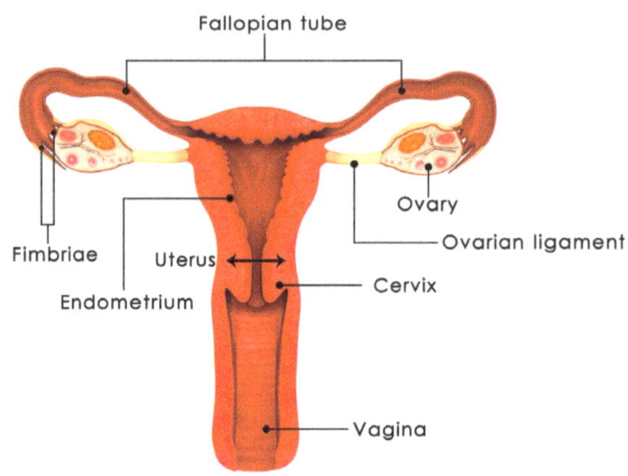

Figure 5.3. Internal female reproductive organs.

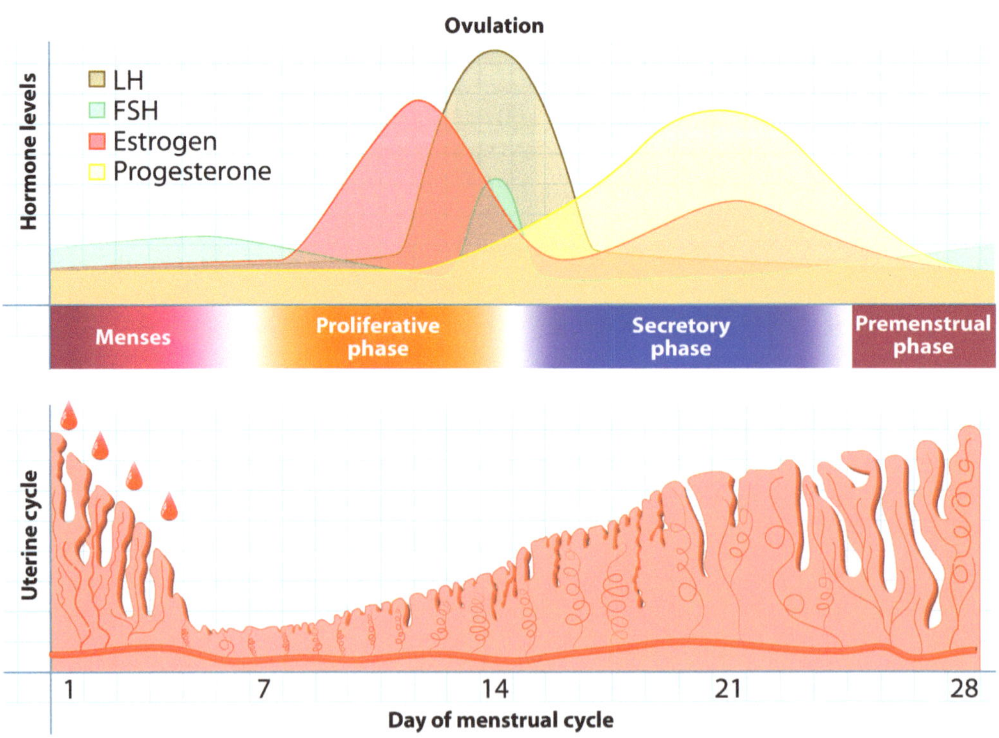

Figure 5.4. The menstrual cycle.

Puberty and Signs of Sexual Maturation

People assigned female grow taller during puberty. They usually reach their maximum height by about Tanner Stage 5—that is, at about age 16, but they *can* still grow taller into their early 20s.

Here are more changes:

- Skin may develop acne (pimples or zits), a temporary change but one that may recur during the hormonal changes of menopause around age 50.
- Pubic hair develops; it is coarse and often curly, and it is usually present by the time periods start.
- Body hair increases, such as underarm hair or hair around the areolas, arms, and legs.
- The body begins to reshape itself with the hips and butt broadening out.
- The face changes also so that a person assigned female starts to look more like an adult woman than a child.

Many times, girls in puberty begin to become more aware of their genitals. They may discover the clitoris, located at the top of the genital area where the vaginal labia come together. Remember how both boys and girls start with the same raw materials when they are little fetuses? Well, the clitoris is the female equivalent of the glans penis ("the mushroom part"), smaller than a penis to be sure but very sensitive.

Stimulating the clitoris by touching it or rubbing it (gently) will likely feel very nice. With continued stimulation of the clitoris, labia, and the breasts, a girl may have an orgasm or climax. Some people assigned female have ejaculations (pass fluid originating from the urethral sponge and Skene's glands) during orgasm. (Look up "G-spot" for more information on this. The G-spot is an area located in the front wall of the vagina that, when stimulated, may prompt the ejaculation response.) As with a person assigned male, the process of self-stimulation is called "masturbation."

It shouldn't be a great surprise that many (most) people do this sometimes. Even babies play with their genitals as soon as they can reach them, and they look quite blissful when they do it!

For more information on sexual enjoyment, see Chapter 22 (Sex and Relationships).

How Would You Describe an Orgasm?

According to the Merriam-Webster online dictionary, orgasm is "the physical and emotional sensation experienced at the peak of sexual excitation, usually resulting from stimulation of the sexual organ and usually accompanied in the male by ejaculation."

Some describe it as a sudden release of physical tension, maybe vaguely like the relief of finally peeing when your bladder is about to burst!

How would you describe orgasm? If it's only a "good sneeze," keep trying. It gets better!

Q Do people assigned female have orgasms also?

A Yup.

Q Does a person assigned female have to have an orgasm to get pregnant?

A Nope (another reproductive inequity).

Here's What Happens in Puberty to Kids Who Are Assigned Male at Birth

People who are assigned male usually start the puberty process a little later than people who are assigned female. Puberty usually happens at about 11 to 13. Like their counterparts who were assigned female, they have also started to have underarm hair and body odor in the adrenal maturation called "adrenarche." Adrenarche is a good indicator that puberty will be happening soon.

The next thing that happens is the growth of the testicles. Testicles measure about 1 inch in length at the onset of puberty in Tanner Stage 2. Through the remainder of puberty, the testicles and penis grow larger and the pubic area fills in with coarse, curly pubic hair.

At around this time, people assigned male begin to produce sperm, so they could create a pregnancy if the sperm meets an egg from a person assigned female. Many times, people assigned male will have sperm come out of the penis during sleep. In medicine, this is called a "nocturnal emission." Everyone else calls this a "wet dream." A person assigned male may not be aware this is even happening, although they may notice a splotch where fluid has dried on their sheets or their underpants or pajamas.

Many people assigned male will discover that masturbation (stimulating the penis, usually by rubbing it in some fashion) will cause the penis to become hard or erect and that this will result in a sexual climax (or orgasm) as sperm leave the penis in a milky fluid called semen.

As we've discussed before, the whole process of getting an erection has to do with blood flowing into the penis and filling the two tube-like structures called the "corpora cavernosa," which is Latin for "cavernous bodies." When these tubes fill with blood, the penis becomes much firmer and larger than in its flaccid (limp) state. A penis that is erect can enter the body of a sexual partner much easier than one that is not erect. Erections are common first thing in the morning when testosterone levels are at their highest, but they can happen spontaneously at any time. Sexual thoughts can prompt erections; in younger people who are assigned male, it may seem that virtually *anything at all* may prompt an erection.

In many transgender females (male-to-female individuals), erections may be considered a bother, and spontaneous erections often go away when the trans woman is taking testosterone blockers or estrogen.

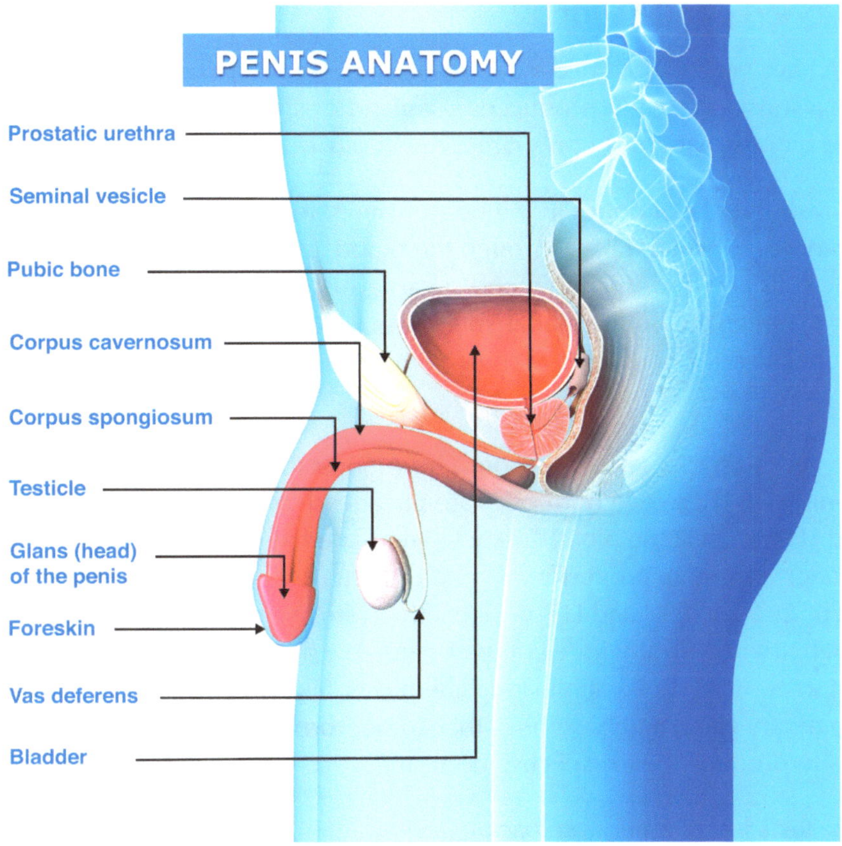

Figure 5.5. Male reproductive tract.

Here are some of the other changes that happen when people assigned male go through puberty:

- Deepening of the voice. It can start with the voice "cracking"—that is, going from low to high with little warning. Or a guy may sound hoarse for a while until his voice settles into a deeper range.
- Growth of the Adam's apple in the neck. This is the enlargement of the thyroid cartilage and we will talk about this more later when we discuss the procedure called a "tracheal shave" or "trach shave" in gender transition.
- Broadening of the shoulders.
- Development of acne.
- Growth in height, with a maximum usually reached by about Tanner Stage 5 or approximately age 17, but kids can continue to grow in height through college age.
- Development of coarse, usually curly, pubic hair.
- Increase in body hair all over, such as the chest, back, abdomen, legs, arms, and underarm area.
- The development of facial hair (sideburns, mustache, beard hair).
- As with people assigned female, the face and body begin to look more like adult males than like boys.

Hormones in Puberty and Beyond

All the changes we have talked about occur as a result of hormones. The scientific definition of hormones is this: A hormone is a substance that is produced by a gland or specialized cells in one part of the body and travels through the bloodstream to act on a target organ or organs in a different location in the body.

And there are many different hormones in the body. Insulin, for example, is a hormone produced in a gland called the pancreas. Insulin travels through the bloodstream to help glucose (sugar) get into cells, thereby nourishing cells and lowering the blood sugar levels. The thyroid gland in the neck produces thyroid hormones that regulate our metabolic rate—that is, the rate at which our cells use energy. There are *many* other hormones in our bodies, and there is a whole medical specialty (endocrinology) that deals with hormones.

For our discussion, let's turn to a set of "directing" hormones: follicle-stimulating hormone (FSH) and luteinizing hormone (LH). These two hormones are produced in the pituitary gland nestled deep within the brain. FSH and LH travel via the bloodstream to stimulate the ovaries in a person assigned female to make more hormones: estrogen, progesterone, and testosterone. In the person assigned male, the pituitary releases the same hormones (FSH and LH) to signal the testicles to release testosterone. If this wasn't complicated enough, there is another area of the brain—the hypothalamus—that communicates with the pituitary by way of its own hormone-stimulating chemicals. So, we have hormones from the hypothalamus that "talk" to the pituitary gland and hormones that come from the pituitary gland that in turn nudge the ovaries or testicles to produce their respective hormones.

Also, the ovaries or testicles communicate *back* to the pituitary and hypothalamus, creating a feedback loop. All of this is happening without us even being aware of it. And all of this happens whether we like it or not.

So, if a person was assigned female *but knows they are a guy and should not grow into a woman*, they need some very specific information to help them. The same is true for a person who was assigned male but knows they are truly female. It is possible to make changes in how puberty progresses. But it takes some special help from people who can give you the help you need (like a doctor like me or one of my colleagues, for example).

One of our trans male patients remembers (at age 36) that getting his period at the age of 11 was the most embarrassing day of his life. *Totally* unprepared for bleeding, he thought he was dying. His mother didn't help; she baked a red velvet cake called the "Becoming a Woman" cake. Real information came from another mom next door.

The Tanner Stages

Healthcare providers use Tanner Stages to describe a person's place in the puberty process. There are five Tanner Stages. Tanner Stage 1 is before puberty starts, when you are a baby or a young child.

In Tanner Stage 2, a person assigned female develops a breast bud under the nipple. Remember that little pinto bean under the areola? That generally happens at about age 9 to 11.

For a person assigned male, Tanner 2 is the stage where the testicles have grown in length to about 1 inch, about the size of an almond in its shell.

Many transgender kids have heard of Tanner Stage 2 because it is in Tanner Stage 2 or 3 that *puberty blockers* are used. Puberty blockers, if used during these early stages of puberty, will put puberty *on hold*. They are given by a healthcare provider as injections or placed as an implant under the skin of the inner upper arm. When the blockers are stopped or removed, puberty chugs along as it was *genetically* programmed to do. When a blocker implant is removed, for example, the person assigned female will continue to develop into a woman and the person assigned male will continue to grow into a man.

Or—*and this is life-changing*—a transgender kid can receive the hormones they know their body should have! In other words, "cross hormones" or "cross-sex hormones" allow a person assigned female but aching to be male to take testosterone and to transition male. And a person assigned male may get estrogen to transition female.

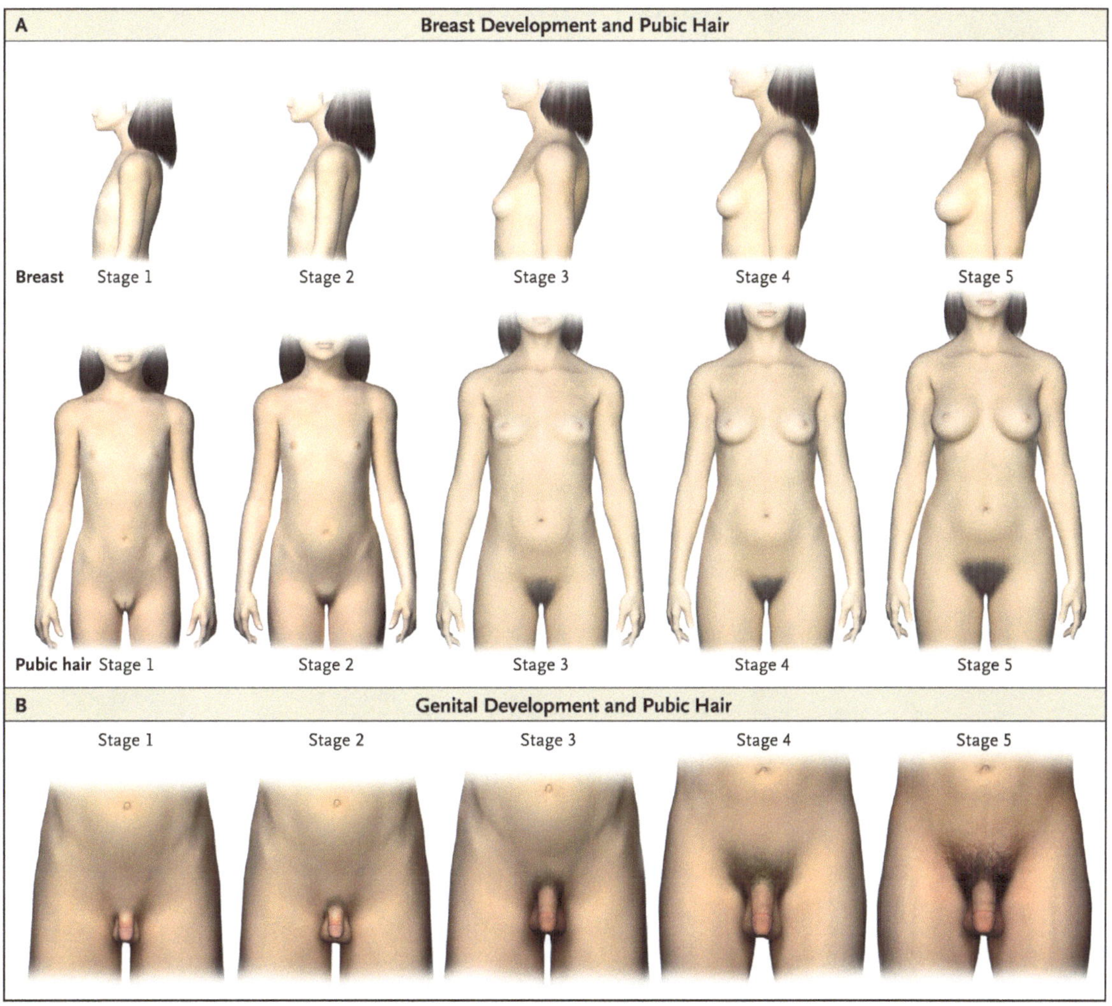

Figure 5.6. The Tanner Stages.

The Tanner Stages diagram can help a young person figure out their current stage of puberty and give a good idea of what is programmed to happen in the future.

Medical Treatment for Children and Adolescents with Gender Dysphoria

We'll cover gender dysphoria more completely in Chapter 6, but I'll discuss treatment for children and adolescents briefly here because I believe it is important for you to have access to this information. We are witnessing transgender adolescents growing up *without* some of the struggles experienced by transgender adults. I have heard many trans adults express an understandable envy toward their younger counterparts.

When I've followed a trans person through their transition, I often ask, "What would you have done differently?"

Almost without exception, I hear the answer, "I would have transitioned earlier."

Unfortunately, transitioning isn't seamless for anyone, even when transitioning at a young age. There are trade-offs either way, as we'll discuss.

What Can Be Done for Very Little Children

Many children, but certainly not all, know from a *very* young age that they belong to a gender other than their birth gender. A little trans person assigned female, for example, may state that they are a boy, beg for a short haircut, play with stereotypically boys' things, wear boys' clothing, and become angry with anyone who challenges them. Or a little trans child assigned male may insist that they are a girl, refuse haircuts, play with stereotypically girls' toys, and wear girls' clothing. A child may beg to use a different name and different gender pronouns.

Some trans kids gravitate to more gender-neutral interests, like animals, music, computers, or video games.

While a child's understanding of their gender can change, we often notice the following three components to early gender identification. World-renowned expert Johanna Olson-Kennedy, MD, medical director for the Center for Transyouth Health and Development at Children's Hospital in Los Angeles, says that kids who identify as gender-nonconforming early tend to be particularly—

- Insistent
- Consistent
- Persistent[10]

These kids are exceptionally clear. They insist that you recognize their correct gender and they keep at it. They are often very angry if you counter their gender understanding.

The gift of selective disclosure is the gift we give with early treatment.

— Johanna Olson-Kennedy, MD

---

10 Johanna Olson-Kennedy, "The Medical Needs of Transgender Youth: Puberty Delay and Cross Hormones," (presentation, Gender Odyssey International Conference, Seattle, WA, August 20, 2015).

For a young child, there's not much that has to be done physically. Parents are encouraged to support the child in their social transition. This may include backing the child's choices in personal clothing and hairstyle and calling the child by a name the child favors rather than their given name. Social transition may involve informing the child's teacher and school administrators, and—most importantly—joining a support group to help everyone in the family in this important process. (See **genderdiversity.org** or **transfamilies.org.**)

Olson-Kennedy points out that, "Adolescents with no prior nonconforming behaviors or indicators may find that their gender dysphoria is unveiled at the beginning of puberty."

The changes of puberty can barrel on like an approaching train! If a kid had any belief that they would somehow mature in their identified gender—and some kids do believe this—puberty proves that isn't going to happen. And puberty can become a crisis time accompanied by depression, anxiety, cutting, or other self-harm behaviors, suicidal thinking, and isolation.

Some kids are compelled to take their gender expression further. Some, for example, try to remove their unwanted genital parts. I have heard of a young child trying to cut off their penis with nail clippers.

I recall one adult patient in my practice who placed their penis and scrotum in a vise; they landed in the emergency room to be cared for by a urologist whom they found to be less than sensitive and probably horrified. Another adult patient of mine shot off a testicle. These two adults survived, but they really might have died.

If you are wishing to have your genitals modified, remember that genital gender-affirming surgery can be done safely by a trained surgeon later on.

Puberty Blockers and How They Work

When parents recognize that their child is experiencing gender dysphoria, puberty blockers can temporarily put the entire process on pause.

We are talking about *puberty* blockers here, not testosterone blockers (like spironolactone), which are used in older teens or adults. Puberty blockers place puberty on a temporary hold until a child, their parents, and the medical team are fully on board. Blockers can buy several years of valuable time for a child and prevent the development of unwanted secondary sexual characteristics that seem to mark a person as male or female forever.

Secondary sexual characteristics include a deep voice and facial hair for a person assigned male, or breast development and menstrual periods for a person assigned female. We know that these characteristics can be modified later, but it often takes multiple surgeries and a lot of time and money to do so.

The medications used for this puberty blockade are called "gonadotropin-releasing hormone (GnRH) analogs." These medications work like the body's own GnRH from the hypothalamus in the brain. When GnRH "talks" to the pituitary gland, it signals the pituitary to send LH and FSH to the ovaries or testicles (whichever the child has). This in turn signals the testicles to release testosterone or the ovaries to release estrogen and progesterone. All of this occurs in a feedback loop, with pulses of the various hormones signaling the next hormonal event.

But with a GnRH analog, the pituitary gland is *flooded* with GnRH in a *steady, nonpulsatile manner.* This flood signals the ovaries to produce more estrogen or the testicles to produce more testosterone.

This change may feel uncomfortable for 5 or 6 weeks in that a person senses the excess of the "wrong hormone." A child may have temporary mood swings or emotional ups and downs. Some kids describe headaches or even mild hot flashes. But after an adjustment period, receptors in the pituitary gland are "down-regulated." This down-regulation temporarily disables the pituitary's feedback loop to the hypothalamus and stops the pituitary from sending out LH and FSH to stimulate the testicles or ovaries. This places puberty on hold and gives everyone a chance to regroup.

Remember, *puberty will come back when the puberty blocker is stopped.* I know this sounds complicated; it is. But think of a puberty blocker as something that temporarily prevents the ovaries or testicles from releasing the sex hormones that produce changes in puberty.

Be assured that puberty blockers have been used for many years to treat a condition called "precocious puberty." This is when puberty starts much earlier than usual. I remember a little cisgender girl in our practice who began to develop mature breasts at age 7. She was placed on injectable puberty blockers to interrupt her early puberty. The blockers were stopped when she reached age 12, and she continued puberty at a more usual time. Why did she even need blockers? When puberty begins so early, a child will stop growing in height long before they should, and they will be short-statured forever. The point here is that puberty blockers are not new. *The medical profession has had years of experience with them, as applied to the condition of precocious puberty.*

How Puberty Blockers Are Administered

Puberty blockers come in two forms: injections or implants. Both forms are typically quite expensive and may require special clearance from a child's health insurance company, if insurance covers the blockers at all. (**Note:** Puberty suppression is an off-label or nonapproved use of these medications.)

Let's look at the injections first: Lupron Depot (leuprorelin) is an intramuscular injection, meaning that it is usually injected into the muscle of the buttocks every 1 to 3 months.

Another form of puberty blocker is the histrelin implant (with trade names of Supprelin LA and Vantas). The implant is smaller than a matchstick and is placed under the skin in the upper arm on the inside (closest to the body), usually in the nondominant side. If you have seen birth control implants like Nexplanon or Implanon, you will recognize that the histrelin implant looks very similar and is inserted in much the same way. And just like the birth control implants, the process can be done under local anesthetic (numbing medicine) in the doctor's office.

In my practice, when I insert an implant, I place a little numbing cream on the prepared site on the inner part of the upper arm. After about a half hour, I then *inject* a little more of a different numbing medicine, although this is rarely felt because the skin is already quite numb. Next, I make a tiny incision in the skin (again, usually not felt at all). Using a special insertion device, I then slip the little blocker under the skin. We put Steri-Strips over the tiny incision and bandage it, and the newly "blocked" kid is good to go.

We teach parents and kids how to feel the blocker under the skin because of the very rare possibility that the blocker could extrude itself or work its way out. Blocker implants are said to last about 12 to 18 months, but I have seen many that have worked for 3 and 4 years. We can do blood tests to monitor the hormone levels of the recipient every few months so that we know when it loses its effectiveness.

Getting a Puberty Blocker

Kids who want puberty blockers need help from willing parents and a willing healthcare provider. We've discussed finding gender-friendly healthcare providers (look up "transgender healthcare for young people in your area"). You may find help through your local children's or university medical center. And you can usually get a solid referral from a local Planned Parenthood.

You will want to be sure your health insurance covers this; otherwise, the cost may be prohibitive (many thousands of dollars).

Remember, though, that the decision to get a puberty blocker is quite straightforward. When the blocker is removed or when blocker injections are stopped, puberty will resume, and the patient will continue to develop in their biologically programmed gender. Except for the cost and small procedural risks, there's nothing really bad that can happen here. The blocker gives a person more time without the onslaught of pubertal changes.

Cross Hormones (Cross-Sex Hormones)

The decision to start cross hormones (from a trans kid's perspective, the "correct" hormones) is more complicated. It must be made by a child and family with the assistance of their healthcare provider and frequently a counselor.

In the Netherlands, where puberty blockers have been available for many years, cross hormones are generally started at age 16. There's nothing magical about the age of 16; it is the legal age of consent in the Netherlands.

Many healthcare providers have come to believe that peer concordance (that is, looking and sounding like your age-mates) has considerable merit. So, we frequently begin cross hormones younger—say, at 12 or 13. Puberty blockers and cross-sex hormones may be used together.

When cross hormones are started, a person begins to experience all the hormone effects of the "correct" gender. For example, a person assigned male and treated with estrogen will develop breast buds as their breasts begin to develop. Their voices will not deepen as they would with male programming. Similarly, their shoulders won't broaden out and their faces will not develop the prominent brow bones, jaw, and thyroid cartilage (Adam's apple) that testosterone would have dictated. They will not begin growing facial hair if it hasn't started. Periods will not begin, of course, because of the child's anatomy (no uterus, for instance).

We now know that uterine transplants have been done. A baby was born by C-section delivery from a woman with a transplanted uterus in the fall of 2014.[11] And a cadaver uterus was successfully transplanted into a person assigned female, with a baby born in 2017.[12]

Perhaps trans women will be able to carry pregnancies one day, but we aren't there yet—a source of significant grief to many transgender adults.

---

11 Susan Scutti, "First Baby Born to Woman with Uterus Transplanted from Deceased Donor," *CNN*, December 5, 2018, https://www.cnn.com/2018/12/04/health/uterus-transplant-deceased-donor-study/index.html.

12 Johanna Olson-Kennedy, "The Medical Needs of Transgender Youth: Puberty Delay and Cross Hormones," (presentation, Gender Odyssey International Conference, Seattle, WA, August 20, 2015).

As trans boys start testosterone, they experience masculinization: a deepening of the voice, increased body hair, acne, the emergence of facial hair, and increased muscle development. Periods will stop if they have already begun. The clitoris will enlarge significantly, and breast development that has already occurred will stop (but not disappear).

Once the hormonal picture is corrected and the child's mind and body become synchronous, many things relax. Gender no longer must be the focus of interpersonal interactions. There's no need to explain or clarify one's gender unless a person wants to!

The Downsides to Puberty Blockers and Early Cross Hormones

When adolescents who are assigned male have puberty blockers that are quickly followed by estradiol, trans girls grow up female, but they *cannot have biological children*. (They don't make sperm.) Similarly, trans boys will grow up male before having the opportunity to have biological children. (They may not have started ovulating yet.)

In other words, kids started on puberty blockers and cross hormones at a young age (before they would be able to bank their own sperm or have their eggs harvested and frozen, usually at Tanner Stage 4 or 5) will generally not have children using their own DNA.

Rather, they may have children by adoption or by other means, such as a sibling donating sperm or eggs to create a pregnancy, or because a partner already has children.

For some people, not being able to parent a child that is biologically related to them is a sacrifice that feels too big. Banking sperm or harvesting and freezing eggs is expensive. It is not generally covered by insurance, and it doesn't always result in a pregnancy.

But if it is *critical* to a kid to be able to have their own biological children in the future, that person is best advised to wait until sperm banking or egg harvesting can be done before starting on cross-sex hormones.

> **I remember one of my adult patients lamenting that their gender transition wasn't possible earlier. "If you'd transitioned as a teenager," I commented, "you wouldn't have had your amazing kids!" Tough argument.**
>
> *— Linda Gromko, MD*

The downside of waiting? By Tanner Stage 4 or 5, secondary sex characteristics have developed, which can make a gender transition more difficult and more expensive.

Another area of *potential* concern in young trans girls who later wish to have gender-affirmation surgery (vaginoplasty) is the actual amount of tissue that is available to use in the construction of the neovagina. In an adult trans woman, the vaginal canal is usually constructed from the penis, and the labia are formed from the fully developed adult scrotum. In adults who have *insufficient* genital tissue for a standard vaginoplasty, surgeons will graft tissue from other parts of the body. I've seen beautiful results, for example, when tissue from the lateral waist area is used as a tissue donor site. Another option is the peritoneal pull-through vaginoplasty, where the neovagina is lined by the peritoneal membrane in the abdomen. (You can read about this and colovaginoplasties—and even about new materials used to create the vagina in Chapter 11.)

I believe that trans women who have a smaller amount of tissue because they never developed adult-sized genitalia may well require graft tissue from other areas of their body. And while this may be a factor to consider in these patients, it would certainly not seem to be a reason to avoid puberty blockers or cross hormones in most patients.

What's Done for Trans Teens Who Are Already Well into Puberty But Haven't Had Puberty Blockers

We've already discussed what happens with puberty blockers and early cross hormones. If a person is already in Tanner Stage 4 or 5 (just about fully mature), a healthcare provider may move directly into cross hormones.

Your healthcare provider will hopefully ask you if you want to have your own biological children later in life. If you were assigned male, you may be able to bank sperm. If you were assigned female, you may be able to harvest and freeze eggs. Such procedures are known as "fertility preservation" and will be discussed in more detail later in Chapter 21.

It's important to remember that going through fertility preservation does not come with a guarantee of having a biological child. It gives you the *chance,* however, of having your own biological children later in life if this is important to you. Health insurance generally does not cover these options, but we have found that some parents have been more than willing to pay to have their kids' sperm banking or egg harvesting done. Another option for trans males is to stop testosterone when they want to have a pregnancy. Trans men can be impregnated by sperm from a partner or a donor and then carry pregnancies and deliver biologically related offspring (see Chapter 21).

Older teens and young adults do well with hormone therapy and gender-affirming surgeries. And while doing things when you're younger may be better in many ways, we certainly advise that you don't do anything surgical (that is, potentially irreversible) without absolute confidence in your decisions.

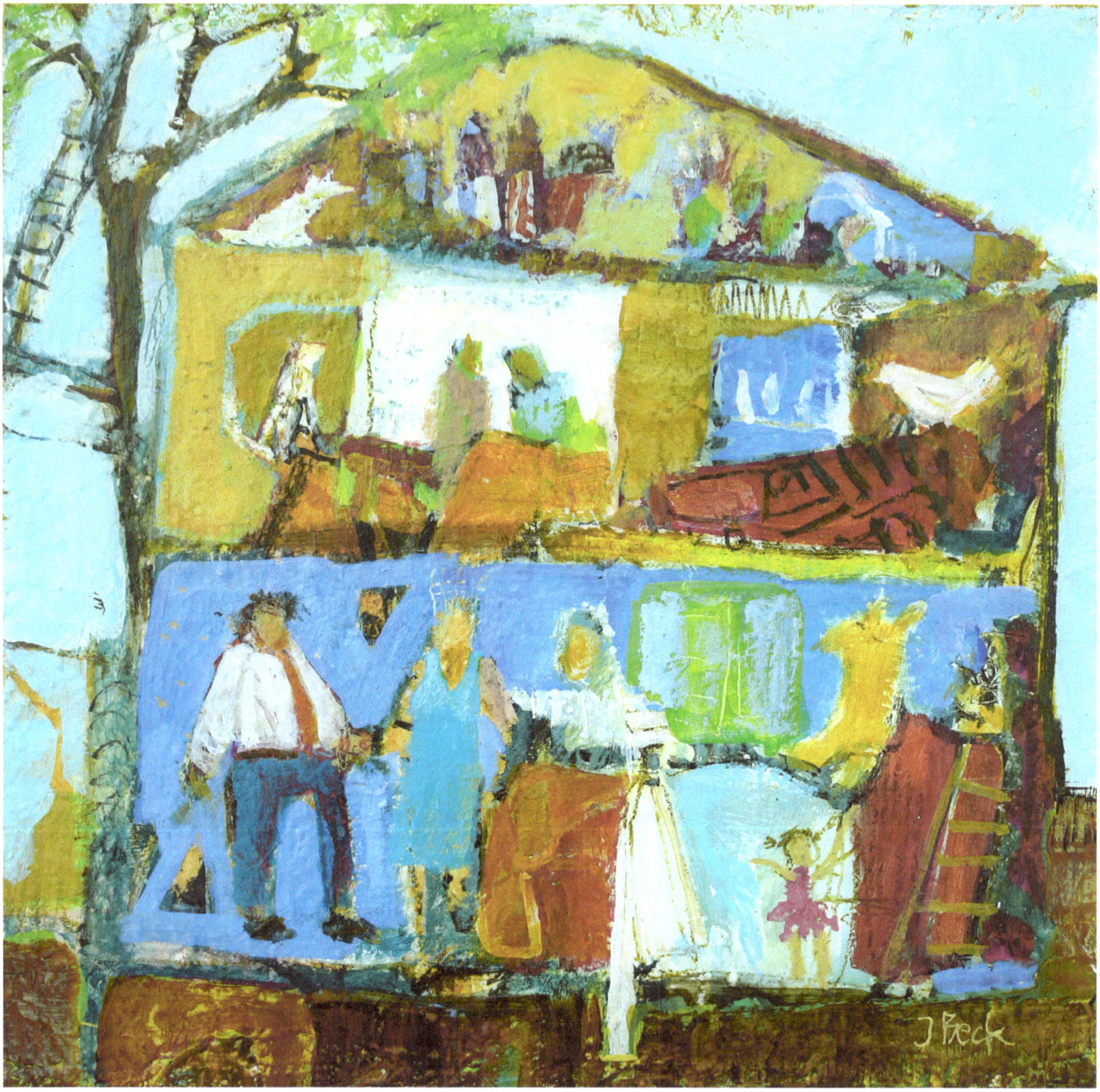

Housework

CHAPTER 6
Gender Dysphoria

By my definition, gender dysphoria is a pervasive sense that a person's assigned birth gender does not match their gender identity, *and a feeling of distress about this mismatch.*

(If you do not feel distress, you don't have dysphoria. Perhaps you've transitioned already, or perhaps you've come to an equilibrium that works in your life. Gender dysphoria is listed in the DSM-5, the American Psychiatric Association's Diagnostic and Statistical Manual of Mental Disorders, 5th Edition, as a clinical diagnosis, not because of being transgender but rather because of the *dysphoria*. A person's gender identity is not considered pathological.)[13]

> **Personally, I don't like the phrasing "female-to-male." That implies I was female until I somehow morphed into a man. I was always male: a boy, he, him, his. The transition was the realization of who I always was.**
>
> — *Adult trans man*

Changing Gender

Can we change our gender? The answer is *yes! Absolutely, yes.*

No matter how young or old you are, many things can be done to help you transition. In my practice, I serve transgender patients from age 5 to 85, all at various stages of transition. We have even seen a few people "detransition" (sometimes called "retransitioning") over the years, although it doesn't happen very often.

I hope that individuals will find their best place along a continuum of gender expression. Some people "dress" only; other people take hormones; others have surgery. Some live in their identified gender all the time, and others do so when they can. There's nothing right or wrong about how or if you transition, but there is likely a "best place" as defined by you.

As you travel along this road, you may find people who firmly believe that there is only one path to gender synchrony. Gender identity and its expression are very personal. Don't get caught up by folks who believe that there is only one true path and follow the "I am more trans than you" mentality! It will only cause you frustration and pain.

Certainly, some things *cannot* be done in gender transition. As stated earlier, we do not yet have the technology to change our chromosomes. We cannot convert someone's sex chromosomes from XX to XY—or from XY to XX. And we really cannot make you taller or shorter.

13 American Psychiatric Association, *Gender Dysphoria*, DSM-5 Update (Washington DC: APA Publishing, 2013), https://www.psychiatry.org/File%20Library/Psychiatrists/Practice/DSM/APA_DSM-5-Gender-Dysphoria.pdf.

But much can be done to help people transition and thereby ease a person's gender dysphoria.

No Conversion Therapy!

Please understand that I have no delusion that one can—or should—"fix" or "cure" someone's gender identity. That's sort of like trying to convert a person who's gay and make them straight. There's nothing to be fixed!

Being gay is just something that *is* and trying to "fix" it is like asking the tide to stay out. Thankfully, measures to "cure" gay people are now illegal in Washington and other states.[14]

In my experience, trying to cure transgender people is equally absurd.

— Linda Gromko, MD

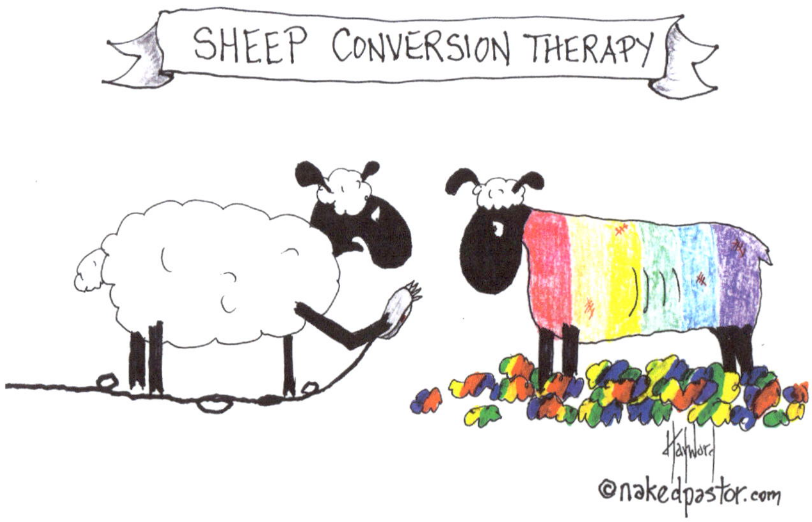

Reducing Gender Dysphoria

Gender dysphoria can be best reduced by first giving careful thought to what you want to see happen. You are more likely to get what you want in any area of your life *if you know what it is that you want.*

There are no magic wands available, of course. But I do know from my practice that gender dysphoria can be reduced, and gender can be modified by using some or all of the approaches on the next several pages.

14 Movement Advancement Project, *Conversion Therapy Laws*, updated July 16, 2021, https://www.lgbtmap.org/img/maps/citations-conversion-therapy.pdf, and Movement Advancement Project, "Equality Maps: Conversion 'Therapy' Laws," accessed July 28, 2021, https://www.lgbtmap.org/equality-maps/conversion_therapy.

Seeing a therapist is probably sound advice for anyone at any stage of life. You may benefit from a relationship with a good therapist as you tackle some of the gender challenges you face. And you will need a therapist's letter (or several) should you proceed to have gender-affirming surgeries. If you don't have access to a gender support group, consider starting your own. Even having dinner every month with a compassionate person who's traveling a similar road can be extremely helpful. You can also find private online groups on social media.

- **A person can take prescription hormones representative of their identified gender and thus reverse some of the effects of the hormones of their birth gender.**
  I've found that even small doses of a person's "correct" hormones can take the edge off of dysphoria. Small doses can be very helpful, especially when a person cannot transition more fully due to work, social, or family issues. If your healthcare provider does not prescribe gender-affirming hormones or if you don't feel comfortable asking them for hormones, search the Internet for "transgender healthcare in (your area)." Many Planned Parenthood clinics prescribe hormones for transgender patients also.

- **A person can adopt many *nonsurgical* approaches to "presenting": appearing and living in their identified gender.**

- **Legal name changes can be done at any time in a person's life, although parental consent is required if one is below the age of majority (18 in the United States).**
  For information on changing your name and executing all of the document changes needed, my favorite resource is transequality.org. Look for the "Documents" section and follow the prompts. Refer also to Chapter 19 in this book.

- **Changing one's gender on a state identification card or a driver's license can be extremely helpful and validating.**
  You will need a form from your state department of licensing or motor vehicles; in Washington State, this form no longer requires a physician signature, and a person can now self-designate the gender of "X" without a physician letter as of November 12, 2019. (See "Changing Your Documents" in Chapter 19.)

- **A person can legally change their name and gender designation on their official documents, including their passport, Social Security record, and birth certificate.**
  Again, go to transequality.org for comprehensive information.

- **Gender-modifying surgeries are becoming much more common as more surgeons are becoming experts and as health insurance is assisting patients in covering the expense.**
  Section 4 of this book covers the major details on surgical approaches to gender transformation.

Trying to Avoid Dysphoria

Many people try to "cure" dysphoria by adopting extreme manifestations of their assigned gender. The following description relates one such person's efforts, although it's something I've witnessed in many people.

I played football on a taped-up knee and torn cartilage. I swaggered with this dead-eye look and tough exterior to ward off bullies and my own feelings of shame, fear, and inadequacy. I got into fistfights, even after getting beat up by a kid who ended up in jail for breaking my nose and caving in my septum.

I went camping in the winter and climbed one of the tallest waterfalls in the country that was iced over. I jumped on horseback without any training and got thrown from two horses. I entered the world of rock-and-roll. That was the most macho world of all. I never felt more like a man. People wanted to hang out with me, people praised me, and a lot of people paid me to play or bought my recordings. Women threw themselves at me.

The more I played, the more the persona and ego took over and the horror diminished . . . until I got off the stage.

— Adult trans woman

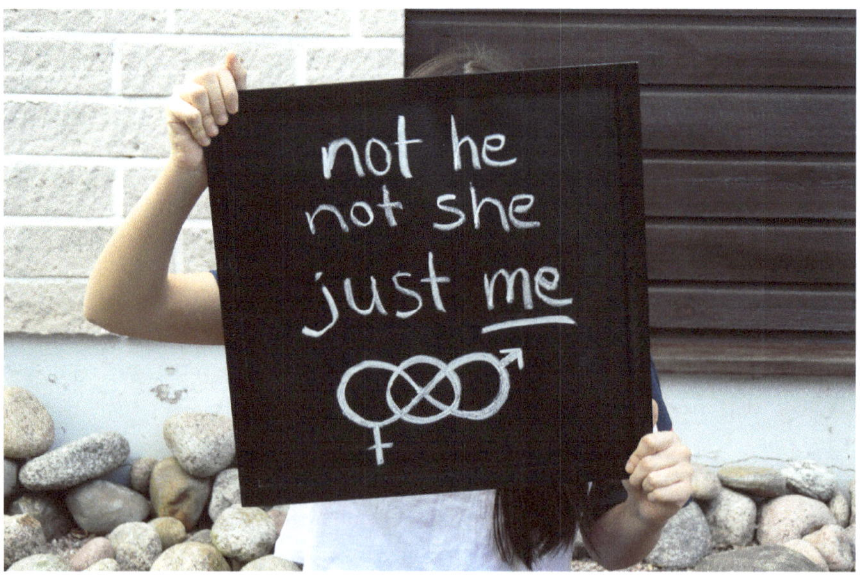

Managing Dysphoria When You Can't Transition

Trigger warning: This frank piece, written by a 67-year-old trans female, deals with raw themes of intense sadness and using drugs and alcohol for relief.

I remind myself that dysphoria is a whole lot better than the trials and tragedies other people are experiencing in war zones and hospitals. It is also far better than having the combined trials of claustrophobia, post-traumatic stress disorder (PTSD), bipolar disorder, depression, tinnitus, eating or sleep disorders, and, worst of all, a huge eye floater that is horrifying to a person who is claustrophobic.

Being transgender is like a back-and-forth ballet. Sometimes I take one step forward, and then invariably, I take two steps back.

On exceedingly rare occasions, I accept being a transgender female. That fades quickly. Very soon, I hate being transgender. Then I love being transgender again because of the relief I felt from getting the diagnosis from professionals I trust. It confirmed my identity and eliminated my fears of all of the other possibilities that could have been worse.

Alpha-state meditation helps. Using an alpha state, I have, over many years and with supreme effort, been able to see myself as female. I still continue to see this image more clearly as other facets of the diamond begin to shine.

My study of so-called "sex-change cases" of past life memories in unjaded children made me appreciate the realistic possibility of reincarnation. The psychological giants who have done this research make me lean toward probability, not possibility. Unless they were religious fundamentalists, any transgender person would find this research exhilarating. At times, reincarnation has been a huge help in managing my condition.

Drugs and alcohol have always been essential for managing my dysphoria. Sometimes, when you're swimming across that metaphorical lake, you get exhausted. Then you spot the raft. You struggle to it, gasping for air. Once on top of the raft, you look up at the afternoon sun, breathe a sign of relief, and feel good…for a time. For me, drugs and alcohol are transgender rafts.

My age is one of my best aids in dealing with gender dysphoria. I am already 67. But if I've suppressed the dysphoria all these years, how much longer will I live?

— Adult trans woman

Planning Your Transition Journey: Holding Your EPPY EGG

(Or More Accurately, Your EPPP-EGG)

By Cynthia Radthorne

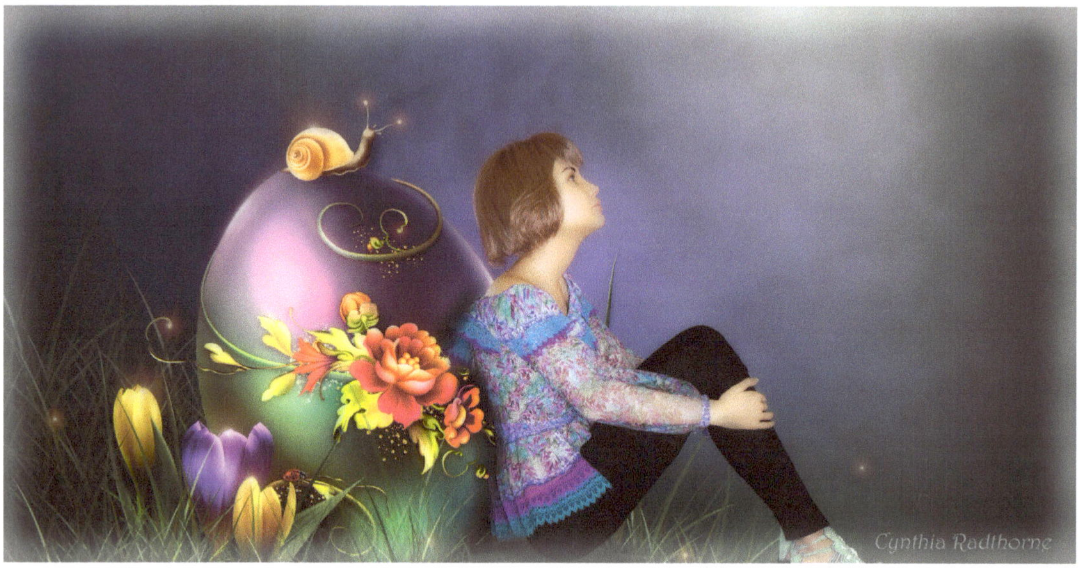

EPPP-EGG is my little acronym for aspects of the transgender journey. It stands for expectations, planning, patience, perseverance, empathy, graciousness, and gifts. While everyone's path is unique to them, there are some principles that tend to be shared by all. And if these are not part of your journey yet, they are perhaps worth considering. So, let's look at your EPPP-EGG.

Expectations

This is well before you do anything else concrete. This is where you are thinking... where you are feeling... where you are assessing who you truly are and what you want your life to be. This is where you take an honest look at what those feelings mean and how they fit into your life or can fit into your life. Will transitioning and living as another gender bring you the serenity and the peace of mind you seek? Will the costs—financial, social, and emotional—be worth it? Before you walk further down the path, know the answers to these questions. And be honest with yourself. This is your life and no one else knows your heart as well as you do.

Planning

So, you've made the decision: Yes, I am willing to change my life, willing to do what needs to be done in order to live as the gender I know I am. Now is the time for serious planning. You don't have to commit yet, and you don't have to disrupt your personal relationships or put your career at risk. You are simply researching: What are the laws in my state?

What practical things can I do and how do I do them (name change, driver's license, Social Security card, passport, credit cards, insurance, and so on)? Where can I obtain assistance (therapists to help you navigate your needs, doctors who treat gender issues and are willing to prescribe hormones, surgeons who handle gender-reassignment surgery if that is your path, and vocal coaches if transitioning male to female), and how will I pay for these things?

How much time will I need for growing out hair if desired (longer locks for male to female, for instance, or facial hair for female to male) or for electrolysis for removing hair? Where can I obtain the wardrobe I seek? And most important of all in your planning, beyond the practical: What will be the effect on my relationships and my work? How will my spouse, my children, my parents, my friends, my coworkers, and my boss react to such a dramatic change? These questions are much harder to answer, but you need to be prepared for them and have an understanding how you will navigate them all.

Patience

Once you begin your journey, you need to be patient. You will feel the urge to get it all done *right* now. But things take time: the legal steps, the physical steps, and most of all, the emotional steps—not just yours but for those around you. You may have been thinking about this all your life but those around you have not. To some of them, this may be a bolt out of the blue. So, exercise patience and follow your plan while you are following your heart.

Perseverance

At times, you will feel discouraged. Roadblocks may appear, and institutions or individuals may not initially accept or support your change. Now is not the time to give up. If you've made it this far and have taken these steps, you really can't put the toothpaste back into the tube. Celebrate each little victory and savor them to offset the roadblocks. And keep your eye on the far side of the bridge.

Empathy

While this is your journey, you are not walking it alone. You do not live in a vacuum. You have family, friends, coworkers, and people in your life who, even if they support you 100 percent, cannot *know* what you are feeling and what you have experienced in becoming *you*. Be empathetic to *their* journeys with you, for they must travel a path too. They may experience their own sense of loss or discomfort or frustration. It is up to you to be as understanding of them as they are, or are trying to be, of you.

Graciousness

Transitioning gender in our current society is not easy and there will be people who may reject your change and others who may just be uncomfortable. But for each of those types of people, there are others who will accept and some who will embrace the new you. Be aware that these allies need *your* support as much as you need theirs. Acknowledge their kindness. Thank them when they treat you with respect. Sometimes, even the best of allies may slip with a pronoun; this does not mean they do not support or believe in you; it just means they are human. Grant them that imperfection, be understanding of any minor slips, and consider the bigger picture of where you are and how far they have come with you.

Gifts

While the road can be difficult in becoming the gender you know you are, at least in our present day, there *is* a road. This has obviously not always been the case. We may feel it should be a right to do so, but the reality is that society is still catching up. If you look upon your transition as a gift rather than as a right, then each successful step will be a happy affirmation rather than a hurdle. And the journey will have been across a bridge to your own personal paradise rather than a slog up a mountainside.

SECTION 2

HORMONES

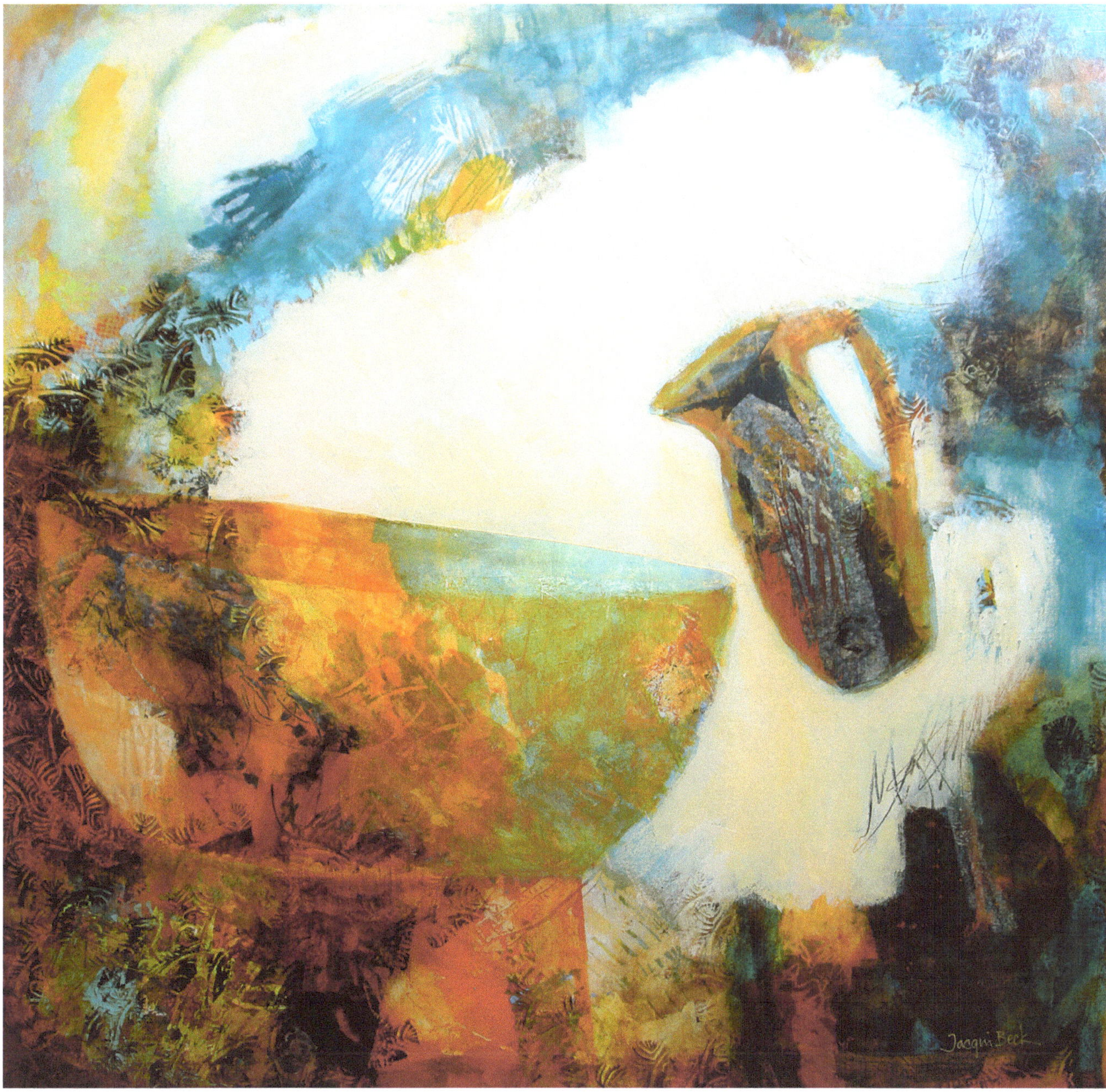

To Fill

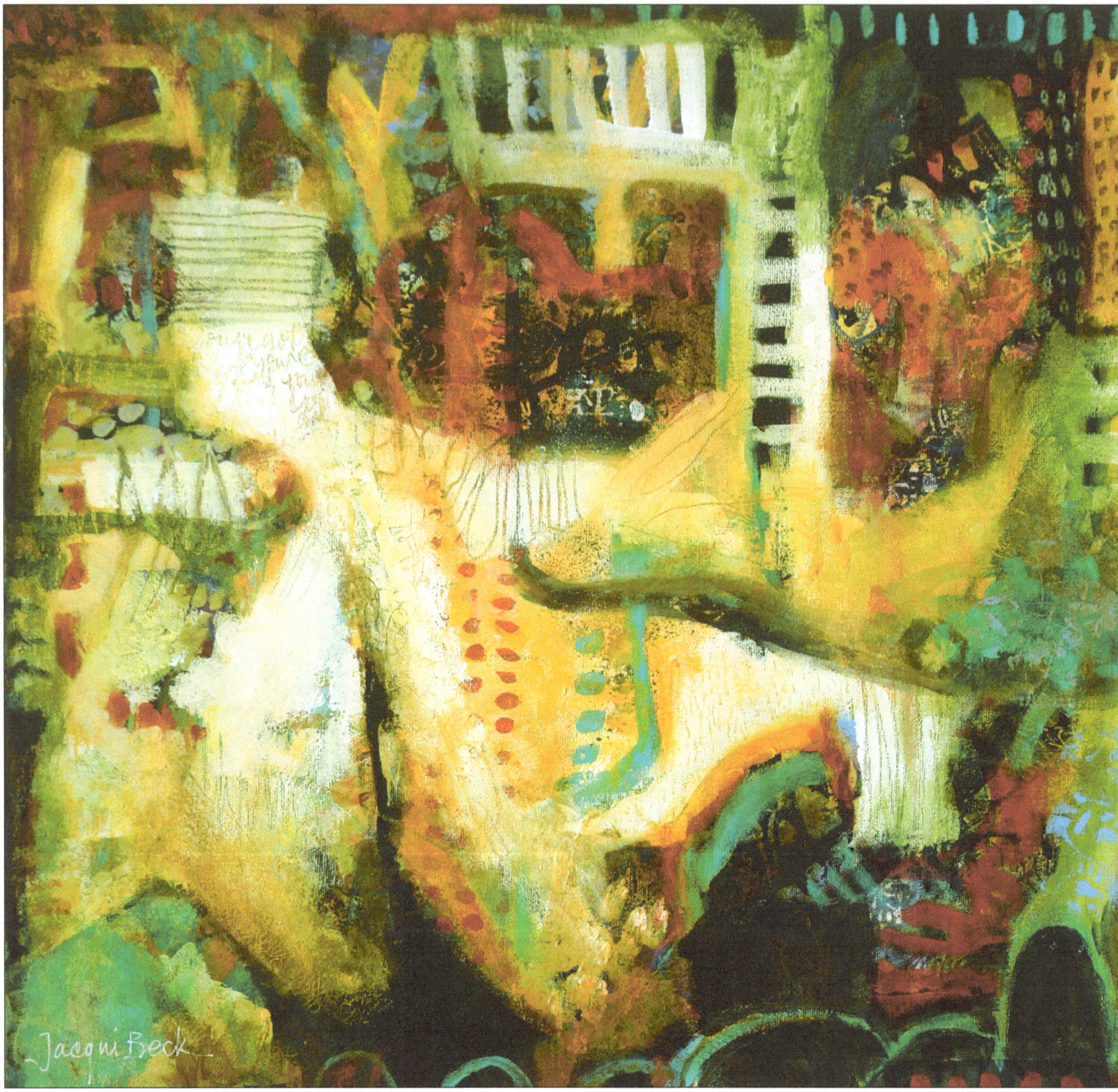

Finding Our Way

CHAPTER 7

Starting Hormones

In this section, you will notice that I don't discuss doses or specific medication protocols. Your healthcare provider will help you with this.

There are protocols published on the Internet, though. Here are good examples:

- Vancouver Coastal Health in British Columbia: **phsa.ca/transcarebc/Documents/HealthProf/BC-Trans-Adult-Endocrine-Guidelines-2015.pdf**
- Center of Excellence for Transgender Health in San Francisco: **transcare.ucsf.edu/guidelines**
- Fenway Center in Boston: **lgbtqiahealtheducation.org/wp-content/uploads/COM-2245-The-Medical-Care-of-Transgender-Persons-v31816.pdf**

Guidelines for Getting Started

Starting sex hormone therapy (basically estrogen or testosterone) is often a first step in gender transition. As with anything else in medicine and life, there are risks and benefits associated with taking hormones. It's important that you know what you want to see happen with hormone therapy, and that you know where potential problems lie.

It's human nature to compare your progress with that of other people who are taking hormones. But keep in mind that everyone responds differently, even to identical medical regimens. Know also that some providers start feminization with estradiol and others begin with spironolactone. They're just different ways to accomplish the same goals.

Here are some of the guidelines I use when dealing with hormones in gender transition. (Skip ahead if the pharmacology content isn't helpful to you.)

There are many regimens—recipes—for starting hormones. And while approaches differ, it doesn't necessarily mean that one way is correct and another is wrong. There are often several ways to arrive at a desirable and safe endpoint.

In medical school, I learned that with medications, it's best to "start low and go slow." By this, we mean start with a low dose and increase it gradually. In general, this is reasonable advice. When you think about puberty, hormones naturally start with lower levels and progress to adult levels as a person matures.

Hormones can be administered in a variety of ways. For example, hormones can be administered as—

- Injections into the muscle (IM or intramuscular injections)

- Injections placed under the skin, but not as deep as into the muscle (SQ, sub-Q, or subcutaneous injections)
- Hormone patches stuck onto the skin with a built-in adhesive (also called transdermal hormones)
- Compounded gels, creams, or lotions—usually for testosterone
- Pills swallowed or dissolved under the tongue (taken sublingually) for estradiol
- Pellets inserted deep under the skin of the buttocks for estradiol or testosterone, and sometimes both

A person may use a variety of routes for taking their hormones based on their age, ease of use, safety, and so on. (We see some patients needing to change routes due to the shortages in injectable hormones that occur from time to time.)

Hormone injections are generally given every week or every other week. I have some patients inject three times a month (on the first, tenth, and twentieth day of each month). The frequency of injections is determined by a person's hormone experience. Specifically:

- Is the hormone user getting the desired feminization or masculinizing effects?
- Are blood levels acceptable?
- Does the patient feel tired or crabby for several days before their injection is due? (In which case I may recommend every 10-day dosing rather than every 14-day dosing.)

I feel it is logical to assess a person's hormone levels periodically by taking blood samples (also called serum levels), but not all providers agree. Some do not measure hormone levels at all. Here are some guidelines I use:

- Remember that hormone levels in the blood vary from day to day and even minute to minute.
- I try to measure hormone levels in the blood consistently—that is, ***I draw blood levels at the same time in relation to dosing every time levels are measured.***
- A "pharmacologic steady state" describes an equilibrium of a medication in the bloodstream when the amount of drug coming into the body is approximately equal to the amount of drug being eliminated. A steady state can be measured after five "half-lives" of a drug have been given and just before the sixth dose is administered. A half-life is the time between the maximum serum level and half of the maximum serum level. In real life, a half-life is approximately the same as *one dosing interval—that is, the time between doses.*[15]

Let's look at an example: If intramuscular injections are given every other week, the steady state would occur at the trough—or "nadir"—after the fifth injection. To measure the steady state, we would get a serum (blood) level of the hormone at the trough level after Dose 5, immediately before Dose 6 is injected. Make sense?

With oral or sublingual meds, you could theoretically get a steady state serum level right before the sixth tablet. (For practical reasons, I may measure blood levels of tablets after a month or so.) I tend to measure these steady-state levels after starting a medication or after making a dose adjustment. These measurements help me increase the dose if the level is low, or decrease the dose if the level is too high.

15 C. Fookes, "Drug Half-life Explained," *Drugs.com*, March 8, 2019, https://www.drugs.com/article/drug-half-life.html.

Not all physicians agree about when the blood draw should be done. If you draw levels at the trough or nadir, remember that the blood level would have been considerably higher at the peak—that is, in the first 24 hours after the dose was given—particularly in a hormone injection.

There's a phenomenon we see where a serum level of a medication is climbing predictably along when suddenly it rockets up to a frighteningly high level. If we can stay below this "inflection point," we find a sweet spot where the drug level is effective but not so high as to theoretically pose additional risks.

Measuring drug levels is imperfect at best. If I get a result that seems higher than expected, I might ask the client if they just took an injection right before the blood draw rather than getting the blood level at the trough. If the level is lower than anticipated, the patient may have run out of medication. And, the tests themselves aren't perfect! The patient may have done everything exactly right and the level is still off. So, we look at trends.

In interpreting levels, I aim for numbers that fall within the physiologic range for the patient's appropriate gender. But this gets tricky, and I don't pretend to represent a consensus view. Here's essentially what I do:

- For trans male adults, I aim for something within the physiologic range of a cis male—that is, in our lab, a total testosterone of 350 to 900 ng/dL. A level of around 600 to 700 ng/dL is generally acceptable to my clients. (There's also a measurement for "free testosterone." This is testosterone that is *not* attached to a sex hormone binding protein or sex hormone binding globulin, or SHBG).
- For trans female adults, the target (estradiol) is more complex as the physiologic estradiol range in cis females runs from 11 to 500 (pg/ml), depending on where a person is in the menstrual cycle. Estradiol levels in early pregnancy run in the 4,000 range. So, in general terms for a trans woman, a level somewhere in the range of 100 to 300 pg/ml is probably acceptable, provided that the patient experiences appropriate feminization and is not experiencing medical complications.

A dominant sex hormone, whether it is estradiol or testosterone, can be important in maintaining optimal bone health.[16] Sometimes we see folks who have grown weary of taking sex hormones after having had excellent surgical and presentation outcomes. We may need to remind people that even though their transition is essentially completed, living bones must be maintained with adequate hormones. (The risk of not maintaining your bone health is osteoporosis, with its danger of fractures.)

An individual's risk of osteoporosis is variable, however. We can get a better assessment of osteoporosis risk by measuring bone density through a DEXA scan. The DEXA (dual-energy X-ray absorptiometry) routinely measures bone density at the lumbar spine and the hip. If your bone density is low to begin with, the lack of sex hormones may impact you more than someone starting with a higher bone density. People who were assigned male at birth (AMAB) will typically have higher bone densities to begin with. If a person is taking no hormones after transition, getting a DEXA scan would be a reasonable part of that individual's health assessment. If the bone density is acceptable, that person may be fine without continuing hormones.

Males and females, cis or trans, have both estradiol and testosterone in the bloodstream, as these hormones are produced in the adrenal glands that sit on top of *all* human kidneys.

16 "Sex steroids regulate skeletal maturation and preservation in both men and women, as already recognized in the 1940s by Albright and Reifenstein," as quoted from K. Venken, F. Callewaert, S. Boonen, and D. Vanderschueren, "Sex Hormones, Their Receptors and Bone Health," *Osteoporosis International* 19, no. 11 (November 2008): 1517, https://doi.org/10.1007/s00198-008-0609-z.

Taking Hormones for Feminization

Many providers recommend a combination of two types of medications to produce feminizing effects: estradiol and a testosterone blocker. (You will recall that a testosterone blocker is different from the *puberty* blocker used in kids just starting puberty and wanting to hold it at bay for a few years.) Many people use the feminizing hormone progesterone as well.

In general, I try to start only *one* new medication at a time. That way, if a person reacts poorly to something, I have a better idea what caused the problem. (It's the same concept we use when feeding babies: Add one new food at a time, see how the baby gets along, and save combos for when a baby has experience with each component in the combination. That way, you don't need to go back to square one when the baby gets a rash, leaving you to guess what the culprit was.)

People who are assigned female at birth (AFAB) produce two main hormones in the ovaries: estrogen and progesterone. Generally, when we discuss hormones for feminization, we are speaking of estrogen in the form of estradiol. But I have patients who take progesterone also, and we'll get into that later. We'll also get to the different forms that hormone medications come in, but first, let's look at estrogen's expected effects.

Here's What You May Notice When Starting Estradiol

- **Breast development starts with a "breast bud."**
  This is a small, tender lump you feel under the areola (the colored part of the nipple).

  As the breast develops, you will see the areola form into a cone shape. Later, glandular tissue and fat fill in under and around the areola as the mature female breast shape emerges. You can probably expect maximal breast development by about 3 years of hormone use, but remember that this process is also influenced by genetics. So, if you come from a family of small-breasted women, you may end up on the smaller side too. (You're best advised to start researching surgeons who perform breast augmentations anyway if you are hoping to develop very large breasts.) And don't be stunned if one of your breasts develops more quickly than the other. This happens in people assigned female also. Everyone has some asymmetry from one side to the other.

  It's helpful to remember that breast size has possibly been modified by people assigned female since time began. Breast forms, bra design and padding, and surgery can all modify breast size and shape, and we'll talk about all of these in later chapters (refer to Chapters 8 and 11).

  Many trans women find that the hormone progesterone can help with breast development. In my observation, this is true in some—but not in all—trans women who try it. In my opinion, if you give it a reasonable try and it helps, great. But why take extra medications if you don't see any difference?

- **Your overall mood may change.**
  Many trans women tell me that they feel calmer and more relaxed on estrogen. (Some of this calm may be attributable to the relief of finally getting hormonal assistance, but I hear this all the time.) Many women say they cry more easily at movies and puppies—anything that evokes a sentimental response.

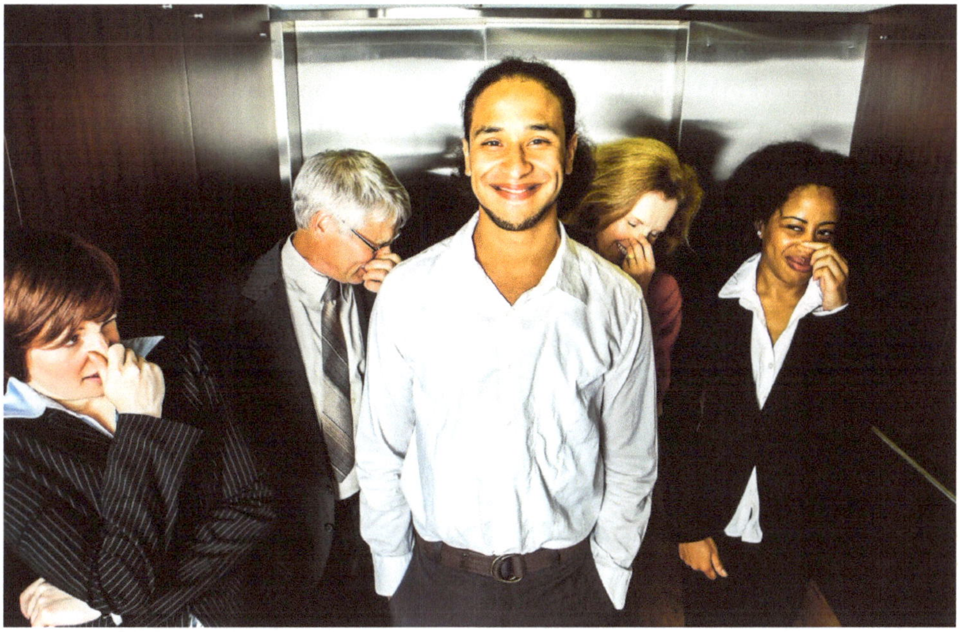

- **Your body odor will change.**
  People assigned male and people assigned female do smell differently; that is, they give off different scents. When one of my patients stopped estrogen as required right before her gender-affirming surgery, she complained, "I smell like a *guy* again!"

- **Your skin may feel softer.**

- **Your body hair may thin out.**
  Your scalp hair is another matter. Estrogen won't prevent your hairline from receding, and it usually doesn't bring hair back to a significant degree. Estrogen won't save you from baldness if that's what you are genetically programmed to do. (Read on; we'll address this in Chapter 8.)

- **Your libido (sex drive) may decrease.**
  But this is quite variable. Sometimes gender transition invites an examination of sexual orientation. While gender identity and sexual orientation are independent of each other, you may find that you are attracted to people differently. You may be attracted to both genders, and you might identify your sexual orientation differently than you did before. If your sex *drive* decreases and that is a problem for you, talk to your healthcare provider.

- **You will likely have fewer morning erections and fewer random erections.**
  Taking estradiol and spironolactone (a testosterone blocker) will likely result in fewer erections, which is a great relief for many of my patients.

  Many people want to continue to have erections, but *when they want them*. If you are having difficulty in this area, talk to your healthcare provider. We prescribe medications like Viagra (sildenafil), Cialis (tadalafil), and Levitra (vardenafil) with some regularity, so don't be shy about asking (see pages 62 and 66).

The science behind these drugs is amazing—actually, Nobel Prize material.[17] Viagra and its cousins allow blood to flow into the corpora cavernosa (the "pontoons" of the penis) and then to stay there, thus causing and maintaining an erection. Erections are generally stronger and longer lasting than without the medications. Following ejaculation or climax, the blood flows back out of the corpora, and the penis becomes flaccid (limp) again.

One of the barriers to using these medications has been cost, but with generic varieties now available, these medications have become much more affordable.

Important Facts about Viagra (Sildenafil) and Its Cousins

- **Sildenafil works with the stimulation of the penis; the penis doesn't just spring to life.**
- **Each of the medications has its own duration of action: Viagra is the shortest-acting and works for about 4 hours. Higher-dose Cialis is the longest-acting and works for up to 3 days.**
- **Sildenafil and related medications are available by prescription only, and some people should not take them! For example, a person taking nitrate blood pressure medications like isosorbide can faint or lose consciousness when combining their blood pressure medication with sildenafil. (This is not a problem with the testosterone blocker spironolactone, which is also a blood pressure medication.)**
- **If chest pain, faintness, or a problem with vision or hearing occur while taking the medication, get medical help right away and do NOT repeat the medication.**

Read the package insert or online information before you take medication of any kind.

- **When you're on estrogen and you have an ejaculation or climax, the fluid coming out of the penis may change in character.**
  It's not uncommon for the semen to change from milky to clear and to decrease in amount. You may even stop ejaculating, although you will still experience orgasm. While the semen may contain fewer sperm or even no sperm, we always recommend safe sex practices, including latex condoms to prevent an unplanned pregnancy or sharing of sexually transmitted infections (see Chapter 22).
- **Your testicles and penis may shrink.**
  Sometimes, they shrink quite a bit, even enough for people to worry if they'll have enough tissue to use in vaginoplasty surgery later. (There are ways, such as skin grafts or surgical techniques other than the penile inversion vaginoplasty, to make this work if there is a lot of shrinkage or if you weren't particularly well-endowed in the first place.) I think it's a courtesy to let people know that their genitals may shrink.

17 Peter Gorner, "Work That Led to Viagra Wins Americans a Nobel," *Chicago Tribune*, October 13, 1998, https://www.chicagotribune.com/news/ct-xpm-1998-10-13-9810130307-story.html.

- **Your physical strength will likely decrease.**
  Know this in advance, particularly if you have a physically active job or lifestyle. You can certainly maintain your fitness with exercise, but your muscles will not "bulk up" as much as they did under the dominant influence of testosterone. You can still do weight training, of course, but you may want to choose lighter weights and higher repetitions if you don't want to bulk up.

- **Your voice will probably NOT change.**
  Unlike trans males on testosterone, trans females do not enjoy a change in voice pitch with estrogen. This inequity always strikes me as unfair; voice deepening is such a rapid and confirmatory change in trans men. Voice change can happen for trans women, but only with practice, coaching, and sometimes surgery (see Chapter 8).

- **Your scalp hair will likely continue to do what it was genetically programmed to do.**
  If you are moving toward baldness, estrogen will not save you. But ask your healthcare provider about medications like minoxidil and finasteride; these can minimize hair loss. If you are planning to have facial feminization surgery (FFS), a scalp advance is a commonly used technique to move the hairline forward toward the face; it is often combined with brow bone contouring to produce a more feminine hairline and forehead shape.

  Hair transplants have become much more elegant over the years. If you are a boomer, you may remember when transplants looked like the little plugs of hair in a Tiny Tears or Betsy Wetsy doll. Today, hair follicles are transplanted as units of one to four follicles at a time for a much more natural appearance (refer to Chapter 8 for more about hair).

Ways to Take Estradiol

Estradiol comes in a variety of forms, and all are effective in producing feminizing changes. Some people may experience better results (as measured by blood levels of the hormone and bodily changes) with one form of estradiol as compared with another. But here's the menu of available estradiol forms:

- **Oral pills that are swallowed**
  The estrogen in birth control pills is *ethinyl* estradiol rather than estradiol and carries with it a higher risk of blood clot formation. ***It is considered risky to take birth control pills for gender transformation.***[18]

- **Oral pills that are dissolved under the tongue (taken sublingually)**
  This thereby minimizes the "first-pass effect of a medication" (see page 64). Annoyingly, available estradiol tablets are not engineered to dissolve quickly.

- **Injections given intramuscularly (into the muscle, usually of the buttocks or the thigh)**
  These require a longer needle to get into the muscle and are usually given weekly or every other week. Many of my patients learn to self-inject.

- **Injections given subcutaneously (into the superficial tissue between the skin and the muscle)**
  These require a shorter needle that is usually thinner, but know that estradiol is a thick solution and may be more difficult to inject with a smaller needle. Subcutaneous injections are usually given weekly.

---

18 Madeline B. Deutsch, "Overview of Feminizing Hormone Therapy," Transgender Care, University of California-San Francisco, June 17, 2016, https://transcare.ucsf.edu/guidelines/feminizing-hormone-therapy.

- **Transdermal patches applied to the skin of the abdomen or buttocks in most cases**
  The hormone is delivered *through* the skin. Transdermal patches are designed for perimenopausal cis women. In my experience, the dose required for a trans female is at least four times the dose required to manage menopausal symptoms in a cis female. And you may need more surface area on the skin to achieve the desired effect in transition.

  Athletic women may find that they sweat the patches off. Many women are also bothered by the lint borders the patches accumulate. (The trick? Wear them on the buttocks or lower back.) And some women are irritated by or are allergic to the adhesive.

- **Pellets inserted deep under the skin but over the muscle of the buttocks**
  (I started offering pellets prepared by compounding pharmacies during an estradiol shortage when many of my patients were unable to get their hormones.)

  After numbing the area with injected anesthesia, the provider places the pellets with a trocar—a device that deposits the pellets in the desired location. The hormones in the pellets release slowly over 2 to 6 months. In my practice, we try not to place pellets into "hormone virgins"—that is, people who have not used hormones before. Why? Because we really cannot get the pellets back out! The hormone effect will dissipate in time, of course, but it can take months. So, it could be uncomfortable for a while if you don't like the effect of the hormones.

- **Creams or lotions prescribed through a compounding pharmacy**
  I see these used with testosterone. (I'm not sure why this isn't done as much with estrogen, but I suspect it has to do with the physical amount of cream or lotion required to produce a feminizing effect.)

The "First-Pass Effect" of a Medication

When you take a medication in the form of a cream or lotion, an injection, an inhalation, a rectal suppository, a pellet, or a transdermal patch, the medication is absorbed directly into the **bloodstream**.

On the other hand, when you swallow a medication in pill form, it goes into the stomach where **it is first partially absorbed** by the blood vessels of the portal system associated with the liver. Part of the medication then continues from the stomach into the small intestines, where it is further absorbed into the systemic (total body) blood circulation.

The implication here is that delivery methods that avoid ingestion will have less impact on the liver, particularly if used over the long term.

Dissolving a pill under the tongue allows the medication to be absorbed by the mucous membrane of the floor of the mouth, where it goes directly into the systemic blood circulation. So, the sublingual use of pills minimizes the "first-pass effect," but it does not eliminate it completely, as some of the medication **is inevitably swallowed.**

Information on Needles, Syringes, and Sharps Containers

Needles

Needle size is identified by gauge. For example, if you use a 22-gauge needle, its barrel diameter measures 1/22nd of an inch. A 25-gauge needle measures 1/25th of an inch in diameter.

Needle length is obvious. A 1-inch needle is 1 inch long. The needle must be the right length for the route of injection to be used. Generally, we use a 1-inch needle (or maybe a 1.5-inch needle) for an intramuscular injection. Because a subcutaneous injection must go in more shallowly, we might prescribe a needle that's 5/8 inch in length.

Examples
For intramuscular (IM), use 1-inch 22-gauge needles.
For subcutaneous (SQ), use 5/8 inch 25-gauge needles.

Transfer needles are used to draw up medication from a vial. These larger-gauge needles (18-gauge) draw up the medication quickly. You then switch out the 18-gauge transfer needle for the needle you will use in your skin. Why do you use a transfer needle anyway? For one thing, it's faster. I've also been told that poking a needle through the rubber stopper of a vial can dull the needle, making an injection more painful. (One of my patients used the transfer needle to inject into their skin. It happened only once, as an 18-gauge needle looks like a pipe! It probably felt that way too.)

Syringes

Syringes come in a variety of sizes. We use mostly 1-cc (ml) and 3-cc (ml) syringes as these are commonly available.

One cubic centimeter (also called 1 "cc") is identical to 1 milliliter (also called 1 "ml"): 1 cc = 1 ml.

What is more important, however, is the tip of the syringe. I specify Luer Lock tips because they are more secure. You screw the needle hub into the Luer Lock tip and it stays put against the pressure needed to inject the hormone.

With a "slip tip" syringe, you push the needle onto the tip. With enough injection pressure, the needle can pop off the syringe. Nobody is happy when that happens, so ask your healthcare provider to specify the screw-on (Luer Lock) tips. Remember that nothing horrible happens if the apparatus comes apart. It may alarm you, certainly. But just start over and inject the remainder of the hormone dose or call your healthcare provider if you are unsure.

Sharps Containers

A "sharps container" is essential for anyone needing to dispose of used needles and syringes. These well-marked containers are made of sturdy nonpenetrable plastic. You can buy them at your pharmacy or online. There will be a modest medical waste disposal fee paid before or after returning your container to a pharmacy.

For further information on disposal, visit "How to Get Rid of a Sharps Container" at **fda.gov/files/medical%20devices/published/How-to-Get-Rid-of-a-Sharps-Container--Printable-Version.pdf.**

Testosterone Blockers

My usual protocol has been to start the testosterone blocker first (before estrogen), but that evolved from a personal bias only. I think it is equally fine to start estradiol first, particularly when that is the preference of a patient. (My concern was that I'm more likely to see a blood pressure drop or an electrolyte imbalance with the testosterone blockers, so I wanted those folks to see me sooner so I could detect a problem. Returning to the clinic for estrogen is motivating.)

In the United States, we tend to use spironolactone (Aldactone) to block testosterone. Spironolactone (pronounced "SPY-roe") has been used for many years as a blood pressure medication. It is still used for blood pressure control, but there are many newer blood pressure meds now available and often with fewer side effects. That said, if a trans woman needs blood pressure control, she may get a "two-for-one" by experiencing both testosterone blockade *and* blood pressure lowering from the same medication.

It has long been recognized that spironolactone has an antiandrogen effect—that is, it counteracts the effects of male hormone. Perhaps you've heard of spironolactone used in smaller doses to treat acne. Why? Because acne requires two factors to blossom: bacteria (specifically *propionibacterium acnes* or *P. acnes*) and testosterone to stimulate oil production by the sebaceous glands. Blocking the testosterone helps reduce acne. (Doesn't this make sense when you think of how trans men beginning on testosterone often seem to develop acne? It's partly due to the testosterone's effect on sebaceous glands, stimulating them to produce more oil.)

People who were assigned male and who take spironolactone may experience decreased erections, particularly those nagging morning erections that occur when testosterone levels are at their highest. But it was also found—and reported as a side effect—that people assigned male and taking spironolactone may develop breast enlargement (gynecomastia). For my population of trans women, decreased erections and an increase in breast tissue are real crowd-pleasers.

Certainly, many trans women still want to have erections, but on *their* terms—that is, not spontaneously. We may prescribe medications like Viagra (sildenafil), which is available in generic form and also called Revatio, Cialis (tadalafil), or Levitra (vardenafil). Ask your provider if this is a problem for you; medication may help. (Please don't self-medicate with these drugs; as stated earlier, some folks experience life-threatening complications using Viagra and other such drugs in conjunction with certain other medications.)

Spironolactone: How It May Work to Decrease Testosterone Effects

Face it: It all comes down to biochemistry. Look at these chemical drawings of the spironolactone molecule and the testosterone molecule.

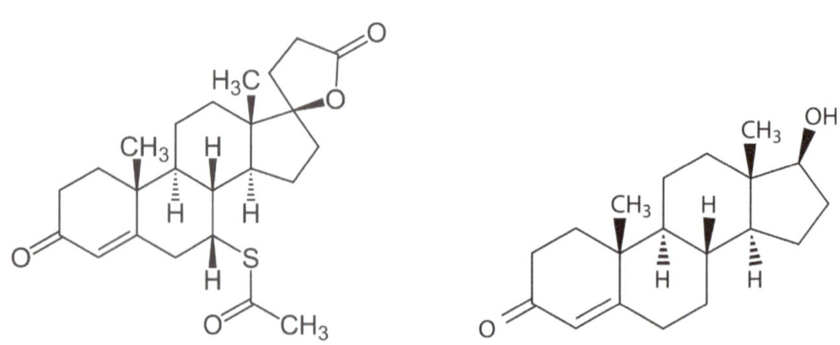

Figure 7.1. Spironolactone molecule (left) and testosterone molecule (right).

Thankfully, we don't have to be biochemists to appreciate that the two molecules look similar. The differences are that spironolactone has a thiol aldehyde functional group and an ester functional group. These functional groups allow spironolactone to bind to testosterone binding sites, but more strongly than testosterone does. As the spironolactone clings to testosterone receptor sites instead of testosterone, the testosterone receptor is not activated. Spironolactone, then, is a receptor antagonist (rather than a receptor agonist), so we do not see the same testosterone effects. As spironolactone binds preferentially to testosterone receptors, testosterone floats freely in the bloodstream and is excreted more readily. It also allows testosterone to be converted to estradiol (aromatized) in fat cells.

How Spironolactone Lowers Blood Pressure

Spironolactone also works as an antagonist (a blocker) to aldosterone, a hormone produced by the adrenal glands that sit on top of our kidneys. To be precise, spironolactone is termed an aldosterone receptor antagonist, but here, we're splitting hairs. Knowing what it does is the important thing.

Aldosterone travels through the bloodstream and works *within the kidney* by reabsorbing salt, which in turn, increases our fluid volume and keeps our blood pressure high enough. Aldosterone's maintenance of blood pressure is one of the many protective mechanisms in our bodies. It keeps us alive if our blood pressure drops too much.

When aldosterone is blocked, as it is by spironolactone, the kidneys release more salt (sodium) and water into the urine, thus decreasing our blood volume and lowering the blood pressure throughout the body. Any drug that makes us pee more is called a diuretic or "water pill."

It's important to point out that any medication that can drop your blood pressure could potentially drop it *too* low and you could pass out. That's why I typically start my patients on a small dose and work up to a full dose over a month. If a patient reports that they feel faint, I'll have them drop the dose a bit. And in some patients, I don't use spironolactone at all and they can still transition just fine. (I am beginning to use lower spironolactone doses in my practice. Many people are very relieved to stop this drug when having genital surgery, mainly objecting to the diuretic effect.)

Because you can potentially lose too much fluid with a water pill, it's important to recognize the signs of dehydration or volume depletion. Look for these symptoms:

- Thirst.
- Dry mouth.
- Decreased urine volume.
- Concentrated urine (urine that looks bright yellow rather than pale yellow or water-colored).
- Constipation: I have seen patients who have become so constipated that they developed rectal tears or fissures from passing hard, dry stool.

  Why does this happen? All of our food leaves the stomach in liquid form and moves through the small intestine as a liquid. When it reaches the large intestine (colon), the fluid is absorbed. By the time it reaches the end of the colon and enters the rectum, the stool is usually "formed" or solid. *When more fluid is sucked out because the body needs every drop of extra fluid, the stool gets harder and more difficult to pass.* Hence, constipation occurs, and with it, occasional tears in the rectum. You can reduce constipation by taking in more water and other liquids, but it's true that occasionally a rectal fissurotomy (a surgical procedure) is needed to help heal the rectum.

The Amount of Fluid Humans Need

Most of us need at least 2 quarts of fluid every day. This can be in the form of water, moist foods, fruit, milk, juices, frozen yogurt, or ice cream; anything that is liquid at body temperature counts as a liquid. We lose fluid continually through not only the urine we make, but also through bowel movements, sweat, saliva, and even breathing. (Did you know that we lose about a quart of fluid per day just through breathing? This is called "insensible" loss; we don't even know it's happening.)

Certain beverages like tea, coffee, and colas have a diuretic effect; they make us pee more often and in larger quantities. If you are already taking a diuretic like spironolactone, be careful not to add other diuretics to the mix.

When we lose more salt (sodium) in the urine, we tend to retain more potassium. These two elements have what we call a reciprocal relationship: The more sodium is eliminated, the more potassium is retained. For this reason, spironolactone is sometimes called a "potassium-sparing" diuretic, meaning that serum potassium may be increased when using spironolactone.

Some people worry that taking spironolactone will increase potassium so much that they avoid eating potassium-rich foods like bananas or citrus fruits. Is this generally necessary? No.

Excessive worry about potassium is usually not necessary in people who have normal kidney function. However, I would likely not use spironolactone in someone with diminished kidney function. And I do check electrolytes (sodium, potassium, and so on) and kidney function with a blood test from time to time.

Also, there are two classes of blood pressure medications that do not interact well with spironolactone: *the ACE inhibitors and the ARBs*. ACE inhibitors are angiotensin-converting enzyme inhibitors. And the ARBs are angiotensin receptor blockers. Both types of medication work to lower blood pressure by interfering with our bodies' ability to increase angiotensin, a chemical that constricts blood vessel walls and thereby increases blood pressure. The ACE inhibitors and the ARBs relax blood vessel walls and lower blood pressure. But they can also increase serum potassium. And at very high potassium levels, kidney failure can occur.

Ironically, ACE inhibitors and ARBs can have kidney-protective effects also. Diabetics, for example, may delay diabetes-related kidney problems by using these medications. Do talk with your healthcare provider if you think you may be on these medications now. Your doctor may not know of this potential risk, so ask them about it. (Common generic names of these medications include lisinopril, benazepril, losartan, and valsartan.)

Cautions about Combining Spironolactone and ACE Inhibitors or ARBs

I remember adding spironolactone to the regimen of a diabetic transgender female who took an ACE inhibitor for blood pressure control. Within a week, she wasn't feeling quite right. Her lab tests showed that her serum potassium was climbing and that her kidney function numbers were plummeting. (My late husband was on dialysis at the time because of kidney failure, so these numbers horrified me. Could I have pushed this woman into kidney failure?)

I phoned a kind nephrologist who gently steered me back on course. I stopped the spironolactone, and the patient's lab values quickly normalized. But it was a lesson I'll never forget.

— Linda Gromko, MD

Helpful Tips for Using Spironolactone

- Start with a low dose and move up gradually.
- Be careful when you stand up too quickly; you could get light-headed or dizzy. Light-headedness usually subsides quickly, but check with your healthcare provider if this persists.
- Do not exceed the dose your healthcare provider recommends.
- Be mindful of age-related risks. If you are a young person, such as an adolescent, you may be more prone to fainting than you will be later in your life. For this reason, I often use half of an adult dose when starting spironolactone. And even then, I start with a smaller initial dose and work up.
- Be mindful of timing. Because spironolactone is a diuretic and will make you pee more in volume as well as more often, don't take spiro right before bed. It isn't dangerous, but you may be up all night peeing.
- Be careful of adding extra diuretics (coffee, tea, cola) when you use spiro; these will make you pee even more.
- Add more fluid and fiber to your diet if you find that you are getting constipated (having difficulty passing hard bowel movements). Consider an over-the-counter stool softener like Colace or DOSS. Ask the pharmacist for suggestions.
- Check with your healthcare provider if you are using any other medications that lower your blood pressure, particularly the ACE inhibitors or the ARBs.
- Realize that surgery will change the dosing. Your doctor will likely recommend that you stop taking spiro if you have an orchiectomy (removal of testicles) or vaginoplasty (gender-affirming surgery). With the removal of the testicles, the majority of a person's testosterone is gone.

In addition to spironolactone, other medications can be used as antiandrogens to reduce the effect of testosterone produced by the testicles. These medications work by blocking testosterone receptors at target organs or by blocking production. Typical uses for these antiandrogens include the treatment of prostate cancer, the reduction of androgen-related hair loss, or the reduction of hirsutism (excessive hair growth) in assigned females with polycystic ovarian syndrome. As these medications do not have a diuretic effect, patients may tolerate them better.

Cyproterone acetate, for example, is an antiandrogen commonly used in Europe. Some of my clients get this by prescription in Canada. Be cautious if you hear of using this medication in combination with ethinyl estradiol in a birth control pill called "Diane." We know that *ethinyl estradiol* has a greater risk of blood clots than regular estradiol.[19] Bicalutamide is another example of an antiandrogen, which is used in the treatment of advanced prostate cancer. Fulminant liver failure has occurred in people taking bicalutamide for prostate cancer. Admittedly, a group of older and ill prostate cancer patients is significantly different than a group of healthy trans women. But being cautious, most healthcare providers tend to prescribe bicalutamide less often.

Adding Progesterone

Progesterone is the other female hormone produced in the ovary (besides estrogen). Many trans women request it because it can help enhance breast development in some. Generally, trans women on estradiol experience the most breast development over the first 3 years. So, if we add progesterone *during* those first 3 years and a woman experiences more breast development, it's hard to know if the increase was due to the estradiol or the addition of progesterone. But it does seem reasonable to me that when a trans woman *who is on estrogen* starts progesterone and she notices a *definite* acceleration in her breast growth, we can probably attribute the change in growth to progesterone. Some people believe that progesterone enhances the shape of the developing breast, but I'm not sure how you would know. (I'm not aware of large studies to address this, and we don't have the option of "life rewind.")

How do you take progesterone? It comes in an oral form. Some women take it daily. But some prefer to "cycle" it to mimic the monthly menstrual cycle by taking estradiol for the first 2 weeks, and estradiol *and* progesterone for the third and fourth weeks.

I always thought of progesterone as the premenstrual hormone. I was concerned that I might expose my trans clients to the irritability, moodiness, and breast tenderness of PMS. In my experience, however, these mood fluctuations don't seem to happen often and certainly not to a point where most clients stop using progesterone.

I have been told by some trans women that they insert progesterone capsules into the rectum, although I don't have enough information to recommend this. Progesterone pellets can also be inserted under the skin of the buttocks.

19 Madeline B. Deutsch, "Overview of Feminizing Hormone Therapy," Transgender Care, University of California-San Francisco, June 17, 2016, https://transcare.ucsf.edu/guidelines/feminizing-hormone-therapy.

Assessing and Mitigating Risks through Evidence-Based Medicine

All medical treatments carry benefits and risks, and a prescriber wants to know that a patient understands both. The patient is required to give informed consent when starting treatment, whether that takes the form of a conversation or a more formal signed document.

What Information and Research Should We Trust?

The most reliable clinical information comes from randomized control trials. In RCTs, an investigator identifies a question to be answered and an intervention to be tested. The question must be clearly defined, and there must be a clear tool to measure the desired outcome. Then, there must be study groups that are very similar to each other—so much so that any difference in the outcome is attributable to the intervention (or variable) being studied.

Let us take an example. Suppose you want to learn if depressed patients taking a new antidepressant (drug A) become less depressed than those taking a traditional antidepressant (drug B). You could divide your patients into three matched (very similar) groups, with the first group receiving drug A and the second group receiving drug B. If it is deemed ethical by a human subjects review committee, the third group would receive a placebo—that is, a pill with no active medication at all. The participants would be assigned randomly to their respective groups.

In a double blind study, neither the person who administers the medicine nor the one receiving it would know if the medication is drug A, drug B, or a placebo. Because each group receives an intervention during the same period, and the groups are studied going forward, this type of research is called a "prospective" study. Outcomes, such as the degree of depression, would be measured in all subjects by a standard assessment tool such as the Beck Depression Inventory.

After the experiment is done and the investigators draw their conclusions, they seek to publish their findings in a peer-reviewed journal, where other scientists review their methods and conclusions—and critique the validity of the information.

A prospective, multicenter, double-blind study with matched controls and large numbers of participants is considered the gold standard for answering scientific questions. They are considered superior to retrospective medical record reviews and also far superior to surveys that depend on participants' recollections. They are generally considered more valuable than comparing a variety of similar studies done at various times on various nonmatched groups (such as meta-analyses). Certainly, they are considered preferable to clinical experience or even expert opinion.*

Unfortunately, research on the transgender community has been limited. After all, medical treatment of transgender patients is essentially a twentieth-century phenomenon.

Sometimes we are left to compare apples to oranges—and to make assumptions on the effects of hormones taken from different populations. For example, information about estradiol given to trans women may come from studies on menopausal cis females. Sometimes, the information on estradiol comes from studies on birth control pills, which contain a different and more dangerous type of estradiol (ethinyl estradiol has a greater clot risk than estradiol).

* Izet Masic, Milan Miokovic, and Belma Muhamedagić, "Evidence-Based Medicine—New Approaches and Challenges," *Acta Informatica Medica* 16, no. 4 (November 2008): 224, https://doi.org/10.5455/aim.2008.16.219-225.

In another example, information on testosterone blockers used in trans women may come from protocols for treating prostate cancer in cis males.

In the absence of evidence-based research, a clinician relies to some extent on their common sense and their clinical experience. It is important for patients to be invested in their own care. Assuming that a prescriber is acting in good faith, patients must still ask their own questions and do their own reading about their treatments. (I would also want to point out that Google Scholar at scholar.google.com may be a good resource to search as you do your own reading. You will often find more credible research cited there.)

Learning How to Mitigate Risk

Suppose you understand that a treatment "may" have certain risks. You cannot know precisely how much risk there is for you as a patient. Perhaps you have been told that estradiol carries a risk of blood clots. I found it difficult to nail down exactly what risks a patient now faces. (Protective modifications like using transdermal estrogen and avoiding ethinyl estradiol from birth control pills are now in widespread practice.) And the bottom line for any patient is: "How will this risk manifest in *me*?"

A low risk is not the same as *no risk*. You may have a one-in-a-million risk, but you can still be *the one* impacted. How dangerous is a particular risk? I like to consider a model that I call "low risk, high stakes." For example, you may have a small risk of developing a blood clot that travels to the lung. But if you should be the person who develops a pulmonary embolus, it has the potential to be fatal. Low risk, high stakes means that the risk is small, but if the problem happens, the outcome can be disastrous.

Can we identify factors that increase or decrease the risk to an individual (such as smoking, obesity, comorbidities, genetics, etc.)? Even though we may never know the precise risk for each individual, what can we do to minimize their risk?

Finally, as we consider risks versus benefits, we must recognize that *not* treating a person is an option. But we must be very clear that providing no treatment has its own risks as well.

Possible Risks Involved in Taking Estradiol

For healthy individuals who have no major medical problems and who do not smoke, the risks involved in taking estradiol are quite minimal. But there are some potential risks, and it is important that you know about them.

As in all areas of medicine—and discussed in the previous section—we would want to base our medical advice on scientific research and clinical experience. We would want to reference prospective randomized control trials that involve large numbers of subjects in many study centers. In transgender medicine, however, prospective research studies often have not been done or haven't been completed if they are in progress. While this is changing, our clients are asking for our advice now.

Even with the best of research, we can never predict with absolute certainty whether a specific patient will develop any given problem. We can, however, examine factors that impact an individual's risk—and inform our patients about risks, warning signals, and possible interventions.

> **Remember that nobody's getting out of here alive. But most of us want to live as long as possible and as well as possible. We can help ourselves by knowing and minimizing our health risks—and by knowing the warning signals that help keep us safe.**
>
> *— Linda Gromko, MD*

In this section, we will look at several disease processes that may occur more frequently in people taking estradiol: blood clots in the legs or lungs (deep vein thromboses and pulmonary emboli), gallbladder disease, heart disease, and breast cancer. We'll do the same with testosterone in a later section.

Blood Clots: Deep Vein Thromboses (DVTs) and Pulmonary Emboli (PEs)

Let me start by saying that I have seen *many* DVTs and PEs in my 40-some years of providing healthcare. But only a handful of these have been in transgender women on estradiol. Certainly, some folks are at greater risk than others. Let's sort this out further.

To understand this better, let's look at the basics of how blood circulates through the body (see Figure 7.2 on page 74). The heart forcefully pumps freshly oxygenated blood out of its left ventricle and into the arteries. The arteries have smooth muscle within their walls, helping to propel the blood along. Arteries become smaller and smaller the farther away they are from the heart. When they become very tiny, they are called "arterioles." They then enter capillary beds, which are transition zones between arteries and veins.

Moving out of the capillary beds, the blood then travels back to the heart, first through tiny venules (little veins) and on through larger and larger veins on the way back to the heart, where the whole cycle begins again. (Think of the arteries and veins as a continuous circuit, where the capillary beds are transition zones between arteries and veins.)

In the illustrations, arteries are shown in red and the veins in blue. In real life, the arteries do have brighter red blood, freshly oxygenated from the lungs. The blood in the veins does look darker—almost maroon—as the bodily tissues have consumed a portion of the oxygen carried by the blood.

Unlike the arteries, veins do not have smooth muscles within their walls to propel the blood onward in its flow back to the heart. Rather, they have a system of valves (see Figure 7.2). Blood moves upward from one set of valves to the next. The blood flow is assisted by the muscles *around* (but not *within*) the veins. Wiggling your toes or flexing your ankles and calves provides an external muscle push to help the blood in the veins move toward the heart.

If a person is very still, like on a long airplane flight or during a hospitalization, blood tends to pool in the lower extremities and sometimes in the pelvic veins. This pooling is referred to as "stasis." During a period of stasis, blood tends to coagulate more easily. The resulting clot, also called a "thrombus," can break free and be carried with the venous blood toward the heart. Because veins get progressively larger on the way to the heart, the clot flows freely into the right atrium and right ventricle of the heart.

But then the blood moves from the right ventricle directly into the pulmonary artery and to the extremely delicate—and minuscule—vessels of the pulmonary (lung) circulation. At this point, the clot is called a pulmonary embolus, or PE. PEs are potentially life-threatening because a pulmonary embolus *blocks* the flow of blood into the lung or parts of the lung. How much damage this creates depends on the size and location of the resulting blockage.

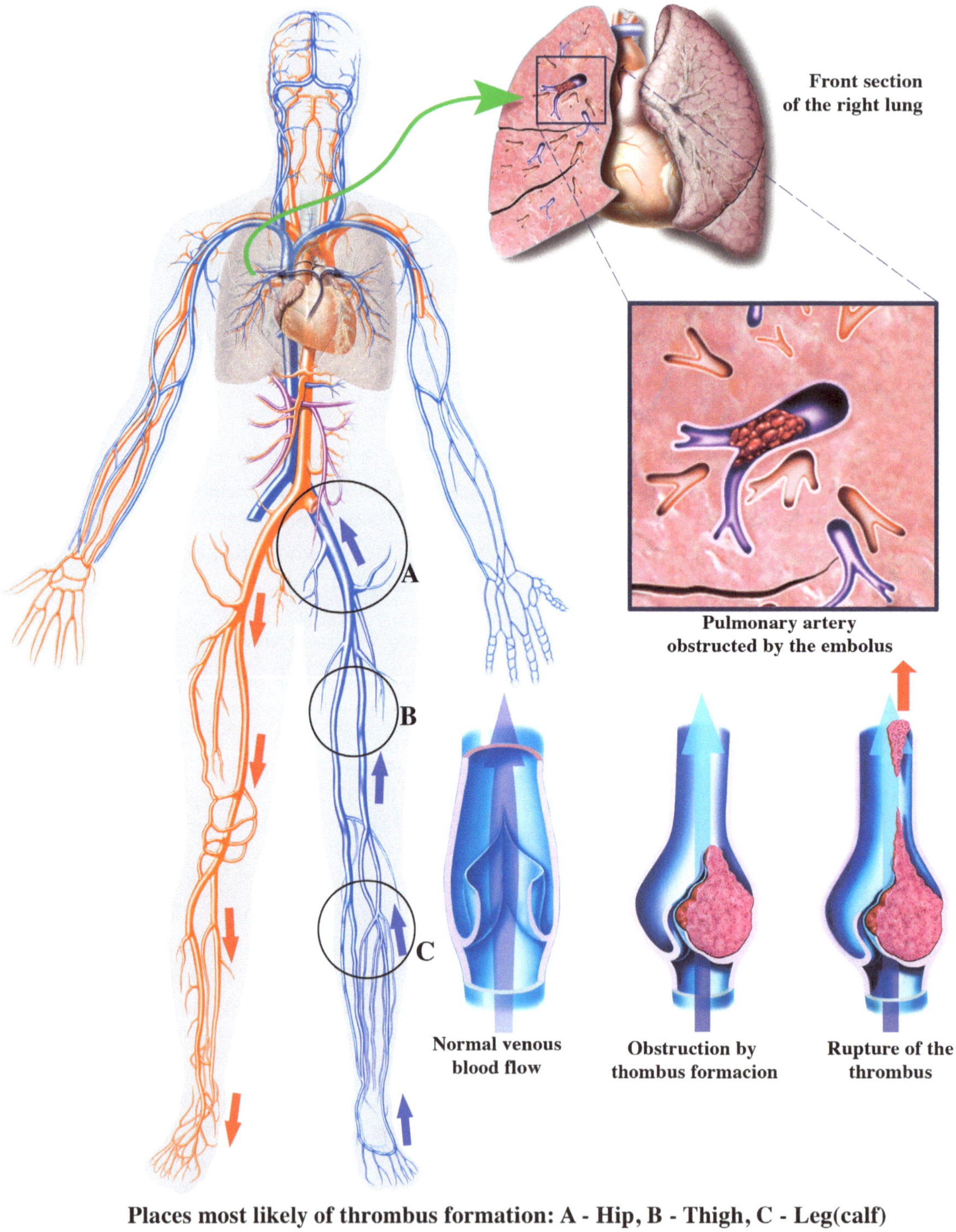

Figure 7.2. Blood clots and pulmonary embolism.

Q What is a hypercoagulable state or thrombophilia?

A A hypercoagulable state is one of several conditions, often inherited, that increases a person's risk for developing deep vein thromboses (blood clots in the deep veins of the leg or pelvis) and pulmonary emboli (blood clots in the lungs that are potentially fatal).

If a blood relative has had a DVT or a PE, ask if one of these clotting propensities has been identified. It may help you get appropriately tested to mitigate your own risk.

Examples of thrombophilias include the following:

- **Factor V Leiden mutation.** You may get one copy of this gene mutation from one parent, or two copies if both of your parents are affected. You have a greater risk of forming clots if you are homozygous (that is, you have two copies of the gene, one from each parent) than if you are heterozygous (one mutation from one parent).
- **Prothrombin gene mutation**
- **Protein S deficiency**
- **Protein C deficiency**
- **Antithrombin III deficiency**
- **Antiphospholipid antibody syndrome** (APS): the presence of anticardiolipin antibodies or antiphospholipid antibodies

Certain Conditions Increase the Risk of DVTs or PEs

You are at greater risk of getting a DVT or PE if you have one of the hypercoagulable conditions or thrombophilias listed above. (The word "thrombophilia" is derived from the Greek, meaning "clot-loving.") Smoking increases your risk of DVTs and PEs. Birth control pills containing estrogen in the form of ethinyl estradiol are associated with more clots, which is why we are careful to warn trans women not to take these medications to self-medicate. Surgery of any type may increase DVT and PE risk, and any form of prolonged immobilization creates stasis, which encourages clot formation.

Some of these risk factors are beyond our control. We cannot control the genetic factors or mutations we inherit. We may be able to identify them, however, if we have a family history of blood relatives with DVTs or PEs. In my opinion, trans women with thrombophilias or prior occurrences of DVTs or PEs should consult a hematologist for more sophisticated advice than I can offer. Having one of these conditions does not necessarily mean you *cannot* take estrogen, but you must make an informed decision. Some people who have higher clotting risks take anticoagulant medications. While anticoagulant therapy is beyond the scope of this book, do talk to your healthcare provider if you think this may apply to you.

Other ways to reduce DVT and PE risk include stopping smoking (see Chapter 10) and avoiding ethinyl estradiol in birth control pills as a substitute for estradiol.

During surgery, your surgeon will ensure that you are using sequential compression devices (SCDs)—a plastic garment fastened with Velcro around each of your legs. The SCDs come with inflatable bladders that are pumped up and down to periodically squeeze your lower extremities and keep your blood circulation moving.

During a long flight (some say more than 4 hours), wiggle your toes, move your feet, and flex your calves. Drink water liberally so you get up to use the bathroom.[20] Also, buy compression stockings online, at the airport, or at a travel store (such as AAA and The Container Store) to wear during your flight.

Deep Vein Thrombosis and Pulmonary Embolism Symptoms

Q What are the symptoms of a blood clot in the leg?

A A blood clot in the leg (deep vein thrombosis or DVT) may cause the following:

- Swelling of one or both legs (usually one leg only)
- A sore lump in the leg that occurs due to a clot within a vein
- A tender "cord" in the leg (actually, a vein filled with clot)
- Pain with walking
- Pain with flexing the foot

Q What are the symptoms of a pulmonary embolism (PE)—a blood clot that travels to the lung?

A A pulmonary embolism (PE) may cause the following:

- Difficulty breathing
- Pain at the top or the deepest part of the breath (called "pleuritic pain")
- Coughing up blood
- Feeling you aren't getting enough air to breathe
- Feeling light-headed or dizzy
- Agitation or intense anxiety
- Rapid heartbeat
- Becoming unconscious

If any of these symptoms are happening, get medical assistance right away. Not getting enough air is worthy of a 911 call.

20 Michèle Cazaubon, "Deep Vein Thrombosis and Air Travel: Risk Management in 2015," *Phlebolymphology 22*, no. 1 (January 2015): 29, https://www.phlebolymphology.org/deep-vein-thrombosis-and-air-travel-risk-management-in-2015/.

Gallbladder Disease

Women on estradiol, including women taking birth control pills, have a greater risk of forming gallstones.[21] See your healthcare provider if you experience the symptoms listed on page 78. Sometimes, a pulmonary embolism (clot in the lung) has symptoms that mimic gallbladder disease. Gallbladder disease (specifically gallstones or slow gallbladder emptying) may have no symptoms at all. You may, for example, learn that you have gallstones as an incidental finding during an ultrasound or abdominal CT or MRI scan done for unrelated reasons.

The gallbladder is a sac that stores fat-dissolving bile from the liver. Triggered by hormones such as cholecystokinin (CCK), the gallbladder empties bile into the duodenum of the small intestine (see Figure 7.3). Gallstones may form by precipitation of cholesterol in the bile, which creates an obstruction when tiny stones become lodged in the duct system. I worry more about the small stones than the large ones. Small stones tend to get trapped in ducts while larger ones are usually too big to enter. Larger stones can cause pain or discomfort, but they don't tend to lodge into the duct system, thus causing pancreatitis and other complications.

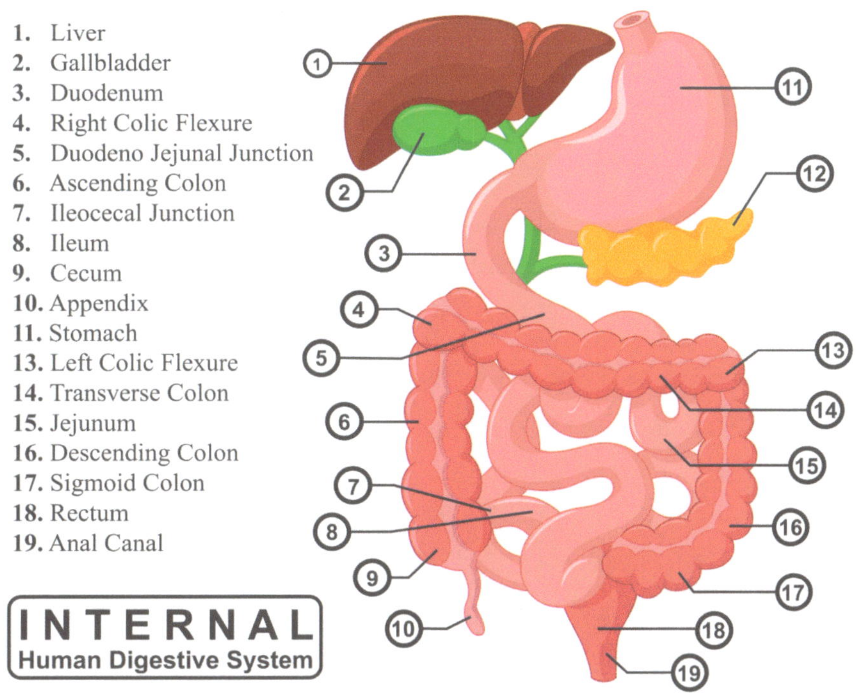

Figure 7.3. The human digestive system.

Did you notice that the yellow organ (12) isn't labeled? Hints: It produces insulin and digestive enzymes; starts with a P; and its cancer produces symptoms late in the disease. The answer is at the end of this chapter.

If you have stones, should you have your gallbladder removed? Not necessarily. Many people simply watch for symptoms and move toward surgery if the symptoms become a problem. As stated earlier, it is worth noting that gallstones aren't always innocent. Trapped in the common bile duct or pancreatic duct, they can provoke serious

21 Dominic J. Cirillo et al, "Effect of Estrogen Therapy on Gallbladder Disease," *The Journal of the American Medical Association* 293, no. 3 (January 19, 2005): 336, https://doi.org/10.1001/jama.293.3.330.

conditions such as choledocholithiasis or pancreatitis. So, if your healthcare provider recommends that you have your gallbladder removed, get all the facts that apply to your situation.

Q What are the symptoms of gallbladder disease?

A Symptoms may include the following:

- Right upper abdominal pain
- Nausea and vomiting, especially with pain and especially after eating a rich meal
- Pain that radiates or refers to the right shoulder, upper back, or the right armpit

Estrogen and Heart Attack Risk in Trans Females

Does estrogen increase the risk of heart disease and heart attack in trans females? There isn't an easy answer to this question. It is a very important question, though, because heart disease is so common. Heart disease is the leading cause of death among American adults, although COVID-19 statistics may temporarily change its ranking.[22]

I started writing about heart disease and admittedly got carried away. I waffled about including this material—but this is lifesaving information. Skip ahead if you like, but if it interests you, move through it carefully. It truly may save your life or that of someone you love.

— Linda Gromko, MD

But First, a Basic Primer on Heart Disease

The main function of the heart muscle is to pump oxygenated blood throughout the body. To carry out this function—beating over 100,000 times per day[23]—the heart requires a robust blood supply of its own. The blood vessels that supply the heart exit directly off the aorta, bringing the most freshly oxygenated blood from the lungs by way of the pulmonary veins. The coronary arteries form many branches that feed the heart muscle from the outside surface of the heart.

When the blood supply to the heart muscle is reduced, the muscle cannot pump effectively and may not be able to keep up with the oxygen demands of the body. The patient may develop angina (chest pain), myocardial infarction (muscle death in parts of the heart), arrythmias that prevent the heart chambers from working together or pumping at all, heart failure (when a poorly functioning heart pumps less blood per heartbeat and cannot keep up with the demands of the body), and ultimately the death of the patient.

22 Centers for Disease Control and Prevention, "Heart Disease Facts," last reviewed September 8, 2020, https://www.cdc.gov/heartdisease/facts.htm.

23 Cardiovascular Surgery of Southern Nevada, "How Many Times Does Your Heart Beat Per Day?" September 25, 2013, http://www.cvsurgnv.com/how-many-times-does-your-heart-beat-per-day/.

One of the most important coronary arteries is the left anterior descending (LAD) artery, the vessel that supplies the powerful left ventricle that pumps blood to rest of the body. If the LAD artery is completely blocked, heart damage can be massive, and a patient may die within minutes. Gender identity aside, the LAD is known in medical circles as "the widow maker"—but it kills both AMAB and AFAB individuals.

Here are some definitions and information about the most common types of heart disease:

- **A heart attack is also called a "myocardial infarction" (or MI).**
  Myocardial refers to the heart muscle (the myocardium) that pumps your freshly oxygenated blood throughout your body. The heart muscle is delivered oxygen by the coronary arteries. When one or more of the coronary arteries is blocked, the myocardium downstream from the blockage gets less oxygen than it needs. The muscle can then become infarcted, or die. This can decrease the heart's overall pumping function, and if the damage is very severe or widespread, the patient may die.

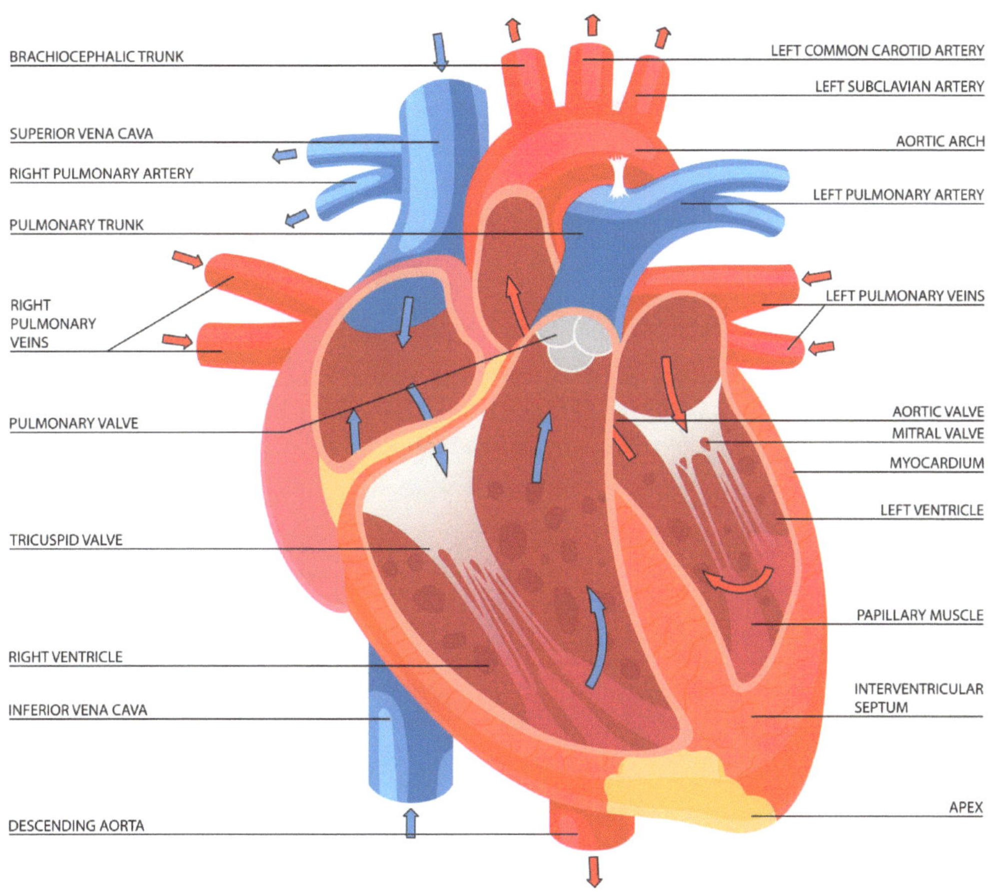

Figure 7.4. The internal anatomy of the human heart. It is very complex, containing four chambers and four valves. Trace the path of blood coming to the heart from the superior and inferior vena cavae to the right atrium, through the tricuspid valve, and to the lungs by way of the pulmonary valves and pulmonary arteries. Blood returns from the lungs via the pulmonary veins into the left atrium and through the mitral valve and to the powerful left ventricle, where it passes through the aortic valve to the aorta.

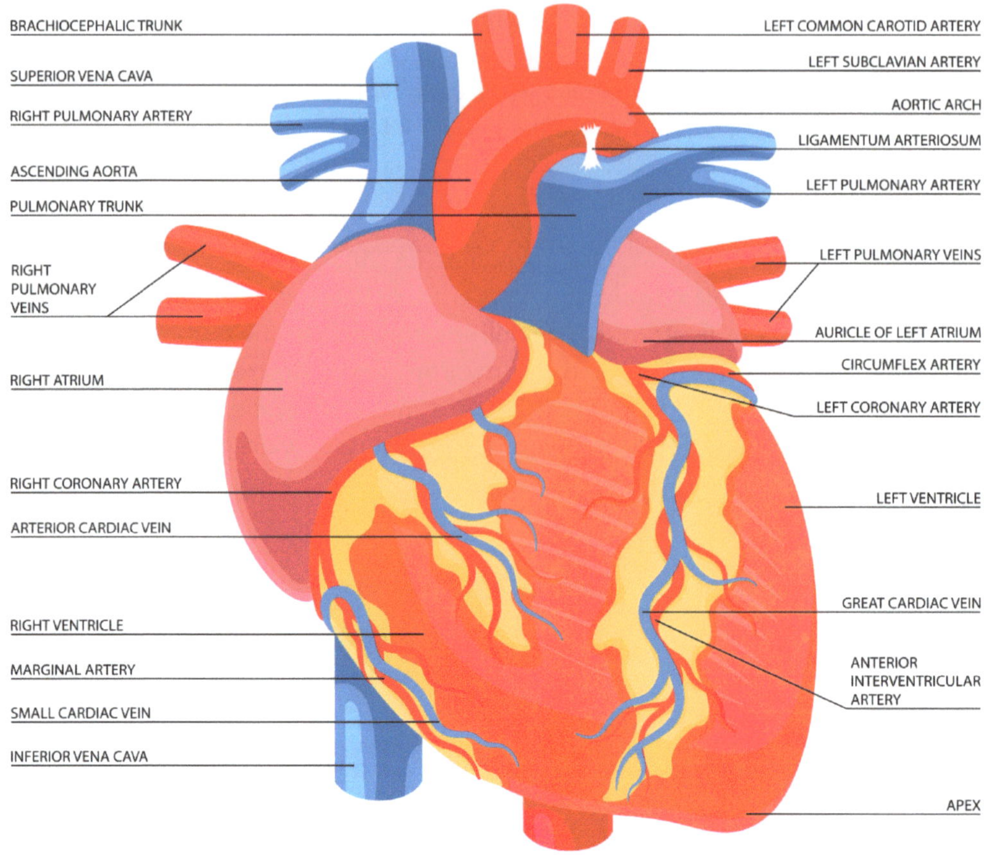

Figure 7.5. External anatomy of the human heart. While they are impossible to see here, the blood vessels that supply the heart muscle come directly off the aorta. Identify the right and left coronary arteries. Here, the left anterior descending artery (sometimes dubbed the "widow maker") is called the anterior interventricular artery.

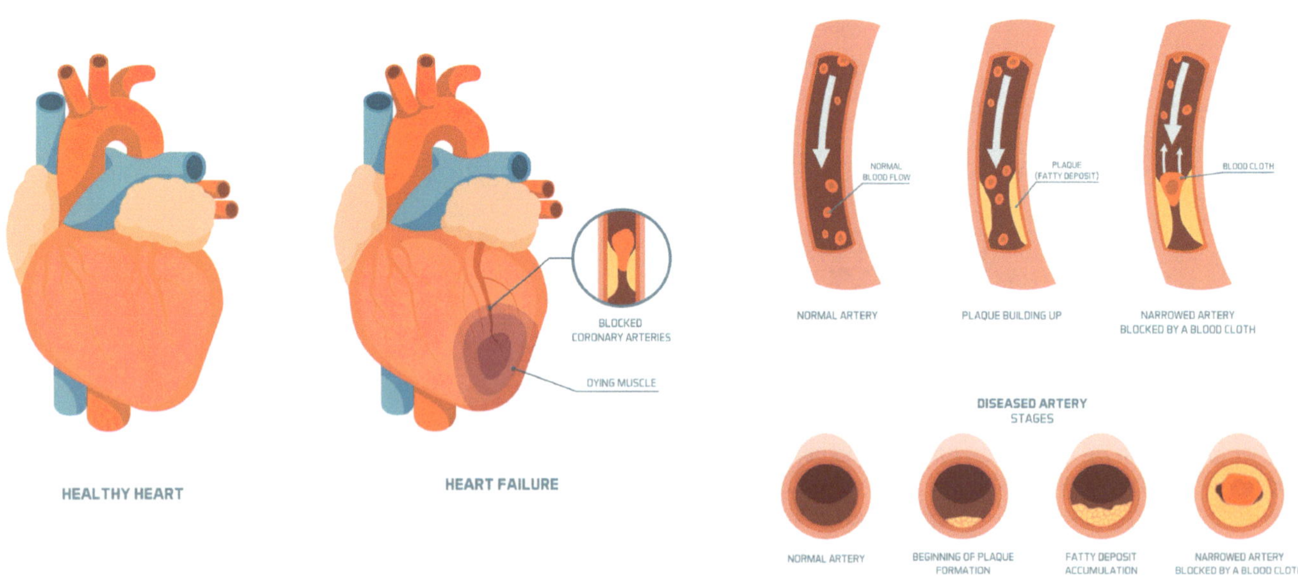

Figure 7.6. Anatomy of a myocardial infarction, or heart attack.

- **How does a coronary artery become blocked and how can it be fixed?**
  The most common scenario involves the formation of cholesterol plaque within the blood vessel. This plaque is made up of cholesterol, fat, cell waste products, calcium, and fibrin. This plaque can narrow the blood vessel, decreasing the blood flow to the heart muscle downstream. A plaque may also break open or rupture, attracting platelets to form a plug that obstructs the vessel completely.

  If a blockage is suspected due to symptoms (see pages 84–87) or because of EKG abnormalities, the blockage can sometimes be opened through a process called angioplasty. Often a stent is placed to buttress the vessel open so that blood flows more freely.

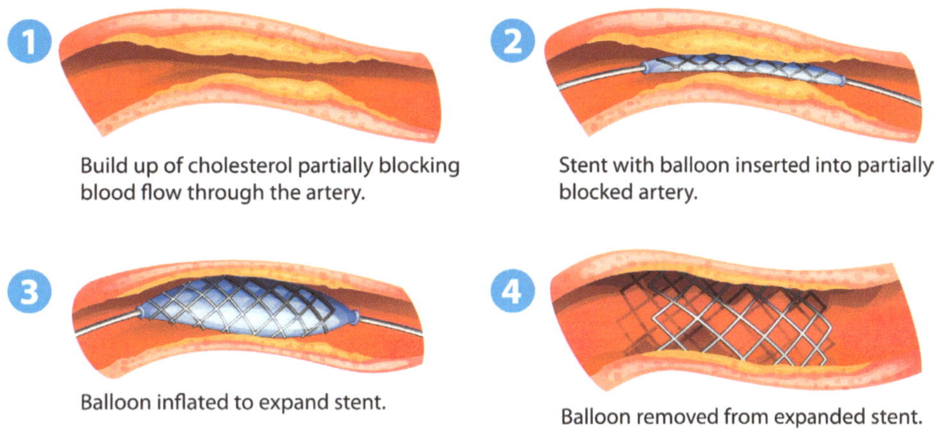

Figure 7.7. Stent with a balloon angioplasty.

When blockages involve several arteries, several stents may be placed. In more severe cases, coronary artery bypass grafts (known in the field as CABG and nicknamed "cabbage") can be performed. Less aggressive approaches include the use of medications aimed at increasing the blood flow and reducing the workload of the heart. The most aggressive intervention, of course, is heart transplantation.

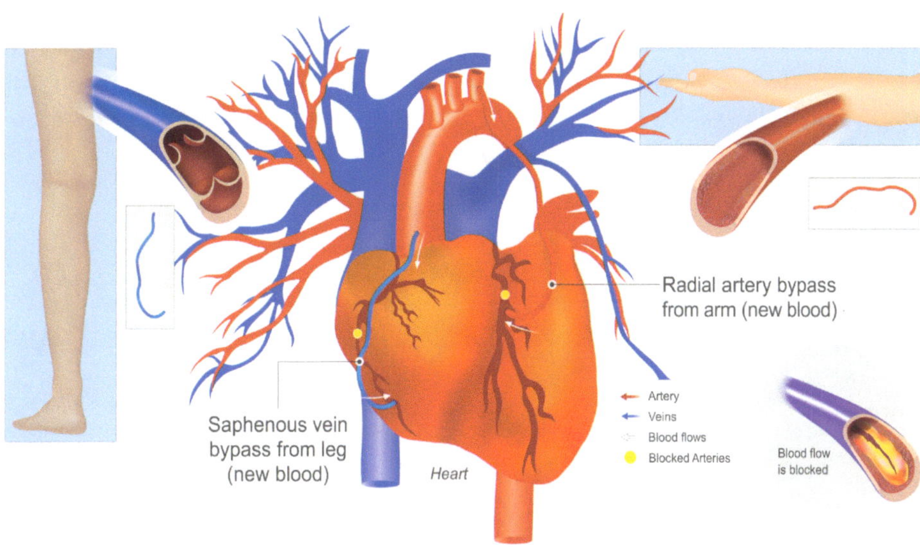

Figure 7.8. Coronary artery bypass grafts (CABG).

What Is a Cardiac Arrest?

A cardiac arrest means that the heart has stopped beating—or stopped beating well enough to circulate blood. In this context, cardiac arrest implies an abrupt and often unexpected stop. Normally, each heartbeat is triggered by an elaborate flow of electrical impulses within the heart. An arrest results from a sudden electrical malfunction. Most of the time, these arrests are related to underlying heart disease, but trauma such as electrocution, drowning, and blood loss can also set off an arrest. The following are two common patterns, known as "shockable rhythms," because they are treated with defibrillation—the sudden shock of an electrical current applied to the chest.

- **Ventricular fibrillation (VFib or VF)** is a chaotic rhythm where the heart muscle simply quivers—rather than beating in a regular pattern that can deliver oxygenated blood throughout the body.
- **Ventricular tachycardia (VTach or VT)** is a rapid rhythm where there is a pattern of beats, but the beats occur so fast that the heart cannot refill with blood in time to pump effectively.

Learn to Perform CPR to Save Lives

With CPR (cardiopulmonary resuscitation), a good Samaritan can temporarily restore the pumping of the heart so blood can circulate until defibrillation can be performed. CPR is simple to learn and it seems to get streamlined every time it is revised. A 911 dispatcher can talk you through CPR technique in an emergency. You can learn how to perform CPR in a free class or online training, and you can get a CPR app on your phone.

There's one app called CPR Tempo that has the CPR compression rate played on a metronome. Easier yet, the proper rate is the same rhythm as the Bee Gee's classic song "Stayin' Alive." Research has verified that pumping to "Stayin' Alive" keeps you on track with a rate of 103 pumps per minute! *

Many songs can lend their rhythm to CPR. If "Stayin' Alive" doesn't speak to you, how about "I Will Survive" recorded by Gloria Gaynor, or "Uptown Funk" by Mark Ronson and Bruno Mars? For a list of other songs that work, see this Spotify playlist at **https://open.spotify.com/playlist/7oJx24EcRU7flVoTdqKscK.**

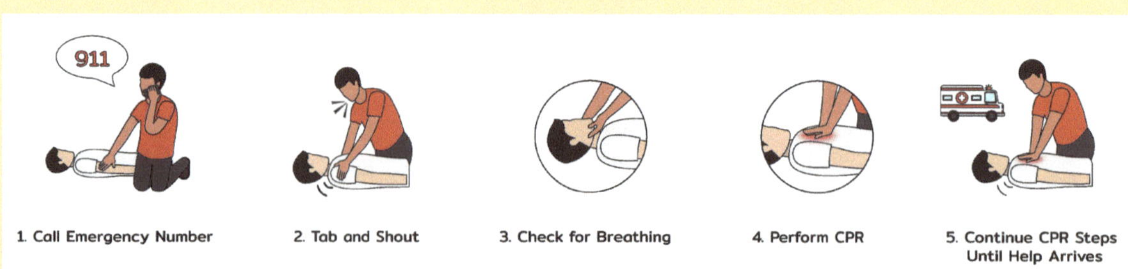

* Martin, Paul, "CPR to Stayin' Alive Beat Helps Keep Proper Rate," *ProTrainings*, last updated October 25, 2018, https://www.procpr.org/blog/training/cpr-stayin-alive-song.

When the heart cannot beat properly and blood flow essentially stops, a patient can die in a few minutes. CPR can take over the heart's pumping function until defibrillation is performed. We have "crash carts" in hospitals with defibrillators and emergency medications. More and more, we are seeing AEDs (automated external defibrillators) in sports stadiums, schools, office buildings, and other places. Now when you take a CPR class, you may be trained in the use of AEDs. If you are not trained, know that AEDs are easy to use; the defibrillator audibly coaches the operator on when to shock the heart!

To be complete, I should mention that there are two "unshockable" rhythms that are seen in a cardiac arrest. These are asystole, popularly known as "flatlining" and "pulseless electrical activity" or PEA. In PEA, you see a rhythm on the screen but feel no pulse in the patient. These rhythms do not respond to defibrillation but may correct when the underlying cause of the rhythm problem (such as low fluid volume, low oxygen levels, and acid-base imbalance) is managed. Medication use is attempted to correct the acute problem and to stimulate the heart (epinephrine or adrenaline).

In medical school, I remember my professor Dr. Mickey Eisenberg saying, "You'll save many more lives with electricity than with medications in the ER." Eisenberg was one of several influencers who advanced the concept of defibrillation in the field, rather than initially in the emergency room.[24]

— Linda Gromko, MD

What Is Heart Failure?

I have never liked the term "heart failure" because it sounds so—well, final. Actually, heart failure is a chronic condition where the heart progressively loses its ability to pump effectively. This function is reflected in what is known as the ejection fraction or left ventricular ejection fraction (LVEF). The LVEF is the portion of blood that is squeezed out of the left ventricle with each beat of the heart. Intuitively, we might expect it to be 100 percent. In real life, a normal ejection fraction ranges from 55 to 65 percent. Heart failure occurs when the LVEF is under 40 percent. This does not mean that the heart stops, but it may not be able to keep up with the body's demands. Heart failure can be treated and improved in many—but not all—cases.

When the heart cannot meet the demands of the body, blood and fluid backs up in the extremities and lungs depending on which part of the heart is most involved. Symptoms may include edema (swelling in the extremities), exhaustion, shortness of breath, and coughing frothy or bloody sputum from the lungs. Heart failure results from underlying coronary artery disease and heart damage from a prior myocardial infarction, but comorbidities such as diabetes and high blood pressure, heart valve damage, cardiomyopathy, alcohol, and other drugs may also be involved. Treatments—well beyond the scope of this book—include optimizing the patient's overall health and treating underlying causes with medications, and today, heart transplantation.

---

24 A. J. Heightman, "Early Citizen Response/CPR/AEDs; Uninterrupted Compressions and Dispatcher-Assisted CPR Emphasized by EMS Experts at CPR Summit," *Journal of Emergency Medical Services*, special report from the Cardiac Arrest Survivors Summit, December 12, 2019, https://www.jems.com/patient-care/cardiac-resuscitation/early-citizen-response/.

What factors increase our risk for developing coronary artery disease? (We'll go through warning signals later.)

- **Family history** (a genetic predisposition to high cholesterol or heart disease in young relatives, "young" generally considered under the age of 60; arrythmias that run in the family can cause sudden cardiac death even if the coronary arteries are reasonably clear)
- **Assigned gender and age** (AMABs 45 and older and AFABs 55 and older are more likely to have heart attacks; we will attempt to discuss gender identity and heart disease further on)
- **Certain autoimmune conditions** (such as rheumatoid arthritis, lupus, psoriatic arthritis, and diabetes)
- **Hypertension** (high blood pressure)
- **Diabetes**
- **High cholesterol, high triglycerides**
- **Metabolic syndrome** (combination of high blood pressure, high cholesterol, visceral obesity—excess weight around the middle—and insulin resistance [diabetes and prediabetes])
- **Smoking tobacco or long-term exposure to secondhand smoke**
- **Stimulant drugs like amphetamines or cocaine**
- **Overweight and obesity**
- **Inactive lifestyle** (risks are higher in people who do not exercise or do sedentary work)
- **Stress**
- **Depression**
- **Loneliness and isolation**

While we cannot control our genetic makeup (yet), most of these risk factors are modifiable. We will examine risk modification in Chapter 23. For more information about the symptoms and causes of heart attacks, visit the websites of the Mayo Clinic[25] and the National Institute on Aging.[26]

What Are Some of the Warning Signals for Heart Disease?

Here are important warning symptoms to know (these can be warnings for other disease processes also—and a person may have heart disease or a heart attack with no symptoms whatsoever):

- **Chest pain or pressure.**
  Be especially aware of pain behind the breastbone, but pain can occur in the jaw, neck, shoulders, upper back, stomach, right or left arm, or even the forearms.
- **Pain varies in character and severity.**
  Heart pain may be described as crushing, squeezing, a "Buick on my chest," a sense of fullness in the chest or abdomen, or a "tight bra" sensation that doesn't stop when you remove the bra. In other cases, you may have no pain at all.

25 Mayo Clinic, "Heart Attack: Symptoms and Causes," *Mayo Clinic*, June 16, 2020, https://www.mayoclinic.org/diseases-conditions/heart-attack/symptoms-causes/syc-20373106.

26 National Institute on Aging, "What Is a Heart Attack?", reviewed June 1, 2018, https://www.nia.nih.gov/health/what-heart-attack.

- **Symptoms may be different in cis men and cis women.**
A cis man is more likely to have the sensation of the elephant on the chest, while cis women are more likely to have atypical, more vague symptoms. Although cis women do have chest pain, they may be more likely to have neck, jaw, shoulder, upper back, or abdominal pain. Fatigue is a common, as are GI symptoms and light-headedness or dizziness. Heart disease is often underdiagnosed or diagnosed later with cis women (thought to be related to factors of bias where women's symptoms are discounted).

Q What about heart attack symptoms in trans males and trans females? Do they differ from those of cis males and cis females?

A We don't know. I ask all the same history questions for everyone and try not to make assumptions. Because we really don't know this yet, I think we are safer to ask "human" heart questions rather than "male or female" heart questions.

- **Heart pain is not likely to be relieved with analgesics like aspirin, ibuprofen, or acetaminophen.**
Heart pain might be relieved by nitroglycerine if you've been prescribed this, but nitro can relieve pain from spasm in the esophagus also.
- **Pain is worsened with exertion and eases with rest.**

In medical school, we were taught that any pain from the nose to the knees should raise the question of heart disease. We also learned that denial was a symptom of heart disease. Don't try to talk yourself out of symptoms. If you have symptoms, get them evaluated. If they are emergent, call 911.

— Linda Gromko, MD

- **Shortness of breath.**
Symptoms may include not getting enough air to breathe, "air hunger," or having to stop exercise that is normally doable. Be especially aware if shortness of breath occurs with exercise, subsides with rest, and restarts with activity. It may be that the exercise places more demand on the heart muscle, but the heart cannot keep up.
- **Extreme fatigue.**
One of my trans feminine patients had no chest pain or breathlessness at all—but she had to rest every few yards while walking slowly through the mall.

- **Gastrointestinal symptoms.**
  Heart disease may cause nausea and vomiting and stomach pain. We know that heartburn or GERD (gastroesophageal reflux disease) originates in the esophagus when acidic stomach contents slosh up into esophagus. It was likely named heartburn because we often feel pain from GERD just under the sternum—people often think they are having a heart attack when they experience severe reflux. GERD pain may be relieved by antacids or acid blockers, while heart pain is not.

- **Clamminess, sweating for no reason, or a gray ashen color to the face may signal acute heart trouble.**

The Value of CPR Training

Should sudden cardiac death ever happen to you, may it happen in Seattle—the home of Medic One, where all of the city's first responders and many thousands of citizens have been trained in CPR (cardiopulmonary resuscitation).

According to the City of Seattle's website: "Since Seattle's CPR Program (Medic II) started in 1971, more than 850,000 Seattle and King County residents have been trained and retrained in the lifesaving technique of CPR. Studies have shown that prompt bystander CPR more than doubles a patient's chances of becoming a long-term survivor."*

* City of Seattle, "CPR Training (Medic II)," accessed July 28, 2021, http://www.seattle.gov/fire/safety-and-community/medic-ii-cpr-training.

- **Palpitations, very rapid or very slow heartbeat, irregular rhythm.**
  Palpitations mean an awareness of the heartbeat—under normal circumstances, we really don't feel our hearts beating. Most palpitations are innocent (look up PVCs or premature ventricular contractions—also called VPBs or ventricular premature beats). While these are generally not associated with heart disease, they can make you feel like your heart is turning over or leaping out of your chest. Some palpitations, however, can be serious, like the following:

  - **Heart rates that are too fast or too slow.**
    When the heart beats too fast or too slowly, the heart may not be able to perform effectively as a pump. These problems may be managed with medication or pacemakers.

  - **Palpitations that go along with dizziness, faintness, or collapse.**
    You may feel faint or pass out if your heart cannot pump enough blood to your brain.

  - **Atrial fibrillation is an arrythmia that carries a risk of stroke.**
    Atrial fibrillation is a rhythm problem where the atria (upper chambers of the heart) aren't coordinated with the beating of the ventricles (lower chambers). This makes the heart inefficient in pumping adequate blood throughout the body. A-fib is also associated with clots: when the atrium quivers rather than beats the way it should, blood settles in the atrium and forms a clot that can travel to the brain. By interrupting proper blood flow to the brain, strokes can cause various degrees of injury—from no damage at all to profound disability and death.

- **Sudden cardiac death.**
  Many people do not experience any immediate warning symptoms. A person has a sudden rhythm abnormality that immediately renders the heart ineffective. Sudden cardiac death is responsible for half of all heart-related deaths. Patients who survive sudden cardiac death may be treated with implantable defibrillators.

Taking a Closer Look at Data

Now that we've reviewed information about heart disease, let's return to our earlier question—does estrogen increase heart disease in transgender females?

There have been reports that estradiol increases heart disease in trans females, as well as the risk of DVT and PE. But it can be difficult to separate facts from rumors. How the data are interpreted can be impacted by people's biases. When a study gets picked up by the broader media, we see other opinion articles piling on to support various agendas. Just as when we gather information from "Dr. Google," we must be discerning, ask good questions, and double-click on judgment!

Let's look briefly at a study by Talal Alzahrani et al. that was reported in April 2019 in *Circulation: Cardiovascular Quality and Outcomes*, a peer-reviewed journal of the American Heart Association. This study was splashed over the media and prompted a fair amount of worry, at least in my clients.

The study concluded that "the transgender population had a higher reported history of myocardial infarction in comparison to the cisgender population, except for transgender women compared with cisgender men, even after adjusting for cardiovascular risk factors."[27] The report went on to say that trans men had a 7.2 percent occurrence of reported myocardial infarction as compared with 3.1 percent in their cohort of cisgender women and 5.6 percent in cisgender men. Trans women had a 7.8 percent occurrence of reported myocardial infarction versus 5.6 percent in cis men and 3.1 percent of the cis women. This implies that for both trans men and trans women, myocardial infarction risk is significantly higher, or perhaps that MI risk increases significantly after transition.

Because we can be more discerning in reviewing a study, let's see what they did. (Remember, I am not a statistician, so my comments will not deal with statistical analysis.) The researchers correctly reported that prior studies looked at younger subjects, so this team appropriately sought out a broader age range. They also acknowledged that health disparities like access discrepancies, psychiatric comorbidities such as depression, and disparate health behaviors such as smoking, obesity, alcohol use, and sedentary lifestyle, are reported to be higher in the trans community. These factors can increase heart risk—and it was fully appropriate to acknowledge these important disparities. But they controlled for cardiovascular risk factors, trying to sift out whether being transgender was an independent risk factor in itself.

Alzahrani's team used data from the Behavioral Risk Factor Surveillance System, a monthly survey of adult US residents that is conducted in a random sampling by state health departments with assistance from the Centers for Disease Control and Prevention (CDC). "The CDC's survey was initiated to collect prevalent data on risk behaviors that can affect health status."[28] The combined data included a total of 1,842,439 individuals over the period of 2014 through 2017, so they examined a large sample size. Of the entire sample, 1,267 were trans men and 1,788 were trans women.

27 Talal Alzahrani et al., "Cardiovascular Disease Risk Factors and Myocardial Infarction in the Transgender Population," *Circulation: Cardiovascular Quality and Outcomes* 12, no. 4 (April 2019): 6, https://doi.org/10.1161/circoutcomes.119.005597.

28 Alzahrani, 2.

While the study controlled for certain heart disease risk factors, they didn't specify what hormone regimens were taken—or even if hormones *were* taken by the trans groups.

Participants were asked, "Do you consider yourself to be transgender?" (I wonder if this question was clear; many times people equate being transgender with being gay.) Transgender, male-to-female individuals were classified as transgender women. Those who identified as transgender, female-to-male individuals were classified as transgender men. Individuals who answered "no" to the question, "Do you consider yourself to be transgender?" were classified as cisgender men if the "Respondent's Sex" was given as male, and they were classified as cisgender women if they did not consider themselves to be transgender and identified "Respondent's Sex" as female.

However, when a subject reported they were "transgender, gender-nonconforming" and reported "male" when asked for "Respondent's Sex," they were classified as "transgender women." And when a subject reported they were "transgender, gender-nonconforming" and reported "female" when asked for "Respondent's Sex," they were classified as transgender men.

So it would appear that "Transgender Men" in the study includes trans men (female to male) plus transgender, gender-nonconforming with "Sex" identified as female. And the category of "Transgender Women" includes trans women (male to female) plus transgender, gender-nonconforming with "Sex" identified as male.

While it is laudable that the researchers even considered gender-nonconforming individuals, I believe the above categorization is confusing. It would have been clearer if identifiers such as AFAB or AMAB were used—or, if the gender-nonconforming groups were reported as separate groups. In fairness, the AFAB/AMAB terminology was early in its use in 2014, and even in the time interval from 2014 to 2017. For my purposes, I would have wanted to see the gender-nonconforming individuals represented separately, rather than being lumped together with transgender men and women.

I also imagine that the transgender, gender-nonconforming individuals made up a relatively small percentage of the total transgender men and transgender women groups (which were not reported in journal article, although likely available from research team). It may not have skewed the data—but we can see where it could.

Cardiac histories were obtained as follows: The respondents were asked, "Has a doctor, nurse, or other health professional EVER told you that you had a heart attack also called a myocardial infarction?" Similarly, respondents were asked, "Has a doctor, nurse, or other health professional EVER told you that "you have diabetes," or "you have high blood pressure," or "your cholesterol is high," or "you have kidney disease?" Admittedly, when we base facts on human recollection, we make less accurate conclusions than we do with long-term, prospective observation.

Other information collected included age, race, smoking status, and reported exercise.

This study looked at the group of transgender men versus cisgender women, and transgender women versus cisgender men:

- 3.1 percent of the cisgender women had myocardial infarctions, but
- **7.2 percent of the transgender men had myocardial infarctions.**

And looking at transgender women versus cisgender men,

- 5.6 percent of the cisgender men had myocardial infarctions, but
- **7.8 percent of the transgender women had myocardial infarctions.**

When I read this, these numbers did not pass the smell test. None of my trans medicine colleagues thought these numbers were consistent with what they saw in clinical practice either.

When we examine raw data, we see significant differences in groups of each year of the study years 2014 through 2017. While the cis men and cis women had steady MI percentages from 1 year to the next (5.4 to 5.9 percent for cis men and 3.1 to 3.2 percent for cis women), there was a significant spread in the rates of MI in the trans groups between the various years (3.4 to 11.3 for the trans men and 6.0 to 9.7 percent for trans women). We really don't know why this might be, but the report states, "the rate of myocardial infarction has increased significantly for transgender men in 2017."[29] This could be a random outlier rather than a trend, as the authors saw it.

A trans person—or their parent or spouse—might be alarmed to read this report. And several my clients were concerned.

What Can I Tell My Clients?

Studies and conclusions vary. In general, studies in general—limited as they are—have not confirmed significant risks associated with hormone therapy. My first rule, when a study's conclusions vary markedly from generally accepted information, is to look for replicating data. As a study is repeated with similar findings, it becomes more credible. I think it is appropriate to gather information from doctors who are involved in your own care—and to get your second opinions from people they trust. When you look for comparative research, go to Google Scholar. But do keep an open mind when interpreting a news splash. (Reread pages 71–72 about assessing and mitigating risks.)

Breast Cancer Risk in Trans Females

Breast cancer seems to be exceedingly rare in transgender women. Here's some information from the University of California-San Francisco's Madeline Deutsch, MD, MPH:

> "A retrospective study of 2,307 Dutch transgender women treated at a single center found an estimated incidence of 4.1/100,000 person-years, in comparison to the incidence of 155/100,000 person-years in the general Dutch nontransgender female population. A retrospective review of 3,566 transgender women receiving care in the US Veterans Administration Healthcare System found 3 cases total, translating to a nonsignificant standardized incidence ratio (SIR) of 0.7 (95% CI 0.03 to 5.57) in comparison to nontransgender women, and a significant SIR of 33.3 (95% CI 21.9 to 45.1) in comparison to nontransgender men."[30]

29 Alzahrani, 5.

30 Madeline B. Deutsch, "Screening for Breast Cancer in Transgender Women," Transgender Care, University of California-San Francisco, June 17, 2016, https://transcare.ucsf.edu/guidelines/breast-cancer-women.

While the risk may be low, remember that *you* are not a statistic. Pay attention if you have a strong family history of breast cancer or if you have certain genetic markers that may indicate you carry a higher risk, such as BRCA1 or BRCA2.

When doctors diagnose a breast cancer in *anyone*, the cancer is analyzed to see if it is stimulated by estrogen and progesterone. If a cancer is hormone-responsive, it may be treated—at least in part—by a hormone blocker.

So, theoretically, a hormone such as estrogen or progesterone could accelerate the growth of a breast cancer that is responsive to a particular hormone. Here are some take-home points:

- **Check your breasts.**
  See your healthcare provider if you find a lump, any thickening, a change in the appearance of the skin, a newly inverted nipple, or any other change that worries you.

- **While breast cancer is generally not painful, it can be.**
  And some people experience itching, tingling, pulling, or warmth (different than the tingling sensation that occurs with the arrival of breast buds early in hormone use).

- **Know your family history to the extent you can.**
  If you have a genetic propensity to developing breast cancer, it doesn't mean that you cannot take hormones, but it may mean that you should be screened more frequently. Be particularly aware of genetic markers in family members. Examples are the BRCA1 and BRCA2 genetic variations.

- **If you are a trans man who has had top surgery, remember that this surgery does NOT promise to remove every breast cell!**
  In fact, some tissue may be left to ensure an improved contour. If you feel something new, especially something that doesn't match the "mirror image" of the other side, get it checked.

Taking Hormones for Masculinization

Here's What You May Notice When Starting Testosterone

Testosterone is the hormone responsible for masculinization. Here are the major effects of testosterone you can expect to experience:

- **Your voice will deepen.**
  This seems to happen quickly, often within the first month or two. At first, you may sound hoarse or like you are coming down with a cold. You may notice your voice cracking like a teenage boy. But after some adjustment, the voice *stays* deep. Testosterone will likely have enough effect on the vocal cords that you will be recognized as male, at least by your speaking voice. Of course, this varies from person to person. You may want to track your vocal frequency by using one of a variety of apps available (Tuna Pitch is one app). If you are not satisfied by the tenor of your voice, consider vocal coaching.

  If you are masculinizing with testosterone, your singing voice will deepen also. If this is an important part of your life or career, you may want to work with a voice therapist during your transition.

A Musical Tribute to the Transgender Community

Find the YouTube video "Home (Cover)—Charlie Peck" for a poignant duet of Charlie and Ruby (Ruby is Charlie before transition). They sing Edward Sharpe and the Magnetic Zeros' song "Home." Peck recorded Ruby's part the day he started testosterone and Charlie's part 9 months into hormone replacement therapy. It's a beautiful song anyway, but the final "conversation" between Charlie and Ruby and the video's conclusion that follows likely had a number of its 396,000 viewers in tears.

> *"No matter how huge a struggle you are facing, don't ever give up. You are never alone. And it gets better. I promise."*

Charlie, who captioned the video "A Tribute to the Transgender Community," stated, "Now that I have the energy to give something back to the transgender community—this is my heart medicine for those in need."

— *Released February 21, 2017,* **youtube.com/watch?v=BVhLD0lNKj0**

- **Your body odor may change as you start to smell "like a guy."**
- **If you have menstrual periods, these will likely stop within 3 to 6 months on testosterone.**
  It is important to remember that if you miss testosterone doses, or even if you take your testosterone late, you may bleed again. For most trans men who are on full testosterone doses and take their medications regularly, there will be no more periods. (Important word of caution: Get evaluated by your doctor or other healthcare provider if you suddenly start having bleeding for no apparent reason. Bleeding can be an important warning signal—even a sign of a malignancy. Get it checked.)

  One of my patients became pregnant while on testosterone; it happens. And in that case, it was a welcomed event. See Chapter 22 for information on contraception if you are a trans man who interacts sexually with "sperm producers."
- **You may notice genital dryness.**
  The vaginal tissue becomes thinner and dryer when estradiol is decreased. It may resemble menopausal tissue. If penetrative sex becomes uncomfortable, use a personal lubricant. Some practitioners prescribe estradiol cream to apply to the area.

  Do be aware that the use of estradiol in trans men on testosterone is not well-studied. We do know that unopposed estrogen (that is, estradiol without simultaneous use of progesterone) increases the risk of uterine lining cancer in cis females—clearly important if you have a uterus. These unknowns, such as the risks to the uterus and ovaries, reasonably prompt many trans men to pursue the surgical removal of the uterus, ovaries, and fallopian tubes. This, of course, would apply to trans men who are not planning to use these organs for fertility purposes.

Pap Tests for Cervical Cancer Screening

Pap tests to screen for cervical cancer are recommended for everyone with a cervix (the lower portion of the uterus). The US Preventive Services Task Force (USPSTF) recommends cervical cancer screening every 3 years beginning at age 21 and ending at age 65. If you have an HPV test along with the Pap, you may reduce the frequency to every 5 years. If you have had a hysterectomy, including the removal of the cervix, you generally do not need further Paps unless you have had a gynecologic malignancy. Check with your healthcare provider.

— *Trans Guys, "Trans Cervical Health Primer,"* transguys.com/ref/trans-cervical-health-primer

- **Acne is common with testosterone use (testosterone + skin oil + bacteria = acne).**
  Acne may not only affect the face, but also the back, chest, and shoulders. There are many over-the-counter remedies. We prescribe topical gels containing antibiotics that may be useful on the face. A larger area like the back or chest may require systemic (total body) antibiotics taken orally. If you develop large, painful acne cysts, you may require a consult with a dermatologist and a more serious prescription medication such as Accutane (isotretinoin). We do see a fair number of men who develop acne initially but then find that it settles down after a few months.
- **You are likely to experience an increase in appetite for food, and you may gain weight.**
  Weight gain may be fine if you are burning calories through exercise and building muscle with a solid protein intake. But remember that increased food intake and little exercise may mean a future of obesity and diabetes.

I'm not trying to "fat shame" anyone. My strong feelings about preventing diabetes are personal. My husband died of diabetic kidney failure after several years on the kidney machine. Many of the struggles he endured might have been prevented by lifestyle modifications made at a younger age.

— *Linda Gromko, MD*

- **You are likely to develop more skeletal muscle.**
  Under the influence of "T," any strength training or resistance training activity will likely result in greater muscle bulk and definition than you've experienced before. Occasionally, my patients tell me they gain muscle without even trying. But you are likely to see better results if you do begin a strength training program. You don't have to be a jock unless you want to be one. Everyone seems to recommend seeing your healthcare provider before starting an exercise program, and this is reasonable advice. Keep in mind that your muscles may develop more quickly than their supporting ligaments and tendons. Back off on exercise or talk to an athletic trainer if you develop joint pain.

If, during exercise, you are experiencing chest pain or pressure, jaw pain or pressure, arm pain, shoulder pain, nausea, light-headedness, or dizziness—

Stop exercising right away and CALL 911!

These may be symptoms of a heart attack. If you try to talk yourself out of symptoms, remember that *denial* is sometimes listed as a symptom of heart disease. You can get back to activity after your heart has passed inspection.

- **Your body hair will likely increase.**
  You may notice this over your legs and arms and to varying degrees over your chest, back, buttocks, and abdomen. The "happy trail" refers to hair growing from the pubic area up toward the belly button.

- **Facial hair will fill in, starting with peach fuzz.**
  Don't expect this to be an early change, although it can be. It varies enormously, and I've seen trans men who have gone for several years on testosterone without significant hair growth. Genetics play a huge role. Dark hair will show more readily than lighter hair. It may also come in patchy, but see Chapter 8 for practical tips.

- **You may start losing scalp hair at your temples, and you may become bald.**
  Hair loss has a lot to do with genetics and your age. Remember that baldness is typically a male characteristic; you are unlikely to be "read" as female if you are bald. But if baldness is not your "look," know that there are medications that can help slow hair loss. And hair transplants, weaves, and extensions can help. Read about transplants for patchy beards, mustaches, and brows in Chapter 8.

I got an unhappy trail: hair in the butt crack. Nobody talks about that!

— Trans man in his 50s

- **Your clitoris will become significantly larger.**
  Refer to the Netter illustration on page 29 in Chapter 5. You may remember that the clitoris is the embryologic equivalent to the glans penis ("the mushroom part"). So, it should be no surprise that it gets larger and more "penis-looking" under the influence of testosterone.

  How much larger? Looking at the clitoris directly (shall we say "head on?"), it's probably the size of the very tip of the little finger in a cis female. On testosterone, it may grow to be the size of the tip of the thumb! Remember also that the clitoris sits atop a shaft—again the embryologic equivalent of the penile shaft. With testosterone, you may be able to follow that shaft to its base, and it can have significant girth. Some trans men stretch the growing phallus with pumps to elongate it (check babeland.com or goodvibes.com/s).

Nobody pees through their clitoris, so if you want to be able to pee through the enlarged phallus, you will need a surgery: specifically, a urethral extension using mucosal tissue from the vaginal wall or the buccal (pronounced "buckle") mucosa from inside the mouth. (Read much more about this in "Masculinizing Surgeries" in Chapter 11.)

- **Your sexual appetite will likely increase.**
  You are channeling that teenage boy! Remember that many factors impact sexual appetite: your work, your mood, whether you are in a relationship, and so on. And it can vary throughout your life. Some people find that their attraction patterns change, so you could be attracted to men, women, or both in a new way.

- **You may notice mood changes, generally for the better.**
  People talk about "testosterone rage," but I don't see that in the trans men in my practice. I suspect that is because we aim for testosterone levels that are physiologic—that is, in the cis male range. You probably see this testosterone rage more in people who are overusing it for bodybuilding. (Did you ever wonder why testosterone prescriptions are so closely regulated? Testosterone is an illicit drug that is sometimes abused in the bodybuilding world.)

  I have asked trans men if they "think" differently on testosterone. And I have heard trans men tell me that they are more linear in problem-solving and that they don't multitask as well. I do believe that trans men become more relaxed on testosterone. But I believe this may be related to not having to struggle so hard against ongoing gender dysphoria.

Pregnancy in Trans Males *Is* Possible

While unlikely, trans men occasionally do have unintended pregnancies. Here are some important rules to consider:

- **Do not miss your testosterone doses.** Even taking a dose several days late can make a difference. You could potentially ovulate, and you could have period bleeding again.
- **Do use birth control if you have sex with partners who make sperm.** Barrier methods like condoms and IUDs may be good choices because they have no estrogen in them. (The Mirena, Skyla, and Kyleena IUDs do have the progesterone levonorgestrel in their stalks and are good for 6 years. The Paragard is a copper-containing IUD and lasts for 12 years. The Paragard has no hormones in it at all.)

You may also want to consider a progesterone-only birth control pill or an implanted progesterone device (look up Nexplanon; it is easily placed by your healthcare provider under the skin of the upper arm and provides 5 years of contraception, as of this writing.)

Language Lesson from GenderCat

When referring to trans guys pumping, most of us prefer to leave out the word "clitoris" and will often call it our "natal penis." I try to be inclusive of nonbinary people who may not identify with having a penis. People usually know what I'm talking about when I say "sensitive parts."

— *Joseph Mudge, Founder of GenderCat, August 2019*

Protecting Yourself and Your Intimate Associates from Sexually Transmitted Diseases (STDs) or Sexually Transmitted Infections (STIs)

Speaking of sex, don't forget that using barriers like latex condoms and latex dental dams can help protect you from contracting various sexually transmitted infections.

Have you heard about Preexposure Prophylaxis (PrEP) against HIV? Preexposure **P**rophylaxis (PrEP) is a single daily pill consisting of two anti-HIV medications (specifically Truvada—emtricitabine and tenofovir disoproxil fumarate—and the newer Descovy (emtricitabine and tenofovir alafenamide).

A word of warning: Descovy has not been studied in people who were assigned female at birth and is therefore not FDA-approved for AFABs.

Taking PrEP every day can drastically reduce your risk for contracting HIV. You might consider taking PrEP if you—

- Have multiple sex partners.
- Would feel more at ease using it.
- Have partners who are known to be HIV-positive.
- Don't know the HIV status of your partner(s), or for that matter, the HIV status of other partners *they* may have.
- Experience penetration as part of your sexual activity. If you are the "receptive" partner—this usually refers to having penetration of the vagina or rectum—you may be at greater risk for contracting HIV because of the surface area of the penetrated vagina or rectum and because of small microtears or tissue injuries that allow the virus to enter your bloodstream.
- Have anonymous hookups or are having sex for money.

For more information on PrEP, go to the Centers for Disease Control (CDC) website at **cdc.gov/hiv/basics/prep.html** and Chapter 22.

How Testosterone Is Given

Like estradiol, testosterone is a prescription drug. Unlike estradiol, testosterone is regulated as a scheduled drug, meaning that it carries more potential for abuse. (Think of bodybuilding here.) The prescription for it must list your birthdate and the prescriber's DEA (Drug Enforcement Administration) number, and it is good for no more than 6 months' duration.

Testosterone can be given in the following forms:

- **Testosterone is injected into the muscle ("intramuscular" or IM) at varying frequencies.** This is given perhaps every week, 10 days, 2 weeks, or even every month.
- **Testosterone is injected under the skin rather than more deeply into the muscle.** Called a "subcutaneous" or SQ injection, it is done weekly—often in the subcutaneous tissue of the abdomen. Many people find this appealing because the needle is shorter and more slender. (Another example of an SQ injection is insulin, which is taken by millions of people with diabetes several times a day.)

> **I have many patients who learn to do their own injections, IM and SQ. Sometimes, a family member or partner will learn to do injections. We give injections at the clinic also but learning to do injections yourself gives you considerably more flexibility.**
>
> *— Linda Gromko MD*

- **Testosterone lotion or gel applied daily.** Be aware that testosterone in lotion or gel form can be transferred from your skin to that of another individual. It's important to make sure the lotion or gel is well-dried on your skin, otherwise the medicine may be rubbed onto someone else. You may unintentionally masculinize your intimate friends!

> **I have seen a number of cis-female patients with substantially elevated testosterone related to their partner's use of testosterone gel. There was no clear intimate contact. I always wonder about applying the gel, sleeping without a shirt, and having the testosterone on the sheets contributing to an androgen increase in the low-testosterone partner. I advised the patient to wear clothing over the testosterone application area or take a shower before bed.**
>
> *— Matt Davies, MD, PhD, endocrinologist*

- **Testosterone in a form designed to be applied under the arm, like an underarm deodorant.**
- **Testosterone patches.** These are expensive and about the size of a silver dollar. They must be changed daily.
- **Testosterone pellets inserted in the gluteal area—just above the muscle of the buttocks.**

These last for 2 to 6 months.

Some information on needles and syringes appears earlier in this chapter on page 65.

Itching or Welts at Injection Sites

Occasionally, I hear about people who take hormone injections experiencing itching, red blotches, lumps, or even welts at the site of their injections.

If this is happening to you, check into the oil used to mix with the hormone. You'll find the name of the oil on the box and it is usually cottonseed, castor, sesame, or mineral oil. I've had good results with using a preparation that contains a different oil.

Naturally, if you are having a serious reaction, such as wheezing, difficulty breathing, or narrowing of your airway, **this is an emergency and you must seek appropriate care—even calling 911—pronto!**

I have also heard that injecting testosterone too quickly may produce itching.

— Linda Gromko, MD

Possible Risks Involved in Taking Testosterone

We will discuss this with the same cautions that were addressed starting on page 72 with estradiol risk in trans women:

- Recognize the limitations in the number of studies and in study design.
- While it is important to recognize a higher risk in a group, the most important information includes—
    - What can be done to reduce the risk for a particular patient?
    - What are the warning signals of a particular problem?
    - What can be done to manage problems that do occur?

Your Red Blood Cell Count Will Likely Increase

Without menstrual periods, a trans man no longer loses blood during periods. But a greater impact comes from secondary polycythemia.

Defining Secondary Polycythemia

The word "polycythemia" is from the Latin *poly* (many), plus *cyt* (cell), plus *hemia* (condition of the blood). Simply translated, this means that there are too many cells in the blood. Polycythemia usually refers to *too many red cells.* (We recall from medical school decades ago that the bone marrow inside of our bones makes red cells, white cells, and platelets.)

Hematologists (doctors who specialize in the blood) break this down to primary polycythemia and secondary polycythemia:[31]

- **Primary polycythemia**
  Also called polycythemia vera or PV, this is a slow-growing myeloproliferative neoplasm, which means it is a form of blood cancer. While polycythemia vera causes an increase in the production of red cells by the bone marrow and therefore an increase in hematocrit, *it is not what we typically see from the use of testosterone*. PV is known to be related to a mutation in the janus kinase 2 (JAK2) gene or the TET2 gene.

- **Secondary polycythemia**
  Refers to an increase in the bone marrow's production of red cells due to a causal factor such as the following:

  - **Living at a high altitude** (you adapt to lower ambient oxygen levels by making more red cells to carry more oxygen)

  - **Medications** (testosterone, but the mechanism is unclear)

  - **Obstructive sleep apnea** (the airway becomes obstructed by the relaxation of the tissues at the back of the throat; the person snores and even stops breathing; the blood oxygen drops until the person gasps and wakes themself, thus correcting their low blood oxygen level)

  - **Heart or lung disease that lowers oxygen levels** (the bone marrow makes more red cells to carry more oxygen to compensate)[32]

Testosterone typically increases the number of red blood cells in the body, although the precise mechanism of this is not completely understood. The kidneys are somehow stimulated to produce more erythropoietin or EPO, which is the kidney hormone that directs the bone marrow to produce more red cells. As stated above, the red cells are particularly important because they carry the hemoglobin molecule, which in turn carries oxygen to our tissues. In the clinic, we would likely notice that a person's *hematocrit* increases after taking testosterone for a few months. The hematocrit is the percentage of blood that consists of red cells.

A Hematocrit That's Too High

How high a hematocrit is too high? Ask five doctors and you may get five answers. Some say a hematocrit is too high at 50 percent; others at 52 percent; others go higher. Part of this decision depends on a man's overall health and other risk factors.

31 For more information, see Fabian P. Siegel and Petro E. Petrides, "Congenital and Acquired Polycythemias," *Deutsches Ärzteblatt International* 105, no. 4 (January 2008): 62–8, DOI: 10.3238/arztebl.2008.0062.

32 Siegel, 63.

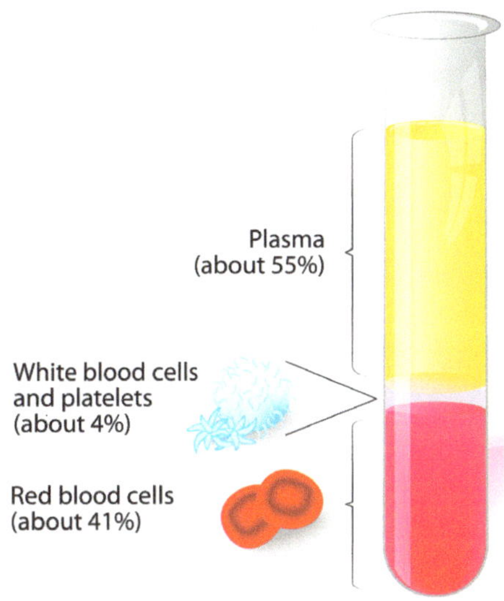

Figure 7.9. Composition of whole blood.

Think of it this way:

- If you take a test tube of a person's blood and spin it in a centrifuge, the blood separates out to three layers: (1) the heavy red cell layer that settles out on the bottom of the test tube, (2) a small "buffy coat" that consists of white cells and platelets, and (3) the top layer of serum or plasma.
- A hematocrit of 40 percent means that 40 percent of the blood consists of red cells and the remaining nearly 60 percent is made of white blood cells plus serum.

If a person's hematocrit becomes very high from the relative increase in red blood cells, the blood becomes more viscous (thicker), which is thought to lead to blood clots that result in strokes or heart attacks.

We may ask a man with an increased hematocrit to drink more fluids to increase the plasma volume, which drops the relative red cell proportion. In some cases, a man may have a therapeutic phlebotomy (a blood draw done simply to remove some of the whole blood volume), or he may be able to donate blood to reduce his blood volume.

Time for a hematologist to weigh in! I asked Dr. Sam Tolman for a quick hematology lesson. Here's what Dr. Tolman had to offer:

Adjusting Testosterone Levels

Polycythemia has always been a misnomer in that only the red cells are upregulated and not the white cells or platelets. That helps us differentiate secondary polycythemia from polycythemia vera—a primary bone marrow disorder which mostly arises from the JAK2 mutation and affects all three lines (red cells, white cells, and platelets) and is therefore truly a polycythemia.

It is also curious that testosterone produces only an erythrocytosis (an increase in red cells), and many feel that testosterone affects lung function in a way that produces erythrocytosis, but this is unproven and as you say, "it is unclear how testosterone drives up EPO."

Regarding phlebotomy (blood draws to remove extra blood) in polycythemia, part of the answer lies in what is "normal" for each individual and therefore how much above normal the patient is, and that is why you get different answers. There have not been good studies in secondary polycythemia regarding thrombosis (clot) risk, but we know it is not as thrombogenic (likely to cause clots) as primary polycythemia. We generally seek phlebotomy for a hemoglobin level of 15 or a hematocrit of 45 in primary polycythemia, based on good data.

By extrapolation, we generally arrive at a hematocrit of 50 to 55 or a hemoglobin of over 17 to 18 for secondary polycythemia, but we also know this is likely overtreatment. I think this is the message: We don't want any thrombosis risk. Baby aspirin (81 mg) in either case is extremely effective at mitigating the thrombosis risk from erythrocytosis. For patients who get a stroke at these levels, there are always other factors and that is also the problem—there are many risk factors for a stroke or heart attack.

Therefore, in my practice, I lower the testosterone slowly while I have the patient on aspirin, following EPO levels and testosterone levels until we arrive at a mutually agreeable target—one where the patient's energy is acceptable (the cis population are on testosterone to boost energy or maybe libido).

In general, I try not to perform phlebotomy more than every 3 months, since we then start to run into iron deficiency.

— J. Samuel Tolman, MD, hematology/oncology specialist

Your Cholesterol (Lipid) Panel May Change for the Worse

This area of information is muddy, but some scientists say that triglycerides increase and HDL (high-density lipids) decreases when you are on testosterone. HDL is the protective cholesterol that removes the so-called "bad" LDL (low-density lipids) from your bloodstream. A low HDL level is thought to be an independent risk factor for coronary artery disease. An article about cardiovascular disease in transgender people on the University of California-San Francisco Transgender Care's website states the following:

> "Direct study of the effects of hormones on lipids and blood pressure in transgender people has been limited. A retrospective study of lipids in 169 Austrian transgender people found trends of poorer lipid profiles in both transgender women and men at 5 years; however, these changes were mild at most, and seemed to be mitigated to some degree by the use of transdermal estradiol. A prospective 6-month study of a young and healthy cohort of 31 transgender women and 17 transgender men in the US found modest overall improvement in lipids in transgender women and only a slight reduction in HDL in transgender men; while statistically significant, the effect sizes were small and of questionable clinical significance."[33]

33 Asa Radix and Madeline B. Deutsch, "Cardiovascular Disease," Transgender Care, University of California-San Francisco, June 17, 2016, https://transcare.ucsf.edu/guidelines/cardiovascular.

What would I recommend? Have your cholesterol panel checked; treat with cholesterol medications if needed but also address nutrition, exercise, and weight management. And stop smoking (see Chapter 10). In my opinion, these interventions are likely to have more impact on reducing cardiovascular risk. *Besides, withholding testosterone from transgender men is like withholding oxygen—we must find another approach!*

Sleep Apnea in Trans Men

If the airway is blocked by the tongue or other tissues of the back of the throat, a person's oxygen level drops during sleep. This may prompt a person to wake up gasping for air. I had one gentleman who told me he was dreaming of suffocation! Over time, this phenomenon increases a person's risk of heart disease, high blood pressure, heart palpitations, elevated serum cortisol levels, weight gain, and even poor mental function. It is known that *low testosterone* is associated with sleep apnea.

Some factors may increase sleep apnea in trans men. Here are some theoretical possibilities as to why:

- Trans men (assigned female at birth) may start out with smaller airway structures to begin with, so these structures of the back of the throat (posterior pharynx) may be easier to obstruct.
- Trans men may develop larger neck muscles under the influence of testosterone, and this can be significant in making the airway more crowded and thus airway obstruction more likely.
- Trans men on testosterone develop more red blood cells, as we've covered above. Their blood becomes more viscous. It is known that hypoxia (low oxygen) from sleep apnea is associated with increased red cell production. (But is increased red cell production a reason for sleep apnea?)
- Trans men may gain weight under the influence of testosterone; if they do, they may be at greater risk for sleep apnea, as obesity is an independent risk factor for sleep apnea.

Heart Disease Risk in Trans Men

We have discussed the limited treatment of heart disease in transgender individuals. Please review the information from the Alzahrani study and my comments about evaluating and preempting heart disease. While the study featured a large study group, its definitions of who is a transgender man or transgender woman are not current. Granted, this was basically a survey (which is not considered optimal for answering scientific questions), but the inference is that trans men have a higher heart attack risk than cis women and cis men. This is certainly not a phenomenon I have observed in my practice.

If lipid changes do occur and if weight gain with visceral obesity is more generalized, cardiac risk factors could rise because of increased metabolic syndrome (the combination of visceral obesity, hypertension, insulin resistance, elevated serum triglycerides, and low HDL cholesterol—which are the high-density protective lipids that remove LDL from the bloodstream). For more information, see the American Heart Association's web page on metabolic syndrome: **heart.org/en/health-topics/metabolic-syndrome/about-metabolic-syndrome**.

The Use of Sex Hormones in Nonbinary Individuals

It is possible for an individual to find a middle ground that suits them. As we discussed before, the most important thing here is knowing what you want to see happen from the use of hormones. But understand that we may not be able to forecast how *much* change will occur with your use of hormones. Nor can you forecast how quickly the changes occur. It's also important to remember which changes are reversible and which are permanent. Let's look at a few examples below:

- Suppose you do want your breasts to develop, but they grow larger than you would have wanted. You can reduce the hormone dose. And you *could* have a reduction mammoplasty or a top surgery. But wouldn't it be convenient to have tighter control?
- Suppose you wanted to masculinize, hoping for a deeper voice and more muscle bulk. But what if *you* are the person who gets more-than-average facial hair and you find that you don't like it? You can have facial hair removed by laser or electrolysis but again, that may not have been your intention.
- And finally, I have had a couple of teenagers in my practice who decided to stop taking masculinizing hormones. Their voices had deepened permanently, making them sound kind of sultry. These changes will be permanent, unless they retrain their voices as many trans women do or have voice surgery. These folks were happy in transition, and equally happy detransitioning.

So, know what you want to the best of your ability. Work carefully with your hormone prescriber to assure that you are getting the changes you want and need. Make sure your provider isn't making assumptions about your gender expression goals. Know which changes will likely be permanent. Be particularly respectful of the fact that surgeries are permanent. While you can have modifications later, it takes considerable time and money to redo an undesired outcome. (See also the information on newer nonbinary surgical options in Chapter 11.)

Answer to the question on page 77: The unlabeled yellow organ is the pancreas. Too bad about the absent spleen.

SECTION 3

PRESENTATION: THE NONSURGICAL THINGS WE DO TO SHOW WHO WE ARE

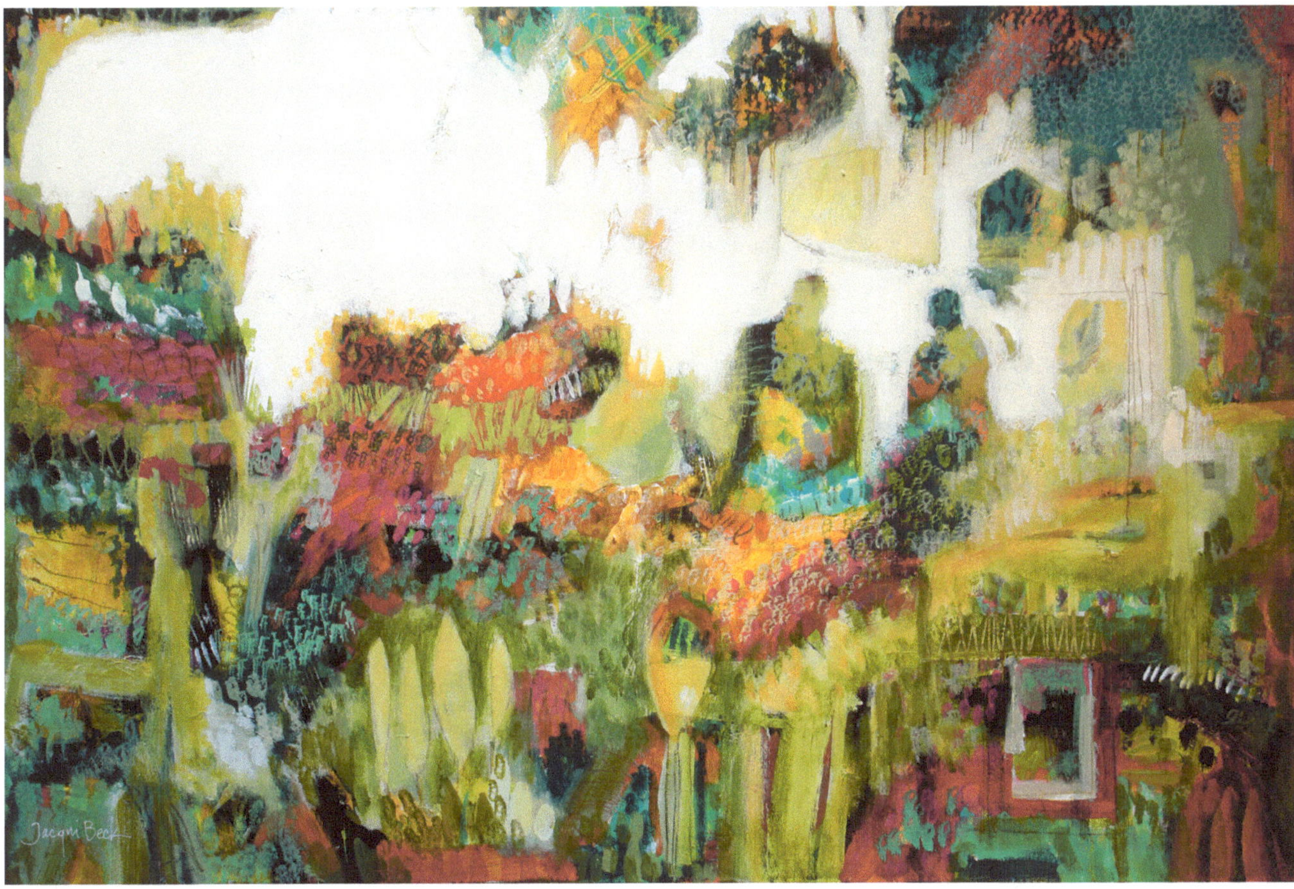

In a Bee Loud Glade

INTRODUCTION

Presentation: The Nonsurgical Things We Do to Show Who We Are

I've often thought that we don't work all that hard to figure out the gender of another person. We simply glance at someone and instantly pick up gender cues:

- Height
- Body type
- Hair length and style
- Body language, posture, and hand movements
- Clothing style and color
- Accessories like glasses, watches, rings, purses, and backpacks
- Shoe style
- A name tag
- Companions (who you're with)

In the blink of an eye, we conclude that the person we are looking at is male or female. This snap judgment isn't *necessarily* a negative. (Of course, it can be very problematic; think about profiling.) We are hard-wired to size people up in an instant to assess whether someone is a threat to us. So, we're skilled at making quick assessments of all kinds.

But, if you are in the process of a gender transition, you may want to help other people "gender" you correctly.

Exploring How You Want to Present

There's no right or wrong way for a person to present, but there may be a best way *for you.*

Give yourself the freedom to consider yourself a work in progress. Try things out in the privacy of your own space. (You may not be fortunate enough to have a personal space for exploration. In Seattle, a trans woman can rent a locker with a changing area, makeup table, and mirrors. Some people carry their femme clothing in a suitcase and change before they go to a transgender support meeting or come to see me in my medical office.)

Watch how other people present to help you define what you would like for yourself. Try conscious people-watching when you're in a mall or surfing the Internet. Notice that many of the tiniest things can convey "masculine" or "feminine." Take eyeglasses, for example. If you are masculinizing, research "eyewear for men." Eyeglass frames "for men" tend to be darker, a little thicker, and more angular. Try the same for "women's" eyeglasses and notice the differences. You can buy reasonably priced frames online to see what works. The same applies to purses, luggage, smartphone cases, jewelry, smartwatches, body art, and piercings.

Presentation involves accentuating the parts of your appearance that you want the world to notice. It also involves minimizing the things you don't want to call attention to. Remember, it's all determined by you and what makes you the most comfortable in your own skin. Giving serious thought to how you present can help minimize some of the gender dysphoria you feel.

Defining Androgyny

The word "androgyny" comes from two Greek roots: *andro*, meaning "male," and *gyn*, meaning "female." Combined, they imply a *mix* of male and female, or perhaps a *neutral* appearance that dominantly conveys neither male nor female.

Androgyny is a good starting position as you examine your own gender expression. Neither strikingly male nor female, it *can* be a comfortable, safe place. You aren't likely to go too far wrong by appearing androgynous. You may have adopted androgyny to some degree if you identify your gender as nonbinary.

Androgyny, however, can be confusing to others. You may get looks that last longer than usual, or rude people who ask, "What *are* you?" Does this matter? Perhaps not, but consider the following comments in the box below. You'll want to give this careful thought.

The Safety of Giving Cues

The time in my transition when I felt the most vulnerable to physical harm was early on when I looked my most androgynous. This was the time when I was approached and challenged the most. What I experienced firsthand was that the world is binary and most people care about whether you are male or female, especially in certain situations like bathrooms, gym lockers, or interacting with their little kids. With their need to feel safe, they need to be able to assess whether you could be a threat, and this includes determining your gender.

So, I knew I was safer if I gave strong cues that I was one or the other. While it was great to be moving away from looking female, I couldn't wait to get out of that anxiety-ridden androgynous phase!

— Adult trans man

Let's take a clothing example. Consider a basic "uniform," which might consist of a cotton T-shirt, jeans, maybe a jean jacket, and athletic shoes. This uniform presents an androgynous look, and it can be worn to convey a gender-neutral appearance that broadcasts neither male nor female.

You can easily buy this uniform from male or female clothing manufacturers. The cut of the garments may vary slightly, and the buttons are sewn on the left half of a "female" shirt versus the right side of a "male" shirt. I see many trans women who are not fully "out" who buy women's jeans but still present male or androgynously. You can take this uniform and tweak it with color and accessories to masculinize or feminize the overall effect.

In our next sections, we will go into detail on **nonsurgical ways to appear more feminine** and **nonsurgical ways to appear more masculine**. As always, read the sections that you find interesting and adopt only the practices that feel right to you.

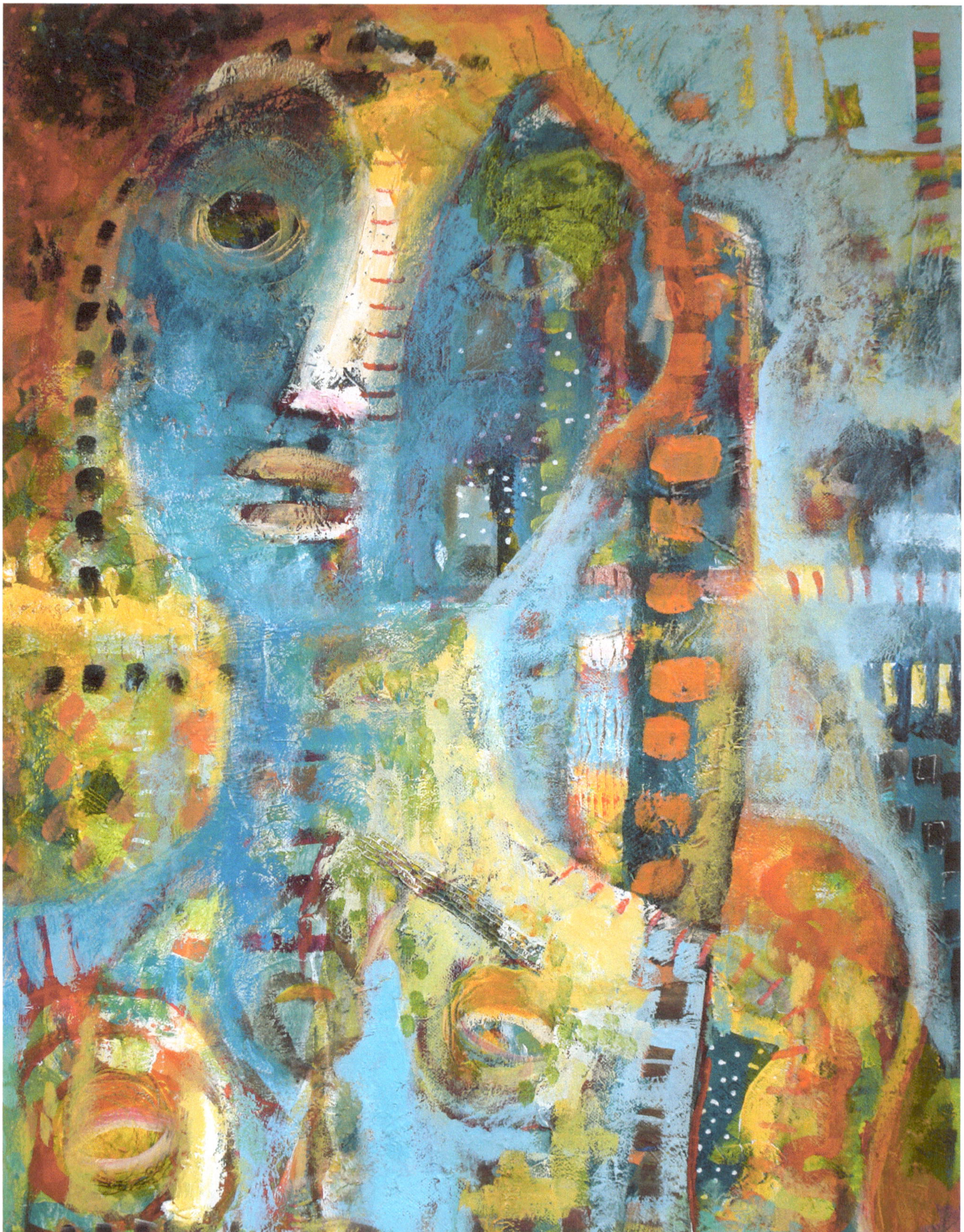

What My Reflection Shows

CHAPTER 8
Nonsurgical Ways to Appear More Feminine

Linda's Disclosure

I have been a feminist since I was a teenager. It makes my skin crawl to think we can **be judged**—and judged harshly—by our appearance. But I know that people may be placed at greater physical and emotional risk when **their appearance causes them to be misgendered by others.**

So, when you hear ***this*** feminist talking about grooming, hair removal, and makeup, please understand that I just don't want anybody to get hurt! I want you to get the job you want, to find friends and partners more easily, and to live the life you are truly meant to live.

I am also exquisitely aware of how expensive it is to feminize even nonsurgically. I am sensitive to the fact that not everyone reading this will have the resources to pursue some of these options. And certainly, not everyone would choose every item on the menu. As always, take what works for you and leave the rest.

— Linda Gromko, MD

If you have given presentation a lot of thought (which I imagine you have), you may have come up with some things you simply cannot change, like your height or your shoe size. But people do many things *without* surgery that can make an enormous visual difference and can make you feel more synchronous with your true self.

Nonsurgical Ways to Make Your Face Look More Feminine

Take a good look at your own face. What features "read" as more feminine—and what features read as more masculine? As in everything related to appearance, maximize the things you want people to notice and minimize the things you want people to ignore. Read ahead to the part on facial feminization surgery (Chapter 11) if this helps you understand this concept more clearly.

Prominent brow bones and an angular jaw tend to convey masculinity. Think about this as you read on. And think about this as you study your own face and observe the people around you. Rounder, softer features convey femininity.

Facial Hair and Hair Removal

Facial hair can be an enormous roadblock for trans women. Sources vary widely, but they seem to agree that there are *thousands* of hairs in a human beard. No wonder it becomes one of the biggest challenges and one of the factors that gets trans women "read" (picked out as assigned male at birth) most often.

So many genetic factors go into the appearance of facial hair. Do you have a dense or a light growth of facial hair? Is your hair darker so that it shows up more easily even when closely shaven? Does your facial hair grow so quickly that you shave in the morning *and* during the afternoon? (See "Grooming" on pages 115–116 for cosmetic tips on concealing afternoon shadow.)

Permanent hair removal or reduction is a costly and time-consuming process, although it is easier if you begin the process earlier in life. There are many over-the-counter options, but you may find that you'll spend less money and experience better results with one of the optimal methods below. I am admittedly biased; these are the services we provide in my medical office. But these are the methods we see working well in our clients.

- **Laser is an FDA-cleared process of permanent hair *reduction*.**
  With laser, the light of a single wavelength is directed at the skin, which targets the pigment melanin at the base of the hair follicle. Over time, the treated hairs fall out. Laser works best on dark-haired people with lighter skin. It tends not to work *at all* on blond, gray, red, or white hair although it may be worth a try if your hair consists of a blend of colors. Laser can be used in individuals with darker skin. However, dark skin may burn more easily; be certain that your technician is experienced in laser hair removal in people with skin that is darker, such as Black, Native American, Mediterranean, and so on. Treatments are spaced out every 5 to 6 weeks; for most people, five to six treatments will provide at least an excellent start; periodic touch-ups may be needed. As they say, "results may vary."

Q **I believe laser turned my facial hair gray! What happened?**

A **Laser treats *only* the brown or black hair. As these hairs are removed, you are *left with the gray hairs you had to begin with*. You may look grayer, but the laser didn't change your hair color. We can remove the remaining gray hairs by electrolysis.**

- **Electrolysis is a meticulous method of removing hairs one at a time, follicle by follicle.**
  We introduce a slender probe into each hair follicle and use an electric current to destroy the follicle forever. Many treatments are required, though, because there are so many hairs! Because hair grows in cycles, you cannot possibly eliminate all hairs at one sitting. The electrologist must see the hair they're removing, and they cannot see those hairs that are still under the skin's surface. There are variations in electrolysis methods and you may want to research this further if this interests you. (My practice website has more information, **queenannemedicalassociates.com.**) Although electrolysis is FDA-cleared for *permanent* hair removal, most people do get periodic touch-ups, sometimes for years.

  Hair removal with laser or electrolysis can be used to remove hair from the chest or back, arms and legs, genitals, and other places. In our office, we also feature "Nose-to-Toes" laser treatments. These take between 2 and 3 hours per treatment and are done about five or six times, generally with excellent results.

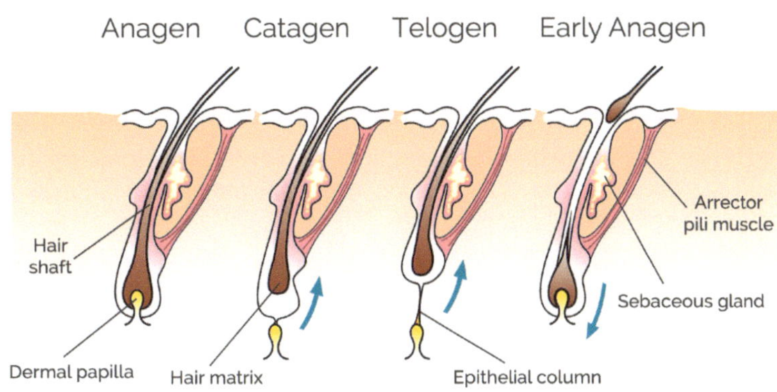

Figure 8.1. Hair growth cycle.

Q What's the difference between permanent hair removal and permanent hair reduction?

A Pardon the pun, but I think sometimes this is "splitting hairs." In electrolysis, an entire hair is removed for good. When you lift a hair out during an electrolysis treatment, you can see the little bulb at the base, and *that* hair won't be coming back (at least theoretically). This is what is meant by "permanent hair removal." With laser, you treat a section or batch of hairs at a time. Because the batch of hairs may be in different phases of growth, you may be eliminating those in the early growth phase, bulb and all. But others may return. It takes a minimum of five or six treatments to complete permanent hair reduction. And there are so many hairs to deal with that it's almost impossible not to require some cleanup from time to time.

Q Do you shave before hair removal?

A You shave before laser hair removal. The laser light is drawn to the melanin under the skin at the base of the hair. Hair that is visible on the surface can attract laser energy to the hair and skin, causing burns. You do not shave before electrolysis because the technician must be able to pick up each hair with tweezers to insert a probe and zap the follicle at its base. You must be able to see a hair to pick it up.

Pain Management during Laser and Electrolysis

Not everyone finds laser or electrolysis to be particularly painful. Not everyone finds it painful to have a baby, either. I found my few electrolysis treatments to the upper lip area to be quite horrible (and I welcomed childbirth anesthesia as a gift from the baby Jesus). Some people describe the pain of laser to be like a rubber band snapping against the skin. But then, some people describe labor as "a little pressure."

My concern in offering laser and electrolysis for hair removal in my medical practice was that if we *didn't* address pain effectively, clients might interpret our treatments to be yet another punishment for being transgender. While we may not be able to take all pain away in every patient, we can do a lot to help. We even see some of our patients sleep through their treatments! Here's what we offer:

- **BLT cream (benzocaine, lidocaine, tetracaine)**
  This is a specially compounded cream can be used 30 to 60 minutes before treatment on the face or genitals. It isn't perfect, but it helps. We usually cover the area with plastic wrap to allow it to absorb better. We include this in our laser and electrolysis treatments—unless, of course, a patient has an allergy to the medications. *(Caution: I use BLT cream only in-house. I have not had patients experience lidocaine toxicity, but it can happen, particularly if applied over a large surface area like a chest or a back. Lidocaine toxicity can produce heart arrhythmias and seizures. That's why we limit the amount and surface area of application.)*

- **EMLA**
  This is another prescription cream consisting of lidocaine and prilocaine. Your healthcare provider may be willing to prescribe this. In my experience, it isn't nearly as potent as the BLT, but it's something! You can also find lidocaine marketed online for tattoo removal.

- **Dental blocks**
  These are for the painful upper and lower lip areas and are the kind of injections that dentists use to numb the teeth and gums when you are getting a filling. Placed inside the mouth, these injections allow our clients to have nearly painless facial hair removal over the sensitive upper lip and chin area. I sometimes must repeat an injection, but they generally work within minutes. If your hair removal provider does not offer this, you may find a nearby dentist who is willing to help you. Your hair removal provider may have already identified a dentist colleague, so ask.

- **Injected field blocks**
  These are game changers for people who are preparing for vaginoplasty. By injecting anesthetic shallowly with a very slender (30 gauge) needle, we can numb the scrotal area well. We do see occasional bruising, but overall, our patients have been grateful for this service. We can use a similar technique for areas of the face that are not covered by a dental block, and we use field blocks for hair removal in the radial forearm or anterior thigh in trans men who are preparing for phalloplasty.

- **Narcotic pain relievers and anxiety medications**
  These are rarely needed, but we use them on occasion.

You may be interested in knowing that health insurance plans of large gender-friendly companies are covering the cost of facial and genital hair removal in preparation for gender-affirming surgery. They sometimes cover the cost of dental blocks and injected field blocks also. Ask your insurance representative, or more specifically, ask to speak to the person *who deals with transgender health services.* Things are changing.

Give yourself plenty of time (about a year) for hair removal in preparation for genital surgery. Hair removal can be done by laser or electrolysis, depending on your hair color and the specific requirements of your surgeon (check with them). If hair is not removed before surgery, you may grow hair inside the vagina later since scrotal and penile skin are used to create the neovagina (new vagina). Likewise, if you do not have adequate hair removal before phalloplasty, you may grow hair on your new penis—or worse—inside the urethra. (One of our trans male clients recommended giving the hair removal process a year and a half, just to be sure.)

To be complete, here are some other methods of temporary hair removal to help you if you are not prepared, financially or otherwise, to begin laser or electrolysis hair removal. ***(Do not use these methods in preparation for genital surgery.)***

- **Sugaring**
  This is the application of a sugar paste over the area to be treated, and the quick removal of the paste and hair with a flick of the wrist. It can be less uncomfortable than waxing or tweezing; it can be worth a try.

- **Tweezing or plucking**

- **Waxing**

- **Shaving**

- **Threading**
  This is an ancient technique of hair removal; you'll find it in East Indian salons and in some shopping malls.

- **Depilatory creams**
  These that can be purchased over-the-counter in a pharmacy or online. I have spoken with trans men who use a depilatory cream placed in the urethra to temporarily remove hair in the urethra after phalloplasty. *Use extreme caution, if you even consider this.* It is most prudent to drink a quart of water 30 to 60 minutes before trying this so you can pee the cream out right away. Talk to other trans men and to your surgeon, of course, before even attempting this.

- **Home hair removal methods**
  These include products such as the No!No! or Epilady.

Remember that people assigned male who have not proceeded far enough into puberty to grow facial or genital hair will have a far easier time with the hair issue. But even people who enter gender-affirming treatment with a heavy growth of facial hair can do beautifully.

Skin Care and Makeup

Starting with Healthy Skin

I appreciate that this sounds elementary, but all facial enhancements work better when we start with a canvas of healthy skin. You can spend a fortune on skin care; as you explore, you'll find that nearly every cosmetic product line has skin *care* products as well. You can try samples of these by visiting a cosmetics counter of a department store. In 1998, Paula Begoun wrote the initial volume of her encyclopedic guide, *Don't Go to the Cosmetics Counter Without Me*. This is a great title—it *does* feel like we need a professional guide just to shop. She can help you make sense of the many products that exist and so can many other experts. As Begoun stresses, you do not have to spend a lot of money if you use dependable products regularly.

Other Basic Principles That Won't Lead You Astray

- **Protect your skin from the inside with good nutrition.**
  We nourish our skin by eating well: fruits and vegetables, nutritious protein sources, and healthy fats like avocado, nuts, and seeds. Junk food contains a lot of salt and can make you look puffy. Too much alcohol and any amount of smoking makes you look older.

- **Drink 2 quarts of water every day.**
  Be especially conscious of this if you take diuretics like spironolactone. Spiro is a testosterone blocker, and it can dehydrate you.

- **Use sunscreen with an SPF rating of 30 or higher.**
  Did you know that malignant melanomas (a type of skin cancer) are more likely to occur on the left side of the face? It's because of the sun exposure we get as we drive. Tanning places you at risk for sun damage and skin cancers, plus it dries out your skin and makes you look older.

- **Cleanse your skin once or twice daily.**

- **Don't go to bed with makeup on.**
  At the very least, remove cosmetics with makeup remover wipes.

- **Avoid touching your face.**
  Your skin gets dirtier and you introduce bacteria and virus particles into your eyes, nose, and mouth. We were reminded during the early days of the COVID-19 pandemic that touching our faces can introduce virus particles into our respiratory tissues.

- **Use a moisturizer of some type during the day and before bed.**

- **Get enough sleep.**

- **Stop smoking now.**
  Smoking accentuates lines and wrinkles, and it delays healing in general. (If you are preparing for a gender-affirming surgery, know that your surgeon will likely not operate on you if you're smoking; a urine test may "out" you as a smoker.) See Chapter 10 for more information on quitting smoking.

- **A variety of skin treatments.**
  Treatments such as facials and microneedling will help you cleanse, exfoliate, and rejuvenate your skin.

Cosmetics

Cosmetics help us accentuate the features we want to play up and also minimize the features we want to play down. You may want to purchase an assortment of brushes; try to keep these very clean. Experts say to buy new makeup at least every several months to reduce the bacteria you inadvertently place on your skin.

Adding up the cost of common beauty products such as foundation, lip color, brushes, and sponges can amount to well over several hundred dollars! Foundation and lip color are good places to start. Be sure to ask cosmetics salespeople for samples. You don't need to buy everything all at once; most cis women buy a little at a time as they learn what they like. As you shop, you may want to ask for a mid-range or lower-priced cosmetics line; but, you can still spend a fortune.

Stop at a cosmetics counter and ask for a makeup lesson or a makeover. Stores want you to buy their products. In the pre-COVID-19 days, you could stop at a cosmetic counter and ask for a makeup lesson or a makeover. The more they demonstrate, the more you are likely to buy. You can also explore YouTube for high-quality makeup lessons.

Become familiar with the basic steps, but remember that there are many ways to apply makeup.

- Start with skin that is freshly cleansed and shaven, followed by a light layer of a moisturizer. (If your skin tends to be oily, you can use an oil-free moisturizer. Experts say that skipping moisturizer will age your skin prematurely.) If your makeup or moisturizer doesn't have sunscreen in it, you can add that also.
- If you have acne, lightly apply a concealer cream over your pimples and cover with your foundation.
- Find a liquid or powder foundation that compliments your skin tone. Blend it well at the edges with a makeup sponge or brush so you don't look like you are wearing a costume mask.
- Ask your cosmetics salesperson for a coordinating highlighter powder or other product to accentuate parts of your face, as well as a contouring product that helps you minimize areas you want to become less noticeable.
- Show off shaped brows by "feathering" them in with a brow pencil or brow powder applied with a brush. Keep this subtle until you are confident.
- Outline your eyelids with a liquid or pencil liner, apply mascara to your lashes, and carefully curl them with a lash curler.
- Apply color to your upper eyelids with a powdered shadow or crème shadow. Earth tones (browns and pinks) are good to start with as you begin.
- Color your lips by tracing their boundaries with a liner pencil or brush. This will keep the lip color in the lines. Then apply your color with a brush or the lipstick itself. Then apply lip gloss over your liner and lip color if you want your lips to shine. And check your teeth to make sure you haven't colored them too!
- Add blush to your cheekbones and touch up any areas with brightener or contour.

Avoid or stop using any products that contain components you are allergic to, and stop anything to which you develop a rash, hives, or other reaction.

Concealing a Beard Shadow

If you have dark facial hair, it may become visible toward the end of an afternoon ("five o'clock shadow"). Many trans women have used the following trick:

- Shave as closely as you can.
- Apply a layer of red crème-based eye shadow or color corrector over the areas that are more densely covered with facial hair. Deep pink or amber works well for some women. (Dermablend makes Quick Fix Color Corrector; check out **dermablend.com**.)
- Apply a moderate-coverage liquid foundation over this and complete your makeup as you ordinarily would.
- Pack portable makeup supplies to take to work if you need to redo your lower face toward the end of your workday.[34]

Accentuate Your Eyes

Focusing attention on your eyes can make you look younger and more attractive, and it doesn't have to be that difficult or expensive. Consider the following ideas:

- **Eyebrow shaping**
  Because heavy, dominant brows can read so stereotypically male, brow shaping can give you striking mileage as you feminize. Invest the $20 to $30 to have a salon professional shape your brows by waxing, threading, or sugaring. A professional will trim your brows, thin them, and remove the unibrow between the brows if you have one. Brows will grow back if you don't like the effect. While you're at it, check out brow tinting (a process of temporarily coloring the brows). In medical school, we learned to "never shave a brow"! (I'm told that shaved brows grow back in a hodgepodge fashion.)
- **Lash lifts**
  This treatment is like having a permanent wave for your upper eyelashes. You can combine this with lash tinting to make your lashes more visible. Plus, if you use mascara, your lashes—and your eyes—will stand out even more.
- **Lash growth promoters**
  Latisse is probably the best known of such agents. Discovered serendipitously when patients using a glaucoma product began growing longer eyelashes, Latisse extends the growth phase of the lashes. Combining this with a lash lift and brow shaping can make a significant difference. Remember that getting people to look at your eyes is a good thing. (When I've given lectures on nonsurgical transgender aesthetics, several people have told me that castor oil applied to lashes also promotes lash growth; you can get this online for much less money than Latisse.)
- **Lash extensions**
  These artificial (or mink) lashes are longer-lasting than traditional false lashes. Extensions are glued one unit at a time, as opposed to a single curved strip of false lashes applied all at once. Lash extensions require a regular time commitment because they must be replaced every couple of

34 See Lucille Sorella's website for styling and feminity tips and guidance at lucillesorella.com.

weeks by a technician or aesthetician. Extensions are not inexpensive, but check them out if they appeal to you.

- **False eyelashes**
  Look for glue-on lashes and newer magnetic lashes, both available online.

Grooming

Whenever we talk about feminization, we should say a few words about basic grooming. If you didn't learn this information as a preteen girl, how would you know it? At its most basic, grooming means tending to our hygiene. Here are some basic tips that cis women learned starting in fifth grade (reinforced by mothers and vigilant big sisters). None of this is intended to offend, so use the information only if it is helpful.

- Take a shower or bath every day or every other day, and more often if you get dirty, have sex, or can smell body odor on yourself or your clothing.
- Use deodorant under your arms. Deodorants are assigned "genders"—that is, they come in different scents and have different names and packaging to appeal marketingwise to male or female customers. Otherwise, they are all pretty much the same.
- Brush your teeth; aim for at least twice a day. You can also buy little toothpicks that have tiny brushes on them to use when you cannot brush. Floss your teeth. Use mouthwash to rinse your mouth, or at least eat crunchy fruits and vegetables to remove debris from between your teeth.
- Shampoo your hair when you shower or bathe. You may want to use a conditioner to make your hair tangle less. You may not need to shampoo your hair every day, but do notice when your hair starts to feel or look oily and shampoo it when it does.
- Carefully tend to facial hairs like ear or nose hair with delicate grooming scissors or a rotating trimmer if this is an issue for you. You can have these areas waxed also.
- Trim and clean under your fingernails and toenails. Get manicures and pedicures if you like them and can afford the money and time.
- Use baby wipes or facial cleansing wipes to clean your perineum if you have difficulty with urine or bowel movement residue getting on your clothing. You can get travel-sized packs of these.
- Get in the habit of wiping from front to back after going to the bathroom; this is especially important if you have a vaginoplasty. (Wiping from back to front brings anal bacteria closer to your urethra and may predispose you to bladder infections. After a vaginoplasty, your urethra will be much shorter, which invites bacteria to move up into your bladder more easily.)
- Consider using panty liners or sanitary pads if you have discharge, especially after surgery.
- Launder your clothing regularly, but particularly when you notice stains or retained odors. (If you are "sniffing out" your underwear, it's time to do laundry.)
- Use fragrance sparingly, if at all, so it doesn't irritate other people or make them wheeze.
- Cleanse and moisturize your face every day, morning and night. Wear sunscreen. Don't go to sleep with your makeup on. Try keeping a pack of facial cleansing wipes or makeup remover wipes (like

Neutrogena or Kirkland brand from Costco) next to your bed so you can at least do the basics if you're just too tired to do one more thing. Most of these products clean and moisturize.

- Don't smoke. Smoking tobacco seems to cancel out a lot of these good grooming habits. For more information on quitting smoking, see Chapter 10.

Body Language

Watch how cis women sit, walk, and move. Watch how they use their hands. Observe their posture and their hand movements. Notice how they cross their legs when sitting. This is all stereotypical, to be sure. But learning from such stereotypes, be they good or bad, may help you feel more comfortable and safer as well.

Voice Training

Unlike trans men on testosterone, trans women taking estrogen do not experience a change in their voice pitch. If you were assigned male and went through male puberty, your vocal cords lengthened and thickened, making your voice deeper. You can feminize your voice through practice.

> **I thought I'd have more trouble on the phone, but I learned to put on my receptionist voice and I have no problem on the phone. I'm more self-conscious in person.**
>
> *— Trans woman, age 30*

> **In my experience, I find that many women have more trouble on the phone, where we typically don't have visual cues.**
>
> **A friend of mine says, "Hello, this is Dr. Jane Doe" rather than "This is Dr. Doe." This gives the listener another bit of information so they are more likely to gender her properly.**
>
> *— Linda Gromko, MD*

Communication Modification Very Slightly Demystified—the Art and Science of Your Voice, Vocal Health, and Information on Vocal Surgery

By Sandy Hirsch

Voice therapist, MS, CCC-SLP, founder of Seattle's Give Voice

The Art and Science of Tuning Your Instrument

I have lost count of the number of times that I have heard a transgender or gender diverse person say, "Changing my voice has been the hardest part of my transition." My clients have said with equal frequency, "When I found my voice, I felt like I really found myself."

More people appear to be choosing a goal and identity of living fluidly along the gender spectrum. As they work on a voice that is comfortable along the spectrum of communication, a number of clients have come to discover that they love their voice and do not feel the need or desire to change it. This is particularly true for adolescents but also for young adults.

To this I say, "Hurray!" Voice is personal, both in our heads and spoken to the world. It is important to develop and live one's own truth regardless of what society might want to impose on us. The journey of voice is circuitous and involves a discovery, whether we are seeking a binary perception or one that is more ambiguous. Sorry to say, there are no quick fixes. But with work and appropriate guidance, there are ways to achieve multiple vocal goals.

The Mindset

If anyone tells you, "All you have to do is…," it means that they have already worked hard to get there and don't remember the hard work, or they have been given talent that is rather rare.

As a singer myself, I know that finding your own voice, nurturing it, and fine-tuning it requires courage, attention, and focus as well as regular practice and patience. Our vocal work is the work of motor memory and motor planning as well as training our ears and retraining our communication habits. The work is equally fascinating, boring, frustrating, and exhilarating. At the end of therapy, one client wrote to me: "When my voice started to click, my identity started to click." She worked hard and with intention to come to this realization.

On these pages, I hope to provide the reader with an overview of the art and science of voice, with some ideas to begin the process of modification and sow the seeds for some healthy head-scratching. It is advised that people seek the assistance of an expert voice clinician or coach in order to develop healthy, sustainable approaches based on clinical evidence and vocal science. I will touch on some foundations and a few exercises that can be used by everyone along the gender spectrum as they search for their own voice.

I wish you courage and patience and joy.

Voice in Transition: An Overview

Basic Vocal Terminology

There are three basic legs to the vocal stool when thinking about voice and communication modification:

- **Pitch**
  Pitch is the term we use to describe the high or low of the voice. It is measured in Hertz (Hz) or cycles per second. Vocal fold vibrations occur approximately 90 to 130 times per second (Hz) for the AMAB mature voice in conversation, and approximately 160 to 230 times per second (Hz) for the average AFAB mature voice in conversation. I am a cisgender woman and my average is about 196Hz. Depending on the day, time of day, and a number of environmental, behavioral, and emotional factors, it is sometimes 220Hz-ish.

- **Resonance**
  Resonance is the term we use to describe the tone or color of the voice, just as we might describe the different tones of color in an artist's palette. A single note sounds different when played on different instruments or in a different environment. The human voice also sounds different coming out of various-size heads and bodies as well as different shapes of mouths. No two voices are the same and one should not strive to sound just like someone else. Every resonance is unique.

- **Intonation and inflection**
  Intonation and inflection are synonymous terms that we use to describe the rise and fall of the voice as it pertains to emphasis. There is no gender difference in where we emphasize a word, since this will be determined by the individual message, but the style of emphasis tends to vary across the gender spectrum. This also varies widely across cultures, as might be expected.

In addition to voice, we might also consider other areas of communication such as body language, language use, and overall communication style. Nonspeech tasks such as laughing, coughing, and clearing the throat might also be addressed as necessary.

Science and Art

When we want to speak, a message from the brain goes to our larynx (voice box) for the vocal folds to vibrate. These vibrations travel on our breath up into our mouth where we shape them into speech sounds. It's all physics! The sound that is released from the mouth is known as the acoustic burst. The sound that we hear is a combination of vocal fold vibrations and the acoustics of the speech sounds. The quality of that sound is affected by myriad subtleties unique to each person, as well as the individual harmonics of speech sounds.

Essentially though, how we "play our instrument" is how we affect sound. The physiological gesture gives rise to the acoustic output. And herein lies the art and science of modifying different voices. We cannot yet do a head transplant, so we need to learn to play our individual instrument to align with our goals and personal identity.

Anatomical and Physiological Challenges to the Larynx during Transition: The Basics

Estrogen does not cause a change in the pitch or resonance (tone) of the voice. If an AMAB woman wants to align her voice and communication with her gender identity, she has to learn a specific skill set to change the pitch, brighten the resonance, and perhaps gently modify the inflectional (rise and fall) patterns used when emphasizing words in conversation for a variety of meanings and messages.

Testosterone usually leads to a lowering of pitch due to changes that come about in the mass of vocal folds, and some cartilage growth to the thyroid. We know from research that this can be highly variable. Testosterone does not change the resonance (tone) of the voice. The length and width of the vocal tract do not change. People taking testosterone often benefit from vocal approaches to allow for easy, healthy voicing while developing a rich, dark, round tone.

It is a myth that people on testosterone cannot benefit from voice therapy. Learning healthy vocal approaches early in the stages of hormone replacement therapy can avoid unhealthy practices. Muscle tension and discomfort are common complaints of transgender men seeking voice therapy after some time on testosterone. Come early, ease on in gently!

Some Foundations and Beginning to Play Your Instrument

Vocal Health

An experienced voice clinician or coach will make vocal health of primary concern during a full voice and communication modification program. Adequate hydration, overall health, and easing into voice change without tension and with appropriate respiratory support are all part of a sustainable, healthy approach. The vocal skill set will be built hierarchically and guidance will be given on approaches to maintaining behavioral change. The latter is the most challenging and takes the most patience. The vocal skill set is actually ***not that hard***. Below and on the next couple pages are a few ways to get started in your thinking toward voice change. I have blended approaches for people along the gender spectrum, as you will note.

What Are Some Things I Can Do to Get Started?

- **Pitch**
  Using a pitch tuner to check where you are (try 185Hz, F#3 as a safe starting point), gently hum or chant that pitch every now and again throughout the day. When you feel you can more easily find it, start gently chanting simple, everyday phrases. When that gets easier, chant a phrase and then *say* the phrase normally without chanting. Can you do it and stay vaguely in pitch? Look around you and just describe what you see or say everyday things that you might say at home, work, socially, or randomly to a stranger.

Tip: Put an earbud in and pretend you're talking on the phone; no one will be the wiser! Even if you aren't raising the pitch, gently humming and chanting can help to settle a lowering pitch for those taking testosterone. Relax. And stay hydrated!

- **Resonance**
  We are told to smile when we answer the phone. The shape of a smiling mouth configures the vocal tract to brighten the harmonics of our tone. Try gently smiling when you speak with that higher pitch. Record yourself and compare a smiling sound with a flat-faced sound. It will be brighter, I promise. If you're on testosterone, try rounding or protruding the mouth very slightly while talking. You will notice that the sound is darker and richer. Record, listen, record, listen. Keep doing that until you hear something you like. Relax, and stay hydrated!

- **Inflection**
  Practice changing the way you emphasize a word or phrase. Take "How are you?" Walk up four steps saying it. When you get to "you," get to the top part of the pitch, and then start back down the steps backward for reaching a logical finish in pitch. You can also build inflection with Legos, put tape on a doorframe, and play with feeling for a pitch change incrementally as you tap up or down. What is your learning style? What works best for your brain? Walk it out, build it, tap it up and down, dance it, use a Theraball to bounce it, and throw a ball in the air.

  If you're trying to flatten your inflection in emphasis, try saying everyday phrases with a finite downward motion. When you say "how are you?", instead of a rise and fall on "you," flatten and go down. Walk down the stairs instead of up, tap on the tape down, instead of up. Drop a ball on the ground instead of throwing it up. Hold your arms out straight and drop them to your sides on "you." Use your brilliant imagination! Record, listen, record, listen, keep adjusting. Relax, and stay hydrated!

A Brief Note on Vocal Surgery

Some people choose to have vocal surgery for myriad personal or perhaps logistical reasons. Surgeries so far have been able to address raising the pitch of the voice fairly effectively. The amount of pitch change varies widely and sometimes not at all. For the most positive acoustic outcomes from surgery, pre- and postsurgical voice therapy is recommended. One might compare this to pre- and postsurgical physical therapy for the best outcomes for a hip or knee replacement. Knowledge and preparation go a long way to enhancing results.

Summary

Have fun with your voice work. Remember, voice is an event, not a product. Play with different approaches but don't try to "nail it." You are discovering your sound; you are not going to the voice gym! Relax and stay hydrated. Seek out a voice expert to help you along the way.

Resources

- **Apps**
  Tuna Pitch for iPhone; Pano Tuner or DaTuner for Android; Voice Analyst for both. This is a very affordable good analyst that allows for measuring, saving, parsing sections of a sample, and bracketing pitches. EVA for transgender women; Voice Up for Transgender Women.

- **Software**
  Praat (free), Estill Voice Training (about $50 for PC and Mac) are my favorites but there are others. Audacity Audio Recorder is a great free recording download for Mac and PC. I use this as my recorder for both desktop and laptop computers.

- **Books**
  One Weird Trick: A User's Guide to Transgender Voice, Liz Jackson Hearns and The Voice Lab, Inc., 2018.

  The Voice Book for Trans and Non-Binary People: A Practical Guide to Creating and Sustaining Authentic Voice and Communication, Matthew Mills and Gillie Stoneham, 2017.

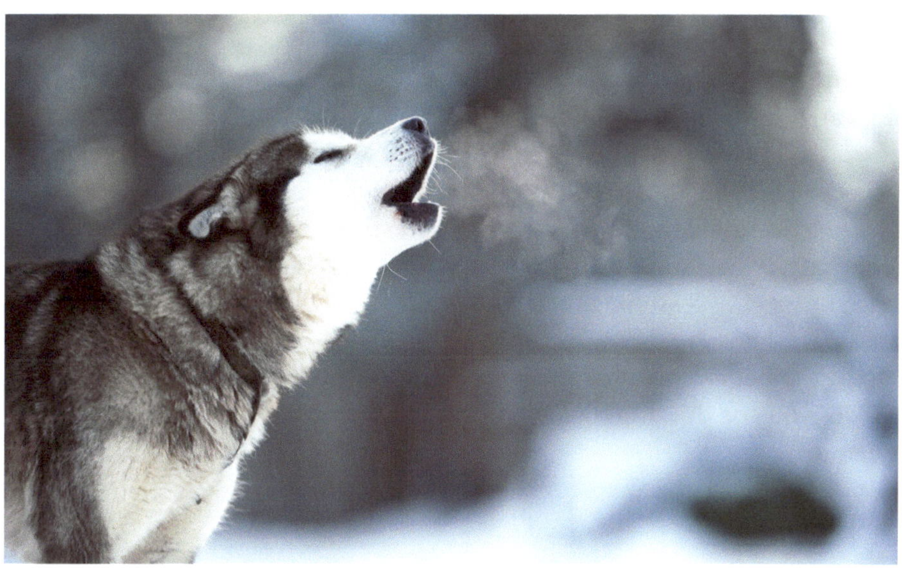

Facial Contouring with Neurotoxins and Dermal Fillers

Many people are aware of neurotoxins and dermal fillers they see advertised to combat the effects of aging. But it has occurred to me and many others that these products can also help you achieve *temporary* facial feminization or masculinization.

Neurotoxins

Neurotoxins like Botox relax treated muscles for about 3 months. They can make you look younger and more feminine. They are most commonly used to treat the following areas:

- **The elevens**
  Wrinkle your forehead like you do when you're angry. You may see two deep vertical grooves (the "elevens") in the middle of your forehead near the inner brows. These develop with repetitive frowning and can make us appear tired, irritated, and older than we are. They develop also with increased computer use and intense concentration. Relax these muscles with injected Botox and your whole face will appear more relaxed—and younger! In people assigned male, facial muscles may be larger and stronger, so you may need more units of Botox if you are a trans woman. The muscles that form the elevens are the corrugator supercilii and the procerus muscles, known together as the glabella. Count on 10 to 40 units to relax these muscles (often 20 units for someone assigned female and 40 for someone assigned male). We generally see results in about a week or less, and the results last for about 3 to 4 months. You'll notice your forehead frowning again when it's time for more Botox.

- **The horizontal wrinkles of the upper forehead**
  These lines emerge due to the movement of the frontalis muscles. Raise your brows to see if yours are prominent. If they are, they can be relaxed with neurotoxins.

- **Crow's feet**
  I prefer the term "laugh lines" for these wrinkles that extend from the outer part of our eyelids. If you don't like them, you can have them relaxed with a neurotoxin.

- **The masseter muscles**
  The masseters are the strong jaw muscles that can make a person look more masculine. Feel yours by placing your fingers over your lower cheeks. Close your mouth and then clench your teeth. The strong muscles you feel are those that help you chew, of course. You can certainly relax these and still eat! But using neurotoxins in the masseters can soften the appearance of a broad jawline. (This is an off-label use for neurotoxins.) And if you have headaches from bruxism (jaw clenching), you may find these headaches lessening too.

Note: If you are noticing the beginning of wrinkles, you can use neurotoxins preventively. You may be able to minimize the wrinkles you see developing in your thirties or forties by using neurotoxins prophylactically (again, a personal decision).

Dermal Fillers

Dermal fillers come in different degrees of viscosity. For example, fillers used over the cheeks are more viscous (thicker), while fillers used in facial lines and lips are less viscous.

I find dermal fillers to be fascinating. Within limits, you can inject volume over the cheekbones to create a much more feminine appearance. You can also inject deeper lines and wrinkles to fill them, although I prefer adding fullness to the cheekbones first. (In our clinic, we use Juvéderm and Voluma, which are both made of hyaluronic acid, a component of your skin already.)

Dermal fillers are used in the following locations:

- **The cheekbones**
  We can add volume to define the cheekbones more clearly. I find that this can be feminizing or masculinizing.

- **The nasolabial folds**
  We can inject filler directly into the nasolabial folds (the lines that run between the edge of the nose and the corner of the mouth) to make these lines appear less prominent.

- **Marionette lines**
  You'd have these vertical lines to move your jaw if you were a puppet, and they can startle you when they show up on *your* drivers' license photo. These are easily addressed with filler, but again, I tend to work on the cheekbones first to create that facial framework. Adding filler can add weight, so we start with small amounts and work up, just like we do with medications.

- **Defining and plumping the lips**
  Lips get thinner as we get older; we can enhance them with filler.

In our practice, we have used dermal fillers in the jaw and brow areas as follows:

- **Defining the angle of the jaw**
  Injecting dermal filler along the visible portion of the mandible (lower jaw) can accentuate it so that it may masculinize its appearance.

- **Defining a brow bone**
  Carefully placed dermal filler can create the appearance of a dominant brow for a trans man (the kind of brow prominence we talk about softening in facial feminization surgery).

Filler prices are set by the syringe—that is, what product is used and how many syringes are used? It is not uncommon to start with a single syringe and divide it between the two sides of the face. We can start with a single syringe, knowing that we are likely to need two or three syringes to create the desired effect. Fillers last anywhere from 6 to about 18 months, depending on the product and your body. Be sure to take before-and-after photos so you can appreciate the differences.

What Could Possibly Go Wrong?

Like anything in medicine, if your provider tells you that neurotoxins and fillers have no possible risk, run away and find a new provider! Read the consent form that you are required to sign. Here are some possibilities to be aware of:

- You may not like the result and even though the changes brought about by neurotoxins or fillers are *not* permanent, you may feel unhappy until the products run their time course. (Naturally, talk with your provider; some posttreatment modifications are possible.)
- Even in the best of hands, you may have an undesired cosmetic outcome. A neurotoxin, for example, can temporarily lower one of your brows, making you look asymmetrical. While it's often correctable and always temporary, we're talking about your face!
- You may have an allergic reaction to a product.
- An injector may inadvertently block the flow of a facial blood vessel. We haven't seen this in our practice, and we take specific measures to avoid it. But it can happen and if it does, it can lead to serious problems—even vision loss and permanent tissue injury.

So, do your homework. Research the products and providers you are considering. And think twice about rushing to take advantage of an amazing bargain coupon from a provider you don't know and trust.

Coolsculpting Can Help Contour Your "Areas of Opportunity"

Coolsculpting is a form of cryolipolysis, and we offer it in our practice. With Coolsculpting, a technician or ARNP applies controlled cooling to a portion of tissue. Popular treatment areas include the upper or lower abdomen, flanks, back, upper arms, chin, three separate areas of the thighs, and the "bra fat" region. Each treatment takes approximately 35 minutes per area, although this can vary. (Treatments are done to the subcutaneous fat only—that is, the "pinchable" fat, not the firmer visceral fat deep in the abdomen.)

It's an ingenious concept: By freezing an area of tissue, we begin a process of apoptosis (programmed cell death). Over the next 3 months, about one-fourth of the fat cells in the treated area die and are eliminated from the body. It's not a diet, where fat cells shrink as we lose weight and enlarge as we gain. When mature fat cells leave the body, they are gone for good. (There are laser approaches to fat cell elimination as well.)

It struck me that we could help feminize or masculinize clients according to their gender goals. We can shape a waistline, for example, in a trans woman wishing to feminize. Or, we can accentuate a triangular torso in a trans man by shaping his flanks. And we can improve the appearance of a double chin, which can help anyone feel more confident about the appearance of the face.

I would never advise clients that Coolsculpting is a substitute for weight loss achieved by good nutrition and fitness. It's not a *weight loss* technique at all. Nor is it equivalent to surgical liposuction! But,

Coolsculpting can help move the needle closer to a person's goals without significant downtime or recovery time. (I'll address surgical body contouring in Chapter 11.)

Hairstyles and Hair Loss

You'll want to consult a trans-friendly hair stylist who can help you with more advanced issues like color and volume. But here are some easy tricks that don't cost anything:

- **Grow your hair longer.**
  Longer hair is generally read as being more feminine and you can cut it if you don't like it.

- **Grow out your bangs.**
  Bangs can hide a high forehead, prominent brow bones, or a receding hairline at the temples. If you don't like the bangs, they'll grow out, although it will seem like forever. (I had one client who said it was either bangs or Botox for concealing her forehead wrinkles; the bangs won out and were certainly less costly.)

- **Part your hair in a way that hides a receding hairline.**
  Parting your hair slightly on one side may conceal a thinning hairline. Try parting your hair in several different ways to discover how best to conceal areas of hair loss.

- **Conceal thinning hair with makeup products.**
  Look for scalp powders that help conceal a widening part. Joan Rivers Great Hair Day is a powder that fills in thinning areas. Toppik is a spray-on product containing static-charged keratin protein fibers that bond to existing hairs and help "fill in the blanks."

- **Talk with your healthcare provider about medications and products that can help slow hair loss.**

  - **Finasteride**
    This is a testosterone blocker that works specifically on the skin and hair. It's a prescription oral medication taken daily and does not impact other testosterone products you may be taking.

  - **Minoxidil**
    This represents one of my favorite stories of medical serendipity. People who were taking minoxidil for high blood pressure were found to be growing new scalp hair where they'd previously lost it. Now it's available over the counter everywhere as Rogaine. Consider the Extra Strength formulation. (**Note:** The generic brands are every bit as effective as Rogaine and a lot cheaper.)

  - **Laser caps**
    These resemble baseball caps, can be purchased online, and are proven to increase growth.

- **Consult a hair transplant physician.**

  - **Hair transplants have evolved tremendously over the years.**
    These days, instead of transplanting large plugs of hair, the surgeon transplants very small, individual follicular units of one to three hairs each. Hair is harvested from the middle section of the back of the scalp and implanted where needed, following the direction and flow of your own hair. The results are very realistic and natural in appearance, especially when compared to the dreaded "doll-hair" effect seen with older hair-restoration techniques.

- **A hair transplant surgeon can advise on treatments that stimulate hair growth.**
  For instance, platelet-rich plasma (PRP) can be taken from your own blood and given by injections directly in the scalp. (See Dr. Robert Niedbalski's website at **hairreplacementsurgeon.com**.)

- **Consult a surgeon who does facial feminization surgery.**
  This topic will be covered in detail in a later chapter, but you may want to consider a scalp advance. In this procedure, the hairline is brought forward, creating a more feminine hairline.

- **Try wigs and hairpieces.**
  If you have already lost so much hair in your younger days that a scalp advance or transplant won't support the style you want, you may want to research wigs or hairpieces. Seattle's William Collier (**williamcollierdesign.com**) has worked with the transgender community for decades. Specializing in alopecia and hormone-related hair loss, Mr. Collier can design and fit you with any number of products. These range from synthetic hair wigs, which may start at around \$300 to virgin hair from Asia or Europe, which may cost \$4,000 to \$6,000. (Virgin means that the hair has had no prior coloring or permanents.)

  In either case, a client is fit according to their head shape and size, and the wig is colored and styled according to the client's desires. Mr. Collier offers complimentary 1-hour consultations and Skype consultations. Clients receive detailed training on how to care for their wigs or hairpieces.

Because hair loss issues are so common in trans women, you are likely to find a resource in many larger cities. (Search the Internet for "wigs for transgender women" and you are likely to find a trans-welcoming provider.)

One Woman's Account of Her Hair Transplant Surgery

I work as an electrician and am transitioning to female. I want to get facial feminization surgery but decided to start with a hair transplant. I have always worried about my hair. My dad lost all his hair at 18. Finasteride and Rogaine have helped me, but I really wanted to take care of it for good.

The transplant was expensive! It was \$14,000 in total. I put \$4,000 down and paid the rest \$1,000 at a time. It was totally worth it.

The procedure took a whole day, starting at seven in the morning. The doctor numbed my scalp, and it didn't hurt after that. He took a strip of my scalp from the back of my head and several technicians separated the hair into two and three follicle parts that were placed in the front of my scalp.

At first, the transplanted hairs fell out—they're supposed to. And I knew that, but it was still a little unnerving at first. It's been 6 or 7 months now and the front hair is over an inch and a half long. It blends in with my other hair, and nobody misgenders me anymore. My hormone doctor says I barely need facial feminization surgery now. I am very happy I did this.

— Trans woman, age 35

Nonsurgical Breast Enhancement

Breast development varies widely in *all* women, cis *and* trans. When they take estrogen, most trans women can expect to see maximal development by about 3 years. Sometimes, we see an acceleration of growth when progesterone is added. Now and then, there's a surge of growth after vaginoplasty (removal of the testicles and creation of a vagina) or orchiectomy (removal of the testicles alone).

How much breast development anyone has depends largely on their genetic constitution. If your relatives who were assigned female at birth are large-breasted, you may grow larger breasts too. If you want breasts that are larger than double-Ds, start looking for your breast surgeon now. In the meantime, here are some helpful ideas:

- **Get an in-person bra fitting.**
  Lingerie departments in larger retailers such as Nordstrom will have salespeople who can do a proper bra fitting for you. At Nordstrom, for example, you'll go into very private dressing rooms where your chest wall measurements are taken under the breasts and at your nipple level. A good bra fitter will consider your breast shape as well. Many trans women have broader shoulders, a factor that's considered when finding the best bra design and fit possible.

  I've heard of only positive experiences at Nordstrom and Macy's. But if you're shy, go at an "off time" when there are fewer shoppers or make an appointment. Zovo Lingerie (**zovolingerie.com**) in Seattle's University Village carries an enormous size range and also gets great reviews from trans women. And research the trans-friendly clothing and fitting options in your area online by searching on "clothing for trans women in my area."

  The Pencil Test (**thepenciltest.com**) is a bra store with locations in Portland, Oregon, and Renton, Washington. They feature bras for larger women (28 to 46, D to K) and offer excellent in-person fittings. (What is the pencil test? It's said that if you can place the stick of a pencil (not the point) under the breast in the inframammary fold without the pencil falling out, it's time to wear a bra!) Many transgender women have large chest wall measurements; we've heard good feedback about this resource.

More Information about Bra Sizing from an Expert

A B cup means (broadly) that there is a 2-inch difference between the under-bust or chest wall measurement and the over-bust measurement taken at the nipple line.

D and DD cups have a 4-inch and 5-inch difference, respectively, between the chest wall and the largest measurement. It is very common in our experience for a trans woman who has been on at least a few months of hormonal therapy to fit into a D or DD cup.

Because bra design is so variable, we think it's important to offer a variety of brands and not limit the selection to a single store brand.

— Holly Powell, founder, The Pencil Test

> Being a plus-size person, I want to look in proportion. I have a natural size 50D, but I still look small in my opinion. I met a wonderful salesperson from the Breast Form Store (thebreastformstore.com) in Vancouver, British Columbia. She was able to assist me in finding the right size form to help me look better. They have both nonstick and stick-on forms in a variety of sizes. My salesperson was very nice and very experienced in helping transgender ladies.
>
> — *F. W., trans woman, age 50*

- **Wear padded bras.**
  Women have always augmented their breast size with padding—even facial tissue or socks. You'll find padding designed into many bras. Padding and good bra design can add at least a cup size to what you already have.

- **Wear breast forms.**
  Breast forms are used by women who have had breast cancer surgery. These soft forms slip into pockets in specially designed prosthesis bras. You can find these at all major department stores. Nordstrom saleswomen have told me they can have a breast form pocket sewn into any bra. You can also buy breast forms online through the American Cancer Society's TLC (Tender Loving Care) Organization at tlcdirect.org. You'll find wigs there also, as they serve women who have had chemotherapy for breast cancer.

  You may find breast forms at fabric stores, and Amazon carries an impressive selection. Nordstrom also carries an insert that you tuck in your bra but under your breasts to create more uplift.

- **Use "chicken cutlets."**
  These breast forms are realistic in their texture and slip into bras to give you more fullness. You can buy them with or without nipples and in a variety of sizes and colors.

- **Look at Knitted Knockers.**
  Barbara, a cis woman in Bellingham, Washington, was heading back to work after a mastectomy for breast cancer. From a medical standpoint, it was too early for her to wear a prosthesis. Her surgeon, recognizing her distress, gave her a pattern to create a knitted breast prosthesis. Since then, she has created a nationwide network of breast cancer survivors who get together and knit "knockers" in all colors and sizes for others in similar situations. You can buy these on Etsy but check out knittedknockers.org for more information and an inspirational story.

Shapewear

The Basics

Perhaps you are too young to remember girdles. People wore them to hold in the stomach area and smooth out the hips. Today we have shapewear. Made of snug-fitting Spandex, shapewear garments can hold in a stomach pooch, smooth out muffin tops, and generally make you look better in clothing. (These products don't help us one bit, though, when we're naked.) Shapewear comes in all varieties, including garments that slim from the waist to the ankles and even long-sleeved pieces that lend a firmer look to the upper arms. You can also find shapewear that adds curves to your hips and buttocks.

Higher-end stores feature more expensive products, but you can find bargains if you look. For example, did you know that Spanx and Assets shapewear garments are both designed by Spanx founder Sara Blakely? You'll find Spanx at Nordstrom and Assets at Target, and they're very similar except in price. Zulily often features reduced-price Spanx and other shapewear products also (zulily.com).

> I have found for myself that a panty girdle is enough to give concealment. But a new line that I have found is from an online company called Shapermint. My favorite product is the Empetua All Day Shaper Panty. It comes in black and taupe in sizes up to 4XL. The other item I have used from them is the Empetua High-Waisted Shaper Short; they are cut a little lower on the thigh. To find them, just go to shapermint.com. At the time of my purchase, they used the code "IAMAWESOME" to save 20 percent. I liked that attitude!
>
> —*F. W., trans woman, age 50*

Tucking and Wearing Gaffs

You may know that the testicles and often the penis will shrink during estrogen treatment. Still, many trans women wish to conceal the contours of the genitals even more. Do you remember from Figure 5.1 on page 29 how the testicles in the embryo first resided in the lower abdomen, later descending into the scrotal sac by way of the inguinal canals in the groin? Particularly as the testicles shrink, they can be carefully tucked back up into the inguinal canals. Women who "tuck" their testicles may also pull the penis downward to create a more feminine contour.

A gaff is genital-concealing padding, often incorporated into a pair of panties. You can get gaff panties with padding over the front of the penis and scrotum. You can order gaff panties with padded buttocks and a range of other features.

Naturally, don't tuck or use a gaff if it hurts or bothers you in any way. Clients ask me if tucking reduces the tissue that is later used to create a new vagina in vaginoplasty. I haven't read or seen any information that convinces me that it does. Certainly, shrinking testicles distend the scrotum less, but I would relate this more to hormone use than to tucking. Since so many trans women tuck, I would imagine we'd be seeing more adverse effects if it was a harmful practice.

Use good common sense. Be rest assured that if you are planning to have a vaginoplasty and you have a smaller penis and scrotum, a surgeon can graft penile and scrotal skin together to create more vaginal depth. Sometimes, a graft is taken from other areas such as the waist, where scars blend into a person's skin lines over time. And new surgical techniques have emerged that use peritoneal or colon tissue to create the vaginal vault (see Chapter 11).

Clothing Choices That Feminize

This aspect of presentation could fill an entire book, but, for our purposes, we'll focus on general principles. As always, check in on the following:

- **What is the desired goal that you want to achieve?**
  Have you heard the expression, "blendable is dependable?" This expression alludes to the fact that you're less likely to stand out if you wear what other women in your environment are wearing. That's not exactly fashion forward! But, do think about what *you* want to project. If you *want* to be noticed, disregard the blendable bit.

- **Does your look and clothing convey something about you that makes you uncomfortable?**
  An important part of fashion seems to be wearing what's appropriate in a particular setting. Deep cleavage won't play well in a business meeting. You may find your business associates staring at your chest rather than listening to your ideas. Baby-doll ruffles and frills might work for you in certain intimate settings, but they're inappropriate at work if you want to be taken seriously.

  If you have any doubts about what you're projecting, make a free appointment with a personal stylist at Nordstrom or other higher-end store. Clothing selection is particularly important if you require a career wardrobe. These personal stylists are familiar with what is considered appropriate in your geographical area and within your business or professional culture. There's no fee; personal shoppers hope you will buy clothing, of course. But you can save money by avoiding costly mistakes.

- **What are factors about your body that you'd like to emphasize?**
  You've probably identified facial and body features on yourself that you like. Emphasize them. You will often be advised to draw the eye up toward your face and eyes. If you like scarves or jewelry, experiment. Perhaps you'd like to accentuate a small waist. Go back to the shapewear department for a garment that smoothes out your belly (and can add a little padding to your hips and butt if you want that). Belts can emphasize a small waist, but they can also create the *illusion* of a small waist, particularly if a sweater or shawl conceals your actual perimeter.

- **What would you like to minimize?**
  There are many tricks to minimize what you may perceive as problem areas! Broad shoulders? De-emphasize them with raglan sleeves or dropped shoulders.

  Do your hands seem large? Keep your nail polish subtle and your jewelry proportionate to your size. (By this, I mean that tiny delicate rings may get lost on larger hands. On the other hand, bright acrylic nails and large rings on every finger with make your hands even more obvious. Many women try to find a middle ground.) And, perhaps in the not-so-distant future, you can change the appearance of your hands through surgery![35]

35 Jasmine Lee et al., "A Review of Hand Feminization and Masculinization Techniques in Gender Affirming Therapy," *Aesthetic Plastic Surgery* 45, no. 2 (April 2021): 589–601, https://doi.org/10.1007/s00266-020-01963-0.

Transgender women have a greater risk of being the victim of a personally violent crime than do cis women. We all know that sexual assault is an expression of anger and power and is not considered a "sexual" act at all. We also know that every human is responsible for their own behavior.

The clothing a person wears *never* justifies being assaulted by another person. Nonetheless, when making your clothing choices, make sure you can get out of harm's way quickly when you need to. Stiletto heels and pencil skirts may be fashionable but may not allow you to get out of an assailant's way fast enough.

— Linda Gromko, MD

Where to Shop for Clothing

Nordstrom (nordstrom.com) is trans-friendly and they have lower-priced **Nordstrom Rack** stores that are wonderful for shapewear, accessories, and lingerie. **Macy's** (macys.com), **Old Navy** (oldnavy.com), and **Land's End** (landsend.com) offer a range of casual and work apparel in large and tall sizes.

Seattle's **Yazdi** (yazdiseattle.com) carries comfortable natural-fiber clothing with an exotic flair. Their adjoining **Yazdi II** caters to plus-size women. And you'll find bold statement accessories from around the world with reasonable prices and great sales.

Searching the Internet for "clothing for tall women," you'll find that **Long Tall Sally** (longtallsally.com) carries a range of styles, with jeans up to a 38-inch leg length and shoes up to size 15. Try stores for larger women like **Lane Bryant** (lanebryant.com) or **Torrid** (torrid.com).

Chico's, with its forgiving elastic waists and easy-care fabrics, has expanded its size range and offers diverse styles and colors (chicos.com). Don't forget about **Recreational Equipment Inc.** (**REI** at rei.com) for casual and outdoor clothing.

QVC and **HSN** (the TV shopping channels) carry many items in tall sizes, including up to 5X.

Many people in Seattle shop at thrift stores like Goodwill or Value Village and at vintage clothing and consignment shops. Try shopping at an online consignment dealer like **ThredUP** (thredup.com). Higher-end, online consignment retailers include **Poshmark** (poshmark.com) and the **RealReal** for designer clothing (therealreal.com). In a consignment store, you won't find many of the same garments, but you can find true one-of-a-kind treasures.

Shopping for Shoes

Trans women in my practice have consistently endorsed **Wide Shoes Only**, located in Edmonds and Renton, Washington, with an online presence at wideshoesonly.net.

Long Tall Sally (longtallsally.com) offers longer, wider shoes from sizes 9.5 to 15 (roughly equal to men's sizes 8 to 13.5). **Avenue** (avenue.com) has been reported to be a good source with reasonable prices for shoes.

Poshmark and the **RealReal** are high-end online consignment stores that also carry shoes. **Nordstrom** and **Macy's** and many of the stores listed in the clothing section carry shoes, although perhaps not with the same size range.

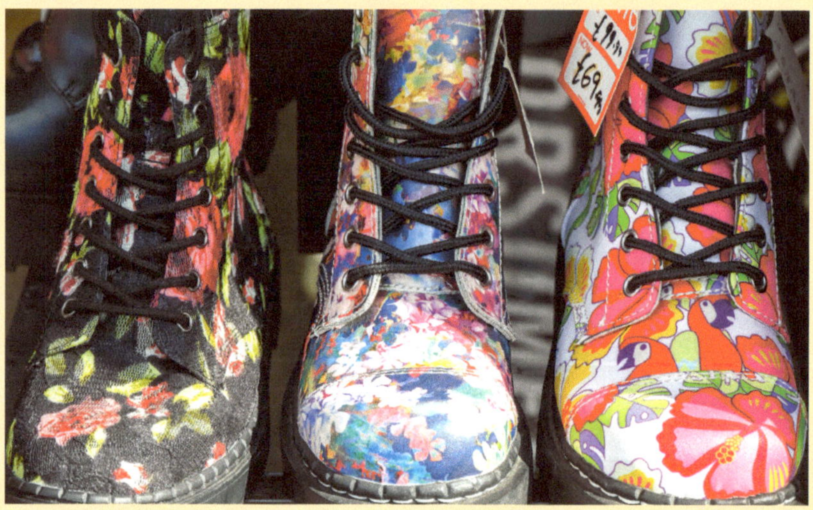

I used to feel uncomfortable shopping in stores for femme clothes. But it's always *someone's* birthday or there's a holiday to shop for. I can't tell you how many times I have been in a store in "male mode" buying a birthday gift—for me!

— *F. W., trans woman, age 50*

Image Makeovers

Head-to-toe makeovers by a consultant who is conversant with transgender concerns do exist. Search YouTube (youtube.com). Seattle trans women have benefited from the makeup lessons and professional application of Carla Petrulli (seattlemakeupartist.com).

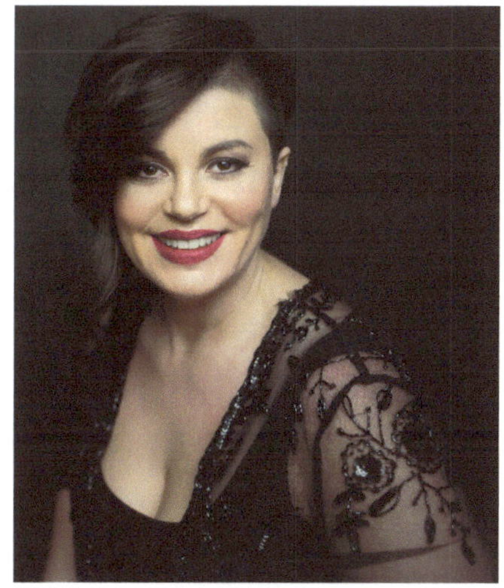

Photographer Erica Sciarretta

Carla can feminize or masculinize a face with extraordinary skill; explore her website for beautiful and honoring transformations. (Please see my interview with Carla on pages 134–136.) Carla works with photographer Erica Sciarretta (sorellaphotos.com) to help trans women assemble professional portraits and personal branding packages. Gorgeous makeup and supportive photography sessions enable women to see themselves as never before. Said one client, "It was more valuable to me than a thousand hours of therapy!"

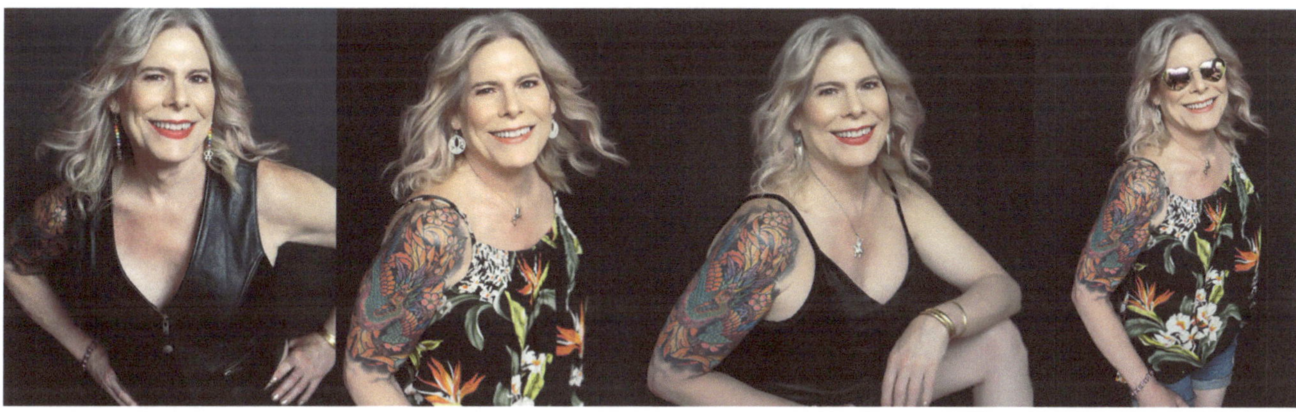

Figure 8.2. Image makeovers. ***Rachel after***

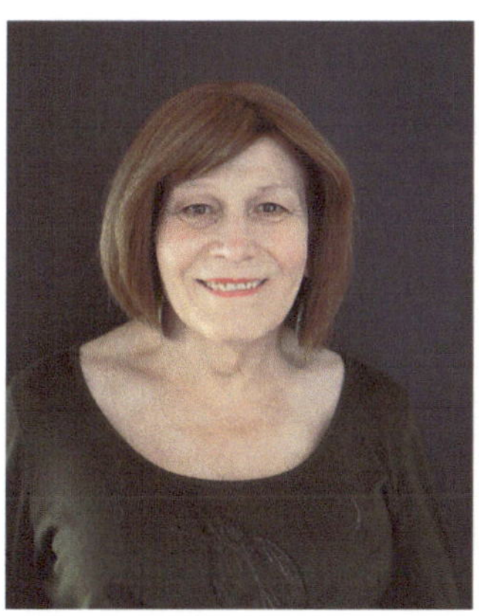

Jenny Robinson before

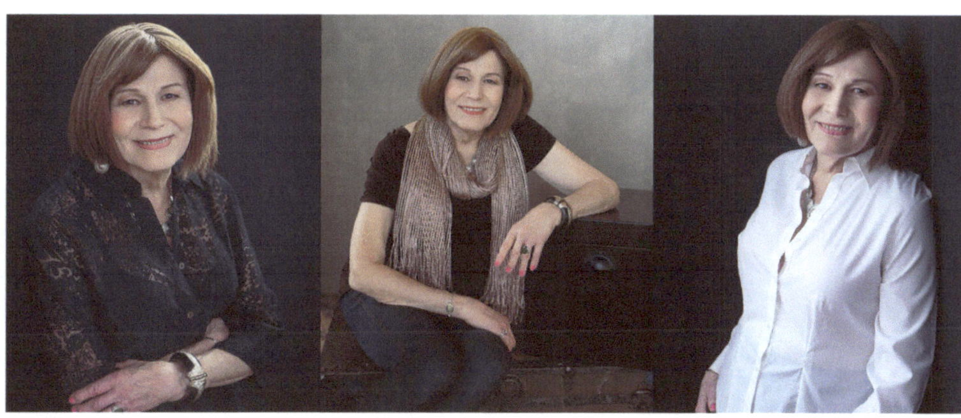

Jenny Robinson after

An Interview with Fashion and Makeup Artist Carla Petrulli

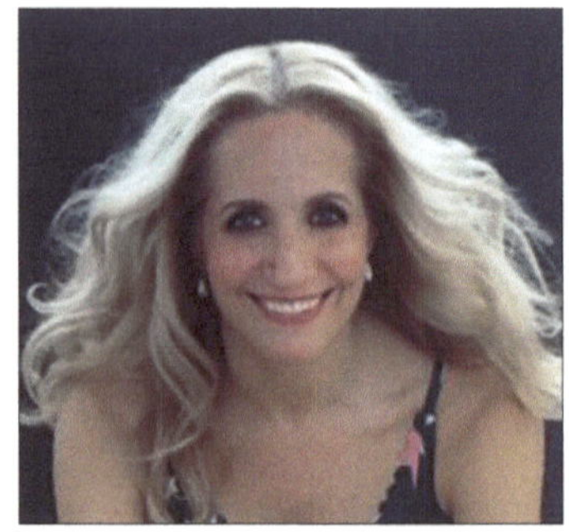

Carla Petrulli

Let me introduce Seattle's expert consultant: Carla Petrulli (**seattlemakeupartist.com**). Carla offers independent personal shopping and teaches makeup lessons to cis and trans women.

Here's our interview:

Linda: Tell me about your background and services.

Carla: I provide makeup lessons and services, plus personal shopping, styling, and even life coaching. A makeup artist for 12 years, I spent 4.5 years on staff with MAC Cosmetics. This gave me exposure to the most diverse clients and types of makeup I had ever experienced. Combined with being a graduate of the Landmark Forum, I am able to be with and hold the concerns of anyone, making space for their truest selves to show up.

I also have a degree in fashion design and over 20 years of experience in jewelry, apparel, and shoes for companies such as Nordstrom and PUMA. I have an innate ability to build an entire look or wardrobe from very little information. Someone can show me a lipstick, or an earring, or a shoe, and I can build an entire look for them just on that. This becomes very important in the styling consultation process, where I ask my clients to create a Pinterest or inspiration board. I think my clients find my background of experience valuable because it allows me to discuss their appearance goals and concerns from several points of view.

Linda: How do you approach a transgender woman when she asks for your advice as a personal shopper?

Carla: When transgender women ask me about personal shopping, I establish some baseline information. I ask about their wardrobe goals, what items they may already own that will be useful to keep, what their top concerns and priorities are, and if they are comfortable to go out shopping or prefer to shop online.

Linda: How do you conceal body areas that may stand out, such as broad shoulders, relatively small butt, tracheal cartilage (Adam's apple), large hands or feet, dominant brow bone, and receding hairline?

Carla: While I work with trans women in all stages of transition, there is a common conversation among most of them about their "structure." Your structure is your frame, including your height and hand and foot sizes, and there's only so much you can do about it. These are all physical attributes that I direct clients on how to soften and minimize—for example, by wearing flat shoes instead of heels, accessorizing their hands with pretty jewelry they like, and having manicured nails in light colors.

Facial and tracheal reconstructive surgeries and breast augmentation are also becoming more common, and I work with my clients based on where they are at a given moment, while also considering where they are headed. If their Adam's apple is still intact, or they have scarring from removal, I like to use scarves and higher necklines. If a client has a small rear end, a belt can help to shape their waist and add more curves.

It's also the case, no matter where a trans woman is in her transition, that accessories *always* personalize their look, making it individualized and memorable. This can include a great pair of boots, a quality handbag, sunglasses, jewelry, belts, and hats. Accessories and a lot of makeup are like my secret magic; they serve to bring certain features forward and minimize others.

For those clients who have not had facial reconstructive surgery, or who may have thin or receding hair, I also provide wig shopping and styling. Sometimes a great solution to a dominant brow bone or patchy hairline can be a wig with bangs in a hue close to their natural color. In makeup lessons, I also discuss how to shape brows to best frame their face and techniques of highlight and contour that can additionally support feminization.

Linda: How do you accent areas that women like?

Carla: When I first meet and work with a trans woman, I find out what's important to her and who or what inspires her. Knowing a bit about her informs what she values, what she loves about herself, and admires in others. When what she wears is grounded in what she loves and values, she will inspire herself and others.

This can look like anything and everything; if she loves her legs, we can focus on skirts, hosiery, and pretty shoes; if she loves her eye color, we will focus on colors in clothing and makeup that make her eyes look bright; if she loves a sense of humor or irony, we can mix funny T-shirts with classic wardrobe pieces and quirky accessories.

The list is endless, and no two women are the same in what they want to accent.

Linda: Are there certain "go-to" recommendations you have that never seem to fail?

Carla: My go-to recommendations that have every woman looking great are to focus on quality skincare, a great haircut or wig that compliments her face shape, and lots of accessories that she can use interchangeably with many outfits.

Linda: Are there things that just don't work to the point that you steer your clients away from them?

Carla: I have very few rules. I style-step with each client to find what is most flattering on them. With that said, I do steer clients away from skirts and dresses that are too short for them mostly because it makes them look like they're trying too hard. I also encourage everyone to go lighter with their eyebrows and hair color as they add more birthdays, because then they look more youthful.

Linda: What stores do you like for finding things that work best for trans women?

Carla: Where I take clients to shop has a lot to do with their budget and wardrobe goals. However, I find that we visit stores with a range of prices and selections. I love both Nordstrom and Nordstrom Rack. In either store, I can work with clients independently and also get personal attention and service if we need it. Both stores also offer alterations, which can be very helpful. I also like stores that have unisex fitting rooms, such as J. Crew, Old Navy, Forever 21, thrift and secondhand stores, and vintage boutiques.

Linda: Are there any things to avoid in working with trans women? Any things that help most?

Carla: Everyone wants to feel heard. I listen for what my clients say and what they don't say, and I reflect them back to make sure I understand correctly. When they work with me, I'm there not only to support my clients but also to challenge them. They don't need me to show them what they already know how to do. As such, I ask all my clients to keep an open mind and try things on that they wouldn't normally pick up. Creating a new wardrobe is like writing a new paragraph about your life, and it deserves time, attention, and detail.

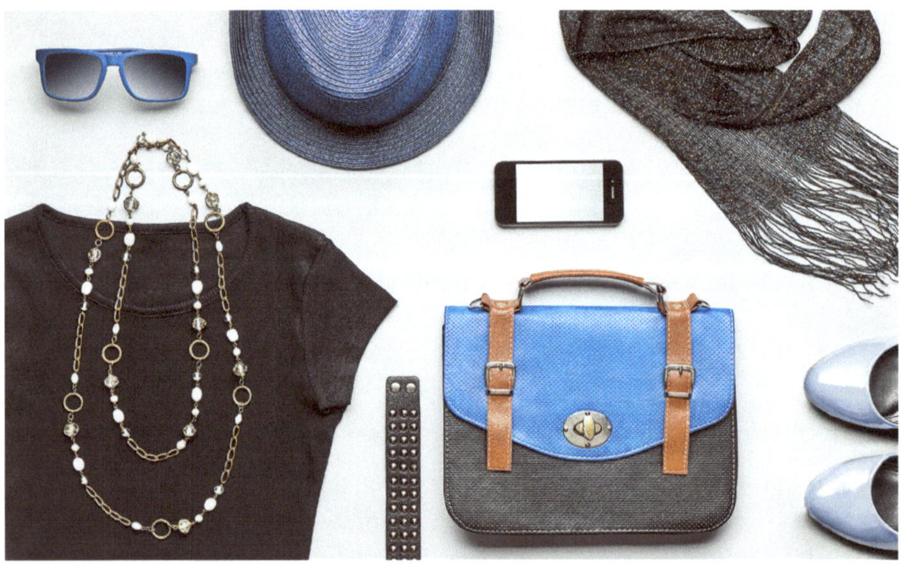

Finding High-End Clothing for an Important Occasion: An Interview with Personal Stylist Amy White

I learned about Amy E. White when Samantha, a friend of mine who is a trans woman, was looking for a suit for a job interview. Samantha was interviewing for a position in executive security, so the suit had to be businesslike, but it also had to be roomy enough to hide a concealed firearm.

Samantha had been ignored by several salespeople in a different store, but while browsing at one high-end Seattle retailer, personal stylist Amy White introduced herself and explained how she might help.

Amy and Samantha worked together for several appointments of shopping and tailoring; the result was a fabulous black suit (jacket and trousers) and a fitted, button-down white blouse. The suit will take Samantha anywhere, both to formal and less formal events, and it is truly elegant.

The most notable part of the visit for Samantha was reflected in her comments: "I *love* the suit. I loved the whole experience. Amy made me feel like every other woman. I didn't feel like I was being treated differently."

So I contacted Amy White and she agreed to be interviewed. It turned out that I had met Amy years before when she managed fundraising and direct services for a YMCA youth program. In the interview that follows, Amy provided very specific information for trans women seeking higher-end clothing.

Linda: How did you go from fundraising to being a personal stylist?

Amy: I have always loved fashion for as long as I can remember. I love working with women like Samantha, and I'm so glad she had a good experience. I started working in handbags and moved to a couple of other departments. But with personal clients, we shop throughout the store.

Linda: How do you assess what would work for a particular client?

Amy: I try to get to know them first. I usually meet them to have coffee, like we're doing now. I ask what they're looking for, of course. Is there a special event you're shopping for? We see a lot of women who are undergoing life changes: weight loss or gain, relationship changes, depression, maybe plastic surgery, births, deaths. There can be tears in the dressing room, both joy and sadness. It's very personal.

We have an intake session and an online questionnaire. I try to find out what people do, where they live, and what their goals might be. I like to include a bra fitting if it's been more than a year since they've had one.

I get an idea of which colors a woman likes and which colors she avoids. I ask, "Who are your fashion icons?" And of course, what is the budget? A woman doesn't have to buy anything; I look at this as starting a relationship.

Linda: What tricks do you use to camouflage broad shoulders?

Amy: I tend to avoid shoulder detailing and set-in sleeves. If sleeves are set-in, they have to be dead-on to look nice. Drop-shoulder tops and raglan sleeves work well. I also find that the right neckline can bring the eye in toward a woman's center. A deep V-neck is great because it draws the eye downward and away from shoulders. Scoop necklines and boatneck shirts work well. A dark top with a lighter bottom can camouflage broad shoulders.

Linda: What helps in women with smaller hips or butts?

Amy: I like to use three types of skirts: a "skater" skirt, an A-line, or a "fit-and-flare" design. All of these flare out and "flow" more. You can find these styles in dresses too, of course. With pants, I avoid tapered pants and stick to full-length or straight pants. Boot cuts work well with jeans.

Linda: What are your go-to recommendations for a business suit or a job interview outfit? And how much would a woman spend for a high-end suit?

Amy: The brands I reach for are Hugo Boss, Akris, and Lafayette 148 New York. These are beautiful. It's hard to spend less than $1,000—that is, year-round. You can find things for less, depending on the season. I usually look for tailored blouses, but some women prefer a sleeveless shell, or a patterned blouse, or even a delicate sweater under a jacket.

Most of the suits I go to are constructed to be tailored. For example, if a trouser is made of four separate panels, you can tailor a pant to go a full inch larger. When sleeves have to be lengthened, that is often done from the shoulder; the shoulder needs to be redone. So, it's important to figure in tailoring costs. All of these suits will need to be dry-cleaned, so that is an extra expense. But when something is so beautiful and it fits perfectly, you never go back! By the way, these garments can be tailored here at the store for the life of the garment.

Linda: How do you arrange for tailoring?

Amy: We do it in the store. For Samantha, I spoke to the tailor first, just to make sure that the tailor understood Samantha's needs.

Linda: I do that too. If I have a trans client who needs to see a specialist, for example, I'll be certain the specialist is trans-friendly. Cultural competence makes a difference. How does your sizing work?

Amy: We have petite through plus sizes. Size inclusion is very important to me. All women can look beautiful in clothing that fits them well.

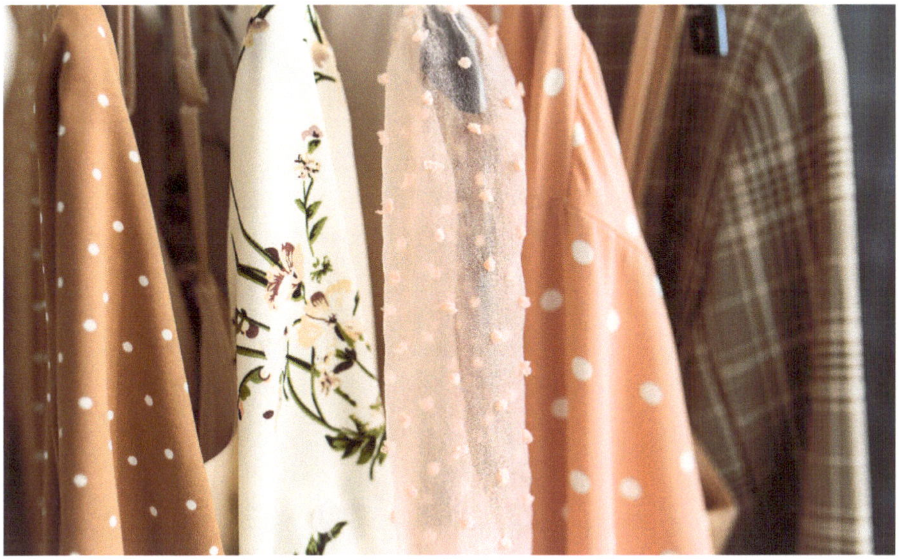

Linda: Do you have any tips for accessory choices?

Amy: For necklaces, I like anything that is long and draws the eye downward. I like longer earrings for that reason. I don't tend to belt jackets much. Jewelry is so individual. Some of the art museum gift shops have very unique pieces.

Linda: What do you think is most important in working with transgender women?

Amy: It is so important to establish a connection with any client. To gain confidence and trust. You and I do similar work. You establish a connection and trust and know medicine; I gain confidence and trust and know fashion! It's very personal work.

Joanna's Story

by Joanna Watson

Hello, I'm Joanna Watson and I'm a 41-year-old transgender girl, originally from Michigan. I began transitioning at 37 after finally looking up "transgender" and discovering why I've always felt different all my life. I moved to Seattle after being a cross-country truck driver for over 9 years, in hopes of helping others within the local trans community. I've also been writing my story, since I have a different perspective than most. I also support local businesses and make donations to food banks and homeless shelters whenever I can. In this essay, I would like to briefly touch on a few of the most common issues.

What Defines You?

In my experience, many trans people fall into the trap of thinking they that they are defined by their gender. But that's only one piece of the large puzzle that is you! Who are you outside of gender? I touch on this because many trans people focus on it so much as to go to one extreme or the other on the gender spectrum. Insecurity tells them they aren't feminine or masculine enough. But sadly, at such extremes, they aren't being true to themselves and are left wondering why they still aren't happy.

Everybody is their own unique mixture. I know it's difficult to think of ourselves outside of gender, but the important thing is that you do what makes you happy. Be the best version of yourself that you can be. Be true to yourself, asking what you need or want. When you do this, the gender part sorts itself out. You know who you are and that is what's most important. If you don't know who you are, it will come in time with patience and self-love.

Let Your Voice Be Heard

One of the biggest obstacles of transitioning is changing one's voice. There are a couple of different surgeries you could undergo to shorten your vocal cords, each with their own pros and cons. Or you could see a speech pathologist for vocal training. The route I chose was to do my own vocal training. I observed cisgender women and adopted speech patterns that I like. I sang along to music by female singers, trying to match their patterns and pitches, being careful to not overdo it. (This method should be used with caution; you don't want to cause permanent damage to your vocal cords.)

If you experience pain or discomfort, give yourself a break. Lower your volume as you raise or lower your pitch outside your usual range. Drink plenty of water and do breathing exercises, breathing from your diaphragm. Try to avoid using throat lozenges, especially in excess. Excessive use of lozenges will have a laxative affect. If you're a trans girl, practice speaking in softer tones and don't be afraid to ask friends how your voice sounds along the way. Be patient with yourself. The changes won't happen overnight, but you can do it with enough perseverance. Eventually, speaking in your new voice will become habit! It will, however, sound different if played back in a recording or heard over a loudspeaker.

This is because when you speak, the acoustics in the skull lower the frequency of the sound waves in your voice, so you perceive your voice as being deeper—which can be troubling for everybody, including cisgender people.

The recorded version of your voice is how you really sound to everyone else. You may cringe at this but it's okay; you're just not used to it. If your friends say you sound feminine or masculine or that you have a nice voice, trust them! They can be a great barometer for how you're doing on your journey! I've been working on mine on and off for 2 years and still cringe when I hear it played back, no matter how many times I'm told that I sound feminine. But this is normal.

When You've Got to Go

Public restroom visits can be unpleasant. Many of us just use the one that best matches how others see us rather than the one that fits our gender. I've gotten dirty looks in the women's room, then reverted back to the men's room until I started making them uncomfortable. "What's a woman doing in here!?"

Now my throne is in the women's room once more. The struggle is real, but thankfully, the horror stories we hear about in the news rarely come true. Most people won't cause a scene by overtly confronting you, assaulting you, or calling the police. They are more interested in just leaving so they can get on with their day. If you're ever feeling insecure and unsure of which public restroom to use, it can be helpful to ask an employee of a business where the restroom is and see which one they direct you to! They also make good barometers.

What to Wear

If you're looking for nice clothes and shoes at cheap prices, look no further than Ross, Burlington, and Goodwill. Or a local thrift store. Sometimes, browsing the clearance sections of high-end stores can be fruitful. For example, if you need a bathing suit, start looking in early fall when they are trying to make room for warmer clothes. You could get a fancy, high-end one way below retail price. Leggings can be cute, but many trans women worry about the bulge in front. This can be concealed with a short skirt or dress.

I'll end this chapter with a quote from Zig Ziglar:
Difficult roads often lead to beautiful destinations.

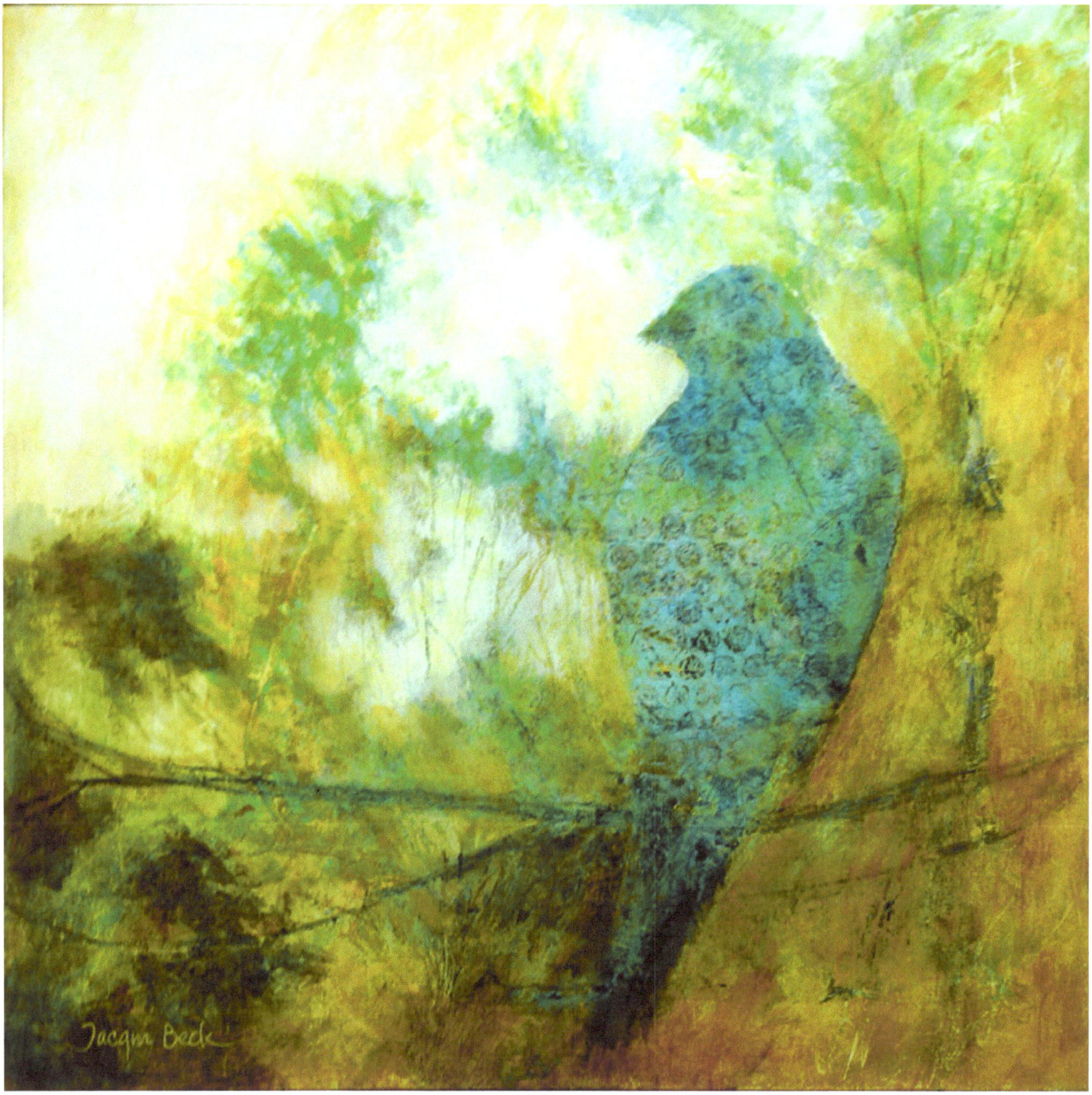

Perched

CHAPTER 9

Nonsurgical Ways to Appear More Masculine

Whenever you make any change, start by sizing up where you are and what you hope to achieve. Know what you want, and you are much more likely to get there.

As always, remember that people don't work too hard to discern your gender but they do look at a composite of cues to make a snap judgment. You can use this to your advantage, as many things can be quickly changed to make you look more masculine right away.

You can increase your muscle bulk through strength training, particularly under the influence of testosterone. You can lose weight if you feel you need to. You can learn to position your body in a more "male"-appearing stance. That's what body language is about.

Testosterone Will Help You Look and Sound More Masculine

Testosterone will deepen your voice, usually starting within several months of beginning hormones. A deep voice is one of those nonnegotiable cues that says "male."

If you are not happy with the depth or tenor of your voice on testosterone, consult a voice therapist. As in teaching trans women to adopt the nonverbal cues that convey femininity, voice therapists can help you learn how to look and sound more male also.

Q What was it like when your voice deepened?

A For the first time, I hear *me.*

— *Trans man, age 55, newly on testosterone*

Stereotypical Body Language Patterns That Declare "Masculine"

Body language, gait, posture, and hand gestures can help us appear more masculine or more feminine. Do you remember the scene in the classic movie *Birdcage*, where the magnificent Robin Williams was trying to teach Nathan Lane to eat in a more masculine way? "Men don't spread mustard [on their toast]," Williams's character admonished. "Men *smear.*"

Men typically sit differently than women do. Men cross their legs with one ankle over the other knee. They don't worry about keeping their knees together to hide the crotch as women are taught to do from when they were toddlers.

Men tend to walk with a broader, striding gait. Walking faster may appear more male. Men are encouraged to stand with "shoulders back, head up!" This may be difficult to do if you developed a large chest and are in the habit of rounding your shoulders to hide it (refer to Chapter 9 for nonsurgical ways to conceal your chest and Chapter 11 for top surgery information).

Observe the stereotypical behaviors of men you know, or at least the ones you'd like to emulate. Can you dissect what it is they're doing and use them as your mentors?

Get a More Masculine Haircut

Short hair, a shaved head, or a buzz cut (or even a receding hairline) is less likely to read "female." Longer hair and bangs may introduce questions about your gender. What is your desired outcome? If you want observers to make snap judgments reading you as male, make their work easier for them.

Think Before You Buzz

Seattle designer Lancer Forney of Emerson Salon (emersonsalon.com) offers the following cautions:

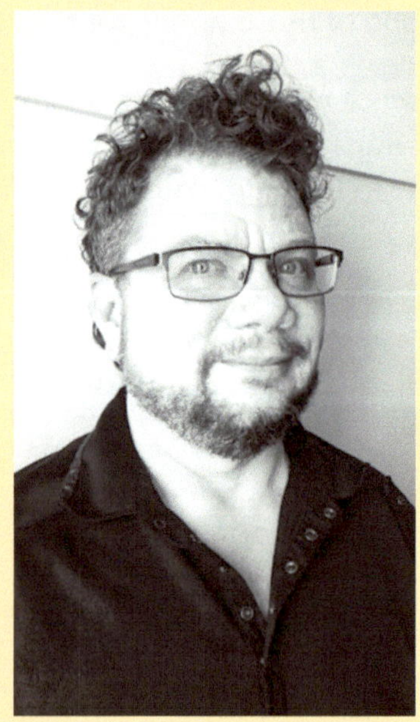

"Shaved and buzzed heads work only if a person doesn't have a round head, a round face, or plump or round facial features. When a person shaves off all their hair, it exposes everything, including scars and irregularities in the contour of the skull. It can show how round the face and head look—not angular like in a cis man. If a person isn't taking hormones and doesn't pass or read as 'male,' then the buzz cuts and tight clipper cuts don't work especially well.

"They do work—over time—later in transition if the transition is medically assisted with testosterone supplementation. Of course, this is contingent on testosterone supplementation being medically and genetically tolerated by the person who is masculinizing. In my experience, I have had clients get shaved or buzzed haircuts and then become upset because they still don't pass as male."

— *Lancer Forney*

Juan Cardenas's Prodigy Hair Studio

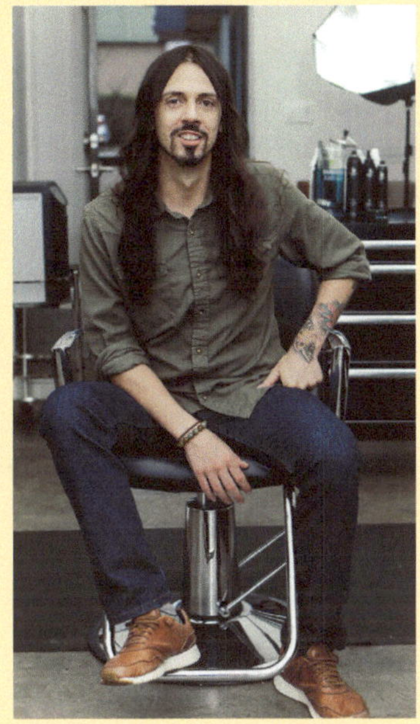

One of my trans masculine clients arrived for his physical exam looking happy and healthy. I didn't realize it, but he was wearing a standout hairpiece. He had purchased a custom virgin hairpiece from Seattle's Juan Cardenas, owner of the Prodigy Hair Studio (**prodigyhairstudio.com**). My client described having a scalp mold made from plaster of Paris and the salon sending hair samples to Cesare Ragazzi in Italy for the creation of a custom design.

Juan Cardenas writes about an early experience with one of his first trans clients:

> "He was looking for a masculine haircut, and every stylist he tried was reluctant to give him what he was asking for. He was young and still early in his transition. I was honored to help him achieve the look he was looking for and learned so much from his willingness to be open. This is also my community and whatever we can do to help someone to feel more comfortable in their skin, whether it's a haircut or an entire hair system, this is what we are here for."

The Seattle studio advertises as being transgender-friendly, and they help clients with all types of hair thinning and alopecia.

— *Linda Gromko, MD*

Eyeglasses

Eyeglasses are gendered. I see trans men wearing thicker, dark-framed glasses even when they don't need corrective lenses. Think of these as accessories that move you closer to being read correctly by others.

Jewelry, Watches, and Body Art

Single loops or ear studs seem to be popular as male statements. Leather strands for necklaces work well; think larger and less delicate pendants.

Watches can help you convey gender also. Wider bands and larger watch faces appear more masculine than stereotypically delicate women's watches. Pay attention to the size of a watch band, as one that's too big will make your wrist look smaller. Gentleman's Gazette (**gentlemansgazette.com/watches-small-hands-wrists**) can guide you to specific watch choices that enhance smaller wrists.

Body art is popular in Seattle. Tattoo art, piercings, and earlobe gauges can all be used to promote your specific gender identity. Just be alert to permanent changes and to changes that might limit your employability. (See **lifehacker.com/these-are-the-most-tattoo-friendly-companies-to-work-fo-1755827988** for employers that do not hold body art or piercings against you.) Also, be aware that tattoos can be removed (we do laser tattoo removal in our practice). A good plastic surgeon can surgically correct large-gauge loops that have split or otherwise outlived their appeal to the wearer.

Grooming

If you were assigned female, you may have been socialized to be well-groomed and "fresh." But if you were not raised with this ongoing critique or want to review the information, refer to the grooming information in Chapter 8.

I never learned about grooming from a mom or big sister. I didn't know how to dress. Nobody told me you couldn't wear white shoes after Labor Day. Or a pink suit in winter. I wore a pink linen suit with my boyfriend's family in the middle of winter. It was the only suit I had, and I was horribly embarrassed by that.

— Cisgender woman, age 50

Skin Care and Acne

Acne is a difficult problem for trans men, especially as they begin taking testosterone. Acne can impact the face, neck, chest, and back. It often improves over time, but it can be difficult. It's that reliable combination: skin bacteria + testosterone-stimulated oil production = acne.

Here are some approaches to acne that we use in the clinic:

- **Clean your skin well twice a day.**
  Be sure to remove any bronzer or concealer you use, particularly before you go to bed.

- **Use an over-the-counter cream or gel containing benzoyl peroxide.**
  This is effective if your acne is mild and confined to your face. Benzoyl peroxide may be somewhat drying; naturally, stop any product that irritates your skin.

- **Consider retinoids (Retin-A, Retinol, Differin).**
  These can decrease oil production, reduce inflammation, and help unclog pores. Different retinoids are available in over-the-counter and prescription strengths.

- **Ask your healthcare provider about prescription products for acne that is more severe but confined to the face.**
  Here are examples:

  - **Differin (adapalene)** is a retinoid that helps skin cells "turn over" faster, and it is available in prescription and nonprescription strengths.

  - **Tetracycline or erythromycin solutions** applied to the face twice a day.

    - **Clindamycin gel.**
    - **A combination of benzoyl peroxide plus an antibiotic.** We prescribe a fair amount of benzoyl peroxide plus clindamycin (BenzaClin), and while it works well on the face, we tend not to use it with acne that covers a more extensive surface area like the chest and back. For larger areas, a systemic (total body) antibiotic tablet may be preferable (see below).

- **Take a prescribed systemic antibiotic daily or a twice-daily tablet if the acne covers a larger area.** This may be more effective, since you'd need more antibiotic in a cream, gel, or solution form to cover affected areas, whereas a tablet will make its way into your bloodstream and impact your whole body.

- **Ask your healthcare provider if your acne has large, painful lumps; you may have cystic acne.** This type of acne responds best to a strong prescription medication called Accutane (isotretinoin). The proper use of Accutane requires regular blood testing to ensure the user's safety. Accutane is teratogenic (dangerous to a developing fetus in utero), so clinicians ask for regular pregnancy testing to ensure that a client is not pregnant. I refer patients who have cystic acne to a dermatologist (skin specialist) for management of this problem.

Brow Treatments

Masculine faces typically have more prominent brows that are fuller and somewhat shaggier. Fuller brows don't have to go ungroomed; a unibrow is rarely a desired look. Try tinting your brows if you feel that darker brows will stand out more.

Did you know that brows can be made fuller by hair transplants? Consult a hair loss specialist if you think this might help you.

The brow bones in males are more prominent than they are in females. We can temporarily enhance the appearance of these by using dermal filler injections (see Chapter 8). Gender-affirming facial surgery would be a permanent approach.

Facial Hair

Precisely *when* facial hair arrives on testosterone varies considerably. Some trans men see facial hair growth within a month or two, while others wait for several years before its arrival.

If your hair growth is patchy, give it time. A patchy start may look less obvious with shaving. I have seen videos on YouTube describing the off-label use of minoxidil (Rogaine) for making facial hair thicker. (I have no experience to recommend its use for this specific purpose.)

If the facial hair growth stays patchy over several years, you may wish to consult a hair transplant surgeon to correct this.

Dark hair tends to be more noticeable than lighter hair. Some of our clients have used brush-on hair color. Just for Men and Blackbeard for Men are brands that darken beard color and conceal gray. And one client used a fiber-containing mascara to thicken a mustache that seemed sparse.

Finding Masculine Clothing That Fits Your Height and Body Shape

We may think that American men average 6 feet in height. In actuality, the average American male is 5 feet 7 inches. Non-Hispanic white males are the tallest group in the US with an average height of 5 feet 9.5 inches followed by African Americans at 5 feet 9 inches. Asian-Americans rank further below at 5 feet 7 inches, while Hispanic and Latino Americans average 5 feet 6.5 inches.[36]

Look for clothing that best fits your height but that also reads "masculine" and "adult masculine" at that. Search the Internet for "clothing for short or small men." If you are shorter, consider shopping in clothing departments for teenagers (juniors) or even for kids. If the styles are the same, it won't matter and the clothing can be significantly less expensive in the teen or boys' departments. If this does matter to you, buy your clothing online.

One excellent blog, *The Modest Man* (**themodestman.com**), contains very practical advice and walks you through finding shoes that fit, brand by international brand. It teaches you how to use lifts, shoe inserts, and thick socks if you have difficulty with even the smallest shoes. *The Modest Man* also covers topics such as dating and building confidence, and features shorter men "the whole world can look up to."

For the Fit (**forthefit.com**) is an online catalog for casual classic styles in smaller sizes. In addition to business casual clothing, you will find underwear, sweatpants, pajamas, and outerwear jackets. They have business casual slacks, khakis, and jeans with inseams starting at 26 inches. For that matter, Land's End (**landsend.com**), J.Crew (**jcrew.com**), Eddie Bauer (**eddiebauer.com**), and Gap (**gap.com**) all carry pants with shorter inseams.

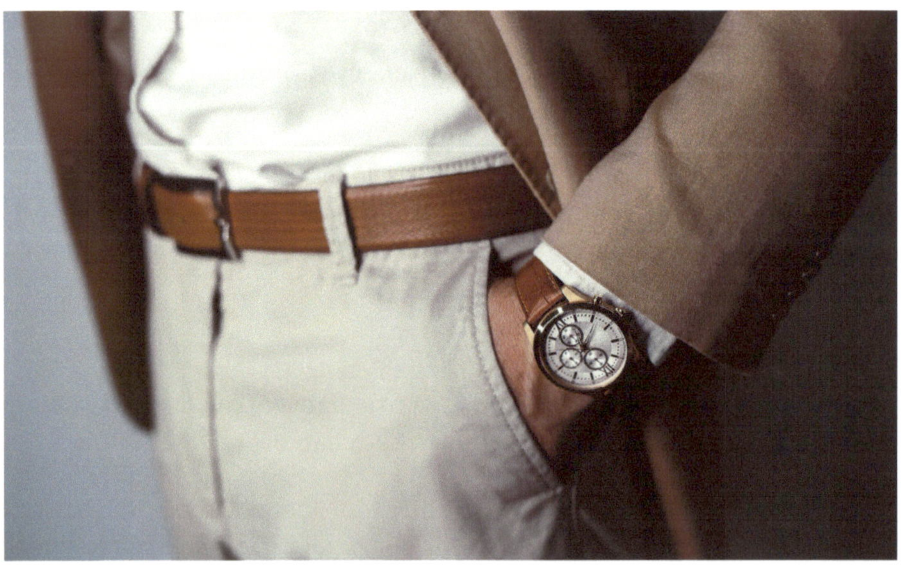

Be sure to look at FLAVNT (**flavnt.com**) for casual clothing, especially for the individual who identifies as nonbinary. If you need a more professional wardrobe or something formal, visit **PeterManningNYC.com**. Their sizes begin with heights of 5 feet 1 inch and weights of 105 pounds. Contact the personal stylist at Nordstrom for similar clothing.

36 Victor Kiprop, "Average Height of American Men," *World Atlas*, March 25, 2019, https://www.worldatlas.com/articles/what-is-the-average-height-of-american-men.html.

Heritage House (boyssuits.com) markets high-end boys' clothing in stock for an online retail experience. They carry silk ties in three lengths (42, 52, and 57 inches) for under $40. Their boys' shoes, including brands like Florsheim and Cole Haan, run to about $60 a pair.

(Note that men's shoes cost a lot more than boys' shoes. There's money to be saved with no apparent sacrifice in style for the man who can comfortably wear a boy's size.)

Look at Boys Italian Suits (boysitaliansuits.com) for ready-made and custom-tailored suits.

Ideas for Looking Bigger or Taller

We cannot physically change our height, but we can—

- Add a lift or insert in a shoe; height-increasing insoles can add 1 to 3 inches to your height.
- Look for shoes in platform styles with thicker soles in brands such as Dr. Martens, Timberland, New Rock, and Lugz.
- Consider athletic shoes like Puma, Fila Disruptors, or Vans that have thicker soles and add height.
- Find Western boots with larger heels.

We cannot make ourselves larger in the short term, but we can—

- Wear clothing and accessories that fit. Have your pants hemmed if you can't or won't do it yourself. A tie that's too long will look "off" and a watch that's too big can make your wrist look smaller.
- Dress in layers.
- Find fabrics that add visual bulk, such as plaid flannel shirts.
- Pay attention to posture; good posture will give the impression of more height. (This is especially difficult if you have been rounding your shoulders to conceal your chest, but you can retrain yourself.)

Concealing the Chest: Binders and Trans Taping

Female breast size and shape do not change with the use of testosterone. Breast size and shape are an enormous source of dysphoria in trans men or nonbinary individuals wishing to masculinize. Even from preteenage trans guys, I consistently hear two priorities: testosterone and top surgery.

Top surgery is the surgical creation of the appearance of a male chest; it is also called a "gender-affirming" or "gender-confirming surgery." It is different from the reduction mammoplasty that cis women get to reduce the size of their breasts while still maintaining a female breast shape. (I see some trans men who have had reduction mammoplasty; they can still go on to have top surgery for a more satisfactory male outcome.) Top surgery will be covered in detail in Chapter 11.

Until a trans man can have top surgery (which is often covered by health insurance and performed on trans males under the age of 18 with parents' consent), he may rely on a binder to produce the appearance of a flatter chest. And certainly, not all folks wanting a flatter chest wish surgery or can afford it, even with insurance.

A binder is a very snug garment that resembles a sleeveless T-shirt, ending above or below the belly button. Binders are usually made of Spandex, but here, think Spandex on steroids. Admittedly, binders can be uncomfortable. These garments are *designed* to be restrictive and to flatten the chest as much as possible.

Binder Tip from Point of Pride

It may be easier to step into a binder rather than pulling it on like a regular T-shirt. Stick your feet in between the shoulder straps and pull it up your body to your chest, then stick your arms through the holes. To make the binding more comfortable and to reduce the possibility of your binder shifting around, some folks wear a light shirt underneath.

— From the Point of Pride brochure, Trans Wellness Conference, Philadelphia, 2019

Binders come in a variety of styles and are produced by a variety of companies. They cost about $40 to $50 apiece. Informally, we hear reliable endorsements from our clients for gc2b binders (**gc2b.co**) and Underworks binders (**underworks.com**).

Trans-Vormer offers a band-like binder without straps. It looks like a tube top and fastens in the back with Velcro, making it quick to remove. (If you look up "Trans-Vormer Binder Band," you will find a variety of sites, including Trans-Missie.com (**trans-missie.com/nl**), which describes Amsterdam products made by Danae. Their band-like binder is fastened with hooks and eyes that can be done in the front or back. Similar binders are listed under BaronHong Lesbian Tomboy binders on Amazon or Etsy.

Shapeshifters (**shapeshifters.co**) offers binders and other garments that are highly customizable for size, style, and fabric. The company asks the buyer for very detailed measurements (such as bust, under-bust, waist, hips, and length). Shapeshifters binders are individually produced, so they require a 5-to-7-week wait. The company's website can inform you which item they're working on at the moment. Shapeshifters's products seem less compressive than binders from other manufacturers.

FLAVNT binders claim to have more "give" than other binders and are "less suffocating." Their Bareskin Binder comes in five different colors, more representative of human skin tones than the usual coal black or optic white. FLAVNT's website (**flavnt.com/need-help-picking-a-top**) displays models who show their actual chest sizes and shapes with and without their binders to give buyers a uniquely helpful idea of what to expect.

You'll find a reasonable variety of binders and other trans-related products on Etsy (**etsy.com**), where individual entrepreneurs market a range of styles. You'll find some made with zippers down the front or on the side of the binder. You'll also find a broader range of colors and styles on Etsy.

Some folks' dysphoria will not permit the suggestion of a sports bra. But if that isn't the case for you, browse through Title Nine's website (titlenine.com) for some of the most compressive sports bra designs available. In years past, Title Nine's Frog Bra was worn by *many* trans men I treated. It resurfaced for a while, but I couldn't find it on my last check in November 2020.

If your chest is smaller, you may find that Spanx for men will provide adequate compression. Search "Spanx for men" on the Internet, and you'll find all sorts of alternatives for smaller-chested individuals. There are compression garments that simulate an abdominal six-pack while concealing the chest at the same time. Esteem Apparel markets gynecomastia garments to conceal "man boobs," but these could also easily hide smaller breasts in AFAB as they transition (esteem-compression-apparel.com/pages/about-gynecomastia).

Binders for Swimming

Look specifically for swimming binders at gc2b or BaronHong. FLAVNT featured a Kickstarter campaign in 2015 to fund skin-tone binders for swimming. TransTape may also be used when swimming.

Getting a Binder

- **Take measurements** with a cloth or paper tape measure; write down your measurements in inches or centimeters across the largest part of your chest and your chest wall underneath. Some sites will also ask you for waist measurements. It will be easier to measure yourself when clothed.
- **Browse Internet sites** like gc2b.co, underworks.com, affirmawear.com, burslfllc.com, etsy.com, and of course, search amazon.com with the key words "transgender binders" or "binders for FTM."
- **Visit the binder vendors** at trans events such the Philadelphia Trans Wellness Conference (mazzonicenter.org/education-and-professional-training). You can talk to people who've used the various binders, get proper measurements, feel the fabric, and try on binders. If you cannot attend, look up the vendors that exhibit at the events and contact them directly. Visit the websites of conference sponsors: gc2b, Underworks, Affirma, B.UR.SLF, Shapeshifters, and others.
- **Source a free binder.** If you cannot afford a binder, go through all the steps above and then go to Point of Pride (pointofpride.org). Point of Pride has donated thousands of free new and lovingly used chest binders to trans people around the world. Gc2b donates hundreds of new binders each month to Point of Pride for distribution. Point of Pride also offers safe-binding pointers and will accept your tax-deductible donations to help "the next person on the waiting list."
- **Look also at Brothers for Binders on Facebook** (facebook.com/Brothers-for-Binders-100598708153456); Thomas Underwood's blog post "A Complete Guide to Chest Binding for Trans Men" (ftm-guide.com/complete-guide-to-chest-binding-for-trans-men); and websites of companies that make binders (such as shapeshifters.co) for binder giveaway contests.

Binder Safety

Binders seem to be designed for compression first and comfort second. Here are some common health issues people report:

- They are uncomfortable. Binders are stifling hot to wear in warm weather or when exercising. This is where a flattening sports bra style may work better if your dysphoria permits.
- They may cause breathing issues. If you have asthma or even a respiratory tract infection, you may find it difficult to breathe with a binder on. Breathing is nonnegotiable!
- They may trigger feelings of anxiety or panic, such as feeling like you are not getting enough air to breathe. Sadly, we were all reminded during the George Floyd tragedy that a person may be able to utter sentences using very small amounts of air.[37] So do not fall back on the old adage that "If you are talking, you are breathing."
- They can worsen GERD, also called gastroesophageal reflux disease; this is an uncomfortable condition where highly acidic stomach contents slosh up into the esophagus, which is less protected. GERD can cause intense upper-chest pain, provoke asthma symptoms, and irritate the throat. Anything that physically compresses the chest—including a chest binder—may intensify the reflux. There are medications that can help you (antacids and acid blockers), but if you suffer from GERD, you may want to minimize your binder hours or try a sports bra or TransTape instead.
- Binders may cause you to develop a skin irritation or yeast infection in warm, moist areas. Ask your healthcare provider to suggest a cream to treat it. Over-the-counter hydrocortisone, clotrimazole for yeast, or a water-proofer like A&D ointment may provide some comfort; check with your provider. Nystatin for yeast comes in a powder as well as a cream, by prescription.

I've found no large controlled prospective studies on binder use as of this writing. Jarrett et al. discussed reported symptoms associated with binding and the low frequency of such symptoms to healthcare providers[38] and Peitzmeier et al. wrote about the health impacts of binding.[39]

I have heard stories about people having broken ribs or collapsed lungs from wearing binders, but I've never actually seen this in my practice. It's hard to know what may be urban legend, and I'd appreciate hearing from people who have experienced these problems firsthand.

37 Law, Anica C., Gary E. Weissman, and Theodore J. Iwashyna, "A Dangerous Myth: Does Speaking Imply Breathing?" *Annals of Internal Medicine* 173 (2020): 754–55, https://doi.org/10.7326/M20-4186.

38 Brooke A. Jarrett et al., "Chest Binding and Care Seeking among Transmasculine Adults: A Cross-Sectional Study," *Transgender Health* 3, no. 1 (December 2018): 170, https://doi.org/10.1089/trgh.2018.0017.

39 Sarah Peitzmeier et al., "Health Impact of Chest Binding among Transgender Adults: A Community-Engaged, Cross-Sectional Study," *Culture, Health & Sexuality* 19, no. 1 (June 2016): 1–12, https://doi.org/10.1080/13691058.2016.1191675.

Common-Sense Recommendations about Binders

How you use your binder will depend on your own dysphoria, but here are some recommendations that may help.

- Consider TransTape or try another style or size if a binder physically hurts you to use it.
- Limit the wearing time of a binder. Take it off when you are at home if you can.
- Don't sleep in your binder.
- Avoid wearing a binder when you exercise if possible.
- Avoid wearing two binders, one over the other. I've seen people do this, but if one binder restricts your breathing, two must be worse.
- Buy a professionally made binder. Don't wear makeshift DIY binders made of Ace bandages or duct tape; these provide inconsistent compression and can tear your skin.
- Try wearing a tank top instead of a binder if you are smaller.
- Be aware that hunching your shoulders forward (as many people do when they are trying to conceal their chest, no matter what their size) can result in back pain and lengthening of the rotator cuff tendons. Consciously remind yourself of your posture to avoid long-term aches and pains.

Information about TransTape

TransTape is *not* duct tape, nor is it a combination of tape and Ace bandages. TransTape, according to its website **transtape.life**, is marketed as a "gender-affirming body transformation system for trans-masculine, trans-feminine, nonbinary, gender-fluid, and gender-nonconforming individuals who are looking for a backless and waterproof alternative to traditional binding." TransTape allows an individual to reduce the appearance of their chest size by the careful application of the tape and respectful attention to skin care to prevent tissue damage.

Invented and marketed by Kaiyote Jackson in 2017, TransTape is made, according to the website, from a "blend of 95 percent cotton and 5 percent spandex with a hypoallergenic, medical-grade acrylic adhesive that is latex-free and nonmedicated." Following written instructions or instructional videos, the user cuts the tape to its proper size and applies it to position the breast toward the side of the body—in some cases, toward the armpit. According to Jackson, the tape can be left in place for up to 5 days, at which time the tape is removed by super-saturating it with an oil-based removal product and gently peeling it off. The removal oil consists of almond oil mixed with tea tree and cedarwood oils that are selected for their stated antimicrobial properties.

TransTape comes in 5-meter rolls of three widths: 7.5 cm, 10 cm, and 12.5 cm. The tape comes in three human colors (light beige, dark beige, and brown), as well as three more festive colors for fundraising purposes. (TransTape donates $2 per roll to the Trans Youth Equality Foundation.)

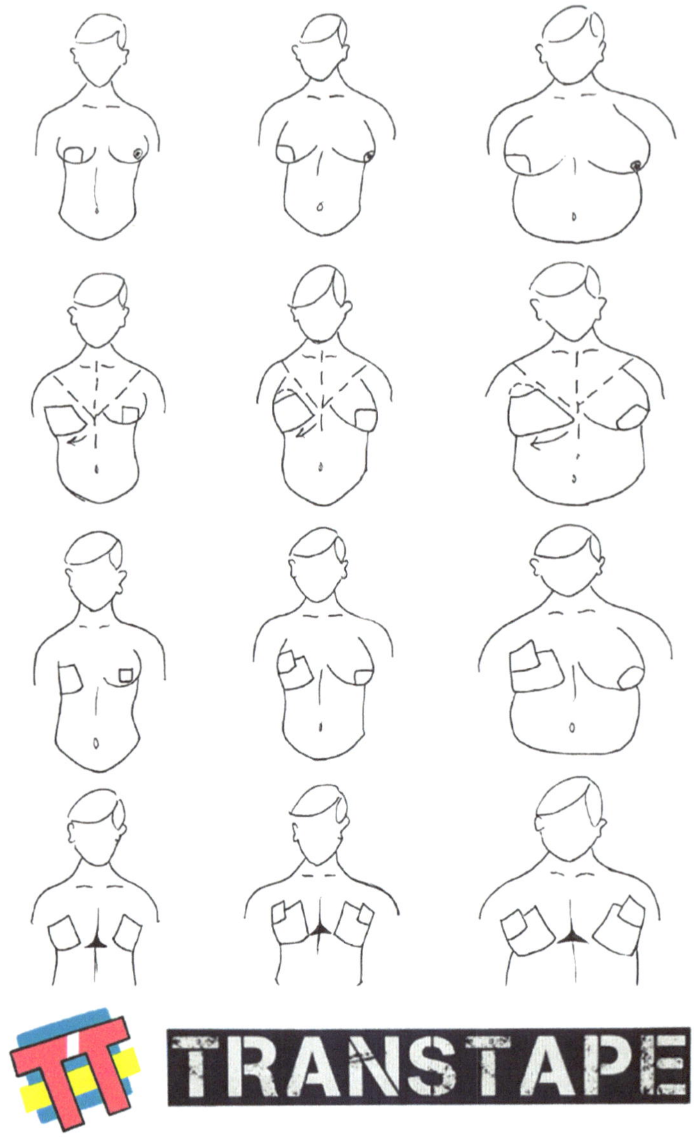

Figure 9.1. Uses of TransTape.

TransTape is, in fact, similar to the KT tape used in physical therapy applications, but it comes in a wider range of widths and more suitable colors. Jackson indicates that the precut sizes of KT tape make it less applicable for chest modification, and that the adhesive used in TransTape is stronger and more appropriate for securing the weight of chest tissue.

TransTape has received variable reviews from consumers online and on YouTube. Those who like the product cite the following:

- TransTape does not resemble a bra, and therefore, there are no shoulder straps or back involved.
- TransTape may be used for 5 consecutive days.
- One can sleep while using it, further managing chest dysphoria.
- Users may shower or swim while using the product.

- There is no chest compression with TransTape; this allows for easier breathing and a comfortable range of upper body movement without overheating.
- It is a temporary, reversible option for individuals not seeking top surgery or perhaps those waiting to have surgery.

Note: The TransTape website indicates that the product can also be used as a gaff or with a packer. While I have clients who are using TransTape to manage chest dysphoria, I have not personally seen clients who use TransTape for genital applications. Please refer to the TransTape site (transtape.life) for further information.

Packing and Peeing

Packing

Many transmasculine individuals use a "packer" (prosthetic penis) to create a bulge in the crotch. In a YouTube video, one man indicated that a packer could define a bulge for the rest of the world to see, or simply give the wearer more confidence and less dysphoria in knowing that it's there.

People have created budget packers with cloth or rolled-up socks for years, of course. Then, there are packers made of silicone, foam, and even fabric. You can buy briefs with a packer pocket sewn in them on Etsy (etsy.com).

Here's a blog post by Aaron Capener describing one way for making a do-it-yourself fabric packer: transguysupply.com/blogs/news/how-to-make-a-packer. And there are a number of knitting patterns for packers; here's a crochet pattern: ravelry.com/patterns/library/drag-king-soft-packer.

The variety of silicone packers is expansive and the anatomical accuracy is impressive. Some packers are circumcised, some are not. Penile length, girth, and texture (firmness) vary and can be made to order. All human colors are available. You can order a packer with or without a scrotum, which in turn can be ordered with or without mobile prosthetic testicles.

In a comprehensive blog post titled "13 Best FTM Packers to Fix Your Dysphoria" (transguysupply.com/blogs/news/top-packers-for-beginners), author Scout Rose describes five FTM packers for beginners, followed by four more advanced products. This outstanding blog post is modified slightly and used with the author's permission. Scout Rose is the founder of TransGuy Supply (transguysupply.com).

It starts with socks, with Rose calling them "the best packer to determine if packing is right for you." Rose explains, "As ridiculous as this sounds, if you are new to the trans community, using socks to pack is a great place to start. It's important to note that not everyone in the community packs. It's not 'required' for you to be trans. This is just to ease the mental struggle of what we call bottom dysphoria. Bottom dysphoria is the uncomfortable feeling that your genitals don't match your gender."

Below and on page 156 is Scout Rose's list of five FTM packers for beginners, as well as more advanced packers.

Beginning Packers

- **Socks: The best packer to determine if packing is right for you.**
  "Some trans guys do not experience bottom dysphoria at all. And some find that packing causes them more dysphoria rather than alleviating it. This is why I recommend starting with something

simple to see if packing is right for you. Try grabbing one of your crew socks and use that for a week or so to see if you enjoy the look and feel. If that helps but you want something more realistic, go ahead and look into other options."

- **Mr. Limpy: The classic starter packer and best cheap packer.**
  "The combination of its low price ($12.95 to $18.95) and realistic look add up to make the Mr. Limpy the most popular packer of all time."

- **Pierre Uncut: The best silicone packer under $55.**
  "'Pierre' is the best-selling intact packer in the United States. This silicone packer features over 100 unique skinfolds throughout the shaft and subtly asymmetrical testicles. There is an ideal Pierre packer for everyone on the gender masculine spectrum."

- **Foam Packer: The best packer for nonbinary folks.**
  "You don't actually have to be nonbinary to love this packer. And it should be noted that some nonbinary folks absolutely love an anatomical packer. However, this foam packer is the perfect packing solution for anyone who wants a nice bulge without the look of an actual penis." Approximate price: $5.

- **Stash-it-Willy: The best anatomical packer for guys allergic to silicone.**
  "This 100-percent cloth packer is incredibly comfortable and can pin to any underwear in your collection. What's more, this company makes swimming-friendly models and is also willing to custom-make a cloth packer just for you." The price is $20 on Etsy.

More Advanced Packers

- **Mr. Right: The best mid-range packer.**
  "Each Mr. Right packer is handmade from 100 percent silicone and comes with excellent detail in the scrotum. Because the Mr. Right is meant to be very realistic, the balls are two different sizes with wrinkles and veins. When considered next to most other silicone packers, Mr. Right is still in the more affordable range. You can generally find this packer for under $70."

- **PeeCock Packer: The best packer company for trans men of color.**
  "If you are (rightfully) annoyed by the lack of color variance you get with other prosthetics companies, you will be pleased to see the expanded skin tone range of the PeeCock Packer. While most prosthetics companies only offer one darker skin tone option, the PeeCock Packer has three. Trans men of color can choose between light brown, medium brown, and dark brown to more closely match their actual skin tone." The approximate price is $90.

- **GenderCat Packers: Hyperrealistic packers with a payment plan.**
  "These packers eliminate the need for straps or harnesses by introducing self-adhesive sheets that affix your packer directly to your body. They are also incredibly customizable. You can choose your own length and level of firmness and even add unbelievably realistic (and movable!) balls to your packer.

  "In addition to being high-quality, GenderCat has what most higher-end prosthetic companies lack: payment plans. You can even choose the amount you pay in your monthly installments, making this packer's high price tag within reach." The approximate price is $269. (Read more about GenderCat's play prosthesis in Chapter 22: Sex and Relationships.)

- **Emisil: Best packer if money is no object.**
  "The Emisil FLO2 (emisil.com/ftm-packer-trans-fl02.html) is basically the Rolex of packers. This packer is known for having three silicone layers made of different softness and when pressing the scrotum, you can visually see the difference in colors between the layers. Like the GenderMender (from GenderCat), it's self-adhesive, but this packer comes in 16 different skin tones and, for an extra cost, you can even add hair. Yes, hair. If money is no object or nothing but the most realistic packer will do, this is the packer for you." The price is over $360.

Mr. Limpy Giveaway for Men under 23

TransGuy Supply offers a monthly drawing for a free Extra Small Mr. Limpy packer.

You must be under age 23 to enter. If you win, your package will arrive discreetly labeled "TG Supply." If you don't win, just enter again (transguysupply.com/pages/ftm-packer-giveaway).

Stand-to-Pee Devices

Many trans men pee standing up and there are a variety of tools to help. Look up transguysupply.com/collections/ftm-stp to find a collection of STP (stand-to-pee) devices. All STPs offer a funnel-shaped collector that is placed over the urethra and surrounding tissues and a tube through which the urine flows out to the campground, urinal, or toilet.

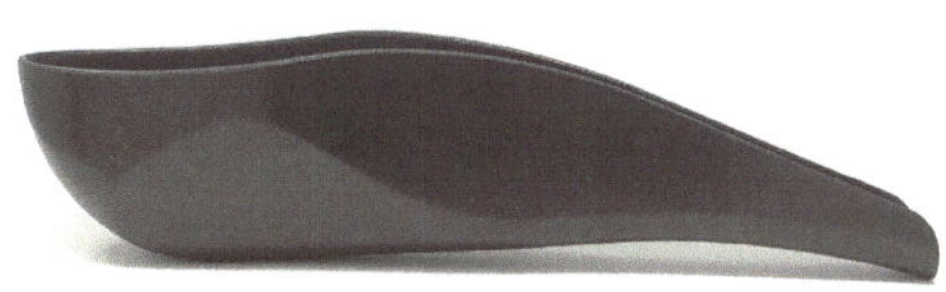

Figure 9.2. The pStyle STP device.

The most utilitarian model offered by TransGuy Supply is the inexpensive "pStyle," which "is like a tiny waterslide for your pee."

In addition to this simple device, TransGuy Supply (transguysupply.com/collections/ftm-stp) carries a range of devices that look like penises rather than funnels. These prosthetic devices are quite lifelike, complete with wrinkles, veins, more or less foreskin, and a range of colors. A true stand-to-pee device will have a hole from the base to the tip. With some, you can insert a rigid rod through the center hole for sexual penetration. The SAM STP device has an insertable rod so you can "pack, pee, and penetrate" (transtoolshed.com/products/internal-rod-for-sam-the-stp). Refer to Chapter 22 on sex and relationships for other similar devices.

If your dysphoria allows, you may want to research REI (Recreational Equipment Inc.). REI (rei.com) sells two devices that are called "FUDs" (female urination devices). Look up the Sani-Fem Urinary Director and the Pibella Travel Female Urination Device from Switzerland, both on REI's website. Both run about $20 and the Pibella is dishwasher-safe! FUDs look like funnels, but they certainly could work, depending on your circumstances and the degree of your dysphoria. Some of our postvaginoplasty clients have used the Shewee (**shewee.com**) or the GoGirl (**go-girl.com**) to help direct their urine stream after gender-affirming surgery; both are available on Amazon.

Using any of these devices takes practice. So, check out YouTube and search STP devices online. Practice at home (perhaps in the shower) until you feel confident.

> **I was with a large group of older physicians on a tour. During the bathroom break when we were all lined up to use the urinals, several men were taking a rather long time to complete their business. Trying to reassure them that they could take all the time they needed, one of the doctors in line said out loud, "no pressure" to which a guy at the urinal responded, "That's the problem!"**
>
> **We all had a good laugh.**
>
> *— Adult trans man*

A Word about Public Restrooms

Public restrooms are a common source of anxiety for trans men. I'm told that there's little verbal communication or even eye contact among men in public restrooms. But I'm also told that trans men may worry about how their urine stream sounds even when peeing in a private stall. Certainly, you can use a stall and sit to pee. But some stalls have shorter doors to discourage criminal activity. And you can be accidentally exposed if a stall door is missing or broken. This is no small matter. Hate crimes do happen in the relative isolation of public bathrooms, so stay alert.

The Restrooms Refuge Site

Restroom insecurity can be a problem. I've known trans men who simply don't pee during the day because of the challenge of finding a safe restroom. To locate gender-neutral, single-stall public bathrooms or family restrooms, go to **refugerestrooms.org** for more information. Your location will pop up followed quickly by little purple toilets springing up near you. To contribute, you can add new bathroom information to the site.

SECTION 4

GENDER-AFFIRMING SURGERIES

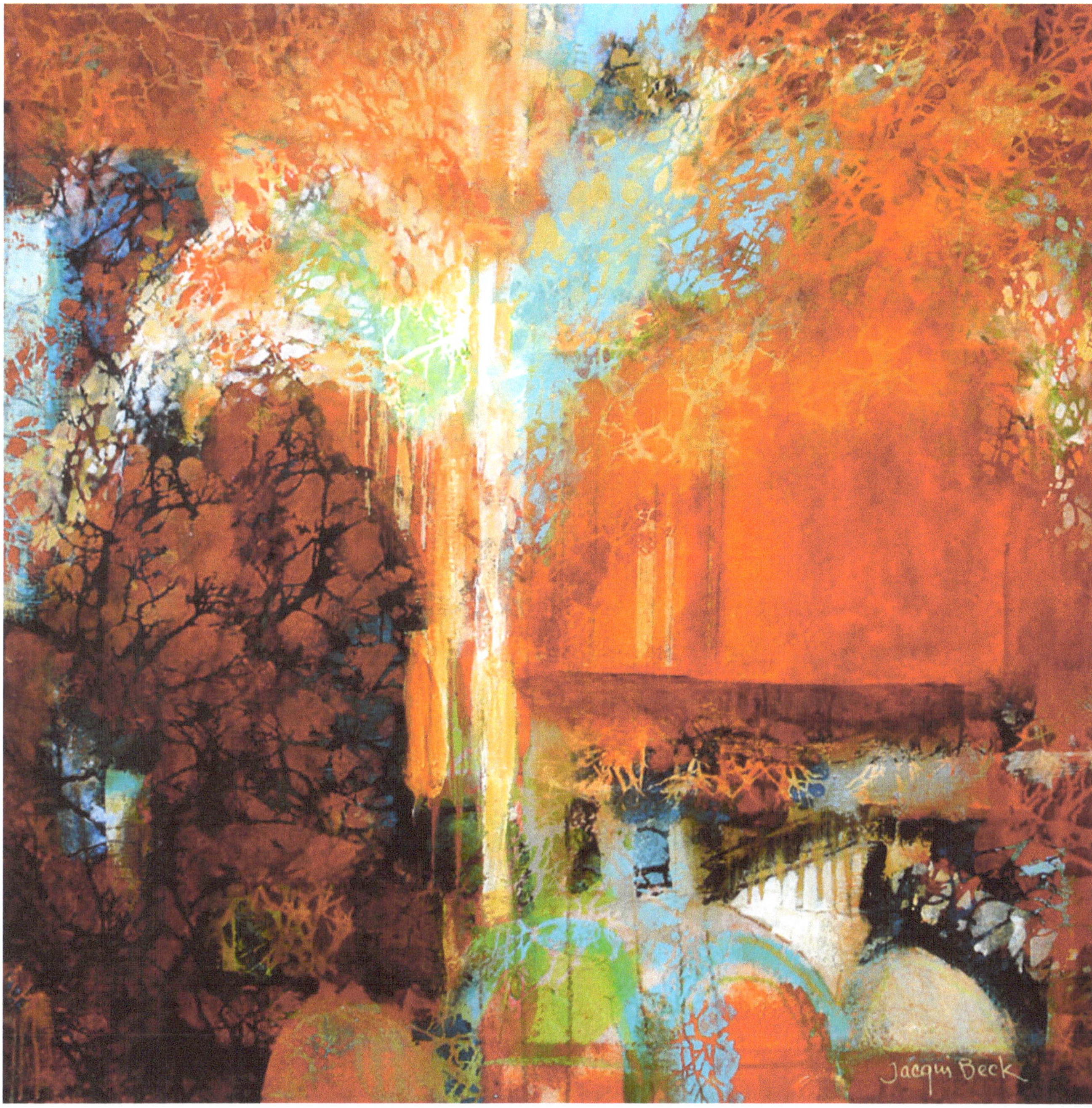

Nature Reflecting

INTRODUCTION

When describing a gender-affirming surgery to a young client, I said, "Remember, now, this surgery is permanent."

My client responded, "But isn't that the idea?"

Fair enough.

— *Linda Gromko, MD*

The decision to pursue a gender-affirming surgery requires careful thought and planning. Most transgender individuals do not have gender-affirming surgeries at all, although the majority of trans individuals state they would want to have them.[40] Some individuals chose one surgery but wouldn't want another. (Many transgender men have top surgery, for example, but may not pursue genital surgery.) Whether or not you have surgery depends on your personal needs and goals, your financial ability to pay or to have insurance pay for surgery, your geographical access to care, and your personal health and life circumstances.

In This Section

- We'll examine practical points to consider and complete in the 1 to 2 years before surgery, knowing full well that you may need to be on a waiting list long before that.
- We'll give you a checklist of things to be sure you do in that critical 6 weeks before surgery.
- We'll take a detailed look at each of the major surgeries for feminizing and for masculinizing. Understand that this information changes continually, and be aware that information provided by your own surgeon far outweighs anything I have to offer.
- We'll examine practical pointers for taking good care of yourself after you have any of the surgeries listed, with more specific details provided for the genital surgeries.

All of this is provided with the intention that you, individually, will be more likely to have a better experience and outcome if you are armed with information. If you are a family member or healthcare provider, perhaps this information will help you advocate more powerfully for your friend, partner, offspring, or client.

40 "In the most robust survey to date, 25% of TGNB respondents report having undergone some form of gender confirming surgery." Ian T. Nolan, Christopher J. Kuhner, and Geolani W. Dy, "Demographic and Temporal Trends in Transgender Identities and Gender Confirming Surgery," *Translational Andrology and Urology* 8, no. 3 (June 2019): 186, doi: 10.21037/tau.2019.04.09.

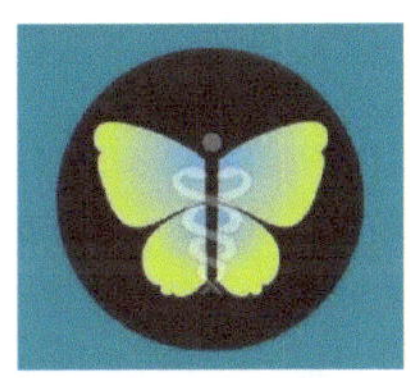

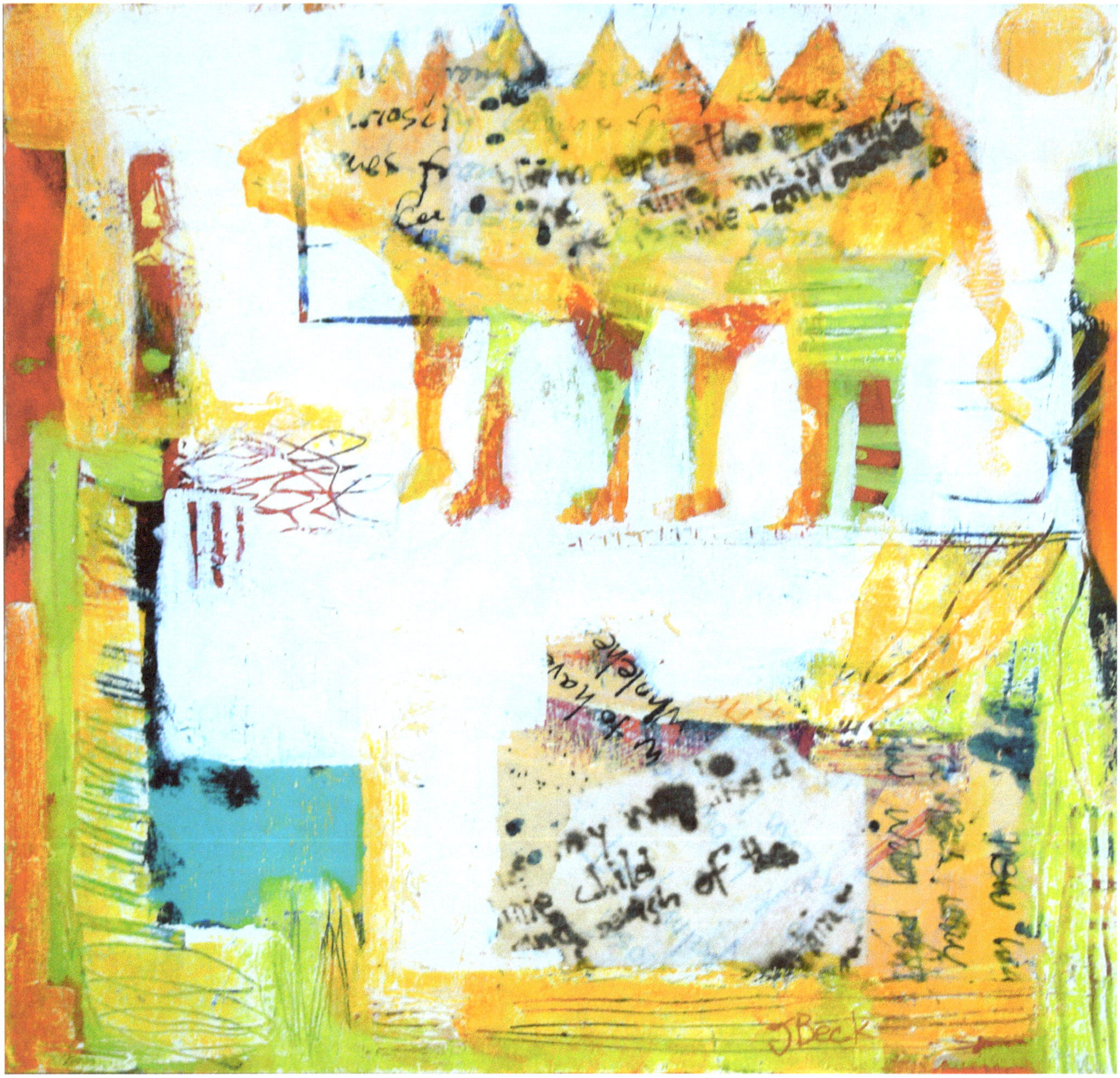

Many Socks

CHAPTER 10

Planning for Your Surgery

Waiting for Your Gender-Affirming Surgery

If you wish to have your gender-affirming surgery performed by one of the country's better-known surgeons, you may have to be on a waiting list for **2 to 3 years**. You can cancel, of course, but you may forfeit your deposit.

And you can ask to be on a cancellation list—that is, to be moved up in line if someone ahead of you cancels. **Fortunately, these prolonged waiting times have lessened as more surgeons have become expert in transgender surgeries.**

The Critical 1 to 2 Years before Surgery

Orchestrating a gender-affirming surgery would challenge the most skilled of project managers. The year or two before surgery is a busy time with much to accomplish and important consequences if details are missed.

In my experience as a clinician, patients undergo a range of emotions in the year or two prior to their surgeries: excitement, frustration, confusion, anxiety, relief, a sense of feeling overwhelmed—you name it. It's all understandable. Arranging and having surgery is a complicated process, and available support is inconsistent at best. If you don't have a therapy relationship already established, this may be a great time to develop one. You'll likely need a therapist to write a supportive letter required for surgery anyway.

Gender-affirming surgery is a major decision. Surgeries are expensive, insurance coverage is variable, and outcomes are never guaranteed (although they are remarkable in most cases). Surgical results are, for the most part, irreversible. That is to say, the only possible way back from a surgical outcome you don't like may be to have more surgery. **And, if insurance doesn't cover a procedure, it may or may not cover a complication or reversal.**

Let's look at some of the factors you will want to consider before having a gender-affirming surgery. Use this chapter as a surgery planner or workbook. Check off what you've already accomplished and make notes as to your questions and to-do items.

Your Personal Goals

What Do You Hope Your Surgery Will Accomplish?

Define your goals as precisely as you can. Examine the detailed descriptions of the various surgeries to assure that you are on the right track. We've discussed that you're more likely to get what you want if you know precisely what it *is* that you want.

How Realistic Are Your Hopes and Expectations?

Arrange for an in-person consultation with your surgeon, or an introductory Skype consultation if you live far away (see "Choosing Your Surgeon" on pages 178–181). After getting to know you better, your surgeon should ask you to define your desired goals of the surgery as precisely as you can. Photos are often helpful. Then ask for an honest and realistic assessment: Can the surgeon deliver the results you are requesting? Everyone comes to the operating room with different "raw materials." One person may require more or different surgeries to achieve the desired results. Don't be afraid to get a second opinion. Experienced surgeons welcome them and are not offended by your wanting a second opinion.

Q **When is gender-affirming surgery required?**

A **That's a question that only you can answer for yourself. Most trans people never have surgery at all, although 75 percent of transgender women say they would want it.**[41]

In working with trans men and women, I often ask, "If money and family were not factors, what would your surgical goals be?" Or alternatively, "If you were completely alone on an isolated island yet somehow had access to gender-affirming surgery, what type of surgery would you have? Would you have surgery at all?"

If You Are Envisioning Multiple Surgeries, Where Will You Start?

Are you planning a surgery such as phalloplasty that requires several steps to achieve the results you need? Different surgeons do the stages in an order based on their experience and preferences. Know the recommended sequence of your surgeries; again, this will require a consultation with the surgeon.

Which surgery is most important to you? Is a large Adam's apple interfering with your comfort in the world? If so, a tracheal shave may be more important than a breast augmentation or rhinoplasty.

41 Per the 2010 *National Transgender Discrimination Survey Report on Health and Health Care*: "Most survey respondents had sought or accessed some form of transition-related care. Counseling and hormone treatment were notably more utilized than any surgical procedures, although the majority reported wanting to "someday" be able to have surgery... Three-quarters of transgender women reported that they desired to have surgery at some point in the future or had already done so. However, it is impossible to know how many would desire or utilize surgery if it were more financially accessible... Genital surgery, on the other hand, remains out of reach for a large majority, despite being desired by most respondents." Jaime M. Grant et al., *National Transgender Discrimination Survey Report on Health and Health Care* (Washington DC: National Center for Transgender Equality, 2010), 10–11, 16, https://cancer-network.org/wp-content/uploads/2017/02/National_Transgender_Discrimination_Survey_Report_on_health_and_health_care.pdf.

I'll say, "Imagine yourself in an emergency room or a nursing home. Would you be okay with your genitalia in those situations?" If you are embarrassed or ashamed of your genitalia in a medical situation, this is something to consider. Your viewpoint may also change with age.

— *Marci Bowers, MD*

Are Your Goals Reachable by Surgery?

Realistically examine with your healthcare provider, your partner, your therapist, or anyone you trust whether surgical treatment even applies to you. Suppose you are seeking to feminize your appearance and feel that your outward presentation is more important than your genital appearance. If so, you may elect facial feminization surgery and perhaps breast augmentation. Genital surgery may not be something you want or need. Except in medical treatment or intimate sexual contact with a partner, who really sees our genitals anyway? (The obvious answer is that *we* do, and genital dysphoria can be severe enough to prompt vaginoplasty or phalloplasty well before outward presentation is addressed.)

Do the Collective Benefits of Surgery Outweigh the Risks for You?

Everyone has their own risk tolerance. All surgeries have risks and you will get a better idea of what these may be as you read the details of respective surgeries in Chapter 11. Only you can make this assessment. Although serious complications are uncommon, would you regret having surgery if you did have a serious complication? Or would you look at the surgery as something that simply had to be done, and manage problems if they arose?

Optimizing Your Personal Health before Surgery

During the 1 to 2 years prior to your surgery, compile information about your own health. This is the time to take stock of your own medical fitness. Here are some things to consider.

Get a Thorough Medical Evaluation

Your healthcare provider will take a medical history and perform a physical exam. Ask for lab tests that reflect your body's level of functioning.

Laboratory Tests for a General Evaluation

Here is a list of commonly ordered blood tests. Ask your healthcare provider which tests might apply to you.

- **CBC (complete blood count)** assures us that your bone marrow is producing normal red blood cells, white blood cells, and platelets. This test can indicate anemia and variation in red cell size.
- **CMP (comprehensive metabolic profile)** measures your blood sugar, kidney and liver function, electrolytes (sodium, potassium, etc.), and reflects your body's acid and base balance.
- **TSH (thyroid stimulating hormone)** is the pituitary hormone that regulates production of thyroid hormone in the thyroid gland. The thyroid hormone regulates your metabolic rate—or how your body uses energy. A high TSH is associated with low thyroid function.
- **Lipid panel** measures your cholesterol level and may signal indicators that place a person at higher risk for cardiovascular disease.
- **HbA1c (hemoglobin A1c or glycosylated hemoglobin)** reflects your blood sugar level during the prior 3 months and may suggest diabetes if it is elevated. It is also used to monitor how well a diabetic is managing their blood sugar.
- **STI (STD) profile** screens for sexually transmitted infections, which used to be called sexually transmitted diseases (I generally include HIV, tests for hepatitis B and hepatitis C, syphilis, herpes simplex type 1 and type 2, gonorrhea, and chlamydia).
- **PSA (prostate specific antigen)** for AMAB individuals age 50 and over.
- **Estradiol and free and total testosterone levels.**

Other Medical Conditions to Be Evaluated before Surgery

- **Make a list of your own ongoing medical issues or concerns—essentially, a "problem list."**
  Your healthcare provider does this routinely. Do your lists agree?
- **Do you have diabetes, heart disease, asthma, depression, systemic skin disease (such as psoriasis) or other conditions that might impact your surgery?**
  If so, get everything "tuned up," so you will be in the best medical condition possible before your surgery. Ask your primary care provider about this perhaps even before you consult your surgeon.
- **Are there specific health benchmarks you must achieve prior to surgery?**
  If so, nail these down now. For example, if you are a diabetic, your surgeon may require a specific hemoglobin A1c level. The HbA1c reflects your blood sugar over the prior 3 months. A normal HbA1c will run under 5.6 percent; as a diabetic, your HbA1c will likely run higher. Your surgeon,

however, may require that you must have a HbA1c of 7.0 or under to qualify for surgery. (A newer way to assess blood sugar is the "time within range," or the portion of time during which your blood sugar is in a normal range. This eliminates the evening-out effect of high and low blood sugars in the HbA1c.) Check to see what *your* surgeon requires and get your blood sugar under good control now—not just for surgery, but for the rest of your life.

- **If you have a heart condition, your primary care provider and your surgeon may ask your cardiologist to clear you prior to surgery.**
  This process may include a cardiologist's examination, a current electrocardiogram (EKG), a cholesterol (lipid) panel, and an echocardiogram to evaluate your heart valves, and your heart's ejection fraction (that is, the "squeeze" function of your heart).

  It's very reasonable to have a presurgical cardiology evaluation if you are a diabetic. It is commonly believed that diabetics have a higher risk for cardiovascular disease.[42]

  If your primary care doctor hears a heart murmur that hasn't been heard or evaluated before, see a cardiologist. (I remember a patient who had a new—and loud—murmur when I performed her preoperative exam. She was found to have a serious mitral valve problem. Her facial feminization surgery was rescheduled; she had to wait for a year after her heart valve was repaired.)

A patient of mine had had a heart attack a couple of years before she scheduled her sexual reassignment surgery in Thailand. She declined the cardiology evaluation I had recommended. When she got to Thailand, though, her surgeon required that she have the same evaluation I had recommended. Thankfully, she passed inspection and had a successful surgery. But suppose she hadn't passed her tests? She would have traveled a long distance only to have her surgery denied. Worse, she might have had a serious cardiac event, cardiac surgery, or death far away from home.

— Linda Gromko, MD

- **Are you up-to-date on generally recommended screening tests, such as colonoscopy screening for colon cancer, a Pap test for cervical cancer, a PSA for prostate cancer, or mammogram screening for breast cancer?**
  Screening is often a controversial topic; the USPSTF (**uspreventiveservicestaskforce.org/uspstf**) publishes recommendations as dictated by evidence-based medicine. Have a discussion with your healthcare provider now about how these recommendations may apply to you. Suppose you found something concerning on a screening test? Take care of it now so there won't be surprises later.

42 New research questions commonly held beliefs vis-à-vis cardiovascular risk assessment in patients with diabetes: "Diabetes has long been considered a 'cardiovascular risk equivalent.' This statement was formerly based in the Finnish study, in which T2DM patients without coronary heart disease (CHD) events showed a similar coronary mortality as nondiabetic patients who had a previous coronary event... [however] Recent evidences indicate that CHD risk in T2DM is not universally similar to the risk of patients with prior cardiovascular disease, but is highly heterogeneous... Type 2 diabetes increases cardiovascular risk in 2 to fourfold, but cannot be considered a risk equivalent due to the high heterogeneity." Marcello Casaccia Bertoluci and Viviane Zorzanelli Rocha, "Cardiovascular Risk Assessment in Patients with Diabetes," *Diabetology & Metabolic Syndrome* 9, no. 25 (April 20, 2017), https://doi.org/10.1186/s13098-017-0225-1.

- **Do you have a blood clotting problem that may increase your risk of a blood clot in your legs or in your lungs after surgery? A venous thromboembolism (VTE) or deep vein thrombosis (DVT) can travel to the lung where it is called a pulmonary embolism (PE).**
  Both conditions are serious; a pulmonary embolism (resulting from a DVT that travels to the lungs) can be fatal. Surgeries carry an increased risk for blood clots in the perioperative period (the time around surgery). Know if you have a condition that increases your personal risk and get your plan in order. For example, **if you've had a prior VTE, DVT, or PE, you may have already been evaluated by a hematologist (blood specialist) to see if you have a "hypercoagulable state."**

  A hypercoagulable state is a condition that increases your clotting risk. If you have a predisposition to blood clots (also called a thrombophilia) or have had a clot before, your surgeon will want you to consult a hematologist prior to surgery. This doesn't necessarily disqualify you from having surgery. But your surgeon and you can make a management plan well ahead of time (that is, using low-molecular-weight heparin at the time of surgery).

  Your surgeon will want you to see a hematologist if you currently take an anticoagulant medication for any reason or have done so in the past.

  Again, this is not an automatic disqualifier, but you and your surgeon will want a perioperative anticoagulant plan to keep you safe. Here are examples of common anticoagulant medications:

  - **Heparin**
    Used in an IV (intravenous) form in patients being treated for a DVTs or PEs; more commonly used in years past.

  - **Low-molecular-weight heparin (Lovanox)**
    Used as a subcutaneous injection twice a day to treat DVTs or PEs. Sometimes used during surgery to prevent a DVT or PE.

  - **Warfarin (Coumadin)**
    An older but less expensive oral anticoagulant used in DVTs, PEs, atrial fibrillation, and so on. Serum levels must be carefully monitored; warfarin interacts with many medications and foods that can move a person's blood clotting indicators out of a therapeutic window. Too little medication, and clots form more easily; too much, and patients can have life-threatening bleeding.

  - **DOACs (direct oral anticoagulants)**
    These more expensive newer agents are taken orally in the treatment of DVTs, PEs, atrial fibrillation, and so on. Monitoring of blood levels are not required as with warfarin. There are many available, such as apixaban (Eliquis), rivaroxaban (Xarelto), and dabigatran (Pradaxa).

  If you are currently taking an anticoagulant for *therapeutic* reasons (that is, to treat a recent blood clot or because you have recently had a coronary artery stent placed), you may be advised to postpone your surgery until later. This is not automatic but be sure that everyone on your surgical and medical teams agree that this is a safe time for your surgery to be performed.

Most anticoagulant therapies can be managed by stopping the oral medications and using a Lovanox bridge without having bleeding problems in surgery. This is obviously done in coordination with a patient's hematologist or cardiologist.

— Toby Meltzer, MD

- **Are there any other medical conditions that might be prudently evaluated before surgery?** Suppose you have a family history or personal history of kidney, urinary tract, or liver disease. Perhaps a physician has recommended you have further evaluation. Now is the time, *before your gender-affirming surgery*, to complete these specialist evaluations.

Modify Any Personal Health Habits That May Impact Your Surgical Risks

Now is the ideal time to examine your personal health habits. Modify any behaviors that might make it more dangerous to have a surgery and recover without complications.

Stop Smoking Now If You Smoke (Tobacco, Marijuana, Hookahs) or Use Tobacco Products

Your surgeon will advise you that smoking impairs your capacity to heal and increases your risk of blood clots. Most surgeons will not perform surgery on you if you smoke. (They'll test your urine before surgery and will cancel your operation if you have been smoking.)

At the second annual WPATH Live Surgery Training course in February–March 2019, several surgeons recommended quitting smoking 3 to 4 weeks before surgery and abstaining until 3 to 4 weeks after. (Better yet, take this opportunity to quit for good.)

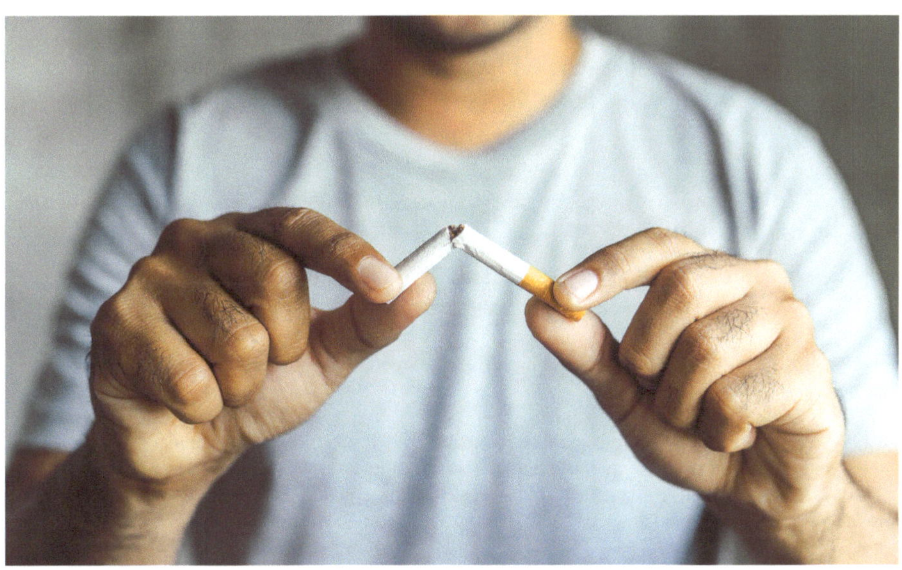

Help with Quitting Smoking

Quitting smoking isn't easy. In fact, nicotine is thought to be as addictive as heroin and cocaine.* But you must stop all forms of tobacco use before surgery. While most people quit cold turkey, there are some powerful pharmacologic agents to help you quit:

- **Nicotine patches** (NicoDerm) and **nicotine gum** (Nicorette) are available without a prescription. These agents occupy nicotine receptors in your brain to help you wean off the nicotine in cigarettes. Some people claim that vaping nicotine may help them transition off other tobacco products; we really don't know this, and we are generally advising that people avoid vaping—particularly in the setting of COVID-19.

  Be alert that all these nicotine replacement products will cause vasoconstriction (constriction of the blood vessels) and impair your ability to heal. In addition, nicotine changes your carboxy-hemoglobin receptors, allowing carbon monoxide to attach to your hemoglobin molecules more easily than oxygen. Plus, they will show up on a urine test. So, use them to help you stop smoking, but stop all nicotine products several weeks ahead of your surgery.

- **Bupropion** (Wellbutrin) is a prescribed antidepressant that shows excellent efficacy in reducing cravings for cigarettes. It is marketed under the name of Zyban for this purpose. If you struggle with depression, you may experience a double benefit in that the medication may help you stop smoking and alleviate your depression as well.

- **Chantix** (varenicline) is also prescribed specifically for smoking cessation. When a person smokes tobacco, the nicotine from cigarettes occupies nicotinic acetylcholine receptors in the brain. This causes the release of dopamine, which we knew as the "drugs, sex, and rock 'n' roll" neurotransmitter in medical school. The release of dopamine in the brain contributes to an overall sense of well-being.

  When Chantix is used, it occupies the nicotine receptors so that the nicotine from smoking cannot occupy them. This in turn results in less dopamine, providing the overall sense of well-being so smoking doesn't have the same effect it used to. While Chantix doesn't work for everyone, I've had some great results with my patients who've used it. Chantix gives the user a clearly outlined path to quitting. Plus, you do not quit on the first day but rather in a few days or weeks into the course. **

  Pfizer, the maker of Chantix, has discontinued an earlier black box warning cautioning users to report psychiatric symptoms such as mood changes, hostility, agitation, and suicidal ideation. Be alert, nonetheless.

* Vanessa Caceres, "9 Best Ways to Quit Smoking," *US News & World Report*, last reviewed February 12, 2021, https://health.usnews.com/wellness/articles/best-ways-to-quit-smoking.

** Per the Chantix (Varenicline) label: "Approaches to selecting a tobacco quit date: May either choose a fixed quit date (i.e., start varenicline, then quit on day 8) or a flexible quit date (i.e., start varenicline, then quit between days 8 to 35). Alternatively, a gradual quit date (i.e., start varenicline and reduce smoking 50% by week 4, reduce an additional 50% by week 8, and continue reducing with a goal of complete abstinence by week 12) is acceptable (Hajek 2011; Rigotti 2020; manufacturer's labeling)." Please see drugs.com/ppa/varenicline.html.

Chantix is a more expensive medication than bupropion; insurance may not cover it or they may require that you try bupropion first.

Here are some other tools:

- Hypnotherapy helps many people quit smoking.
- 1-800-QUIT-NOW (1-800-784-8669) is a phone number that directs you to Quit Smoking programs in your locale.
- *Allen Carr's Easy Way to Quit Smoking Without Willpower* (November 2019) is a useful book that has helped many of my patients. As with Chantix, Carr doesn't recommend that you stop smoking immediately. Rather, he walks you through the process, preparing you to stop. I've seen his approach work for people who've chain-smoked for decades. Find it online.

When you do quit, quit for good. If you slip, recognize that it happens and quit again. As your life gets better, don't shorten it with a technicality like a smoking-related disease.

Manage Your Weight

If you are overweight or obese, your surgeon will advise you what BMI (body mass index) you must have to qualify for surgery.

- **The BMI is a measurement based on height and weight alone.**
  It has nothing to do with gender. You can Google "BMI calculator" and enter your height and weight to find your own BMI. A BMI of over 30 means you are technically obese; if your BMI is over 40, you are severely obese (formerly and rudely called "morbidly obese") or at least 100 pounds above your ideal body weight. Obesity increases your risk of adverse events occurring during surgery as well as your risk of poor wound healing.
- **Learn now what BMI is specified by your surgeon.**
  That way, you'll have a reasonable time to lose weight before surgery. Certainly, there can be some leeway with a BMI measure. For example, if you are muscular from working out, your BMI will be higher than that of a sedentary person with less muscle. Muscle simply weighs more than fat tissue, and a slightly higher BMI in a well-muscled individual may not increase surgical risk.

  The point is that you need to know the standard set by your surgeon. At the second annual WPATH Live Surgery Training course in February–March 2019, I heard BMI limits of 32 to 35, but several surgeons said they did top surgery on severely obese transmasculine individuals. BMI requirements may vary between vaginoplasty, phalloplasty, and chest reconstruction, and genital surgeries have more stringent requirements. Again, find out your surgeon's requirements and be mindful that surgeons set these standards out of concern for your good outcome.

Help with Weight Loss

Just as with stopping smoking, try to lose weight for good, not just for surgery.

Here are some tips we compiled during a weight loss support group we ran in our practice and others from the National Weight Control Registry (NWCR) (nwcr.ws). The NWCR is helpful, as it tracks the habits of people who have lost a significant amount of weight (66 pounds) and kept it off for a significant time (5.5 years).

- Plan to do some exercise nearly every day; walking is the most popular among long-term members of National Weight Control Registry.
- Eat breakfast regularly.
- Limit TV watching to 10 hours per week.
- The best exercise for you is the one you'll actually do.
- Plan your eating and record your daily food intake.
- Drink water freely.
- Limit alcohol; think of alcohol as having calories without nutritional value.
- Focus on fresh vegetables and fruit (nobody gains weight from carrots) and lean protein.
- Limit, but don't eliminate, treats.
- You may choose to eat "normally" on weekends, for example. But realize that like most of us, you may not have eaten "normally" before.
- Use smaller-size plates; you'll eat less.
- Be realistic: "The best way to lose 10 pounds is to lose 5."
- Weigh yourself at regular intervals and keep track of your progress. Made it to your goal? Use a margin of 2 pounds; if you're up 2 pounds, get back to work!

- **If you need to lose a moderate amount of weight, consider Weight Watchers or Noom.**
  Weight Watchers is logical, easy to do, and flexible, plus it can be done online. If you haven't done the program for a while, there have been many recent changes (weightwatchers.com). Noom is quite new and features online and group participation (noom.com).
- **Look at Kathy Abascal's To Quiet Inflammation plan (tqidiet.com).**
  Abascal focuses on portion balance: two-thirds of any size plate is for vegetables and fruit, and no more than one-sixth of the plate is for protein or whole grains. She conducts in-person and online classes. It's a reasonable approach to healthy eating; many followers of the plan report that they lose weight and have fewer symptoms attributable to inflammation, such as skin rashes, joint aching, and bowel irritability.
- **Search for information on the Mediterranean diet for weight loss or maintenance.**

- **If your BMI is over 40 and you have already tried every conceivable way to control your weight, consult a bariatric surgeon.**
  Most people trying gastric bypass surgeries will lose around 100 pounds. There *are* people who learn to "eat around" the constraints of a gastric bypass and gain the weight back. But it may be the most successful route to controlling weight-related conditions such as diabetes and its many complications, degenerative joint disease, and certain cardiopulmonary conditions.[43]

Address Your Alcohol Intake

Excessive alcohol use can complicate your surgical and postoperative course. Be honest with your surgeon about how much alcohol you use, and tell your surgeon if you have alcohol withdrawal symptoms when you stop drinking (shaking, tremors, fever, DTs, hallucinations, and so on). Certainly, it's best to get the use of alcohol other recreational substances under control now if they represent problems for you.

Know Your STI (STD) Status

If you know you have HIV or another blood-borne sexually transmitted infection such as hepatitis B or C, tell your surgeon for their protection. (Of course, all healthcare providers use universal precautions to prevent themselves from becoming infected, but I think disclosing this information is a simple courtesy.) If you are concerned that you may be infected, find out now so you can be completely assessed prior to surgery.

Allow at Least a Year for Hair Removal If Your Surgeon Requires Hair Removal for Genital Surgery (Vaginoplasty or Phalloplasty)

One of my clients recommends 18 months to 2 years for phalloplasty hair removal. Why is this necessary? We can see hair growing in the neovagina postoperatively, as the scrotum is used to construct the vagina. (Is hair in the vagina world-ending? Probably not, but it's hardly the desired outcome. It can also cause odor, irritation, and decreased vaginal depth if a clump of hair rests in the vaginal vault.)

Q **If some of my genital hair grows back, does it mean I had poor treatments?**

A **Not necessarily; there are simply *so* many hairs there, including hairs under the surface that may not have been visible during treatment.**

With phalloplasty, hair must be removed from the donor site (such as the forearm, anterior lateral thigh, or back). If it is not removed, hair may grow on the outside of the phallus, or worse, inside the urethra where it is even more difficult to remove. Hair in the urethra can be dense enough to reduce the flow of urine or cause postvoid dribbling. The hair can also react with urine to form tiny concretions that reduce urine flow. See "Facial Hair and Hair Removal" in Chapter 8. Be sure to check with your surgeon to see which method of hair removal (such as electrolysis versus laser) they prefer. Know also that not all surgeons require hair removal prior to vaginoplasty.

43 Maurizio De Luca et al., "Indications for Surgery for Obesity and Weight-Related Diseases: Position Statements from the International Federation for the Surgery of Obesity and Metabolic Disorders (IFSO)," *Obesity Surgery* 26, no. 8 (July 2016): 1659–96, https://doi.org/10.1007/s11695-016-2271-4.

Dr. Richard Santucci cautions that 2 years of hair removal may serve as a barrier for people seeking phalloplasty. He encourages people to do several cycles of hair removal, but not to delay surgery to get a year or two of electrolysis completed. He reports seeing some hair growth occurring even with conscientious removal.

Optimize Your Physical Fitness

It makes sense that a physically fit body can respond to the stresses of surgery and recovery with greater resilience. You don't have to be a jock, but do get some daily physical exercise, even if it's simply walking. Exercise also increases your collateral circulation: extra blood vessels grow to bring more blood to an area, which is particularly important for phalloplasties.

Check Your Immunization Status

Check your immunizations, particularly if you have a chronic illness (such as diabetes, heart disease, or asthma) or if you are traveling out of the country for surgery. You will be expected to update your immunizations as you get closer to surgery. It's not a "one-and-done" matter.

Paying for Your Surgery

Gender-affirming surgeries are expensive. While insurance coverage varies, it is more common than ever to find that gender-affirming surgeries are covered. Larger employers, particularly tech companies, have been leaders in gender-inclusive coverage. Examples include Microsoft, Google, Facebook, Amazon, Boeing, and Starbucks. Many government-funded organizations, such as the University of Washington, the State of Washington, and the City of Seattle, cover gender-affirming surgeries. A variety of other municipalities do also, such as San Francisco, Berkeley, and San Jose.

That said, if you are looking for a job, why *not* share your skills and talents with an employer that fully supports you as an individual? As of this writing, Washington State's Apple Care through the Health Care Authority and Medicare cover gender-affirming surgeries, although their reimbursement may be so low as to limit the number of surgeons who participate.

- The point of the above is to advise you to carefully check your own health insurance before making any assumptions. When you contact your health insurance company, use the customer service contact information on your insurance card but also ask to speak with a representative who deals with transgender coverage. You may save yourself time, frustration, and misinformation. Insurance may cover presurgical hair removal, so ask!
- Read your insurance plan carefully. You are generally responsible for paying the deductible amount specified by the plan. Then you may have to pay a percentage of the surgery cost.
- If you have an accountant, check to see what noncovered surgical or presurgical expenses (such as hair removal) you may declare for tax purposes.

- If you have a health savings account or a cafeteria plan available as a benefit from your employer, you may be able to use pretax dollars to pay for your portion of a gender-affirming surgery.[44]

Find a Trans-Advocacy Legal Organization to Help You Understand Your Insurance and Get Your Surgery Covered

When attorney Noah Lewis was a student at Harvard Law School, he was able to get his *own* gender-affirming surgery covered, although it had been previously excluded from the Harvard policy. Lewis went on to establish the nonprofit organization Transcend Legal with the aim of helping others get insurance approval for gender-affirming care by appealing adverse decisions and overcoming roadblocks. Lewis produced an informative video series to help individuals understand and navigate the health insurance maze. While Transcend Legal has closed, you can still find Lewis's video series on YouTube (**youtube.com/channel/UC8ufMm0N1n3JjRpJtAuGgPA/playlists**).

Noah Lewis is now affiliated with the Transgender Legal Defense and Education Fund, a 501(c)(3) nonprofit organization "committed to ending discrimination based upon gender identity and expression and to achieving equality for transgender people through public education, test-case litigation, direct legal services, and public policy efforts." While the organization deals with a variety of trans discrimination issues, individuals wishing information regarding insurance denials may contact TLDEF at **tldef.org.**

Surgery Itself Is Only *One* Expense

Remember that the cost of surgery itself represents only a portion of the cost of having surgery. Here are some other expenses that you may incur that are unlikely to be covered by insurance:

- **Living expenses for the time of surgery, the time off for recovery, and postoperative visits.**
    - You may buy more prepared or take-out food.
    - You may pay someone to help you with cleaning or personal care.
    - You may have expenses for items such as wound dressings, pads, or other items you use postoperatively.
    - You may incur rideshare expenses such as Uber, Lyft, or a taxi if you are unable to drive for a while.
- **Travel expenses for yourself (and a travel partner) if your surgeon is not local.**
    - You may have to stay in a hotel or Airbnb when you are not in the hospital. Your travel partner will have additional room and board expenses while your meals and so on are covered in the hospital.
    - If you have a complication after returning home from surgery, it may be difficult to find a local surgeon willing or qualified to help you. Consider having a reserve for extra expenses of traveling back to your original surgeon if additional surgery is needed.

44 "Transition-related medical care is eligible with consumer-directed healthcare accounts, which was a result of the United States Tax Court's 2010 decision in *O'Donnabhain v. Commissioner* which ruled that a transgender woman's medical expenses for hormone therapy and sex reassignment surgery were legitimate treatments for GID and therefore tax-deductible under Federal law. As a result of this pivotal court decision, on November 21, 2011, the Internal Revenue Service (IRS) affirmed that transgender people can deduct the costs of hormone therapy and sex reassignment surgery from their gross income as medical expenses for the treatment of gender identity disorder (GID)." FSA Store, "Transgender Counseling or Surgery: FSA Eligibility," accessed July 28, 2021, https://fsastore.com/FSA-Eligibility-List/T/Transgender-Counseling-or-Surgery-E717.aspx.

- If you are planning to travel out of the country, are there country-specific costs that you might expect? (Don't forget to get immunized prior to leaving the country if this is appropriate. For that matter, update your immunizations even if your surgeon is only a block away.)
- Additional costs for people who depend on your income, such as childcare costs.

Other Ways to Help Cover Surgical and Nonsurgical Costs (Besides Insurance)

You may have to be creative here, and you may not have great options. But here are some options my patients have used:

- **Benefits from an employer.**
  If you have a health savings account or a cafeteria plan available as a benefit from your employer, you may be able to use pretax dollars to pay for your portion of a gender-affirming surgery.[45]
- **Tax benefits.**
  If you have an accountant, check to see what noncovered surgical or presurgical expenses (such as hair removal, travel, and medical supplies) you may declare for tax purposes. This saves you money, but after the fact. Save receipts so you can deduct these costs.
- **Military veterans and active duty personnel.**
  When President Donald Trump tweeted a ban on transgender military service on July 26, 2017, surgeon Dr. Christine McGinn countered that she would offer gender-reassignment surgery pro bono for active duty military personnel. Dr. McGinn confirmed that her Papillon Center (**drchristinemcginn.com**) offers a 15 percent discount on surgical fees for veterans and that she provides pro bono surgery for active duty military personnel.[46] Dr. McGinn, a former Navy flight surgeon, stated in her CNN interview, "If the commander-in-chief won't take care of our veterans, our veterans will." Watch the interview in its entirety at **cnn.com/videos/tv/2017/07/29/trans-ex-navy-surgeon-on-trumps-ban.cnn**.

  On June 19, 2021, the Department of Veterans Affairs announced a reversal of this ban and that gender-affirmation surgery will be covered for military veterans.[47] Hormones and mental health therapy have been provided for some time. Veterans are advised to watch for details in this very recent development.

> **To transgender Americans across the country—especially the young people who are so brave—I want you to know your President has your back.**
>
> **During Pride Month—and all the time.**
>
> — *President Biden, @POTUS, 4:31 PM, June 7, 2021*

45 FSA Store, "Transgender Counseling or Surgery: FSA Eligibility," accessed July 28, 2021, https://fsastore.com/FSA-Eligibility-List/T/Transgender-Counseling-or-Surgery-E717.aspx.

46 Dr. Christine McGinn, email message to the author, September 29, 2019.

47 Meryl Kornfield, "VA Plans to Offer Gender-Confirmation Surgery to Transgender Veterans, Reversing Ban," *The Washington Post*, June 19, 2021, https://www.washingtonpost.com/national-security/2021/06/19/veterans-gender-affirmation-surgery/.

- **Some surgeons offer a significant discount for clients who pay cash.**
  One practice offers a 65 percent cash discount on surgical fees. Ask in advance.

- **Family members may help.**
  For some, this option will be clearly out of reach. But think about your parents and grandparents; they *may* be delighted to help you with your expenses. They may be gracious enough to gift you the funds, but never *assume* they will. Structure any funding as a *loan* that you pay back at fair terms. If you are young enough to be covered by your parents' insurance (usually up to but not including age 26), use it. Expect to do the footwork to find out what's provided.

- **Run a GoFundMe campaign to raise money for your expenses.**
  GoFundMe is a trans-supportive organization that provides an Internet platform for all kinds of fundraising. (GoFundMe has raised a collective $5 billion for various causes over their 8 years in operation, including $27 million within 30 days sent directly to folks impacted by Hurricane Harvey.) You can tell your story internationally and raise money from people who earnestly want you to meet your goal.

  There's no fee to list your plea on a GoFundMe platform and it is simple to set up. Beyond that, GoFundMe takes 2.9 percent of each donation in addition to a 30-cent fee per credit or debit transaction. *You keep the rest of the funds raised.* (On Kickstarter, conversely, you state a dollar goal but keep nothing if you don't make the goal. On GoFundMe, you keep whatever you raise, minus the fees.) You'll find a helpful blog post titled "The Ultimate Fundraising Guide for Gender Confirmation Surgery" at **gofundme.com/c/blog/gender-confirmation-surgery**.

- **Apply for a grant from one of these three organizations:**
  The **Jim Collins Foundation** (**jimcollinsfoundation.org**) provides financial assistance to fund gender-affirming surgeries for qualified applicants. Tony Ferraiolo and Dru LeVasseur started the foundation in 2008 in honor of Jim Collins, who was a licensed clinical social worker and clinical instructor in the department of psychiatry at the Yale School of Medicine. According to the Foundation website, Jim was "an avid supporter and ally to the transgender community, advocating for the right of all people to live their lives with honesty and passion." The foundation receives funds from thousands of individual donors and has been fortunate to use the pro bono services of Drs. Marci Bowers, Christine McGinn, and E. Antonio Mangubat. Applicants must be 18 years of age by the end of the foundation's annual grant cycle. Complete an application online.

  Point of Pride (**pointofpride.org**) is an outgrowth of Point 5cc, a clothing and accessory company that contributes 20 percent of its proceeds to provide funding assistance to trans and nonbinary people needing surgery. In 2016, Point of Pride branched off from the parent organization, becoming its own 501 (c)(3) nonprofit organization. It offers the following programs: their Annual Transgender Surgery Fund, a free chest binder program, a free trans femme shapewear program, and an electrolysis support program. Point of Pride has served thousands of trans folks in all 50 states and over 50 countries in meaningful, life-changing ways.

  Genderbands (**genderbands.org**) is a Utah-based nonprofit founded in 2015 to pay for the founder's top surgery. Now the organization funds gender-related surgeries for others. Genderbands receives sponsorships from several surgeons performing transgender care, sells merchandise, and offers support and social groups for the trans and gender-nonconforming community.

- **Raise money by selling things you don't need.**

Many online services allow you to sell your unneeded things for cash. Investigate OfferUp, letgo, eBay, Facebook Marketplace, thredUP, and Poshmark for selling good used clothing, or Craigslist. Maybe you have an old musical instrument or a car that would bring in some money. Sports trading cards, autographs, and other collectibles may mean less to you now that you're considering gender-affirming surgery. Even old furniture and clothing add up. You take a photo of the item you're selling, write a description, and set a price. Obviously, take *extreme* care if you are having people you don't know come to your home!

- **Get a part-time job.**
  Just when life is complicated enough, do you have time and a vehicle to allow you to drive for Uber or Lyft? Could you add a less-demanding part-time job to bring in some extra cash? Some part-time positions (such as Starbucks) offer health benefits that may cover your surgery.

- **Consider a personal loan.**
  Consider this option only with great caution. Be even more careful if you consider using a credit card. These ideas may lead you into financial hell, meaning poor credit or even bankruptcy. So, be certain about your choices here. Talk to someone you trust, such as a financial advisor who doesn't stand to profit through your decisions.

- **Consider a home equity loan if you have property.**
  Be extremely cautious if you consider this option. A home equity loan or home equity line of credit can be very risky territory. A default on this loan could result in the loss of your home.

- **Use CareCredit.**
  Our office and a variety of surgeons' offices offer CareCredit. This company allows qualified individuals to borrow money for medical procedures. Just be sure you pay it back *quickly*, or the interest rate accelerates over time, increasing the total that you owe.

Choosing Your Surgeon

Choosing a surgeon who is a good match for you is critical. It goes without saying that your surgeon must be competent—preferably excellent. But you want someone who communicates well with you, too. How do you judge? Here are some pointers.

- **Ask your own friends, healthcare provider, or therapist for some names to get you started.**

- **Look up surgeons' names and contact information through WPATH.**
  Then visit their websites and see how they present their services (**wpath.org**). Or in Seattle, check Ingersoll Gender Center's site (**ingersollgendercenter.org**).

- **Ask trans friends and contacts for information on their surgical experiences.**
  Many individuals may be willing to tell you about their experiences or even show you their results. (Of course, we are talking about consenting adults here.) Online contacts through Reddit and through monitored, invitational trans sites may also be helpful to you. Look up transgender surgeries on YouTube and Instagram as well.

- **Go to conferences; many surgeons attend national and regional transgender conferences.**
  Check out the Philadelphia Trans Wellness Conference held every summer, Gender Odyssey (originally in Seattle, but in San Diego starting in 2019), Gender Spectrum in Oakland, First Event in

Boston, Keystone in Pennsylvania, Esprit in the Pacific Northwest, and regional events held by the UCSF Transgender Center of Excellence or by WPATH (wpath.org).[48]

At these conferences, you may have the opportunity to hear a surgeon speak, see slides of their work, and ask them questions directly. Sometimes, they will even arrange an informal consultation with you. This will give you an idea of the surgeon's personality, their willingness to answer questions, and how you feel about them. (A surgeon doesn't have to be your buddy, but you should have a sense that they are sincere and have your best interests at heart. If your gut says, "I can't work with this surgeon," don't.) If you cannot attend these conferences, browse the conference websites to see which surgeons have served as financial sponsors of the event. That's not necessarily a cause for an endorsement, but it's another clue.

- **Read online reviews of different physicians.**
  Keep in mind that all physicians get "Yelped" from time to time and reviewers aren't always kind or fair. A reviewer may blast a doctor without the benefit of knowing or explaining the whole story. I've seen some vicious reviews written about outstanding surgeons.

Ask the surgeons you're researching or their surgical coordinator if they can put you in touch with one or more of their former patients who would be willing to share their experiences with you.

- **Verify that your surgeon is board-certified.**
  In general, surgeons have completed medical school (generally for 4 years after graduating from college) and a residency (an additional 4 to 10-plus years of surgical training). They may have done a specialized fellowship for a year or longer in addition to that. The American Board of Medical Specialties certifies physicians through their inclusion requirements, CME (continuing medical education) requirements, and periodic recertification examinations. A surgeon may approach sexual reassignment surgery from a variety of disciplines: gynecology, urology, plastic surgery, and others. We are now beginning to see fellowships in transgender surgery, such as the Mount Sinai Program in New York City.

- **Research completely.**
  While board certification is a good place to start in your search, go a little further. Ask about your surgeon's education, training, and experience in the procedure you want to have. Ask how long they have been offering the procedure and how many they have performed. A surgeon may be board-certified, but if they perform a specific surgery only occasionally, you may want to continue your search until you are comfortable that your surgeon will deliver the results you want. As stated, we are beginning to see fellowships in transgender medicine and surgery, but it's still early. (At my alma mater, the University of Washington School of Medicine, transgender medicine is still offered as an elective course.)

- **Be aware that volume and experience can make a difference in quality.**

48 Gender Spectrum holds an annual gender conference each July that is particularly popular among trans youth and families. It has grown annually and now attracts hundreds.

Expanding on the point above, research in other surgeries (such as coronary artery bypass grafts, bariatric surgeries, and breast cancer surgeries) has established that surgical volume correlates with better outcomes.[49] According to Dr. Richard Santucci, the Crane Center reported performing a total of 108 phalloplasties and 140 vaginoplasties in 2018 alone. Not a single patient had to go back for a vascular emergency. This is impressive, considering that some centers may do only a few phalloplasties per year.

- **Find a surgeon who knows and works with the trans community.**
  Make sure the surgeon knows the community, uses appropriate vocabulary, and doesn't ask unnecessarily prying questions. Try to make sure your surgeon understands the many issues that trans people encounter. You may learn this by talking to former patients, reading reviews, or getting a "gut sense" when you hear them speak.

> **I had a trans male patient who needed a urologic consultation for recurrent urinary tract infections. The patient had had a metoidioplasty but not a urethral extension. He, therefore, didn't pee through the phallus—but rather through his urethra just underneath it. It was certainly appropriate that the urologist sort out the revised anatomy, but my patient was devastated when the urologist asked, "So, you mean the penis is just for show then?"**
>
> **I'm certain this remark was not intended to injure the patient, but it may have reflected a lack of trans competence. Fortunately, the patient was able to process the remark as a lack of sensitivity on the part of the physician rather than reflective of some personal inadequacy of his own.**
>
> *— Linda Gromko, MD*

- **Check with the surgeon's department of medical licensing.**
  A doctor must be licensed in the state in which they practice. Be certain that the surgeon's license is current and that there haven't been disciplinary actions taken or pending. Even this may not be a deal breaker, but wouldn't you want to know if your surgeon's license had been suspended?

- **Research and understand the potential complications associated with the surgery you are planning.**
  Some surgeons are very open and willing to share their own complication rates for specific surgeries. (If the surgeon says they have had no complications, that's your clue to find a different surgeon.) No surgery is without risk. So, how does a surgeon manage complications that do arise? Many surgeons give patients their personal contact information, like a cell phone number, to use during the postoperative period, or they provide the number for an on-call physician.

- **Make a list of pluses and minuses about that surgeon and their approach after you've met with them and had a face-to-face consultation.**

---

49 Johannes Morche, Tim Mathes, and Dawid Pieper, "Relationship between Surgeon Volume and Outcomes: A Systematic Review of Systematic Reviews," *Systematic Reviews* 5, no. 1 (November 2016): 1, https://doi.org/10.1186/s13643-016-0376-4.

But then, give your heart a vote. How did you feel about this person? How did you feel about the staff? Were there nonverbal messages, like being treated rudely, being put on hold forever, or having your paperwork lost? All of these experiences reflect on the surgeon who sets the tone for the culture in the office. Were they trans-friendly and trans-sensitive? Most importantly, would you want your parent, spouse, or child to be in their care?

Getting Your Presurgery Letters

If you are arranging a gender-affirming surgery, your health insurance company and your surgeon will require letters of support from one or more healthcare professionals. These letters ensure that a candidate for surgery (patient) meets the Standards of Care as set forth by the World Professional Association for Transgender Health (WPATH). WPATH is a nonprofit, interdisciplinary professional and educational organization devoted to the health of transgender and gender-diverse persons. The most recent Standards of Care (SOC-8) were released on July 15, 2022. Download the new Standards of Care (SOC-8) free at **WPATH.org/publications/soc**.

You will find that WPATH Standards are offered as "recommendations" rather than firm requirements. Health insurance companies tend to accept the WPATH Standards of Care, however, and require letters based on these standards. Letter requirements vary among health insurance companies and surgeons.

Practical Pointers to Help You Get Your Letters

- Specific health insurance providers—and specific surgeons—will have their own letter requirements. Know what these requirements are *in your situation*, so you will not face last-minute barriers.
- Genital surgeries tend to require more letters from providers than do breast modifications, facial surgeries, or body contouring. When two letters are required, one letter is to be from a mental health therapist of master's level training. Another may be required from a mental health provider at the MD or PhD level (i.e., a psychiatrist or psychologist).
- Letters must be current, i.e., within one year of the surgical date. If not, your surgeon will require a more up-to-date letter.
- A letter from your hormone prescriber may be required by surgeons and insurance companies. Unless your hormone prescriber is very experienced in writing such letters, you cannot expect them to know what is required. Here is a template that may help: **transline.zendesk.com/hc/en-us/articles/229372788-Surgery-Sample-Letter**.
- More letters will be required for adolescent candidates, as will parental consent (see SOC-8, Statement 13.7).
- More letters will be required for candidates seeking individually customized or "nonstandard" surgeries (see SOC-8, Statement 13.8).

The WPATH Standards of Care ensure that a surgical candidate (patient) is likely to have a positive outcome from a requested surgery. Refer to Appendix D in SOC-8. The Standards also delineate the credentials of the surgeon, ensuring that the surgeon is qualified to perform gender-affirming surgeries. The Standards protect both surgeons and patients. (Refer to WPATH SOC-8, Statement 13.1 for surgeons' credentials.)

Facial surgery is now designated by WPATH as a gender-affirming surgical procedure (see Appendix E in WPATH SOC-8), as are many other surgeries that were not previously covered by insurance. If facial surgery is being done to manage gender dysphoria, the diagnosis must be supported. For a thorough account of the literature surrounding the medical necessity of facial surgery for trans women, see the Transgender Legal Defense and Education Fund's review.[50]

If you do not have a mental health therapist now, this is a good time to find a therapist who will write a letter in support of your having gender-affirming surgery. And since you are about to have a major life event, it might not hurt to have a therapist waiting in the wings. Google "mental health therapists who work with transgender people" in your area.

The Critical 6 Weeks Prior to Surgery

A multitude of things must be clarified, arranged, and purchased before your surgery. Hopefully, you will have a chance to read this chapter before the last minute. Use this as a checklist if it helps.

Confirm Logistical Arrangements with Your Surgeon's Office

- ❑ Double-check the date and time of your surgery.
- ❑ Confirm your arrival time at the surgical facility. Record the facility's address and phone number.
- ❑ Most surgeons require a preoperative visit to go over detailed post-op instructions, write prescriptions needed after surgery (medications for pain and nausea, and typically an antibiotic to prevent infection). Some may show you the post-op dressings and how to use them.
- ❑ Confirm that payment arrangements and insurance billing are in order.
- ❑ Find out how long you are expected to stay in the hospital or if the surgery is considered an "outpatient" or a "day surgery" where you go home on the same day of the operation.
- ❑ If you are traveling out of town for surgery, confirm the length of time the surgeon requires you to stay in town after your surgery for follow-up care.
- ❑ Confirm whether your surgeon has arrangements with an inn, local recovery house, or hotel where you will stay during your convalescence.
    - ❑ If you are to be supervised by someone during your stay at a hotel or inn, find out if the person caring for you has medical or nursing credentials. (Just know what to expect.)

50 Transgender Legal Defense and Education Fund, *Medical Necessity of Facial Gender Reassignment Surgery for Transgender Women: Literature Review*, Washington, DC: Transgender Legal Defense and Education Fund, September 10, 2020, https://transhealthproject.org/documents/34/Facial_surgery_medical_necessity_literature_review.pdf.

    - ❑ Remember also that you must be medically stable enough to go to an inn or hotel. Do not cut corners on your early postoperative recovery or allow someone else to suggest that you do.
    - ❑ Surgeons often say that undergoing surgery is not the difficult part; recovery is. Don't risk jeopardizing your results.
- ❑ If you are staying out of town, find out if you yourself must arrange for a recovery facility or care providers outside the hospital.
- ❑ Record the name, phone number, and email address for your surgeon's contact person, which is who you'll contact if you have routine questions or concerns before or after surgery.
- ❑ Learn how to access the surgeon or their on-call person in an urgent situation. What is their emergency contact phone number and who will you be reaching?

Confirm Medical Arrangements with Your Surgeon's Office

- ❑ Ask the office staff if you need special tests from your primary care provider prior to surgery (such as an EKG, blood tests, and an HIV test).
- ❑ Ask if you will need a preoperative physical exam by your primary care provider. (Is there a form provided for that? How close to the day of surgery should it be completed? Or, how far in advance of the surgery may it be done?)
- ❑ Ask when you are supposed to stop medications prior to surgery and clarify which medications you are supposed to stop.

It is a universal rule to not take aspirin for 10 days prior to surgery. Aspirin impairs your platelet function and can impair your blood clotting ability. NSAIDs (nonsteroidal anti-inflammatories like ibuprofen or naproxen sodium) must also be stopped ahead of time, as must vitamin E supplements.

- ❑ Check with your surgeon's office regarding hormones. Many surgeons will specify no hormones for 2 weeks prior to surgery, but others do not. Know your surgeon's recommendations.
- ❑ Ask when you can have your last electrolysis appointment prior to surgery. (About 2 to 4 weeks is common, but check with the surgeon's office.)
- ❑ Find out what equipment and supplies you will need to buy ahead of time, such as sanitary protection for trans male and trans female surgery or sterile lubricant for dilation (vaginal dilators are provided by the surgeon).
- ❑ Learn the specifics of bowel prep prior to surgery. (This is a regimen of laxatives to clean out the bowel, common in any abdominal or genitourinary surgery.)
- ❑ Find out if there a cancellation list so you may have your surgery earlier if someone else cancels.

- ❑ Ask if there is anything you can do to prepare yourself and your living space for recovery (see Chapter 12).
- ❑ Ask if your surgeon recommends making post-op arrangements for pelvic floor physical therapy. This modality helps people with urinary, bowel, and sexual function after gender-affirming surgery. Ask for a referral.

Dr. Bowers's Recommendations on Stopping Hormones before Surgery

For years, it was considered gospel that all patients undergoing gender-affirming surgeries would stop HRT 6 weeks before surgery. In general, they arrived miserable and basically in menopause or with recurrence of androgenic symptoms. This was never questioned until more contemporary surgeons challenged this notion as lacking evidence and allowed patients to drop to a baseline level of hormone replacement therapy, usually 6 weeks prior to surgery, and proceed with some intraoperative preventative measures such as pneumatic compression devices (sequential compression devices) and low-molecular-weight heparin (Lovanox). Patients were considerably happier and rates of thromboembolism were unaltered.

— Marci Bowers, MD

Note: Follow your own surgeon's advice, of course, but Dr. Bowers's comments may stimulate discussion. Madeline Deutsch, MD, of the University of California-San Francisco, echoed Dr. Bowers' comments in her presentation, "Should Estrogen Be Discontinued Prior to Surgery?," presented at the WPATH 26th Scientific Symposium Surgeon's Program on November 6, 2020.

In a review of available literature on the subject, Deutsch concluded that was no scientific evidence to support routinely stopping estradiol before surgery. (She clarified that ethinyl estradiol commonly used in birth control pills does have a higher rate of blood clotting events.)

- ❑ Ask if there are written post-op instruction sheets that you can read ahead of time. (It really does matter that you follow them. Surgery is a partnership between you, your family, your primary care providers, your surgeon, and the surgical team. Everybody must do their part to keep you safe and comfortable, and to allow you to achieve the best results possible.)
- ❑ Make a list of your medications to take with you. Note the dose of your medication, the dosing schedule (how often you are supposed to take the medicine), and know why you are taking your medications. (Know this information in advance; your providers cannot know what your "little yellow pill" is.) Some people photograph their medication labels. It doesn't matter how you do this, but take the information with you.
- ❑ Most importantly, make a list of allergies and medications you are allergic to so you can inform your medical staff.

- ❑ Get a copy of your EKG to take with you if you happen to have a known heart problem and your primary care provider has taken an EKG. (An old EKG is golden if you have cardiac or respiratory symptoms; comparing the old EKG with a current one provides extremely useful information.)

> ***For facial surgery, hair removal must be stopped 1 month before surgery and cannot be started for 3 months after facial surgery.*** **With the very few infections we've ever had in head and neck surgery (and with maybe one exception), all the patients had electrolysis or laser hair removal within a few months of surgery. Pseudomonas and other bacteria that seem to peacefully coexist within hair follicles don't bode very well if they escape by manipulating the follicle and seeding the circulatory system (during electrolysis, it is possible for bacteria in the skin or hair follicles to move into the bloodstream and cause serious infections).**
>
> *— Jordan Deschamps-Braly, MD*

Confirm Your Travel Arrangements

- ❑ Confirm your hotel or Airbnb reservations.
- ❑ Confirm airline, bus, and train tickets for you and your travel partner.
- ❑ Update immunizations (refer to page 174 in Chapter 10).
- ❑ Confirm that you have your travel documents, such as a driver's license, a US passport, or other appropriate documents for international travel (see Chapter 20).
- ❑ Obtain a "carry letter" if you need one. If you are carrying injectable medications, needles, and syringes, you are advised to get a carry letter from your primary care physician. (I write these on my prescription pad or office stationery, stating that "John Doe is my medical patient and requires injected hormones to treat a medical condition. Therefore, the patient is required to carry the medication, and needles and syringes for administration during travel.")

Confirm Work Arrangements

- ❑ Have you notified your direct supervisor and your human resources department that you will be gone? It's important to consider what information you are giving and to whom; you can be discreet about personal information. Does your company require a note from your healthcare provider? Is a note required for you to return to work?
- ❑ Do you need to arrange for Family and Medical Leave Act (FMLA) paperwork? The FMLA may apply to you if your company employs at least 50 people and you have worked there for 12 months (see **dol.gov/general/topic/benefits-leave/fmla**). FMLA applies to workers in the private sector (provided that the above conditions are met), the government or public sector, or in public or private primary or secondary schools, regardless of the number of workers. FMLA allows you to be away from work due to illness, injury, or surgery—in you or a family member—for up to 12 work weeks. *The FMLA*

does not provide for pay, but it does ensure that you will have your prior job or a comparable one on your return. If you have a travel partner who qualifies for FMLA to care for you, they may apply for FMLA at their workplace also.

Your primary care physician (or your surgeon) is often the one who completes the paperwork. In my office, I do this with the patient sitting right there so there's no question how the absence is represented.

- ❑ Have you confirmed with your employer whether you qualify for sick leave or personal time off, or possibly short-term disability if it is provided by your company? If there is short-term disability, know that it comes with its own raft of paperwork. Don't be caught short because you didn't know.

Being Discreet

Be alert that if you are not "out" with respect to gender issues, your human resources department or supervisor could out you. While I'm not a proponent of lying, your privacy is critical. Here are some examples that have worked for patients of mine when they were asked for specifics:

"I'm having some female surgery." You may find that your supervisor will become embarrassed and look away. Of course, it isn't their business. And you do not have to give them specifics.

"This is quite private, but I'm having a birth defect corrected. I'd appreciate your being discreet about this." Again, it's not their business. If they feel compelled to ask for details, respond, "Like I said, its private. I really can't discuss it further." Or, "This is a painful matter for me to discuss." Say nothing more.

If you are having facial surgery, you won't be able to hide this during your recovery or when you return to work. If you're in a trans-friendly workplace, consider telling a few of your allies what's going on; you don't want to be the target of gossip when you return.

One of my patients was arranging return-to-work details with her employer, a large software company. She was very concerned about having to perform vaginal dilation three to four times per day—but her workplace was trans-friendly and did know the details of her upcoming absence.

So, she asked if her company might provide a quiet room with a recliner and a locked door for the purpose of dilating at work, but in private. The company was happy to oblige. After all, nursing mothers frequently have a private place to pump their breasts after they give birth.

— Linda Gromko, MD

Other Preoperative Considerations

Most of the people I treat are very excited before their surgeries; many are anxious. I think any range of emotions would be completely normal before a gender-affirmation surgery. Allow yourself some time and room for whatever emotional reaction you have.

It is important to think about your own postoperative care well in advance. If you are having a genital surgery where people won't be able to see what you've had done, you would likely get more sympathy and unsolicited support with a cast on your leg! We'll discuss all this in more detail in Chapter 12.

A temporary disabled parking permit may help streamline your postoperative recovery, particularly if you're having a more extensive surgery. You may not need one, but if you do, you'll be grateful you thought of this ahead of time. Download the form for your state's permit and take it to your doctor. (For Washington State, go to dol.wa.gov/vehicleregistration/parkingtemp.html.)

Your healthcare provider will sign this and give you a prescription indicating the diagnosis prompting the need for the parking permit, such as "Needs disability parking placard for postsurgical recovery."

— Linda Gromko, MD

Before you have your surgery, consider the following:

- ❑ Try to get your living space cleaned and organized before you leave; you're starting a new chapter. Change the sheets; wash your towels. Having some control at home can help you move through the disruption easier should you experience that.
- ❑ Buy frozen foods, pantry items, and nutritional snacks in advance—things you can keep in the refrigerator or freezer for when you get home. Know that you need extra protein to heal wounds, even surgically created ones. Think chicken, beef, pork, eggs, protein bars, peanut butter and other nut butters, and Greek yogurt. (Refer to "Postoperative Nutrition" in Chapter 12.)
- ❑ Be prepared in advance with the postoperative supplies. For vaginoplasty, they include sterile lubricant and sanitary protection. For phalloplasty, it's sanitary protection (look at "Guards" in the male sanitary protection aisle, although you may want to have some women's sanitary pads on hand, as the size of the neophallus may be too large for a conventional pad). I have had patients who appreciated having a pack of Depends (disposable incontinence underpants) at home.
- ❑ Have personal care supplies on hand in advance: clean towels and washcloths, baby wipes for cleaning, facial towelettes—anything to make you feel more comfortable.
- ❑ Think ahead about easy clothing to wear. No fancy underwear (you will leak).

- ❑ Buy a pair of knee-high compression hose to wear during flights or long periods of immobility. These prevent swelling and may prevent DVT (blood clot) formation.
- ❑ Look online for a peri bottle if you are having vaginoplasty. This is a plastic bottle with a special nozzle that you fill with warm water to rinse your perineum from front to back. The nozzle is to direct the flow of warm water, not to insert into the neovagina. (Check with your surgeon, of course.)
- ❑ Have perineal ice packs with machine-washable cloth enclosures on hand to provide postvaginoplasty relief (check online).
- ❑ Buy a curved neck pillow to sit on (the kind you find in airport kiosks) if you are having vaginoplasty. This can help keep pressure off the perineum when you're healing. (Some people do find these pillows to be aggravating; don't use one if it bothers you.)
- ❑ Buy a NutriBullet, Vitamix, or other blender that can crush ice cubes, no matter what surgery you're having. This will help you in making high-protein smoothies.

Helping Others Help You

If you are fortunate enough to have a supportive group of people who wants to check on your progress, consider designating a point person for communication. You may not want to handle a barrage of phone calls or texts; your point person can do that. Use a password-protected communication system, like the ones below:

- **Caring Bridge can help you update concerned friends (caringbridge.org).**
  This service enables people to post details about someone dealing with a surgery or illness. All concerned individuals may simply log onto the site with their password. Plus, they can make encouraging comments to support you.
- **Lotsa Helping Hands can help you organize.**
  You may find yourself in the enviable situation of having people who want to help you but don't know how to help you most effectively. If you anticipate needing extended support for meals, rides to appointments, grocery runs, and so on, look at **lotsahelpinghands.com/about-us.** This service allows you or your point person to set up a temporary website in advance to help you coordinate the help that you might need.

Shopping Lists for Surgery

You won't need all of the following, but review this list as you make your own plans.

- ❑ Protein-rich foods (turkey, chicken, beef, tuna, shellfish, peanut butter, cheese, cottage cheese, string cheese, Greek yogurt, eggs, protein bars). If you are a vegan, search online for "high-protein vegan foods" and you'll find plenty of options.
- ❑ High-fiber foods like fruits, vegetables, and bran muffins help to reduce or prevent constipation.
- ❑ Frozen and pantry meals
- ❑ Protein powder for smoothies
- ❑ A blender that can handle ice cubes (NutriBullet, Vitamix, etc.) for making protein smoothies
- ❑ A "grabber" device that allows you to reach items without getting up and moving around (**amazon.com/grabber/s?k=grabber**)
- ❑ Phone chargers with longer-than-usual cords
- ❑ Compression travel stockings from a travel store or airport kiosk
- ❑ A fever thermometer
- ❑ A neck pillow or other travel pillow to sit on
- ❑ A peri bottle for rinsing front to back (get approval from your surgeon first)
- ❑ Extra washcloths and baby wipes
- ❑ Chux pads (also called "incontinence pads," "under pads," or "puppy training pads")
- ❑ Tucks pads for hemorrhoidal care (soothing witch hazel pads for your perineum)
- ❑ Sanitary pads
- ❑ Depend Guards for Men, Depends, or sanitary pads after phalloplasty
- ❑ Sanitary pads and panty liners after vaginoplasty
- ❑ Sterile lubricant (water-based sterile lubricants like Surgilube, Slippery Stuff, or McKesson)
- ❑ Perineal ice packs (look online)
- ❑ Medical and dressing supplies: A comprehensive list of supplies is outlined on the following blog post designed for postphalloplasty care. Many of the supplies listed are appropriate for postvaginoplasty care as well. The list will familiarize you with the various products, and you won't need all of them, but it may help you organize: **myphalloplasty.wordpress.com/2016/09/28/medical-supplies-packing-list** (and compare it with your surgeon's office list).

If you are having a radial forearm phalloplasty, your surgeon may ask you to get a protective garment from a medical supply or burn center. Ask ahead of time if they provide this.

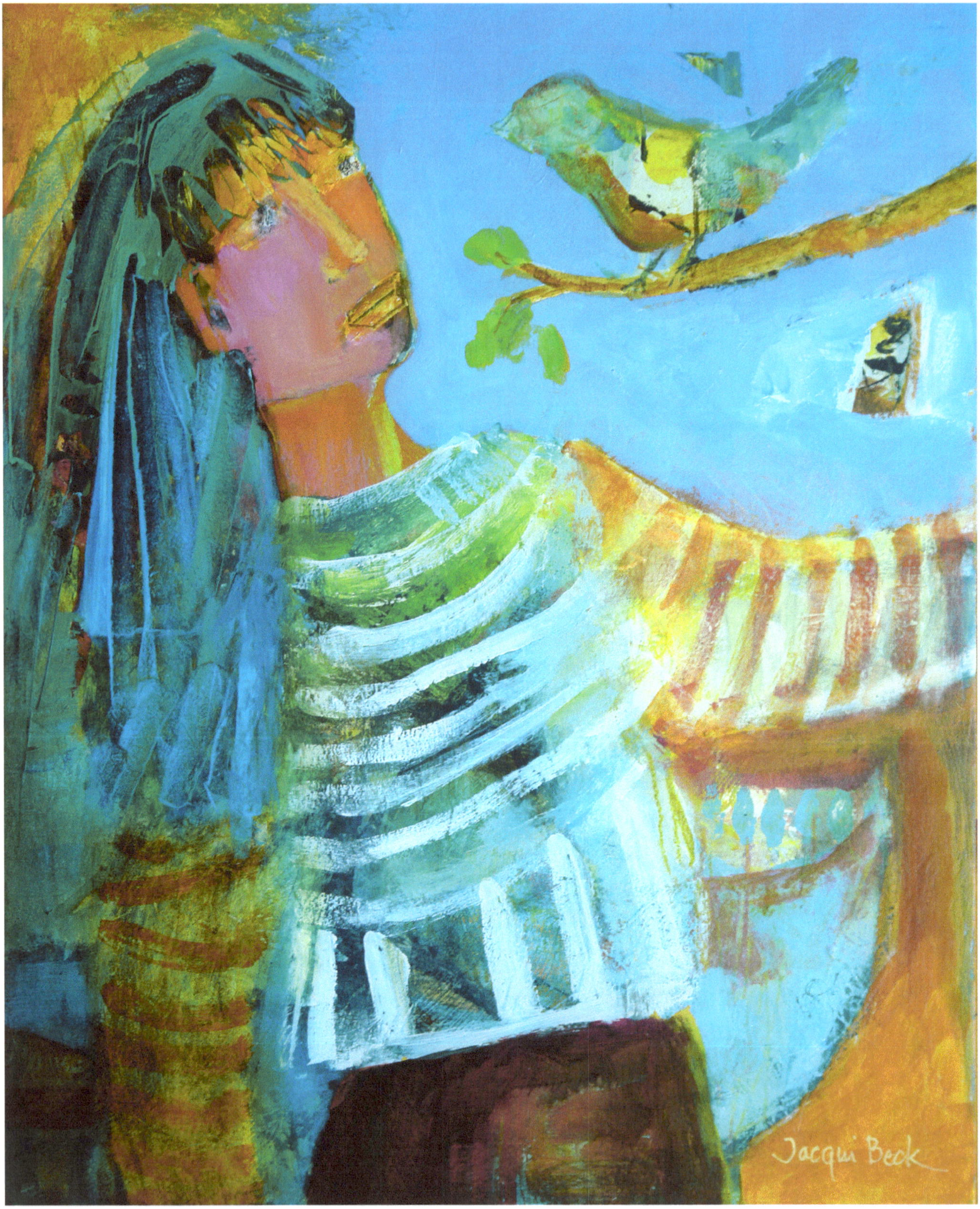

Conversation

CHAPTER 11
The Surgeries Themselves

For no specific reason, we will begin by discussing feminizing surgeries and follow with masculinizing surgeries.

Keep in mind that all surgeons do even the same surgeries slightly differently. If a surgeon has developed a style of doing a procedure, it probably means that they have found specific ways that work best for them and for their patients. *It doesn't mean that one way is right or wrong or that one doctor's approach is the only way to perform a given surgery.*

Surgeons and patients alike can be quite opinionated when it comes to styles of surgery. Just keep an open mind as you read and gather your own questions in advance to prepare yourself in the best way possible.

In this chapter, we will discuss each of the gender-affirming surgeries available (or at least most of them). In Chapter 12, we'll go into the postoperative period in general, emergencies, and postoperative information for specific surgeries.

Disclaimer

The information provided here is intended to give you an overview on gender-affirming surgeries. It is not intended as medical advice for you personally.

For medical advice pertaining to you specifically, seek your answers from your surgeon and their surgical team. They are the obvious professionals who will have the answers pertaining to your body and your circumstances. Information provided by them must be given more weight than my input.

You will also note that I am not including photos of surgical outcomes. They are widely available on the websites of the surgeons.

FEMINIZING SURGERIES

Facial Feminization Surgery

When we think of facial feminization surgery (FFS), it is more accurate to think of FFS as a *collection* of surgeries that feminize the head and neck. Individuals may be advised to have several or all of the surgeries discussed. Changing one area of the face almost always impacts the appearance of adjacent structures and the overall proportions of the face. A surgeon experienced in gender-affirming surgeries will likely appreciate these subtleties and be able to discuss them with you.

As we begin to discuss facial feminization surgery, let's look at the common differences between the facial structure of people assigned male at birth (AMAB) and people assigned female at birth (AFAB). These are the facial features that declare "male" or "female" from across a room. Remember that most people don't work all that hard to figure out another person's gender, but they do respond to reliable, stereotypical clues.

Remember that children's faces start out essentially the same. Assigned male faces develop differently under the influence of testosterone beginning in puberty. Look at the following photos of stereotypically male and female faces, and notice the following differences (we know *nothing* about the gender identity of these models):

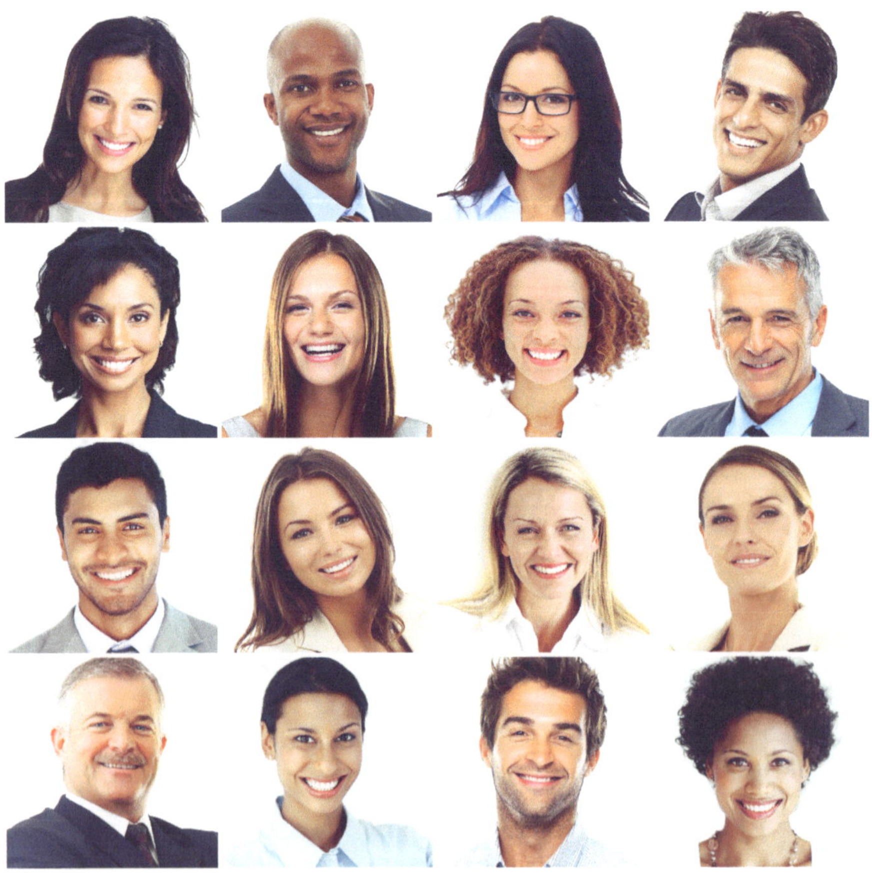

Figure 11.1. Stereotypically male and female faces.

- Brow bones—that is, the bone of the central forehead above and between the brows—tend to be more prominent in males. So are the bones over the outer brow and above the eyes.
- Brows tend to rest lower on the supraorbital ridge (the bony rim on the upper part of the eye socket) in males. In females, the brows appear higher and more arched.
- The male forehead may appear higher or longer from the brow to the hairline.
- The male hairline tends to be squarer or more peaked with less hair in the temples, while a more feminine hairline is rounder in shape.
- A receding hairline or baldness is likely to be read as male.
- Cheekbones are stereotypically less defined in males than in females. This difference is more the result of soft tissue than of bone volume. Other factors, such as racial and genetic differences, may influence cheek structure also.
- The male nose tends to be larger and longer, with males having a less defined tip and females having a slightly curved tip.
- The male upper lip tends to be longer from the bottom of the nose to the top of the lip.
- The male lips (upper and lower) are often less full than in females.
- The male jaw appears larger, broader, and more angular.
- The male chin appears longer, wider, squarer, and more forward than the female chin.
- The Adam's apple may be quite prominent in the male. The Adam's apple is made of thyroid cartilage, and both assigned males and assigned females have them. As with other changes, it is the influence of testosterone that makes the prominent Adam's apple recognizable as a male trait.

> **All of these are general guidelines for attractive males or females who fit within an ideal of aesthetic norms. I think it is helpful to explain that these are not absolute criteria and that a person shouldn't be compelled to change a part of their face that they like or want to preserve. Sometimes they like a feature because it is similar to that of a parent, brother, or sister.**
>
> *— Toby Meltzer, MD*

Examine these photos of the skulls of assigned males and assigned females. You'll spot the bony differences easily.

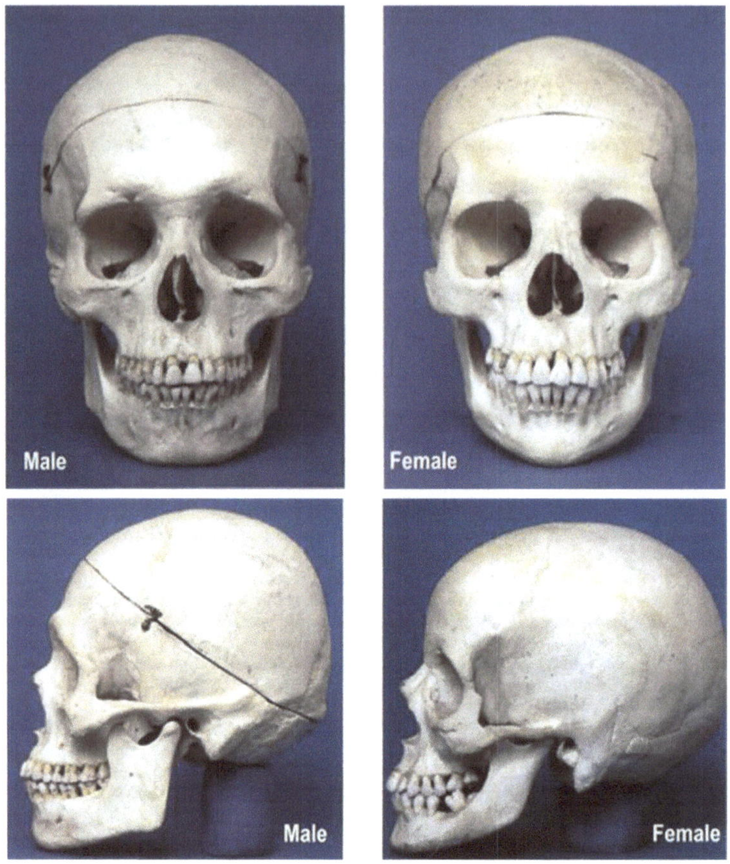

Figure 11.2. Differences in the skulls of assigned males and females.

When you consult a surgeon regarding FFS, the surgeon will examine your facial structures carefully. Images of the face, such as CT scans, CT scans with 3D reconstruction, cephalometric X-rays, or MRI scans, may be used to define your facial bones precisely. Your surgeon may ask to see photos of other females in your family. They will also ask about your personal objectives, such as what *you* want to see happen as a result of your surgery.

The surgeon will make recommendations based on your facial structure and your goals. As stated earlier, FFS is best represented as a *collection* of surgical procedures. Some women will be advised to have all of the components of FFS, while others to have relatively few. Remember that when you change one part of your face, the rest of it may appear off-balance unless other portions are changed as well. This truly calls for an expert opinion, and preferably from a surgeon who does FFS routinely.

Surgeons vary from one another in how they evaluate a face prior to surgery. For instance, the surgeons of Facialteam in Spain use CT scans with 3D reconstruction. A 3D printer can be used to create personalized cutting guides for surgery on the lower jaw. If forehead work is to be done, a 3D reconstruction from a CT scan informs the surgeon of the exact boundaries and the size of the frontal sinuses in the forehead.

FFS Is a Collection of Surgeries

In many facial feminization surgeries, you'll see the following modifications:

- **Brow bone reduction**
  The brow bone may be shaved and rounded. There are several approaches.
  - One surgeon says, "Shaving with a burr [a drill bit that cuts bone] is possible in about one-third of patients. In the remainder, the anterior wall of the forehead is removed, reshaped, and put back down. Bone over the outer brow is frequently reduced. Bone from the orbit around the eye is frequently removed to shape the eye."
  - Another surgeon comments, "Burring alone tends to be sufficient in about 2 to 3 percent of patients."
- **Scalp advance**
  This brings the hairline forward and makes the forehead appear less pronounced. An added benefit of a hairline advancement is often a brow lift that further feminizes the face.
- **Hair transplants**
  Harvested from the base of the skull, the transplants fill in areas of androgynous alopecia (male pattern hair loss), often one to three follicles at a time. Keep in mind that to gain the hair density required for a female hairline, most patients require two to three transplant procedures. (See one patient's experience with hair transplantation in Chapter 9.)
- **Brow lift**
  This elevates and shapes the eyebrows, creating a feminine arch.
- **Rhinoplasty (nose job)**
  This creates a smaller, more feminine-appearing nose. A female nose is often more delicate and upturned than a male nose; it is often narrower and more "refined."
- **Cheek implants**
  These accent the cheekbones. Implants imply that solid silicone, Gortex, or a type of hard plastic is inserted, while grafts are transfers of fat or bone from other parts of the body.
- **Lip lift**
  This reduces the distance between the lower edge of the nose and the upper lip, rotates the upper lip upward and outward, and creates a shorter, more feminine appearance. By shortening the lip, you create more dental "show," which also creates a more female appearance. Lip contouring with implants may also help to make the lips look fuller.
- **Chin and mandible contouring**
  The chin is rounded and the angles of the jaw are softened and reduced. The jaw bones are usually accessed from inside the mouth. Some surgeons make an exterior incision so it can be hidden, such as under the chin. The jaw can also be reduced with a technique called "reduction genioplasty." In this procedure, the chin may be reduced vertically in length and horizontally in projection.
- **Tracheal shave**
  The thyroid cartilage (Adam's apple) is shaved down to make it less prominent. The incision is hidden below the chin or in a neck crease. It is common to see this procedure done alone without other facial feminization procedures.

- **Facelift**
  Excess skin is removed and the lower and midface are tightened and repositioned to provide a more youthful appearance. Incision lines may be camouflaged immediately in front of and behind the ears and the hairline. A separate incision, similar to a tracheal shave incision below the chin, is used to tighten the neck. This is commonly done in middle-aged and older individuals.
- **Fat grafting**
  This adds contour or fullness to areas such as the cheeks, lips, and nasolabial folds.

Q Is it possible to do FFS on a teenager?

A It is medically possible. Dr. Daniel Simon and Dr. Luis Capitán of the Facialteam stated at the WPATH 26th Scientific Symposium Surgeon's Program in 2020 that one could perform FFS on a teenager. However, in addition to imaging the face, they would recommend performing a bone age test to confirm the closure of the growth plates.[51]

In addition to the above, we may see implants placed in the lips, the chin, and the sides of the temples—in other words, a *combination* of surgeries customized for each individual patient. The Facialteam in Spain has published a protocol that describes the sequence in which they perform FFS.[52] They begin by contouring the Adam's apple and move upward to reconfigure the lower jaw. Then they perform forehead reconstruction; next, they do rhinoplasty. They finish with the more minor aesthetic procedures, such as blepharoplasty, lip lifts, implants, or injections.

Vocal feminization surgery, specifically cricothyroid approximation and feminization laryngoplasty, which are approached through the front of the neck, can be done at the same time as the tracheal shave. Endoscopic vocal cord shortening is done through the mouth and leaves no external scar. This is done during a separate surgery that allows plenty of healing time before an endotracheal intubation is performed. (See "Vocal Feminization Surgery and ET Tubes" on page 198.)

FFS isn't easy to go through, according to most of my patients who have had it. Most people experience pain, bruising, and temporary swelling. But it can make the biggest possible difference in a person's *outward* presentation.

I cannot overemphasize the importance of not smoking. The face has a rich blood supply that promotes healing. But you will always heal better and faster if you don't smoke. Stop smoking—or using *any* tobacco products—today if this is an issue for you. Ask your healthcare provider if you need help in quitting, or refer to Chapter 10.

— Linda Gromko, MD

---

51 Luis Capitán, "Management of Complex Revision Frontal Sinus and Forehead Cases," (presentation, WPATH 26th Scientific Symposium Surgeon's Program, November 6, 2020).

52 Capitán et al, "Facial Gender Confirmation Surgery: A Protocol for Diagnosis, Surgical Planning, and Postoperative Management," *Plastic and Reconstructive Surgery* 145, no. 4 (April 2020): 818e–28e, https://doi.org/10.1097/prs.0000000000006686.

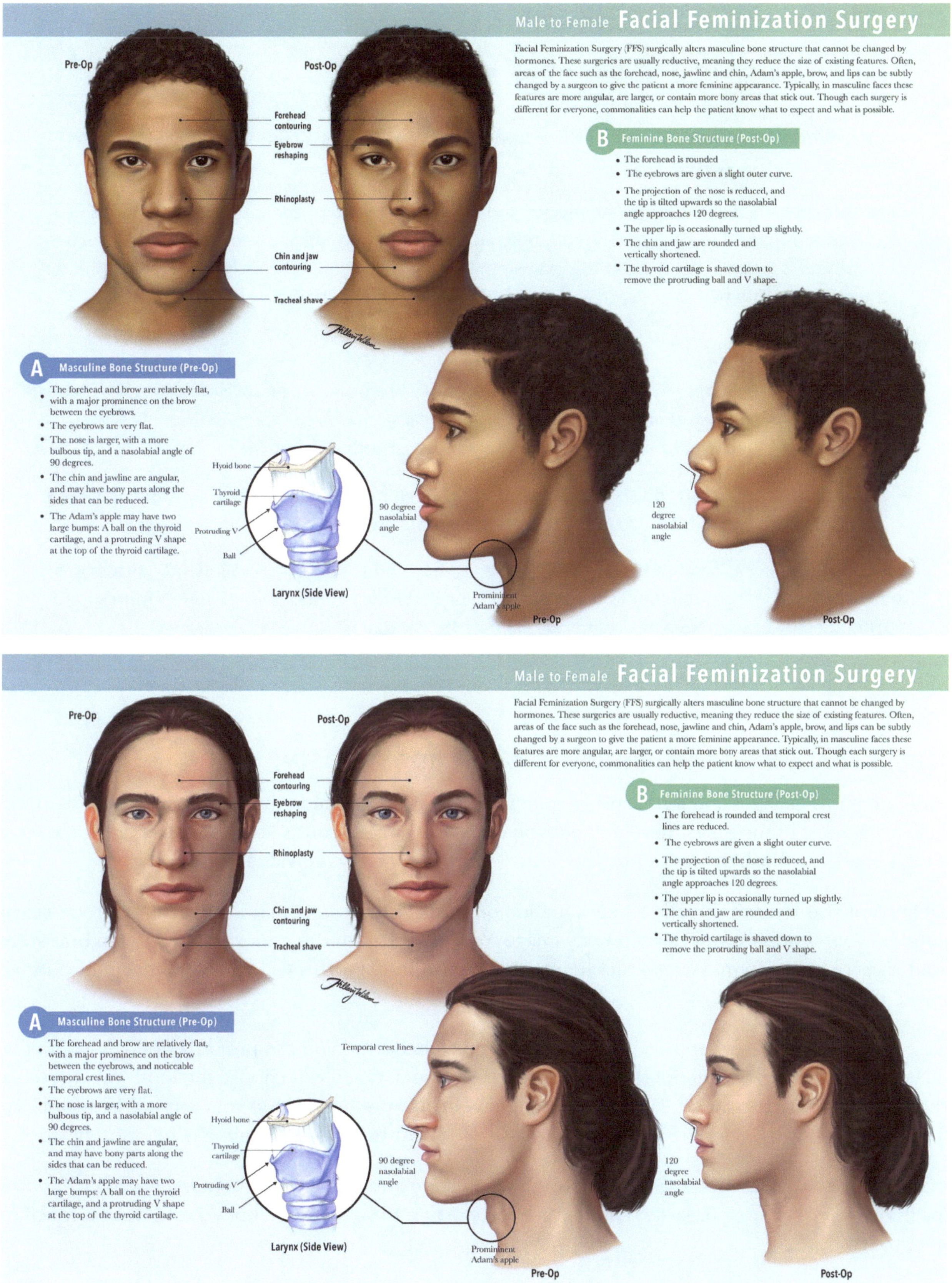

Figure 11.3. Facial feminization surgery.

Vocal Feminization Surgery and ET Tubes

Vocal feminization surgery is beyond the scope of this book. However, the following abbreviated information may be useful.

Most surgeries are done with anesthetic gas and oxygen provided by an endotracheal tube (ET tube). The ET tube is placed through the mouth, beyond the back of the throat, and between the vocal cords before it lands at the base of the mainstem bronchus where the bronchi move out to the left and right lungs. The patient, of course, is sedated with IV medication before this is done.

There are two main approaches to vocal feminization surgery:

- **The cricothyroid approximation and laryngoplasty** are done via an incision that goes through the front of the neck. This surgery tightens the vocal cords by changing their angle with respect to other structures, such as the thyroid and cricothyroid cartilage.
- **The endoscopic glottoplasty (Wendler glottoplasty)** is done via an endoscopy tube that is placed in the back of the throat; the vocal cords are sutured together to shorten them.

Intubation can occasionally damage the vocal cords. Care must be taken to allow the vocal cords to heal before any subsequent intubations. A smaller endotracheal tube or a different form of anesthesia (such as laryngeal mask anesthesia) may be needed.

Breast Enlargement (Augmentation Mammoplasty)

Breasts come in all shapes and sizes, and people have very strong opinions as to what's best for them. You will likely get most of the breast development you can expect after about 3 years on estrogen. Some women see additional growth when progesterone is added, but this is highly individual.

What implant size is best? There is a wide variation of normal breast sizes in humans. The "correct" size will depend on your vision of your desired body image. You will be given the opportunity to try on bras with various sizes of breast forms (sizers) tucked into the cups of the bra. This will help give you an idea of what size you like best.

Make sure that you wear appropriate clothing to the consultation so you can properly evaluate your new look. Wearing a sweatshirt will not show your proper contours. Once you choose the look you like, the size of the implant will be measured. Taking into account your size preference and your chest dimensions, you and your surgeon will determine the best implant size for your body to achieve the results you desire.

Implant sizes may be described in terms of volume and are expressed in cubic centimeters or cc.[53] It often helps think of your desired breast size in terms of proportion to your overall body, rather than a specific number of cc.

53 For reference, there are 30 cc in an ounce and 240 cc in a liquid measuring cup. In one small study, implant volumes for trans women ranged from 350 cc to 700 cc, with an average breast implant volume of 520 cc (480 cc is 1 pint).

Talk about your breast size preferences with your partner or a good friend who will tell you the truth. Bigger isn't always better. Large breasts are heavier and may result in soreness of your upper back and shoulders. Take your surgeon's recommendations seriously and listen to the other people whose opinions you value. But remember, the final decision about what *you* want is yours.

— *Linda Gromko, MD*

Since many trans women have broader shoulders and a wider chest than cisgender women, a trans woman may be able to accommodate a larger cup size and implant size without looking out of proportion. This is where a surgeon who is highly experienced in the subtleties of trans surgery may be a better choice than a plastic surgeon with less transgender experience.

In general, breast implants are composed of a silicone shell that is filled with either saline (basically, saltwater) or a cohesive silicone gel. Note that the latest generation of silicone implants is filled with *cohesive gel* silicone rather than liquid silicone. In the event of a rupture, cohesive silicone gel stays together, rather than leaking out into the surrounding tissues.

The implants may be placed into the chest—

- over the pectoralis muscle (one of the chest muscles) as in the drawing on the left, or
- under the pectoralis muscle as in the drawing on the right.

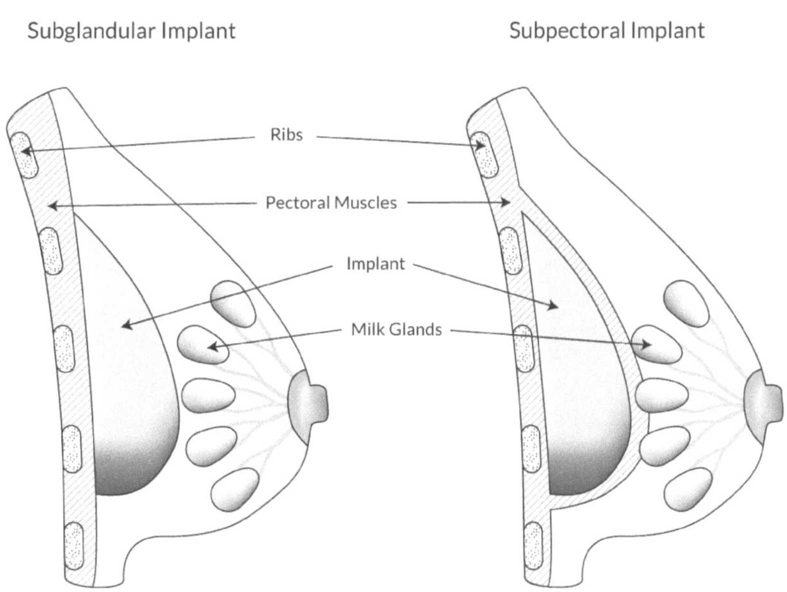

Figure 11.4. Breast implants over the pectoralis muscle (one of the chest muscles)— also called a "subglandular" implant, as in the drawing on the left—or under the pectoralis muscle, also called a "subpectoral" implant, as in the drawing on the right.

In both techniques, the implants are placed under the actual glandular tissue of the breasts. If the over-the-muscle technique is used, a woman must have enough breast tissue to camouflage the implant beneath it. Otherwise, you will see the margins of the implant and it will look unnatural. For many trans women, placing the implant under the pectoralis muscle is more favorable because it provides enough soft tissue coverage to create a smooth, natural-appearing breast. Placing the implant under the muscle may also reduce the risk of a complication called capsular contracture.

Incisions for augmentation can be placed as follows:

- In the armpit (axillary approach)
- Under the lower crease of the breast (inframammary incision)
- Along the lower margin of the areola (periareolar)
- Transumbilical breast augmentation (TUBA). This is the newest of the approaches listed. An incision is hidden in the hood of the umbilicus (belly button) and tunneled into the chest area. As of the time of this writing, this technique can be done only with saline implants because they can be inserted completely deflated and then filled with saline after proper placement. For more information, refer to an article by Dr. Richard V. Dowden, "Transumbilical Breast Augmentation Is Safe and Effective."[54]

Augmentation mammoplasty is typically performed as an outpatient surgery (also called short-stay, ambulatory, or day surgery) under general anesthesia.

The Rice Test: Determining Breast Size and Breast Implant Size

Note: Dr. Scott Mosser makes the following information available to his clients so they can explore breast implant sizing at home.

Dr. Mosser will let you try on implants during your consult. The breast implants are usually tried on underneath a sports bra or in a regular-type bra. Dr. Mosser may suggest that you try on different sizes at home using the "Rice Test." Even though it is widely known as the Rice Test, we have found many materials that work better than rice for measuring volume. Particularly good is quinoa (although it's expensive), but other options that are light and a bit better than rice are oatmeal, potato flakes, and grits.

Instructions

Fill knee-high hose (or cut-off pantyhose) with the desired amount of rice, using the cc conversions listed below. Avoid using zipper-lock bags because of their pointed corners. Once you have the hosiery filled, try on the "implants" under a sports bra or under a somewhat snug underwire bra that is sheer and has no padding at all. A sports bra is helpful, especially if you plan on having your implants placed under the muscle. The sports bra compresses the breast implant sizers much like the

54 Richard V. Dowden, "Transumbilical Breast Augmentation Is Safe and Effective," *Seminars in Plastic Surgery* 22, no. 1 (February 2008): 51–9, https://doi.org/10.1055/s-2007-1019143.

muscle will compress the real implants. If you are going under the muscle, you'll need to add about 15 percent more to the amount that you like.

For example, if you like the way that 400 cc looks under the sports bra, you need to add 15 percent to that amount (which equates to 460-cc implants) to achieve the look you see with the 400-cc implant sizers in the sports bra.

How to Measure for CC Amount with the Rice Test

The conversions below (from cups to cubic centimeters) are approximate and will help you when doing the Rice Test.

- 1 cup = 236 cc
- ½ cup = 118 cc
- ¾ cup = 177 cc
- ¼ cup = 59 cc
- 1/3 cup = 78 cc
- 2/3 cup = 156 cc
- 1/8 cup = 30 cc

Do ***not*** weigh the rice. The rice must be measured as **volume** using the system above. The measurements above can be used in different combinations to achieve the cc amount you desire. It's important to remember that you should not solely rely on cc amounts just based on the photos of other patients with different body types. For instance, if you like the way that 400 cc looks on one person, that does not mean that 400 cc will give you the same look.

This is due to several things, including—but not limited to—the amount of breast tissue, shape of the chest wall, deformities of the chest wall (such as pectus excavatum and pectus carinatum), and overall body weight, to name a few. Therefore, you should do the Rice Test to give you an idea of how many cubic centimeters you may need to get the size you want.

Please remember that the Rice Test is not an exact science and is meant only to give you a rough estimate.

Possible Complications Associated with Breast Implants

Anesthesia-related complications and allergic reactions are rare, but they can occur in the perioperative period, as with any surgery. These include allergic reactions, low blood pressure, aspiration pneumonia, and peripheral nerve damage (from spinal or epidural anesthesia).

Other potential complications include infection, malposition or migration of implants, formation of hematomas (collections of blood), or rarely, seromas (collections of clear serous fluid under the skin). Hematomas and seromas may resolve spontaneously or require draining by the surgeon.

A capsular contracture occurs when normal scar tissue around an implant begins to contract and squeeze the implant, creating a firm, unnatural feel. The exact cause of contracture formation is unknown. They occur about 10 percent of the time; 90 percent of patients have the expected soft result. Contractures are graded according to the Baker Grading Scale as follows: Grade I (perfectly soft), Grade II (firm but retaining a natural appearance), Grade III (firm and misshapen), and Grade IV (firm, misshapen, and painful). A distorted appearance often requires another surgery to repair it, increasing the risk of another contracture.[55]

> **Although there is no solid evidence that any postoperative treatment can decrease capsular contracture, external massage, certain oral nutraceuticals (milk thistle and vitamin E), and the asthma medications montelukast (Singulair)[56] and zafirlukast (Accolate) have been reported to decrease contractures. It is important to understand that capsular contractures are not 100 percent avoidable and may require another surgery.**
>
> *— E. Antonio Mangubat, MD*

Another complication is implant rupture (a tear in the outer shell of an implant). When saline implants rupture, the breast deflates completely and the breasts appear asymmetric. Modern silicone gel implants are semisolid and do not leak like the older liquid silicone implants did (liquid silicone was used before 2000). With any leak, the semisolid silicone tends to remain within the implant capsule. The condition can be confirmed by magnetic resonance imaging (MRI).

Some patients with breast implants have reported systemic (total body) symptoms such as fatigue, memory loss, rash, joint pain, and brain fog—collectively termed "breast implant illness" or BII. This poorly understood syndrome continues to invite investigation, and the FDA requests adverse event reporting should such symptoms occur (1-800-FDA-1088) or online at MedWatch (**fda.gov/safety/medwatch-fda-safety-information-and-adverse-event-reporting-program**).

> **An important mindset to have when getting breast augmentation is that this type of surgery may require maintenance. If any of the complications above occur over the course of your life, you may require surgery to address them. Implants do not need to replaced preemptively, but they do need to be replaced if they rupture, become infected, or develop capsular contracture.**
>
> *— Thomas Satterwhite, MD*

55 US Food and Drug Administration, "Risks and Complications of Breast Implants," updated September 28, 2020, https://www.fda.gov/medical-devices/breast-implants/risks-and-complications-breast-implants#Capsular_Contracture.

56 Catherine K. Huang, and Neal Handel, "Effects of Singulair (Montelukast) Treatment for Capsular Contracture," *Aesthetic Surgery Journal* 30, no. 3 (July 2010): 404–8, https://doi.org/10.1177/1090820x10374724.

Breast Implant-Associated Anaplastic Large-Cell Lymphoma (BIA-ALCL)

A possible association between breast implants and anaplastic large-cell lymphoma was identified by the US Food and Drug Administration in 2011. The World Health Organization designated breast implant-associated anaplastic large-cell lymphoma (BIA-ALCL) as a T-cell lymphoma that can develop following breast implants. This condition is not a breast cancer but rather a type of non-Hodgkin's lymphoma (a cancer involving the immune system).

Symptoms of pain or swelling, often occurring years after implant placement, should be evaluated. BIA-ALCL has been reported with both saline and silicone gel implants, although textured surfaces of implants are thought to carry a higher risk. Implant removal, chemotherapy, and radiation treatment are used to treat BIA-ALCL. For more information, read the FDA report as well as common questions and answers at fda.gov.*

* US Food and Drug Administration, "Questions and Answers about Breast Implant-Associated Anaplastic Large Cell Lymphoma (BIA-ALCL)," updated October 23, 2019, https://www.fda.gov/medical-devices/breast-implants/questions-and-answers-about-breast-implant-associated-anaplastic-large-cell-lymphoma-bia-alcl.

Body Contouring

Body contouring is basically an aesthetic procedure or a set of procedures that reduces fat from some areas and adds a contouring material (such as transferred fat, implants, or dermal filler) to other areas.

Nonsurgical Body Contouring

Available for both feminizing and masculinizing are a variety of *nonsurgical* techniques for removing fat, including CoolSculpting (cryolipolysis or freezing fat) and LaserLipo (a technique for removing fat by melting it). These techniques work on fairly small areas like an abdominal pooch or flanks.

To reduce a double chin, you may want to explore CoolSculpting or Kybella injections. Kybella consists of several injections placed directly into the fat under the chin. Kybella is deoxycholic acid, a chemical that dissolves fat when injected directly into the fat under the chin. (Don't plan your photo opportunity for the next day, however; many people experience significant under-the-chin swelling before the fat lessens.)

These procedures are generally less effective than surgical contouring in that they are best suited for smaller areas and cannot claim to have the results of the surgical techniques. That said, clients who cannot afford the downtime or expense of surgery may find them to be very acceptable alternatives.

Surgical Body Contouring

If you are looking for a more extensive body modification rather than focusing on a limited area, you will likely have better—and even less costly results—from a combination of *surgical* techniques.

Liposuction can remove unwanted fat from specific areas. That fat can be recycled by sterilely processing and reinjecting it to enhance other areas of one's own body (but there's no possibility of fat donations to other people!). This is commonly done to enhance the buttocks, face, and even the breasts. You can appreciate how this requires an artistic eye and a surgeon experienced in working with gender-variant individuals.

Tumescent liposuction is the cornerstone of surgical fat removal. Here's how it works:

1. After the patient is relaxed (by general anesthesia or IV sedation), fluid is injected into the area to be treated.
2. The injected fluid consists of a mixture of saline (sterile saltwater), lidocaine (an anesthetic), and epinephrine (adrenaline). Lidocaine reduces postoperative pain. Epinephrine constricts blood vessels, significantly decreasing blood loss and postoperative bruising, and permits time to sculpt the areas of liposuction.
3. Using a variety of techniques, the fat is liquified and suctioned out using a cannula (tube) in the planned areas of fat reduction.
4. The harvested fat is processed by separating it from the other fluid. It is then recycled by reinjecting it into another area where the patient wants more volume, or it can be discarded.

After the surgery, the patient wears a compressive support garment around-the-clock for a prescribed number of weeks. Following this period, the garment may be worn less, perhaps only at night. Patients should take some downtime—such as about a week off work—and avoid heavy lifting and strenuous activity.

A return to normal activities generally depends on a person's comfort level. One surgeon's rule-of-thumb: "You may drive your car if you do not require pain medications." Some patients require no pain meds; others medicate for 2 weeks. The average postoperative medication period is about 5 days.

Tumescent liposuction can be applied in any area with superficial fat: face, neck, "bra fat," back, arms, abdomen, waist, hips, buttocks, and the legs, including the thighs, calves, knees, and ankles. It can be used on the mons area (fat above the pubic bone). Trans men in particular may seek liposuction to remove feminine-appearing fat around the hips and buttocks. Some ask that the harvested fat be transferred to the waist to camouflage a more feminine curve or placed in the chest to augment the pectoralis muscle. And some physically fit patients request sculpting their six-pack abs.

Tumescent liposuction can be combined with skin removal following massive weight-loss procedures (such as bariatric surgeries that result in the weight loss of 100 pounds or more). Tummy tucks, body lifts, and thigh lifts are commonly requested. You may also have the opportunity to create a waistline and to spot-reduce arm fat and bra fat that really cannot be exercised away.

While the fat cells that are removed from your body are gone forever, if you gain weight, your remaining fat cells can enlarge. Your results will always be better if you exercise and maintain healthy eating.

Risks of Tumescent Liposuction

Tumescent liposuction carries risks of infection, bleeding, bruising, damage to tissues, asymmetry, and contour irregularities (lumpiness). You could have an allergic reaction to the medications used, including anesthesia and pain relievers. You won't lose cellulite, and your results may not be as flawless or as symmetrical as you had hoped. You will incur expenses that are not likely to be covered by insurance, and you'll bear the cost of an enforced time away from work, if that is a concern for you.

Doing the Math: Is an Aesthetic Procedure Worth It?

Body contouring and other aesthetic procedures may be covered by insurance at times and be considered reconstructive in the setting of gender confirmation surgery. But suppose your insurance doesn't cover it. Can you afford it? Let's do some math.

Suppose you're contemplating a surgery that costs $15,000. You are 50 years old. Your parents lived to be 85 and 95. You are generally healthy and don't smoke or participate in risky activities that could shorten your life. Let's calculate the procedural cost but spread it out over your anticipated lifespan—maybe 40 more years if you live to 90 years of age. (Of course, this does not count the potential growth of this money if used in other ways.)

Cost = $15,000 divided by (40 years) = $375 per year of your life

Cost per day of remaining life: $15,000 divided by (40 years x 365 days/year) = $1.03 per day ($2.05 per day if you lived 20 years)

Q Isn't this just a rationalization for spending a lot of money on appearance?

A Perhaps, but what is the cost of living for years with something that makes you uncomfortable every single day?

Q Doesn't this sound like something reserved for the "privileged?"

A In the past, plastic surgery was the exclusive domain of the privileged. But we are beginning to see these surgeries covered by insurance for the medical treatment of gender dysphoria.

More Body Contouring: Lifting and Filling

We have already discussed breast augmentation, which is an excellent example of filling an area that requires more volume. The breast contour is enhanced by using saline or silicone implants that are placed by way of the armpit under the breast, under the areola, or through the navel.

Here are other examples:

- **The Brazilian butt lift (BBL)**
  Estradiol helps to feminize the body shape to some extent. But if you want a fuller, rounder butt and want tissue sculpted away from the waist, flank, or abdominal area, it may be possible to have a fat transfer. Fat is removed by tumescent liposuction (described earlier on page 204) and injected into the buttocks in sections via a large syringe and cannula. Because the fat tissue is a person's own fat, there is no risk of an immune reaction to a foreign substance—that is, no rejection. This is a popular surgery in AMAB individuals, as their buttocks are quite flat. Additionally, one can have contouring to slim the waist, which emphasizes the butt contour even more. This combination of reduction and augmentation in the same setting has been popular and successful.

- **Butt-contouring implants**
  Silicone implants can be used to add volume to the butt. They are placed through a vertical incision in the gluteal crease (the crack in the butt) under the gluteus maximus muscle so you do not sit on them. This is particularly suited for patients with little or no fat to harvest. Getting implants, however, carries the added risks of discomfort, malposition, and infection.

- **Injections to increase volume**
  Various injectable fillers may be used to add volume. These are considered temporary and are also "off-label"—that is, not FDA-approved for enhancing butt volume.

Be an Informed Consumer

Because of a number of deaths related to fat emboli, Brazilian butt lifts are controversial and have been banned in some areas. (A fat embolus is similar to a pulmonary embolus from a blood clot, except that the blockage results from transferred fat landing within a large vein and traveling north to the heart and the blood vessels in the lungs.) This is more likely to happen if large volumes of fat are injected into muscle tissue with large blood vessels. Do check with your surgeon about complications and practices aimed at reducing fat emboli before you sign up for a larger butt.

An Important Warning about Liquid Silicone Injections*

Although we don't see this much in the Pacific Northwest, many trans women have been seriously harmed by illegal silicone injections for body contouring. I'm not talking about off-label use on an otherwise FDA-approved product but about industrial chemicals, like the silicone caulking found in hardware stores and other products like paraffin and glue that black-market "pump" doctors use to inject their "patients" (victims) in hotel rooms.

Long-term effects include disfigurement of tissue, infection, and the spread of silicone to other parts of the body, producing kidney damage, stroke, and pulmonary emboli. Free or discount-cost silicone injections to any part of the body to add volume are **not** recommended.

* US Food and Drug Administration, "FDA Warns about Illegal Use of Injectable Silicone for Body Contouring and Associated Health Risks," November 13, 2017, https://www.fda.gov/news-events/press-announcements/fda-warns-about-illegal-use-injectable-silicone-body-contouring-and-associated-health-risks.

Feminizing Genital Surgeries

Orchiectomy

Bilateral orchiectomy refers to the surgical removal of the testicles. This may be performed as a surgery separate from vaginoplasty. Orchiectomy may be requested in a woman who simply wishes to stop taking testosterone blockers, or a woman who wants a surgery that is less extensive than vaginoplasty. After a bilateral orchiectomy, a person will have a flatter-appearing scrotum but still have a penis and scrotum. (Bilateral orchiectomy is a routine part of vaginoplasty in gender-affirmation surgery.)

Orchiectomy is more commonly performed as part of the treatment of testicular or prostate cancer. When it is performed to treat gender dysphoria, WPATH standards are observed (meaning the medical standards set by the World Professional Association for Transgender Health, a nonprofit, interdisciplinary professional and educational organization devoted to transgender health). Orchiectomy is performed as an outpatient surgery under local anesthesia with sedation, or under general anesthesia.

Surgeons remove the testicles and spermatic cords by way of a midline incision in the scrotum. (Groin incisions on either side are not needed and create unnecessary scars. If your surgeon is nonnegotiable about this point, get another opinion.) Care is taken to minimize tissue loss, as the scrotal tissue is used in vaginoplasty. (The scrotum looks smaller after the testicles are removed because it is no longer distended by them.)

After orchiectomy, an individual no longer takes a testosterone blocker such as spironolactone or cyproterone acetate. This simplifies a trans woman's medical regimen and in the case of spironolactone, eliminates the diuretic effect.

Vaginoplasty

Vaginoplasty (basically, "building a vagina") goes by several names and will likely have more names in years ahead. **The current hot term is *gender-affirming vaginoplasty* (GAV).** But it is also commonly called gender-affirming surgery (GAS), gender-reassignment surgery (GRS), or sexual reassignment surgery (SRS). The term "sex change" is outdated.

Before getting into the details, it is important to mention just how far genital surgery has come. Years ago, surgical results were not nearly as elegant as they are today. In years past, trans women seeking genital surgery often had no choice but to sacrifice their sexual responsiveness.

> In the 1980s when I transitioned, there was no easy way to find out if you had a good surgeon or not. There were no before-and-after pictures or reviews by former patients to fall back on. The surgeon my psychiatrist referred me to was my only choice. When the surgery was done, I was ecstatic!
>
> When the swelling went down, I started to see the work he did in more detail and noticed that there was no clitoris, or none in the right place, and no real labia minora. When I went in for my next post-op checkup, I complained that my new vagina wasn't very anatomically correct, to which he replied, "Turn off the lights, nobody will notice."
>
> I had no recourse or legal rights back then, so I had to bite my tongue.
>
> — *Trans woman who transitioned in the 1980s*

While they might have had an acceptable genital appearance, many sacrificed the ability to orgasm. But because of advances in surgical techniques, trans women are now able to look and respond like the women they *are*. A good sex life should never be a "frill," so this is a significant development.

Let me explain how the newer surgeries have made sexual response possible.

Once again, let's go back to embryology and how we developed before we were born. As embryos, our genitals grow from the same basic structures whether we are genetically male or female. The sensitive head of the penis (glans penis) is the embryologic equivalent of the natal female clitoris, although the clitoral head and shaft are much smaller. The natal scrotum is the embryologic equivalent of the labia majora in the natal female. And the perineal raphe (ridge) is analogous to the natal female labia minora. Note that these structures may be open or fused and yet still be analogous. Dr. Frank Netter's illustration in Figure 11.5 on page 209 color-codes these various structures, making it easier to understand which ones are analogous to others. So when the glans penis is transformed into a clitoris, the same neurologic pathways persist and sexual responsiveness is preserved.

While not shown in the Netter illustration, the testicles are analogous to the ovaries located deep in the female pelvis. Naturally, both genders have urethras to pass urine from the bladder to the outside of the body, and rectums through which the bowel movements travel to the outside world.

If you are not medically trained and do not speak medicine as a second language, stop for a moment before you go on. The following information about genital surgeries gets quite complicated. Don't get discouraged as you read. If you find this difficult, remember that it is complex information, but it is manageable.

It's *my* problem as the author if I cannot make it understandable! *Read slowly* and look up words you don't know.

— Linda Gromko, MD

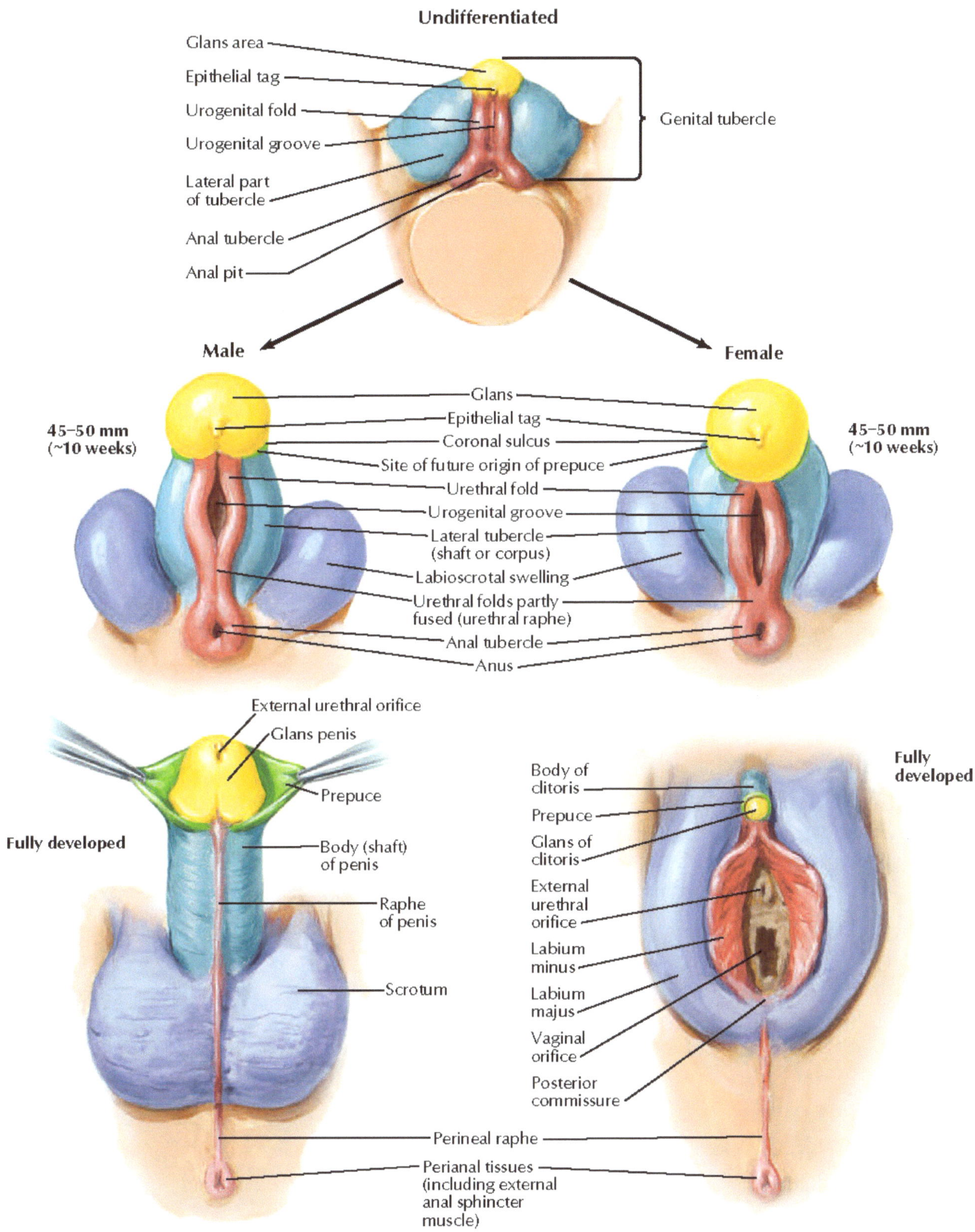

Figure 11.5. Embryologic equivalents in male and female external genitals.

Learning about the Feminizing Genital Surgeries

- Read the information out loud to another person or an animal. (I remember a medical school classmate who would tell her tiny daughter "stories" about the anatomy of the heart. Kids want to hear your voice and don't care as much about content.)
- Stop after every paragraph and be sure you're still on track before going ahead. Otherwise, you may get lost, anxious, and overwhelmed.
- Don't give up!
- If you're more of visual learner, look at a picture, a medical illustration, a diagram, or a video. Visit YouTube (youtube.com) and search on the terms "sexual reassignment surgery," "vaginoplasty," or "MTF sex change."

Animation Videos of Vaginoplasty

Sexual reassignment (vaginoplasty) animation (youtube.com/watch?v=SH-j3r_Rwsw or youtube.com/watch?v=zGkiC3Y8kk0). While other sites show the actual surgery being performed, start here. It's simply illustrated, but it's still complicated. Know also that vaginoplasty techniques may vary, so start with these basics; they'll hold you in good stead.

Animation illustration by Rebecca Betts (youtube.com/watch?v=6J9-QORp8To). Most importantly, if you are reading this to prepare for your own surgery, be certain that you know exactly what you are having done. Speak to your surgeon, their ARNP or PA, the clinic coordinator, or someone else ("To whom may I talk with to get my questions answered before surgery?") Do not sign up for a surgery that you do not understand!

One-Stage Penile Inversion Vaginoplasty

Penile inversion vaginoplasty for gender affirmation was pioneered by surgeon Georges Burou in the 1950s and used more generally after his address to Stanford University in 1973. Early references to a "sensate vaginal pedicled spot" demonstrate earlier attention to sexual responsiveness.[57]

There are many variations in technique from surgeon to surgeon and from region to region. Obviously, a one-step vaginoplasty is designed to be completed at one time. In a two-step vaginoplasty, the hood of the clitoris and labia minora are completed during a second stage, usually several months later. (Some women do not go on to have Stage 2, as they are satisfied with their results of Stage 1.)

You may want to watch a YouTube animation as we go through the basics of the one-step procedure (youtube.com/watch?v=SH-j3r_Rwsw or youtube.com/watch?v=zGkiC3Y8kk0).

Or follow the medical illustrations of Hillary Wilson as you walk through the narrative below and on the next few pages. Remember that the procedure varies somewhat from surgeon to surgeon, but Wilson's color-coded illustrations will help you understand the basics.

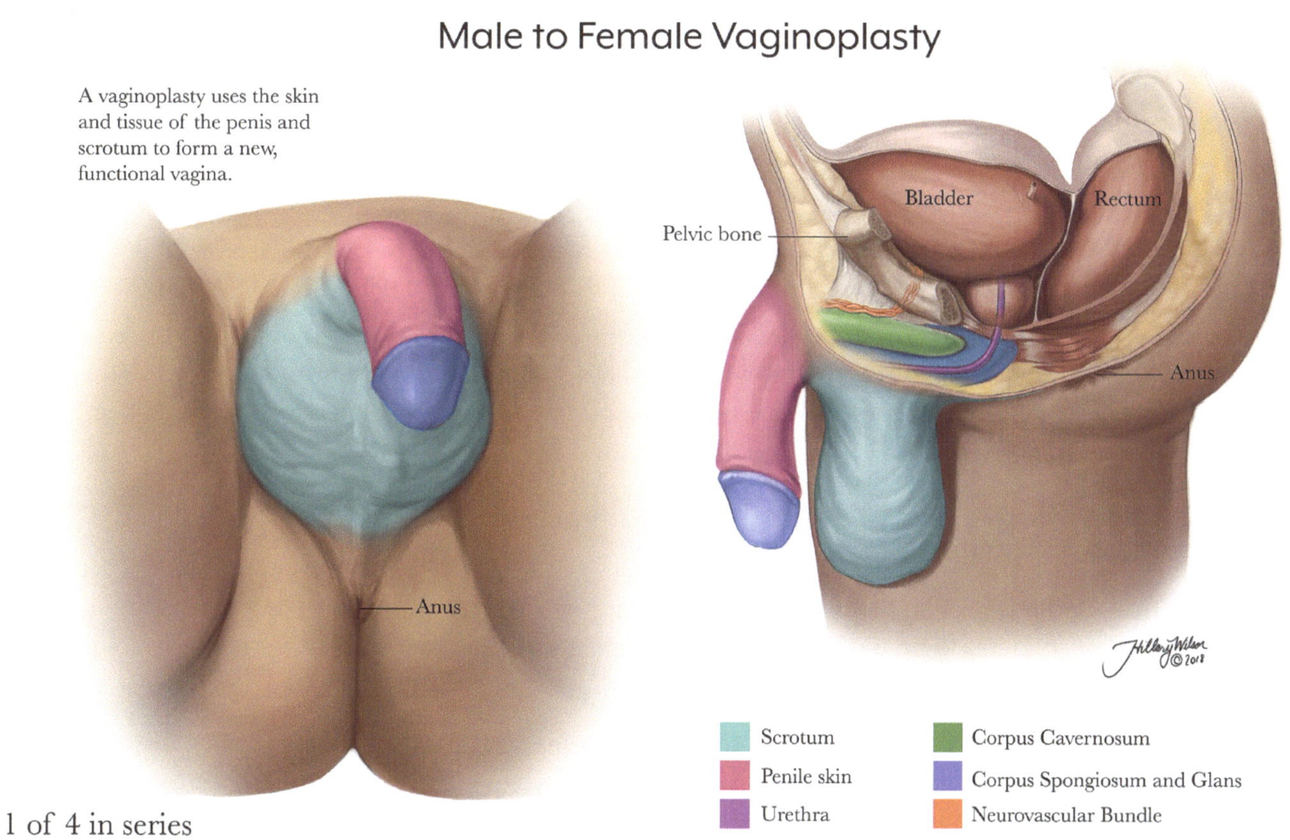

Figure 11.6. Vaginoplasty 1 of 4: The starting point.

57 Robert C. J. Kanhai, "Sensate Vagina Pedicled-Spot for Male-to-Female Transsexuals: The Experience in the First 50 Patients," *Aesthetic Plastic Surgery* 40, no. 2 (February 18, 2016): 284–7, https://doi.org/10.1007/s00266-016-0620-2.

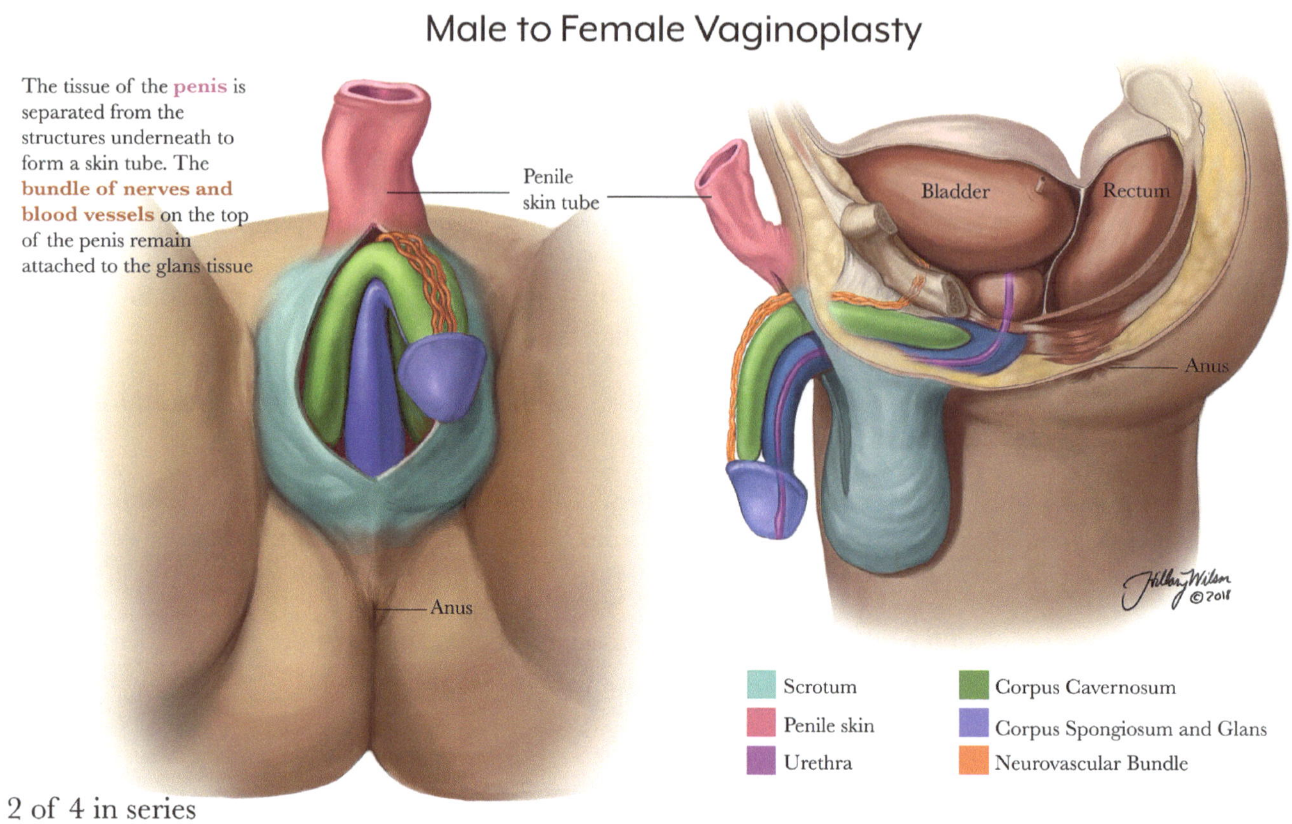

Figure 11.7. Vaginoplasty 2 of 4: The testicles are removed, and the penis is disassembled.

- The testicles are removed through an incision in the scrotum. ("Removed" means forever, which is why we emphasize sperm banking for fertility preservation before you even begin hormones or testosterone blockers.) The scrotal skin may be used to add more vaginal depth if needed, or to create the labia.
- The penis is dissected into its component parts. This is critical to retain urinary and sexual function. Here are the basic steps:
    - The skin of the penis is incised around the base of the glans (mushroom part). This skin is then pushed to the base of the penis. It will be inverted later and used to create the lining of neovagina (new vagina).
    - The neurovascular bundle—that is, the nerves, veins, and arteries that serve the glans penis—are dissected apart from the underlying structures. The neurovascular bundle remains attached to the glans penis at the dorsal surface.
    - The urethra is separated away from the cavernous bodies—the two pontoon-like structures that fill up with blood during an erection.
    - The corpora cavernosa or cavernous bodies are removed and discarded. To be precise, they are sent to the hospital's pathology department for examination and disposal (incineration).

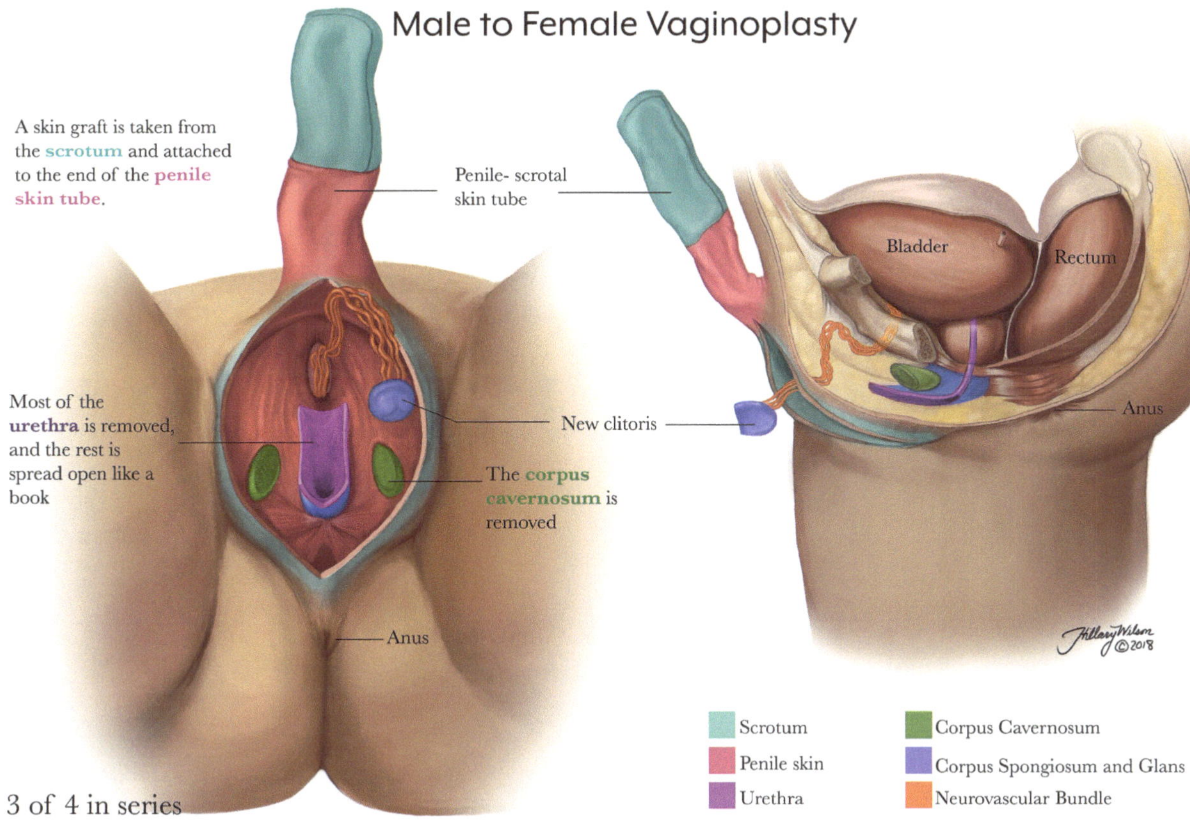

Figure 11.8. Vaginoplasty 3 of 4: The glans penis is reduced and reshaped to become the neoclitoris.

- The glans penis is reduced in size and rounded to become the neoclitoris, still keeping it as the sexual pleasure center. Because the nerves are still intact, stimulation of the neoclitoris will generally result in orgasm in people who had orgasms prior to surgery. Creating a clitoris of the "correct" size is important: if it is too small, the neoclitoris will be hard to find, and too large, it will look just like a small penis. Urine does not flow through the clitoris as it would in the penis. Rather, the urine will flow through the urethra, which will open below the clitoris.

- The urethra is shortened. Urethral tissue no longer needed for a shorter female urethra is splayed out to line the vaginal vestibule.

- The internal vaginal space is created by blunt dissection. This means that the tissue planes are separated with the surgeon's gloved fingers rather than scalpels, scissors, or cutting cautery. Other surgeons dissect the canal sharply using cautery or scissors. The vaginal space is created between the bladder and the rectum. (Said another way, the bladder, urethra, and prostate gland will remain in *front* of the space of the neovagina, and the rectum sits behind it.)

- The skin of the penis is inverted and directed into this newly created vaginal space. The inverted penile skin lines this space and is held in place by vaginal packing or is anchored to the ischium (part of the pelvic structure) or deep sacrospinous ligaments. In most cases, the inverted penile skin does not provide enough tissue for a vagina with adequate depth, so the surgeon uses scrotal skin as a graft at the apex of the canal.

- The inversion of the penis into the new vaginal canal begins the process of closing the surgical site. It brings the apex of the exposed surgical site down to join with the base of the surgical site, revising it from an open oval to a curved incision line.

Think about this carefully: The surface skin on the *outside* of the original penis becomes the lining skin on the *inside* of the vagina. It is different tissue than cisgender vaginal tissue in that it is not a mucous membrane and does not provide lubrication during sexual arousal. Added lubrication in the form of a surgical or personal lubricant (such as Surgilube, Slippery Stuff, Sliquid) will be needed during dilation or sexual penetration to prevent microtears that can make a person more susceptible to infection.

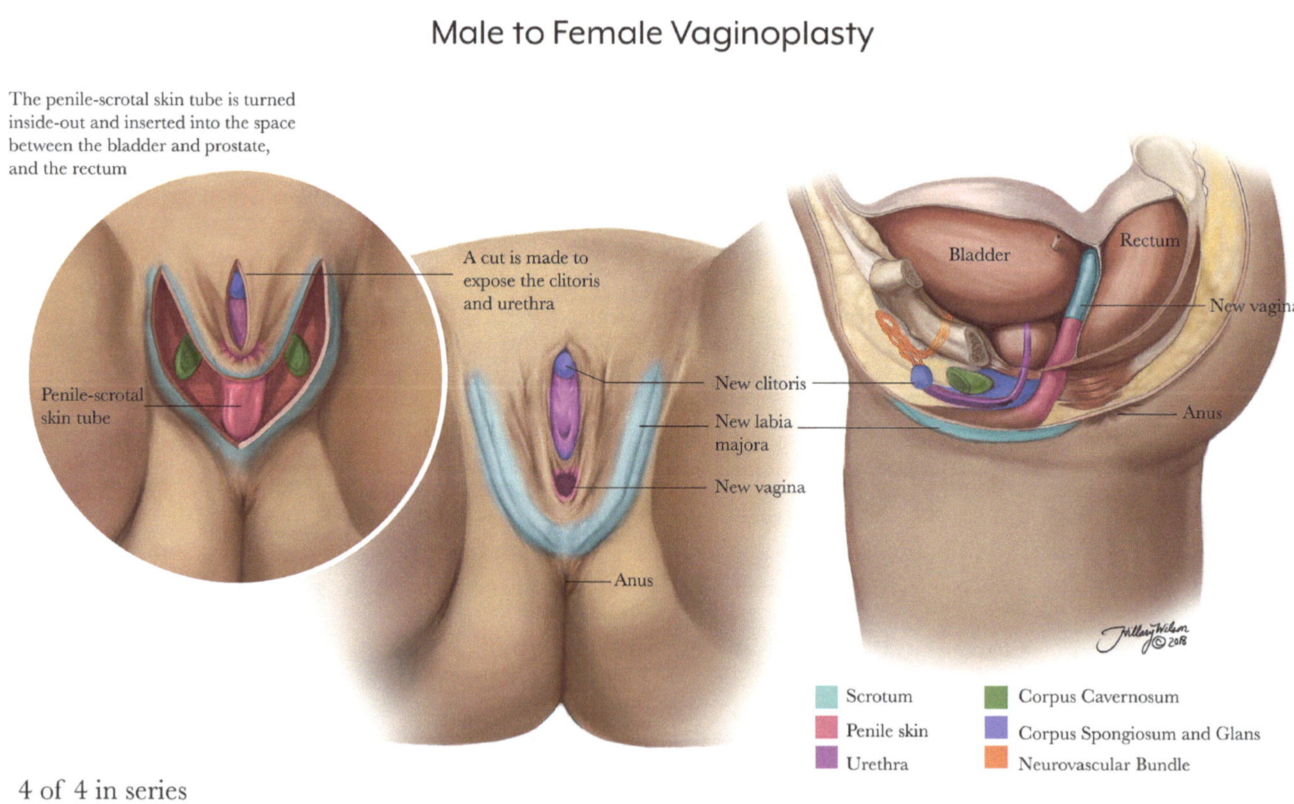

Figure 11.9. Vaginoplasty 4 of 4: Completion of the neovagina and creation of the labia.

- External openings in the skin below the pubic bone are created for the neoclitoris and for the urethra right below it. The urethra will appear slightly lower in position than in a natal female.
- Labia are created by using tissue from the inverted penis and the scrotum, depending on the technique being used. If the neoclitoris is not "hooded" at this time, it will be completed as part of Step 2 in a two-step procedure (Step 2 is also called a "labiaplasty").

After the vaginoplasty is completed, a urinary catheter is placed in the urethra and vaginal packing is inserted to minimize bleeding, to hold the neovagina in place, and to maintain vaginal patency (that is, to keep the vagina from closing in on itself). The catheter and vaginal packing are removed by the surgical staff about 5 to 7 days after surgery, marking the beginning of the routine of vaginal dilation to maintain vaginal depth and girth. (See pages 278–281 in Chapter 12).

What Happens to the Prostate?

The prostate gland is left in its original location, "wrapped" around the urethra at the base of the bladder. It is generally smaller after exposure to estradiol, so an enlarged prostate in a trans woman could be worrisome. The examiner palpates (feels) the prostate through the vagina; it is just on the other side of the anterior (front) vaginal wall. When examining a male, I palpate the prostate during a rectal exam. With my patient leaning forward over an exam table, I feel the prostate through the rectum, and just on the other side of the anterior (front) wall of the rectum.

Two-Stage Vaginoplasty (Penile Inversion Vaginoplasty plus Labiaplasty Done Later)

Some surgeons perform vaginoplasty as a two-step procedure, with the second stage performed about 3 to 4 months after the initial vaginoplasty.

Not all clients go on to have the second stage performed, as they may be fully satisfied with the initial vaginoplasty results. However, the labiaplasty may increase a woman's comfort, particularly if the exposed neoclitoris protrudes to the extent where it is irritating.

Labiaplasty allows a surgeon to refine thinner labia minora and to create a more defined hood over the clitoris. A vertical incision is used in the procedure. Labiaplasty can be done as a day surgery. If there are other refinements or revisions to be done, these can be performed at the time of the labiaplasty.

> **If you look up the word "labiaplasty," you are likely to find information about a cosmetic procedure to improve the appearance or tightness of a vagina. It is sometimes advanced as a treatment for rejuvenating the aging natal vagina. This is a different category of labiaplasty altogether, and the two are not performed for the same reasons.**
>
> *— Linda Gromko, MD*

The Limited-Depth or Zero-Depth Vagina

Limited-depth vaginoplasties are also known as zero-depth vaginoplasties or vulvoplasties. (The term "vulva" refers to the external genitalia, including the labia majora and minora. You will notice that I often use the term "vagina" to refer to these structures—and this is not really accurate. "Vagina" refers to the internal genital structure. I am aware of this, but I use "vagina" because it is better understood and therefore communicated more clearly.)

Particularly for women who do not plan to have vaginal penetration, a limited-depth procedure provides for the removal of penis, scrotum, and testicles; the creation of a neoclitoris and labia; and the relocation of the urethra. In essence, the limited-depth vagina looks like that of an assigned female except that there is no vaginal "vault." Sometimes, a small depression or dimple is created. A limited-depth vagina allows a woman to urinate like other females and to orgasm since she has a functional clitoris.

Hair removal may not be required prior to the limited-depth vaginoplasty, but confirm this with your surgeon. Vaginal dilation is not needed.

As the surgery itself is less lengthy, a limited-depth procedure may be an excellent option for a woman with medical factors that would make it more difficult for her to weather a more extensive vaginoplasty and recovery period.

Vaginoplasty with Limited Graft Tissue

In a penile inversion vaginoplasty, the neovagina is created from the inverted penis and often a graft derived from scrotal tissue.

Particularly with the use of puberty blockers in transgender adolescents, we are likely to see more young people coming to vaginoplasty with less genital tissue. If histrelin or a Lupron-Depot blockade is initiated in early puberty and the adolescent goes on to use cross-sex hormones, the penis and scrotum do not grow to full adult size.

Circumcision (the removal of infant foreskin that is done on most babies assigned male at birth in the United States) can also limit the amount of available skin.

Full- or partial-thickness grafts may be derived from the lateral flank or abdominal areas at the waist. In this technique, scars are concealed within the skin lines at the waist and covered by underpants or a swimsuit. It may also be possible to do a peritoneal pull-through vaginoplasty, where the peritoneal membrane from the abdomen is used to line the upper vaginal vault, or a colovaginoplasty, where colonic tissue forms the neovagina.

The Peritoneal Pull-Through Vaginoplasty

More recently, there has been the development of the peritoneal pull-through vaginoplasty technique. Dr. Davydov popularized this technique in the mid-twentieth century as a solution for cisgender women with vaginal agenesis (a birth defect involving the absence of or an incomplete vagina), and it is now also being used in gender-affirmation surgery.

After the same initial steps of the penile inversion technique, an abdominal procedure, which can be done laparoscopically or as a robot-assisted laparoscopic procedure, is performed to obtain peritoneal grafts that then line the neovagina and attach it to the epithelium at the perineum or lower vagina. All external genitalia and the vaginal opening are fashioned from penile and scrotal skin. The peritoneal graft can be used for a primary vaginoplasty, a secondary salvage vaginoplasty, or as an adjunct to penile inversion to add additional depth to the neovagina.

The risks include all those associated with the penile inversion technique—that is, possible stenosis (narrowing of the opening) and graft rejection—as well as those with abdominal laparoscopic surgery. In cisgender women with vaginal agenesis, the benefits include some natural lubrication, less need for dilation, less need for douching, and adequate depth. There are currently no data on long-term outcomes for the peritoneal grafting procedure in transgender individuals.

— Heidi Wittenberg, MD

In the peritoneal pull-through procedure or series of procedures, an individual first undergoes an orchiectomy (removal of the testicles). A vaginal vault is developed in the perineum and lined with a portion of the *peritoneal* membrane that encloses the abdominal organs. This tissue is brought down from the abdomen by way of robotic-assisted laparoscopy. Here, the peritoneal membrane becomes the lining of the neovagina.

Alternatively, in the full-thickness skin graft technique, a graft is typically taken from the abdomen and used as the lining for the vaginal canal. The skin graft is harvested using an abdominoplasty incision (a horizontal incision like you would see with a tummy tuck). The advantage of this approach, of course, is that you can get a tummy tuck at the same time. The disadvantage, when compared to the peritoneal-pull through, is the presence of a potentially long horizontal scar on the abdomen. Scrotal tissue is used to form the vaginal labia.

Perineum versus Peritoneum: Big Difference!

According to the Merriam-Webster dictionary, the perineum is "the area between the anus and the posterior part of the external genitalia." It is also defined as "an area between the thighs that marks the approximate lower boundary of the pelvis and is occupied by the urinary and genital ducts and rectum." (We sit on our perineums.)

The peritoneum, on the other hand, is an internal abdominal membrane that consists of two layers: the parietal peritoneum that lines the abdominal and pelvic cavities, and the visceral peritoneum that encloses the stomach, most of the small and large intestines, and the liver, gallbladder, and spleen.

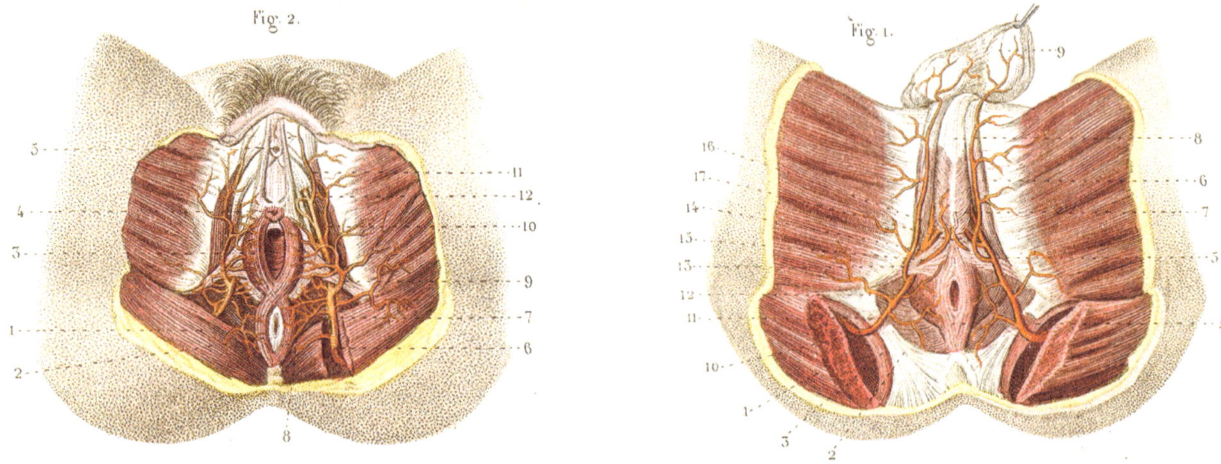

Figure 11.10. The perineum in an AFAB (left) and an AMAB (right).

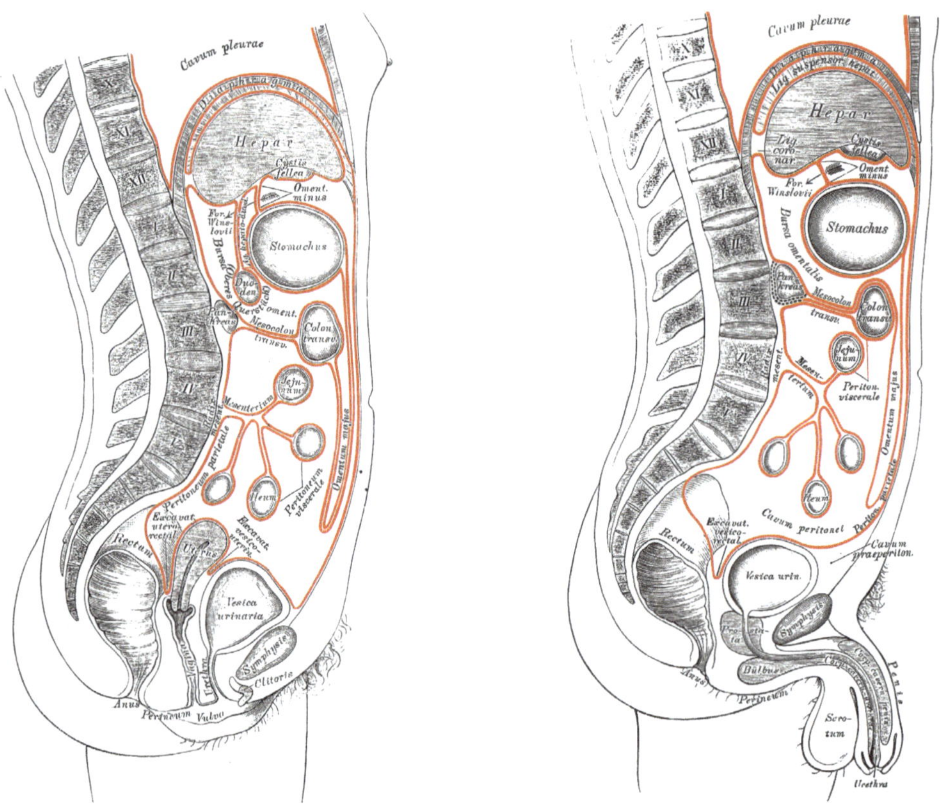

Figure 11.11. The peritoneum in an AFAB (left) and an AMAB (right).
Trace the peritoneal membrane as it encloses the various abdominal organs (red lines).
The peritoneum consists of two layers, with a "potential space" in between.

In AFAB individuals, the fallopian tubes and ovaries are included within the visceral peritoneum. The top of the uterus indents the peritoneum but is not enclosed by it. The kidneys, the upper part of the ureters, adrenal glands, the aorta, and the inferior vena cava are retroperitoneal. This means that these organs sit behind the peritoneal membrane and are not enclosed by it.

The parietal and visceral peritoneum lie immediately on top of each other, but can glide over each other since they're lubricated by secretions containing water, protein, and electrolytes. The area between the peritoneal layers is referred to as a "potential space." It is normally not a space at all, but it can be filled by pus, blood, or other fluid in states of infection, trauma, or malignancy.

For information on the penis/phallus-preserving vaginoplasty, refer to the newer nonbinary options below and on the next several pages.

Vaginoplasty Using the Sigmoid Colon (Rectosigmoid Vaginoplasty)

The rectosigmoid vaginoplasty[58] is rarely used in the United States, except in "salvage" or reconstructive surgeries in the event of vaginoplasty complications. First performed in 1904, the use of sigmoid and rectal tissue to create the neovagina has theoretical appeal for several reasons:

- The sigmoid colon self-lubricates with mucus.
- The length of the vagina created is not limited by the length of the penis (although this is circumvented by using scrotal or other tissue).
- Hair removal is not required preoperatively.
- Rectosigmoid surgery can now be done laparoscopically or robotically; in the past, an abdominal incision was required.

However, rectosigmoid surgeries have disadvantages as well:

- The lubrication produced by the sigmoid colon is *very* abundant.
- Colonic lubrication is continuous.
- Colonic secretions may have an associated odor.
- The neovagina still requires dilation.
- Dehiscence (the spontaneous opening of sutures) of the colonic repair can occur and may have life-threatening complications such as sepsis (bloodstream infection) or necrotizing fasciitis.
- The vaginal opening may look like colon tissue, even resembling a stoma in a colostomy rather than labia. This is not correctable by plastic surgery.
- Prolapse (out-pouching of the neovagina) can occur, but it is correctable.
- Screening an individual for colon cancer would require examining the neovagina as well as the colon; otherwise a colon cancer could go undetected.

Rectosigmoid vaginoplasty is widely used throughout the world, although penile inversion vaginoplasty has surpassed it in popularity.

58 "Bowel vaginoplasty was first described by Sneguireff in 1892 using the rectum in the treatment of vaginal agenesis. Later, in 1904, Baldwin reported the use of ileal segment in the treatment of congenital vaginal absence, but also suggested that the sigmoid colon might be used for the same purpose… In male to female transsexuals, first mention of intestinal vaginoplasty dates from 1974, when Markland and Hastings used cecum and sigmoid transplants." Marta Bizic et al., "An Overview of Neovaginal Reconstruction Options in Male to Female Transsexuals," *The Scientific World Journal* 2014, Article ID 638919 (May 26, 2014): 8 pages, https://doi.org/10.1155/2014/638919.

Vaginoplasty Using the Right (Ascending) Colon: aka Right Colo-Vaginoplasty

Note: Information about this surgery is provided by Geoffrey Stiller, MD.

See Figure 11.12 below. As you look at the drawing, remind yourself that the "right colon" refers to the *patient's* right. Remember that the ascending colon begins with the cecum, which is where the appendix originates. The stool is liquid when it moves from the small intestine into the cecum and ascending colon. It then travels upward to the hepatic (liver) flexure, where the colon turns at a near-right angle and travels horizontally to the splenic (spleen) flexure on the left side of the body. The colon takes another near-right angle turn as it becomes the descending colon and ultimately, the sigmoid and rectum.

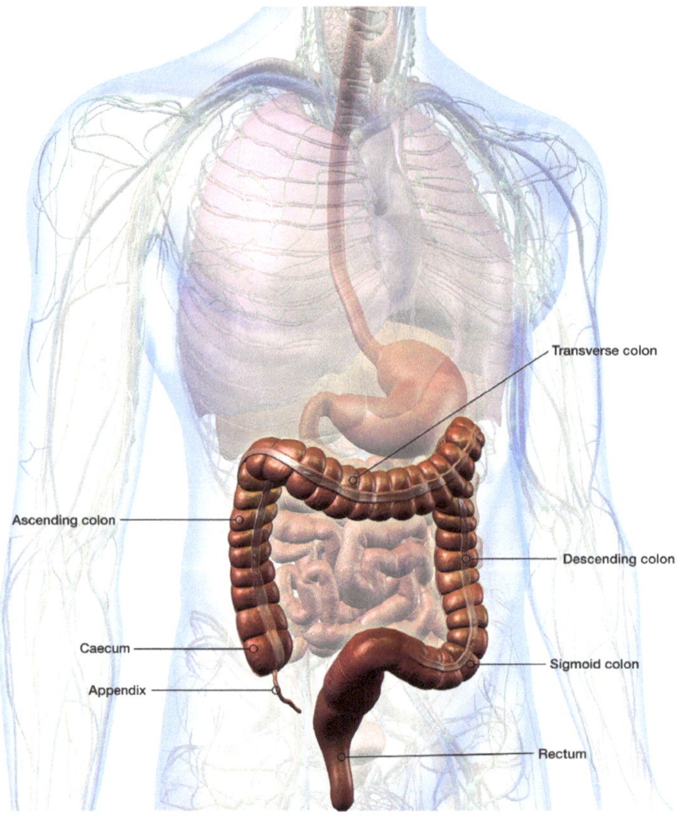

Figure 11.12. Anatomy of the colon.

The main function of the colon is to absorb fluid from the liquid stool, transferring it as a solid stool to the sigmoid colon and rectum—from which it is eliminated.

Another—and newer technique for vaginoplasty—uses the right or ascending colon rather than the sigmoid colon to create the vaginal vault. The right-colon vaginoplasty is offered as a primary procedure as well as a salvage operation for the revision of complications.

Right-colon vaginoplasty may be done in two separate surgeries. The first surgery is the creation of a zero-depth vagina using penile and scrotal tissue to create the labia. After a recovery period, the patient returns for the creation of the vaginal vault. Here, the right colon is moved to join the perineum at what will become the opening to the neovagina.

Because the full right colon is mobilized, vaginal depth can be generous (such as 9 inches), regardless of the patient's penile and scrotal size. The mobilization of the right colon can be done laparoscopically.

Potential Advantages of the Right-Colon Vaginoplasty

- The size of the right colon allows for a generous neovaginal depth, regardless of penile and scrotal size. This may be helpful in patients who are less well endowed, including those individuals who had puberty blockers and thus developed a smaller volume of genital tissue.
- The appendix can be removed at the time of this surgery, eliminating it as a potential site of inflammation (appendicitis) in later life.
- The blood supply of the right colon is generous, since several branches of the mesenteric vessels feed it. The sigmoid colon has a more complex arterial network with shorter branches.
- The colonic tissue is moved to the vaginal site, carrying its blood supply with it.
- No electrolysis is needed preoperatively, as the penis and possibly part of the scrotum are not inverted to create the internal tissues of the neovagina. This means no hair in the neovagina! We recognize that genital hair removal is expensive and time-consuming and can be painful.
- Using the penis and scrotum for the vaginal labia may result in a superior cosmetic result; simply, there is more tissue to use.
- The right colon lubricates, providing lubrication for the neovagina.
- If a patient is satisfied with Step 1—the creation of the zero-depth vagina—she can stop there.

Potential Disadvantages

- There are usually two surgeries, with exposures to two rounds of anesthesia. Two hospitalizations can mean more cost and more exposure to nosocomial infections (infections that a person contracts in the hospital, perhaps from sturdier, more drug-resistant bacteria).
- There may be an odor for roughly 6 months.
- Screening for colon cancer may become more complex. In a screening colonoscopy, a scope is introduced via the rectum so the examiner can see all the way along the colon to its beginning—that is, the cecum of the right colon. If a portion of the right colon becomes the neovagina, the vagina must also be scoped to perform a full exam of the colon.

> I would prefer that a colonoscope was used for screening; however, if a vaginal speculum can expose the entire vagina, that may be fine. If my patients have a hard time finding a gastroenterologist who is comfortable doing a vaginal scope at the time of their colonoscopy, then I would be more than happy to do their colonoscopy.
>
> — *Geoffrey Stiller, MD*

Dr. Alvaro H. Rodriguez Introduces Vaginoplasty Grafts from Tilapia at the WPATH 26th Scientific Symposium Surgeon's Program

Tilapia is the common name for a species of freshwater fish that is farmed all over the world. Plentiful and inexpensive, Nile tilapia were first used to graft burn injuries in human and animal skin in Brazil in 2015.

At the WPATH 26th Scientific Symposium Surgeon's Program on November 7, 2020, Dr. Alvaro H. Rodriguez presented a new use for tilapia—as a graft in vaginoplasty.[59] Rodriguez, a Colombian reconstructive surgeon specializing in gender-affirmation surgery and creator of the technique, stated,

> "After several years of research, we found that tilapia skin shares the same type of collagen as human skin, and it has almost the same strength. Because it is a fish, tilapia has DNA that is different than in humans. We think that is why tilapia skin is not rejected by human tissue."

Rodriguez went on to explain that after grafting the tilapia to line the neovagina, the tilapia skin is absorbed completely, leaving only the collagen.

> "This works as a matrix for the growth of new epithelium that looks like the vaginal mucosa both macroscopically and histologically."

Rodriguez showed pictures of tilapia skin with a prominent scale pattern. He explained that the fish skin is prepared by sterilization to be sure it is free of bacteria, and that the scales leave a tattoo pattern on the skin even though the scales themselves do not remain.

Dr. Rodriguez and colleagues are preparing their results for publication and are examining other uses of tilapia grafts that may serve the transgender community. Read more about Dr. Rodriguez's research and contact him at cecmcolombia.com.

In addition to Dr. Rodriguez, the tilapia research was conducted by Universidade Federal do Ceará professor Edmar Maciel Lima Júnior MD, coordinator of the research and head of the studies on the use of tilapia skin for burn treatment at the Instituto José Frota in Fortaleza, Ceará, Brazil, as well as Universidade Federal do Ceará professor Leonardo Bezerra PhD, coordinator of research in gynecology. Dr. Bezerra is also a pioneer of the treatment of vaginal agenesis (Mayer-Rokitansky-Küster-Hauser syndrome) with tilapia skin xenograft.

59 Alvaro H. Rodriguez, "Male-to-Female Gender Affirming Surgery Using Nile Tilapia Fish Skin as a Biocompatible Graft," (presentation, WPATH 26th Scientific Symposium Surgeon's Program, November 7, 2020).

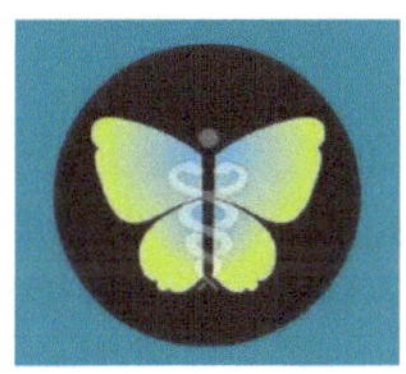

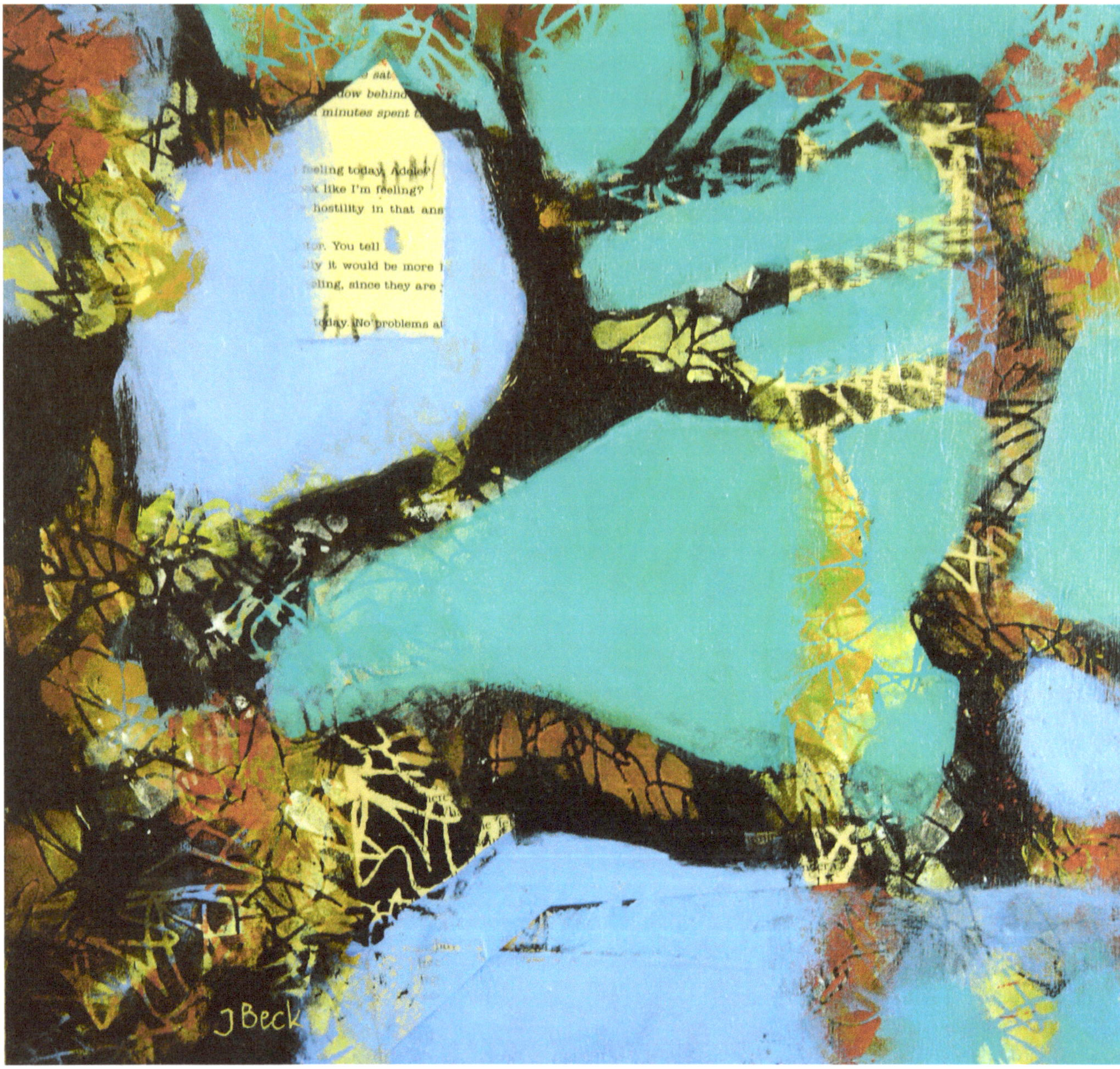
dow behind
minutes spent
feeling today, Adele?
like I'm feeling?
hostility in that
You tell
it would be more
since they are
today. No problems
J Beck

Birdhouse

MASCULINIZING SURGERIES

Disclaimer

The information provided here is intended to give you an overview on gender-affirming surgeries. It is not intended as medical advice for you personally.

For medical advice pertaining to you specifically, seek your answers from your surgeon and their surgical team. They are the obvious professionals who will have the answers pertaining to your body and your circumstances. Information provided by them must be given more weight than my input. You will also note that I am not including photos of surgical outcomes. They are widely available on the websites of the surgeons.

Facial Masculinization Surgery

A first case of *full* facial masculinization surgery (FMS) was performed by Dr. Jordan Deschamps-Braly in 2015. Many of the techniques used resemble FFS in reverse, but Deschamps-Braly also introduced the technique of the Adam's apple implant using a cartilage graft from the patient's rib.

The rib cartilage is harvested through an inframammary incision, below the breast. The cartilage is then shaped to resemble a Y and implanted over and slightly below the patient's existing thyroid cartilage. Two notable points: (1) The rib cartilage is harvested via an *inframammary* incision that many trans men already have from top surgery, and (2) the cartilage graft is autologous, meaning that the patient will not reject their own grafted tissue.[60]

In more recent years, the practice of facial masculinization surgery has expanded, both in cis and trans males. As with FFS, facial masculinization surgeries represent an aggregate of separate procedures done together or in stages. Performed together, these surgeries may take 6 to 12 hours to perform.

You may want to review the part on facial feminization surgery earlier in this chapter to examine the basic differences between AFAB and AMAB faces. Generally, male faces have more prominent brow bones and larger, more angular jaws. Male-pattern hairlines appear squarer and more angular, particularly at the temples.

A typically "male" feature is the Adam's apple (thyroid cartilage), and it does not usually enlarge with the addition of testosterone in transition. Trans men do show facial changes while on testosterone. Some changes are likely due to a change in fat distribution, age, and changing hair patterns.

While others disagree, I believe bony changes are visibly evident also. I see it in our trans male patients, and you'll see some impressive chronologies on YouTube. I did not find scholarly documentation for facial bony changes in trans men on testosterone, but bone is living tissue and it does undergo remodeling.

60 Jordan C. Deschamps-Braly et al., "First Female-to-Male Facial Confirmation Surgery with Description of a New Procedure for Masculinization of the Thyroid Cartilage (Adam's Apple)," *Plastic & Reconstructive Surgery* 139, no. 4 (April 2017): 884e, https://doi.org/10.1097/prs.0000000000003185.

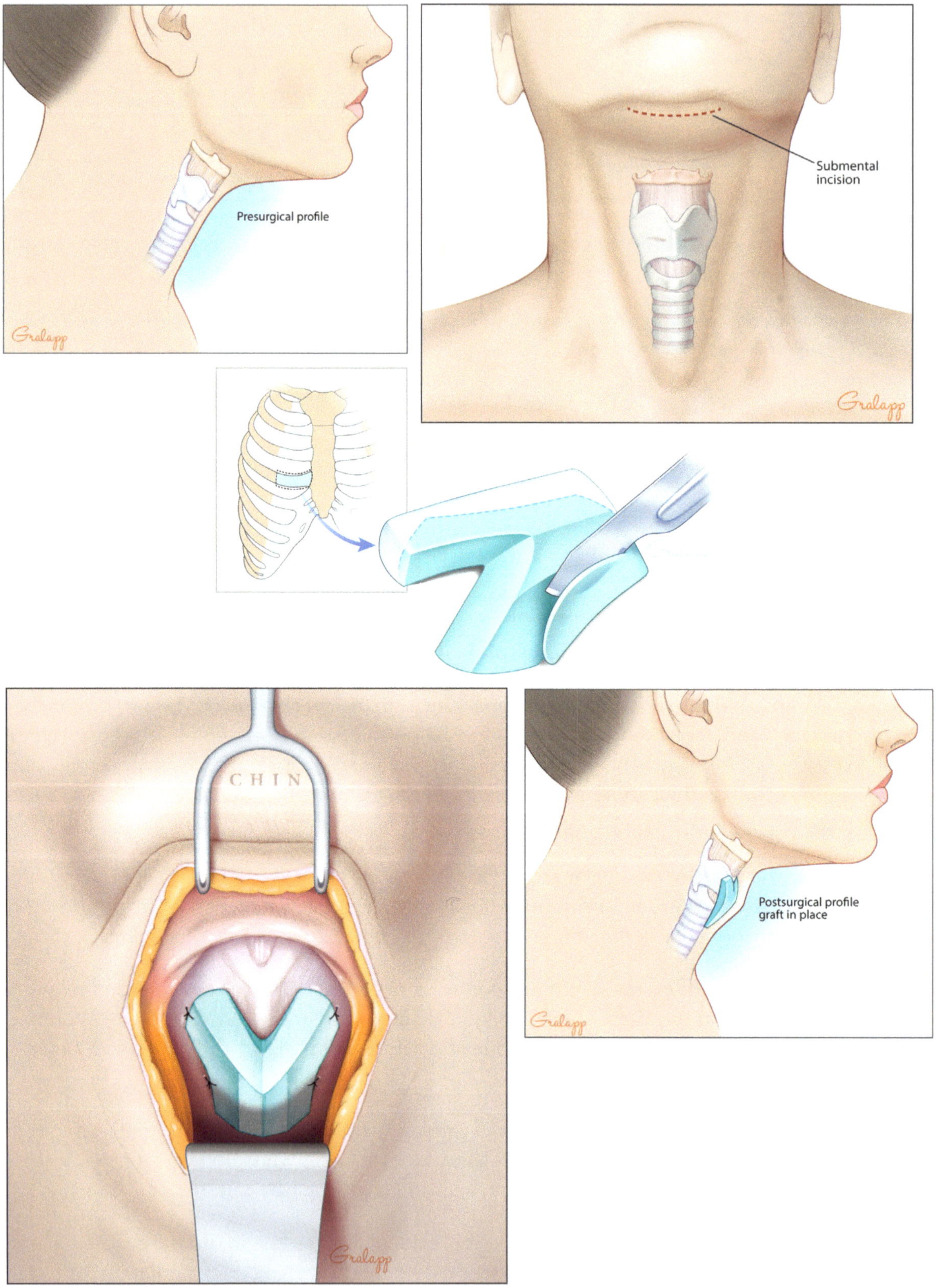

Figure 11.13. Tracheal augmentation.

As in FFS, your surgeon will want to know *your* desired outcomes. What would *you* like to see happen to enhance your facial masculinity? The surgeon will examine your head shape, hairline, face, and neck and offer their recommendations. It's important to remember that a single change in one part of the face will impact not only the appearance of adjacent structures, but the entire face. Because of the facial subtleties of gender, it is wise to seek out a surgeon with experience with transgender individuals.

FMS Is a Collection of Surgeries

In facial masculinization surgeries, you may see the following modifications:

- **Brow bone enhancement**
  The male brow bone is typically prominent (referred to as brow "bossing"). In FMS, the brow bone is augmented with implants or sculpted with a biologically completable chemical to create a ridge above the brow.

- **Forehead elongation**
  Male foreheads tend to appear higher, with more distance between the brows and from the brow to the hairline. In FMS, a higher forehead can be accomplished by lifting and moving the scalp backward, placing an implant between the brows, and revising the orbital sockets.

- **Hair transplants**
  Hair is harvested from the base of the skull, often one to three follicles at a time. The transplants fill in areas of androgynous alopecia (male pattern hair loss). But, do remember that balding is almost always read as male.

- **Rhinoplasty**
  This surgery, otherwise known as a nose job, creates a larger, more masculine-appearing nose. A male nose tends to be longer and not as upturned as a female nose. Rib cartilage can be used to enlarge the bridge of the nose or extend its length. Most importantly, the nose must balance the face.

- **Cheek implants**
  Implants accent the cheekbones. Implants imply that silicone or some other compatible material is inserted, while grafts are transfers of fat or bone from other parts of the body.

- **Chin and mandible contouring**
  The chin may be squared by lengthening it, and the angles of the jaw are made more prominent with a custom implant. The jawbones can be accessed from inside the mouth. Some surgeons make an exterior incision, such as under the chin, so it can be hidden.

- **Adam's apple enhancement**
  Although both males and females have an Adam's apple (thyroid cartilage), it is typically much more prominent in natal males. As stated earlier, Dr. Jordan Deschamps-Braly described his technique of harvesting and shaping rib cartilage and placing it over the existing thyroid cartilage to create a visible Adam's apple. The harvest of the rib cartilage is made at the inframammary crease, often through an existing scar from top surgery.[61]

61 Deschamps-Braly et al., 884e.

- **Facelift**
  As in females, excess skin is removed and the lower and middle parts of the face are tightened to provide a more youthful appearance. However, if done in the same way as female faces, it may actually feminize the face. The techniques vary with males and should be approached in the same way as in cis men. Again, it is important to choose a surgeon who is expert in transgender facial variations. Incision lines may be camouflaged immediately in front of the ears or behind them. This is commonly done in middle-aged and older individuals.

Gender-Affirming Chest Reconstruction (Top Surgery)

Nothing seems to impact the overall life experience of individuals seeking to masculinize like top surgery does. It is a commonly performed surgery that is frequently covered by insurance (sometimes even in adolescents), and it grants trans men freedom from wearing chest binders.

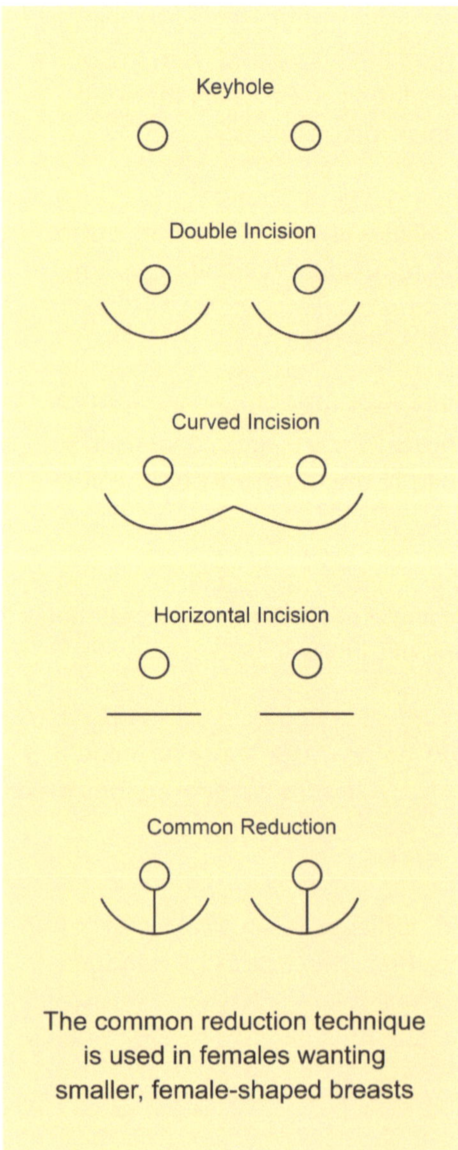

Figure 11.14. Top-surgery scars.

The goal of top surgery is to create a *male* chest contour, not to create *smaller female-appearing* breasts. Look at the diagram at left to see the differences between the scars after a reduction mammoplasty and typical gender-affirming top surgery.

Postsurgical Scars in Reduction Mammoplasty versus Top Surgery

There are two general types of top surgeries, and they both depend on the size of the breasts before surgery.

Most trans men will have a *double incision surgery*. The double incision refers to the two nearly horizontal or curvilinear scars that follow the borders of the pectoralis muscles. In the double incision technique, most of the breast tissue is removed, while some remains to create a masculine contour. Sometimes, instead of having two separate incisions, the double incisions are connected into a single curvilinear incision. The effect of each type of top surgery is to create the appearance of a "cut" (fit or "buff") pectoralis muscle.

In the double incision surgery, the areolas (or more properly, the nipples and areolas) are removed and reshaped. (Aerolas are the colored parts around the nipples.) Male areolas are considerably smaller than female areolas. The nipple and areolar complex are grafted back onto the chest at the end of the surgery, and a medicated gauze stent or bolster is sewn on to secure the areola. After about 5 to 7 days, the nipple stents are removed. The nipple grafts must be kept moist with petroleum jelly or Aquaphor for the next 2 weeks. By the time the stents are removed, the blood supply from the chest is serving the reattached nipple directly. This is a critical step and the reason surgeons are so insistent that a patient does not smoke.

A surgeon told one of my clients:
"If you don't stop smoking, your nipples may fall off like dried cornflakes."

— Linda Gromko, MD

Bidding the Girls—but Not My Personality—Goodbye

After top surgery, my level of self-confidence is amazing. I now walk with my head held high, but with a humble spirit. Because for me, stepping into manhood is NOT about going shirtless or so-called "masculine swag." It goes much deeper than that. It's becoming one with ALL of me. I'm finally embracing and celebrating ALL of who I AM: my Sacred Self; the wounded child; the strong-willed, fiercely independent but scarred woman; and the sensitive, soft-hearted man who isn't afraid of his feminine attributes. Becoming a man has allowed me to homogenize all of my Sacred Souls into that of a healthy, well-adjusted male.

Since taking this journey, I am being forced to confront all of my demons and embrace my quirks and flaws while opening my heart and mind to ongoing healing and growth.

Setting the Record Straight

Becoming a man wasn't about me finding "happiness" or peace of mind. I had to do the road work before entering the ring. Hence, after 4 years of weekly therapy, I was able to arrive at a place of psychological and emotional contentment BEFORE I was rolled into the surgical suite. This is because I've never believed top surgery and hormones to be a panacea or quick-fix—it was only to align my physical body with my inner truth.

So, What *Was* It All About?

My journey into manhood was not about being macho, chasing women, wearing three-piece tailored suits, finding happiness, escaping depression, hanging with the boys on a Saturday night, building large muscles, or gaining brawn. It's about acquiring emotional maturity, dignity under pressure, greater calmness in the midst of chaos, and gentleness and compassion toward myself and others. It's also about being accountable, having increased patience, having strength during those moments when I want to just let it all go, and pursuing continued spiritual development along with service to others.

For me, this is what becoming and being a man is all about. Have I arrived yet? Not yet, because I am a Designer's Original that is an ongoing work in progress.

— Harlowe Rayne Thunderword-Cohen

Areolar pigmentation may change in the process of top surgery. The areolas may appear mottled, with patches of hypopigmentation or even no pigmentation. Sometimes the nipple itself will not protrude as prominently as a patient might have hoped. Time and patience can remedy both of these conditions. Pigment often returns to the areola slowly over time. If all areas have not filled in by a year or two, tattooing may be used to fill in the hypopigmented (pink) parts. If the nipple projection is not enough, 3D tattooing can also be done using shading and highlights to create the appearance of a protruding nipple (see page 285).

Individuals who have less chest tissue may have keyhole surgery. For this surgery to be successful, the patient must have a relatively small amount of breast tissue and no excess skin. Additionally, the nipples and areolas must be small and they must naturally be positioned higher on the chest near the edge of the pectoralis muscle. If these requirements are not met, a person may have a more satisfactory result with a double incision procedure.

> **What does a keyhole have to do with this? "Keyhole" is a confusing term as it implies a vertical incision so it looks like an old skeleton keyhole or a lollipop. Most surgeons have a different idea about what a keyhole approach actually is. It really should be called a periareolar or transareolar surgery.**
>
> — *Toby Meltzer, MD*

With the keyhole technique, the surgeon enters the breast by making an incision under or around the areola. Most of the breast tissue is removed and the incision is sutured together. If the nipples are relatively large, they will be reshaped as in the double incision surgery.

> **As a reminder, top surgery does not eliminate the possibility of breast cancer, so chest exams done by a transmasculine person and their healthcare provider are important. Evaluation of any lump is critical, as is special attention to those men with cancer-provoking gene mutations such as BRCA1 and BRCA2.**

Hysterectomy and Bilateral Salpingo-Oophorectomy

Many—but certainly not all—trans men have their uterus, cervix, fallopian tubes, and ovaries removed.

Hysterectomy and bilateral salpingo-oophorectomy can be accomplished through the abdomen or the vagina. But today, these procedures are often done using minimally invasive surgical techniques such as laparoscopic and robot-assisted procedures. These enable the surgeon to make much smaller incisions. The organs are clearly seen, as a camera (the laparoscope) is placed through the belly button, and photographs are projected on large screens opposite the surgeon and assistant. In robotic surgeries, the surgeon actually manipulates the "hands" of the robot and the camera remotely via computer, while the assistant holds and retracts the laparoscopic instruments so the surgeon can see the surgical field.

> **After the hysterectomy, I could feel that something was missing. But it was something that never should have been there in the first place.**
>
> — *Trans man, age 55*

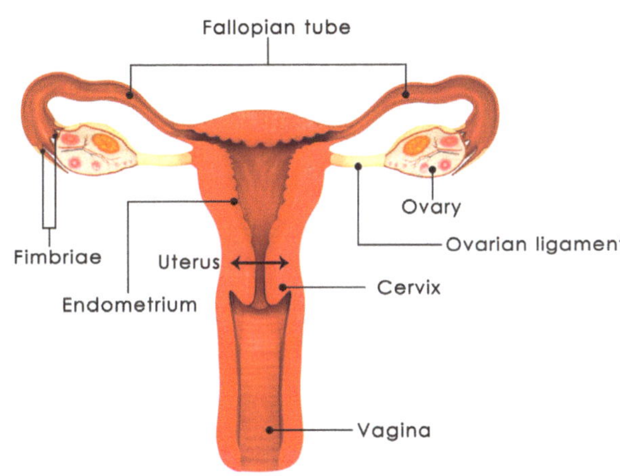

Figure 11.15. Internal female reproductive organs.

This surgery is done in preparation for phalloplasty, and removing these organs accomplishes the following:

- It allows for the definitive treatment of benign pathology, such as uterine fibroids, and essentially eliminates the possibility of cancer of the uterus, cervix, ovaries, or fallopian tubes. (Fallopian tube cancer is very rare but can occur in people who have the BRCA1 or BRCA2 gene mutation that also increases the risk of a person getting breast, ovarian, peritoneal, or pancreatic cancer.)[62] Typically, cancers of the ovary, fallopian tubes, or peritoneum have subtle symptoms that are recognized late in the disease process. Particularly for trans men who are reluctant to seek out gynecological care, removing these organs can be prudent.
- Eliminates the possibility of the vaginal bleeding that occurs when people run out of their testosterone, forget to take it, or are prescribed a dose that's too low. Bleeding can also occur due to a disease state, such as—and most importantly—with cancer. That's why bleeding that doesn't stop with hormone adjustments must be evaluated further.

A hysterectomy and bilateral salpingo-oophorectomy can be combined with procedures that reduce incontinence of urine or stool. This can be helpful for trans men who have had vaginal deliveries before transitioning.

62 Nancie Petrucelli, Mary B. Daly, and Tuya Pal, "BRCA1- and BRCA2-Associated Hereditary Breast and Ovarian Cancer," in *GeneReviews*, ed. Margaret P. Adam et al. (Seattle: University of Washington, 1993–2021, September 4, 1998), updated December 15, 2016, https://www.ncbi.nlm.nih.gov/books/NBK1247/.

Monsplasty

The mons pubis is a fatty area that lies over the pubic bone. It tends to be more prominent in assigned females, especially after having a baby, and there is no amount of physical exercise that can be done to get rid the mons specifically. It typically "reads" female.

By liposuction or via an open horizontal incision, mons tissue is reduced to create a flat mons rather than a pooch. This surgery can be combined with other male reconstructive surgeries such as metoidioplasty or vaginectomy.[63]

Learning about the Masculinizing Genital Surgeries

This is a repeat of information shared earlier: If you are not medically trained and do not speak medicine as a second language, stop for a moment before you go on. The following information about genital surgeries gets complicated. Don't get discouraged as you read. If you find this difficult, remember that it is complex information, but it is manageable. It's my problem as the author if I cannot make it understandable.

— Linda Gromko MD

- Read slowly and look up words you don't know.
- Read the information out loud to another person or an animal. (I remember a medical school classmate who would tell her tiny daughter "stories" about the anatomy of the heart. Kids want to hear your voice and don't care as much about content.)
- Stop after every paragraph and be sure you are still on track before going ahead. Otherwise, you may get lost, anxious, and overwhelmed.
- Don't give up!
- If you're more of visual learner, look at a picture, a medical illustration, a diagram, or a video. Visit youtube.com and search on the terms "sexual reassignment surgery," "phalloplasty," "metoidioplasty," or "FTM sex change."

Most importantly, if you are reading this to prepare for your own surgery, be certain you know exactly what you are having done. Speak to your surgeon, the ARNP or PA, the clinic coordinator, or someone else in their office ("To whom may I talk with to get my questions answered before surgery?"). Do not sign up for a surgery you do not understand!

63 Osama Kamal Zaki Shaeer, "Shaeer's Technique: A Minimally Invasive Procedure for Monsplasty and Revealing the Concealed Penis," *PRS Global Open* 4, no. 8 (August 29, 2016): e1019, https://dx.doi.org/10.1097%2FGOX.0000000000001019. See also the video graphics at https://www.ncbi.nlm.nih.gov/pmc/articles/PMC5010356/figure/F9/.

Masculinizing Genital Surgeries

Masculinizing genital surgery is also known as male sexual reassignment surgery, lower surgery, or bottom surgery. In this part, we will review the different types of masculinizing genital surgeries. Within each type, there are wide variations in style and technique. A phalloplasty, for example, may really incorporate three or four individual operations done in a series. These surgeries can be very complex, and surgical complications are not uncommon.

Male sexual reassignment surgeries have evolved tremendously over the past 20 years. Until recently, masculinizing genital surgeries were not covered by health insurance. Today, they are covered more commonly, particularly with larger group policies.

Each of the broader types of masculinizing surgeries has a different outcome—that is, it meets a different goal. It is critical that a person knows exactly what is important to them and to be clear about wanting genital surgery at all.

We have reviewed that embryonic genitals in assigned males and assigned females are virtually identical (refer to the Netter Embryologic Equivalents illustration on page 209 for a refresher). The clitoris and its shaft are the embryologic equivalent of the penis. Under the influence of testosterone, the clitoris enlarges and looks very much like a small penis. Many trans men find this clitoral enlargement (clitoromegaly) to be very satisfactory without *any* surgical intervention.

Certainly, many trans men don't want to risk the possibility of surgical complications. Many do not have financial access to surgery or regional access to a qualified surgeon. And I often hear from my clients, "I'm going to wait for another 10 years to see how these surgeries evolve."

Needless to say, it is important to do your homework. Talk to people who have had the various surgeries performed *on them*. Go to conferences, follow online groups, and explore reddit.com for candid information on trans male surgeries. Examine the photographs on the websites of various surgeons.

Deciding on the Best Type of Masculinizing Genital Surgery for You

Answer the Following Questions about Your Own Goals

- **Is it the *appearance* of my genitals that matters most to me?**
  (I'm told that many men really don't stare at one another's genitals in bathrooms or locker rooms, but surgery can make you feel more comfortable in these day-to-day situations.)
- **Is it important for me to have a *bulge* in my crotch?**
- **Is it important for me to have a scrotum?**
- **Is it important to have testicles that can be felt in the scrotum?**
- **Is it important that I am able to *stand* to pee?**
- **Is it important that I can pee *through* the end of my penis?**
- **Do I want to be able to use my penis to have sex with a partner?**
  Stated another way, is it important for me to be able to *penetrate* or enter my partner with my penis during sex? If so, am I seeking a particular size of penis?

Read through Table 11.1 below to help you sort out your own goals and match them to the various types of genital masculinizing surgeries available.

Deciding on a Type of Male Genital Surgery						
Surgery Type	**Looks like a Penis**	**Can Stand to Pee**	**Can Pee through the Penis**	**Can Use the Penis for Penetration**	**Bulge in the Crotch**	**Can Feel Testicles in the Scrotum**
Metoidioplasty	Yes	Not through the phallus	No	No*	Unlikely	No
Metoidioplasty and urethral extension (lengthening)	Yes	Maybe**	Yes	No*	Unlikely	No
Metoidioplasty and scrotoplasty	Yes	Maybe with urethral extension**	With urethral extension	No*	Yes	No
Metoidioplasty and scrotoplasty and implants	Yes	Maybe with urethral extension**	With urethral extension	No*	Yes	Yes
Delayed pedicle flap phalloplasty only ("shaft only")	Yes***	No	No, unless modified with separate urethral lengthening	With an erectile pump	Yes	With scrotoplasty and implants
Phalloplasty with radial forearm or anterior thigh flap and urethral reconstruction	Yes	Yes	Yes	With a pump or malleable rod	Yes	With scrotoplasty and implants

Table 11.1. Deciding on a type of male genital surgery.

* Metoidioplasty is generally not advertised for penetration, but many trans males state that they can penetrate partners. This is highly individual, so do not assume that penetration will be possible with metoidioplasty as you make your decision.

** Standing to pee is dependent on a person's overall size. If obese, a person may not be able to stand to pee after metoidioplasty with a urethral extension. A metoidioplasty phallus may not be long enough to clear a zipper, meaning that you may have to lower your pants to pee standing up.

*** Probably less "classic" appearance; can be modified.

Remember: You will not pee through a phallus without a urethral extension; nobody pees through a natal clitoris without urethral extension (urethral lengthening)!

Metoidioplasty (Also Known as "Meta")

The word *metoidioplasty* is derived from its Greek roots: *meta* (toward), *aidoia* (male genitals), and *plasty* (formation).

There are a number of variations on the metoidioplasty procedure, and which surgery a person selects depends on their overall goals.

In a basic metoidioplasty, the clitoris—which is already enlarged by the effects of testosterone—is released from its supporting ligaments. (Released, not removed!) The ligaments involved here are the suspensory ligament that connects the clitoris to the symphysis pubis (pubic bone) and the supporting ligaments of the labia minora. This type of metoidioplasty can also be called a "clitoral release." Tissue from the underside of the clitoris or the labia minora may be used to increase the "bulk" of the neophallus.

The effect of metoidioplasty is to make the clitoris appear longer, protrude farther, and look more penis-like. Metoidioplasty creates a phallus that measures about 4 to 6 centimeters. Given that 2½ centimeters equals 1 inch, you might have a phallus of about 2 inches in length. As stated above, sometimes girth *can* be augmented by using labial tissue.

Talk to your surgeon and be as specific as you can about what you want to see happen. Your surgeon should be able to give you an idea about how much length and girth you can expect. If you want to be able to pee through the penis, read on about metoidioplasty with urethral extension (urethral lengthening). Going back to embryology, nobody pees through the clitoris but assigned males pee *through* the urethral opening in the glans penis; so, the clitoris must be modified to make this possible.

Metoidioplasty with Urethral Extension (Also Called Urethral Lengthening)

Metoidioplasty with urethral extension is sometimes called a *metoidioplasty with a urethral hook-up*. The urethra (the tube through which you pee) is elongated and directed *through* the phallus. The skin used to elongate the urethra is often the buccal (pronounced "buckle") mucosa from inside the cheeks of the mouth, or skin from the inner lining of the vagina. This is a more complex procedure than metoidioplasty alone, and it has a greater risk of complications.

Other names may be used to describe various techniques. A ring metoidioplasty uses vaginal wall tissue and tissue from the labia minora to connect the urethra and the neophallus. The Centurion technique uses the round ligaments of the labia majora to add girth to the phallus. (See **healthline.com/health/transgender/metoidioplasty**.)

Any surgery that creates a new tube-like structure or elongates an existing one carries a risk for stricture, or narrowing of the newly created tube. The place where a new tube attaches to an existing one is called an "anastomosis" (connection). Anastomoses are particularly vulnerable to stricture or the formation of a fistula (an opening where it doesn't belong).

If a person has a stricture, he may be looking at several possible solutions, including dilation to widen the neourethra or a surgery to revise the urethral extension.

It is possible that a stricture can stop the urine flow entirely. The bladder continues to fill up with urine but the flow is obstructed. Should this happen, a man needs to be evaluated right away to dilate the stricture open and catheterize the urethra. If this cannot be accomplished, a suprapubic catheter can be inserted.

A man may require two catheters while the neourethra heals after surgery: one in the urethra and another placed in the suprapubic space that drains the bladder through the lower abdomen.

Q How does a man recognize that a stricture is developing?

A As the neourethra narrows, urine flow slows and it takes longer to pee. A man will also have to push harder to get the urine out.

Another complication of metoidioplasty with urethral lengthening is fistula formation. A fistula is a hole where there shouldn't be one—in this case, a new opening in the underside of the phallus. This causes dripping, or more than one urine stream appearing during urination. Fistulae may resolve spontaneously, or they may require a surgical repair. Today, because men who have had vaginectomies have significantly fewer fistulas and strictures, most surgeons do not perform urethral lengthening without vaginectomy.

A metoidioplasty with urethral extension enables a man to pee through the penis. It also allows a man to pee standing up, although this works best for trans men of normal body weight (not obese). As with trans women who have had a vaginoplasty, post-op trans men may have a urinary stream that may vary in direction for several months.

Metoidioplasty and Scrotoplasty with or without Testicular Implants

A scrotum can be created by fusing the labia majora in the midline. Adding well-vascularized fat grafts (fat has a rich blood supply) can add fullness to the neoscrotum. If a person elects, prosthetic testicles may be implanted into the neoscrotum. This gives more fullness and the appearance and feel of mobile testicles.

Sometimes, the scrotum is enlarged by placing tissue expanders in the neoscrotum to allow for larger testicular implants. Tissue expanders are fluid reservoirs that are placed temporarily within the scrotum. The owner injects gradually larger amounts of sterile water to gently stretch the tissue at designated time intervals. (Injection ports sit outside of the scrotum, so a man injects through the ports, not directly through his scrotal skin.)

Expectations for Metoidioplasty and Its Variations

These procedures provide for an excellent genital appearance. The phallus looks like a classic penis, although smaller. And in cases where the urethra is elongated and directed through the phallus, they allow for a trans man to pee standing up (although, as stated earlier, this works best for trans men who are not obese). Some men will have to lower their pants when urinating, as the phallus may not clear the zipper.

Metoidioplasties do not interfere with sexual sensation or orgasm. There is virtually no scarring, and recovery time is comparatively short. They can be combined with the more extensive procedures of hysterectomy (removal of the uterus), bilateral salpingo-oophorectomy (the removal of both ovaries and fallopian tubes), and vaginectomy (sealing of the vagina and closure of its perineal opening). These additions require more surgical time, a longer recovery, and more money.

If you are the kind of man who wants to keep his options open, know that you can have *all* the procedures described above, or even some of them, and still have a phalloplasty later on.

> One of my experienced trans male patients had a metoidioplasty and scrotoplasty several years ago. He was helping a younger trans man after his brand-new metoidioplasty and scrotoplasty.
>
> "Wow," said the younger one, "I can't believe I have a scrotum."
>
> "Yeah," said the veteran, "just wait 'til you get your balls!"
>
> *— Linda Gromko, MD*

Phalloplasty

Some Important Surgical Definitions

Knowing the difference between a graft and a flap is important in understanding these complex surgeries. Take your time to go through this information because it will make it much easier to comprehend what happens in the various phalloplasty techniques.

Skin Grafts and Flaps

Before we get into the details of phalloplasty, let's start by discussing the types of skin grafts and flaps that are used to build the neophallus (new penis). Grafts and flaps both serve the same two functions in phalloplasty: One function is to create the phallus itself; the other function is to physically cover the site where the penile graft or flap came from. This should become clearer in "Radial Forearm Flap Phalloplasty" starting on page 240 and the paragraphs that follow.

As you learn about grafts and flaps, refer to Figure 11.16, the anatomical illustration of the skin, on page 239 to further your understanding of the differences.

Definition of a Graft

In a graft, tissue is removed from one part of the body and reattached directly onto another site to cover a wound or a tissue defect from trauma. The donor site is the place where a graft is taken or removed. (The donor human and recipient human are the same person, so tissue rejection is not a problem.) **Grafts must rely on the blood supply at the site of attachment,** as opposed to flaps, where the blood supply is carried to the new site along with the flap tissue.

- **Full-thickness graft:** This refers to a graft composed of the donor skin's epidermis (outer or top layer) and the entire dermis (the layer below the epidermis that contains elastic fibers, connective tissue, hair follicles, nerves, and tiny blood vessels). The subcutaneous tissue, which contains fatty tissue, is not included. A full-thickness graft must be closed surgically.
- **Split-thickness graft:** This refers to a graft composed of the donor skin's epidermis and part of the underlying dermis. Thinner than a full-thickness graft, a split-thickness graft will heal on its own without being sutured onto the recipient site.

Definition of a Flap

In a flap, tissue is removed from one site and surgically repositioned to another location, carrying its blood supply along with it. In a flap, there must be at least one robust artery to supply blood to the site and several veins to allow blood to return back to the heart. A flap may consist of skin only, but it can be skin plus muscle and even bone. The blood supply is always carried with a free flap or pedicle flap.

- **Free flap:** In a free flap, tissue is moved from a donor site to a distant recipient site. Moving the tissue this far requires disconnecting the artery and vein completely from the donor site, then reconnecting the artery and vein at the recipient site. Making this reconnection of vessels to supply blood flow is done using microsurgical techniques. An example is the radial forearm flap (RFF), which will be explained below.
- **Pedicle or pedicled flap:** Tissue is relocated by way of a tissue bridge rather than isolated blood vessels. This does not require microsurgical joining of one blood vessel to another. (They are not separated, so they do not have to be reattached.) An example is the anterior lateral thigh flap phalloplasty (ALT), discussed below.
- **Delayed pedicle flap or delayed pedicled flap:** This refers to a flap where tissue is repositioned to cover a nearby site, leaving a "corner" or a bridge of adjoining tissue through which the blood vessels travel. This does not require microsurgical joining of one blood vessel to another. (They are not separated, so they do not have to be reattached.) In a delayed pedicle flap, the surgery requires multiple steps done at intervals of 1 to 3 months.

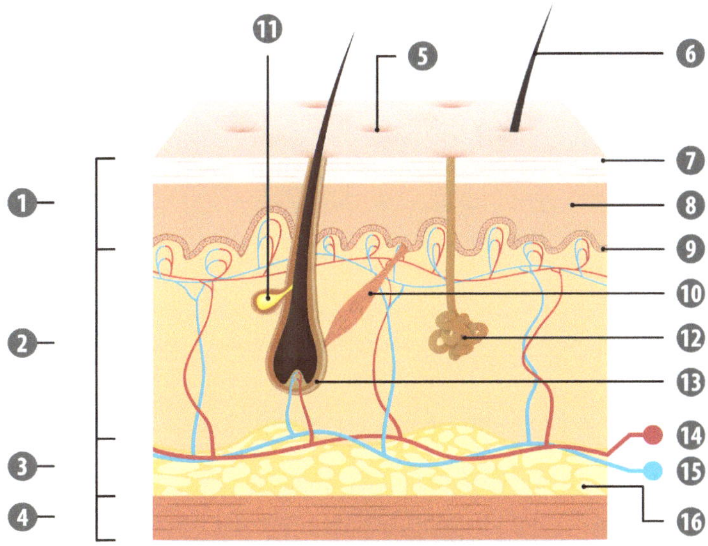

1. Epidermis
2. Dermis
3. Hypodermis
4. Muscle
5. Pores
6. Hair shaft
7. Stratum corneum
8. Squamous cells
9. Basal cells
10. Arrector pili muscle
11. Sebaceous(oil) gland
12. Sweat pore
13. Hair follicle
14. Artery
15. Vein
16. Adipose tissue

Figure 11.16. Structure of the skin.

Phalloplasty Options

The word *phalloplasty* is derived from the Greek and means "building a penis." Phalloplasty is much more complicated than metoidioplasty and its variations.

In practical terms, phalloplasty is far more expensive, more time-consuming (usually performed in several surgical procedures over 1 to 2 years), more difficult for a surgical team to perform, and more likely to have complications that will require surgical correction than other masculinizing genital surgeries.

All that said, phalloplasty creates a much larger penis, a penis that can penetrate a partner, and in many cases, a penis you can pee through. Here are the main categories of phalloplasty performed in the United States:

- **Radial forearm flap (RFF) phalloplasty**
  A free flap procedure where the neophallus is created from the radial forearm. (The radial forearm refers to the part of the forearm served by the radial nerves and blood vessels; "radial" refers to the radius bone on the thumb side of the wrist.) The forearm site is resurfaced by a split-thickness graft taken from the thigh.

- **Anterior lateral thigh (ALT) flap phalloplasty**
  The ALT phalloplasty is actually a pedicle flap phalloplasty where a flap from the thigh is carried by a bridge of tissue to form the neophallus. A split-thickness skin graft (also taken from the thigh) is used to resurface the ALT donor site. Donor tissue can also be taken from the side of the back using the latissimus dorsi muscle area. And there is another technique using the fibula (bone in the lateral lower leg) and nearby tissue. The latter two techniques are less common in the United States.

- **Delayed pedicle flap phalloplasty**
  In this technique, abdominal or groin tissue is used to create a nontubular (closed) cylinder, which is separated from its base at one end only. This creates a larger penis than with metoidioplasty. Penetration is possible with an implanted pump or malleable rod. A urethra may be reconstructed later and requires a microsurgical procedure. The delayed pedicle flap phalloplasty is done in several steps and is described on pages 246–247.

All Phalloplasties Require Several Steps

Most people coming to phalloplasty have already had a hysterectomy and bilateral salpingo-oophorectomy performed. As stated before, this is the removal of the uterus, cervix, ovaries, and fallopian tubes. A hysterectomy can be approached through a vaginal incision, a lower abdominal incision, or by way of robotic-assisted or laparoscopic techniques that add tiny incisions in the lower abdomen and belly button. If you have not had a hysterectomy done, you generally start with this. You may have a vaginectomy performed at the same time, but do talk to your surgeon about the technique and sequence they recommend.

In a vaginectomy, the vaginal lining tissue is removed so it can heal with one vaginal wall adhering to the opposite side. This causes the vagina to seal up and close the perineum so there will no longer be a vaginal opening at all. Particularly for nonbinary individuals, preservation of the vagina may be desired, along with creation of the phallus, although vaginectomy reduces the risk of fistula formation.

Please refer to these excellent medical illustrations done by artist Hillary Wilson. While the technique and the order of the steps may vary, these illustrations will give you a good idea of the basics of phalloplasty, complex as they are. Follow along with the illustrations as you read on.

Radial Forearm Flap Phalloplasty (RFF)

First Stage: Phallus Creation

- **The radial forearm site is prepared ("radial" means it is on the thumb side).**
  Generally using the patient's nondominant arm (that is, if you are right-handed, your left forearm will likely be used), the surgeon uses a template to trace the shape of the radial forearm flap. The flap is then surgically removed from the underlying tissue as a full-thickness flap, which includes the radial artery and veins as well as the lateral antebrachial sensory nerves and superficial veins. After this flap is removed, the donor site on the radial forearm will be resurfaced with a split-thickness skin graft harvested from the thigh.

  This patient will have already had electrolysis hair removal over the donor area. This is important, as the "tube in a tube" (which creates the penis) will have hair-bearing surfaces on the *outside* of the penis as well as on the *inside* of the urethra. The outside surface can be treated with electrolysis later if necessary. But hair on the *inside, lining the urethra itself*, is much harder to treat after the fact. (Allow 12 to 18 months for the electrolysis process to ensure adequate hair removal before phalloplasty.)

- **Removing the full-thickness radial forearm flap and then resurfacing the area with a split-thickness skin graft leaves a scar that closely resembles a burn scar.**
  Because this "forearm burn" is becoming so recognizable as a phalloplasty scar, some people worry that their scar may "out" them as transgender. Some men chose the ALT phalloplasty because the donor site scar on the thigh is more easily concealed by their clothing. (You may be able to minimize scarring with proper postoperative care of the donor site.)

  - **The new urethra is created by wrapping one side of the detached forearm flap around a urinary catheter.**

  - **The outside of the penis is created by then reversing the direction of the "wrap"** as the flap is wrapped the other way. Look very closely in the upper left portion of Wilson's illustration in Figure 11.17; you'll be able to appreciate this wrap and reverse-wrap.

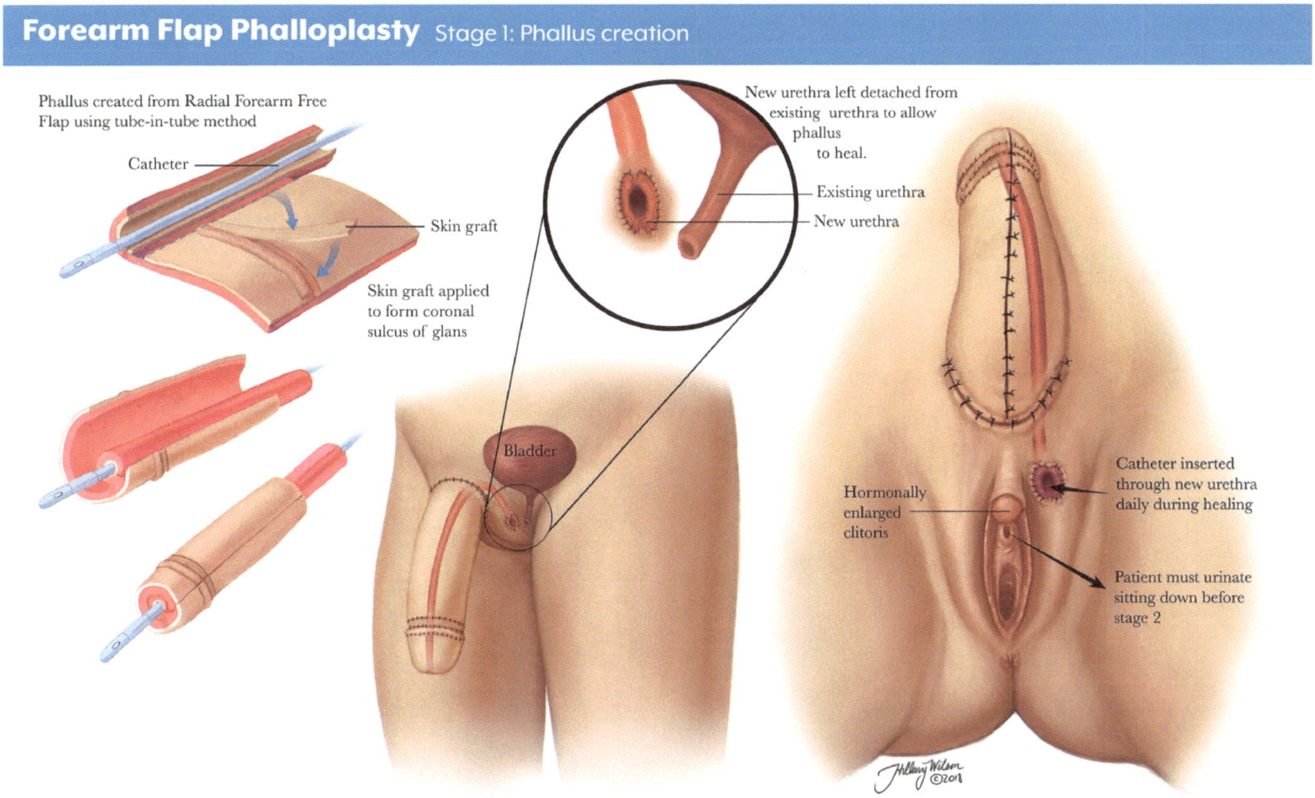

Figure 11.17. Forearm flap phalloplasty, Stage 1: phallus creation. Note in the upper left, the closeup of the neophallus creation from the radial forearm free flap using the tube-in-tube method.

Note also that different surgeons' techniques and sequences will vary. In the Wilson illustration, glansplasty is done at the initial surgery. Glansplasty is a plastic surgery technique. (One technique is to create two circumferential incisions parallel to each other at the end of the penis. The distal—more distant—incision is rolled under itself to create a "hem," creating the appearance of a circumcised penis (or the end of a noncircumcised penis with the foreskin drawn back.)

- **The end of the penis is sutured with delicate stitches to bring both layers of the "tube-in-a-tube" together.** This rounds out the end of the penis.
- **The neophallus is attached to the lower suprapubic area.** In the technique illustrated, the patient will pee sitting down through their original urethra for a while as the neourethra heals. Care is taken to keep the neourethra patent (unobstructed) by regular saline flushes (irrigations) through its catheter.
- **The free flap site at the radial forearm is covered by a split-thickness skin graft taken from the thigh.** This requires special care to facilitate healing: A wound VAC device or surgical compression bandages used for third-degree burns, and physical therapy are commonly used to protect mobility in the hand and wrist.

Second Stage: Urethral Lengthening and Scrotoplasty

Note: There is considerable variability from surgeon to surgeon. Some do vaginectomy in Stage 2. Some do glansplasty in Stage 2 or in a separate and brief outpatient surgery. Your surgeon will have their own reasons supporting their preferences for your surgery. Just be certain you know what you are having done.

Forearm Flap Phalloplasty Stage 2: Urethral lengthening and scrotoplasty

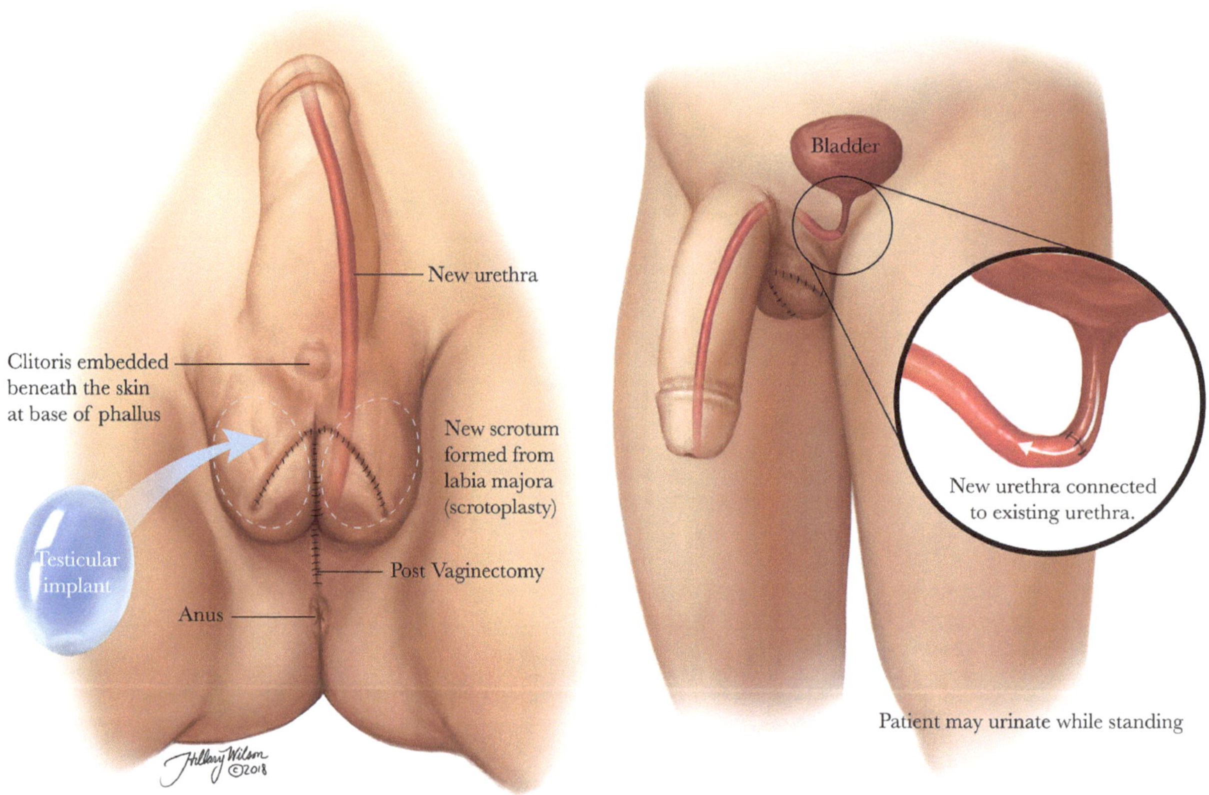

Figure 11.18. Forearm flap phalloplasty, Stage 2: urethal lengthening and scrotoplasty.

- **The clitoris is tucked under and *inside* the base of the penis, or it remains exposed and positioned *below* the base of the penis.**
  The nerves that serve the clitoris are then connected to nerves in the free flap. (More precisely, one of the dorsal nerves to the clitoris is preserved, and the other is connected to the nerves in the radial forearm flap.) This way, the primary erogenous sensation still originates in the clitoral tissue and orgasmic ability is maintained. Remember that the glans penis in phalloplasty will not have the same sensation as in a cis male; after all, the glans is newly constructed from the skin of the forearm (or the thigh in ALT phalloplasty).

- **A scrotoplasty is performed using the labia majora.**
  In Wilson's illustration, note the midline vaginectomy incision below the scrotum. Prosthetic testicles are placed in the scrotum, then or later. If more scrotal space is required to accommodate larger prostheses, tissue expanders might be placed first. The testicular prostheses replace the expanders later on.

As in anything in medicine or surgery, there is some controversy about the use of tissue expanders. Dr. Richard Santucci, citing the complications of eroded or infected scrotal tissue, stated, "I make the largest scrotum I can and at the 6-month mark, I can place bilateral testes implants… the weight of the scrotum acts as a sort of ersatz tissue expander."

- **The patient's original urethra is then connected to the neourethra.**
  If more urethral tissue is required, it may be grafted from buccal tissue in the mouth or from the free flap. The connection site, like anastomoses in general, may be the location of troubling complications such as urethral strictures or stenoses (narrowing), even to the point of obstruction. (**Note:** The terms "stricture" and "stenosis" are often used interchangeably.)

  If a stricture or stenosis occurs, the urine flow will slow down. It may require the use of a urethral dilator or a catheter on a temporary basis. In some cases, the urethra must be repaired surgically: "filleted" open at the site of the stricture, relined with buccal mucosa, and fully repaired 4 to 6 months later. The patient passes their urine through a suprapubic catheter in the abdomen as the urethra heals.

  Fistula formation, if it occurs, tends to happen at the "seam line" on the underside of the penis, particularly at the base or the tip of the penis. When a fistula forms, urine can leak out from the fistula as well as the opening at the end of the penis. These usually heal on their own but they can require surgical correction.

Third Stage: Erectile Implant

- **Erectile devices, such as an erectile pump or a malleable rod, are placed at least 8 to 12 months after the phalloplasty.**
  Initially, the new penis lacks sensation as the nerves are regenerating. What would happen if penetration was attempted too early with a pump or malleable rod in place? As the man pushed against a partner, the erectile device could poke through the penis! And the owner might not be able to feel it to recognize that this was happening.

  Wilson's illustration shows an inflatable erectile pump. Note that the pump device resembles a single corpus cavernosum. Also note the abdominal reservoir that holds saline before it is pumped into the device. And finally, notice the pump mechanism that is placed on one side of the scrotum. A prosthetic testis occupies the opposite side. Cis males with erectile dysfunction have used such devices for decades.

  While not illustrated, a malleable rod may be placed in the penis instead of a pump—again, after 8 or 9 months have passed. The rod can be moved from a downward position "at rest" to an upright position (or a 90-degree angle) for penetration.

Forearm Flap Phalloplasty Stage 3: Penile Prosthesis

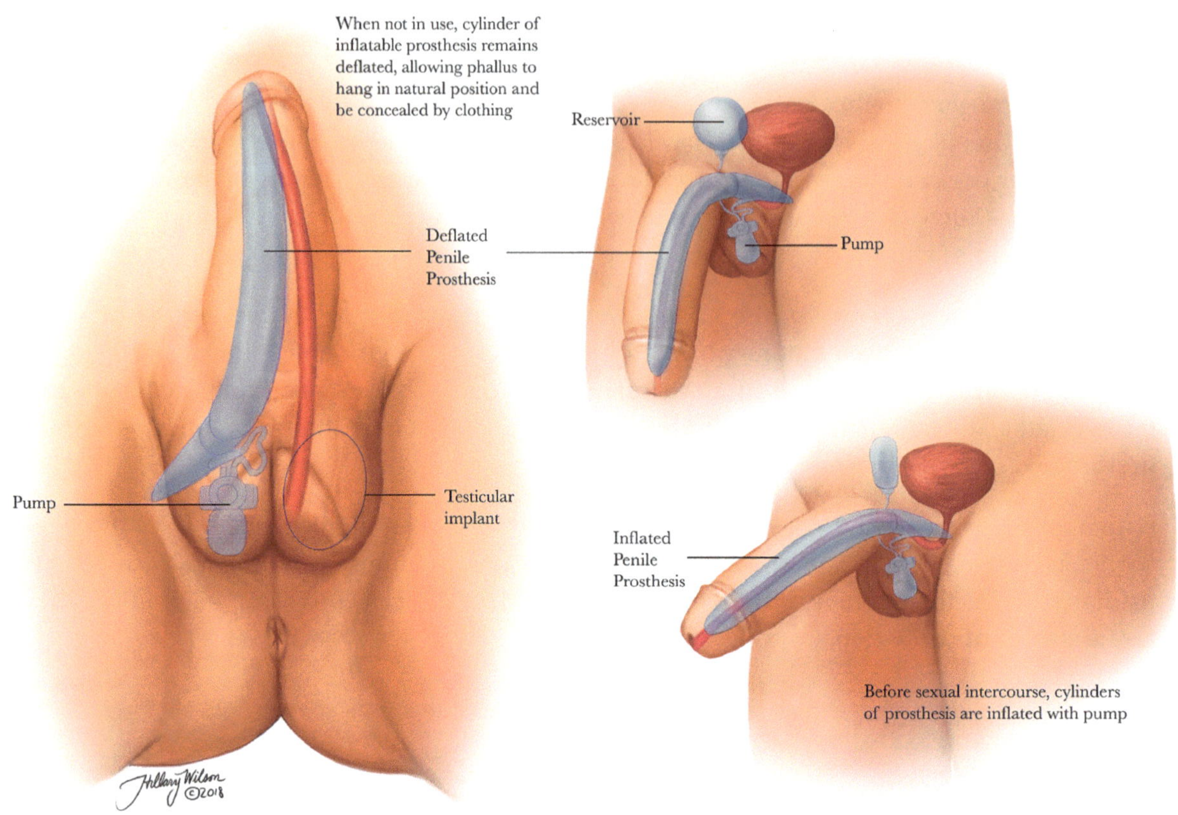

Figure 11.19. Forearm flap phalloplasty, Stage 3: penile prosthesis.

Shower or Grower?

A trans man with a phalloplasty is a ***shower, not a grower***! This expression means that the ***shower's*** penis size is the same whether it is flaccid (limp) or erect.

Many cis males experience enlargement of the penis as it becomes erect (they are ***growers***); the penis becomes longer and thicker. In a trans male, firmness occurs but growth in penile length and girth do not.

Anterior Lateral Thigh Flap Phalloplasty

- **The anterior lateral thigh flap site is prepared.**
  As before, electrolysis would have been completed, allowing 12 to 18 months for full clearing of the hair. A template is used to define the flap area and remove the flap from the donor location.

- **With its blood supply attached, the flap is moved under the groin muscles and through a groin incision to its anatomically correct position.**
  The ALT flap with its blood supply attached can be moved to a nearby location without interrupting its blood flow. The remaining steps are performed similarly to the techniques described in the part on radial forearm flap phalloplasty.

- **The skin of the ALT flap is thicker than a forearm flap, so it produces a penis that is very large (nearly the diameter of a soda can).**
  This phallus can be resized with liposuction later on, whereas the radial forearm flap is right-sized at its creation. Surgeon Richard Santucci points out, "A reality of ALT: If you have a thigh with a lot of fat, you will have a fat penis." Surgeon Toby Meltzer says, "An ALT flap is most suitable for a very lean male who has very thin skin over the thigh. Even then, it can be very large with a tube-in-a-tube design."

- **The ALT flap donor site must be covered with a split-thickness skin graft.**
  Care is similar with the ALT site, although mobility is much less of a concern than in the radial forearm, which requires physical therapy to ensure full wrist function later on.

- **If used as a shaft-only phalloplasty (no urethra), excellent results with normal girth and aesthetic appearance can be achieved.**

The Delayed Pedicle(d) Flap Phalloplasty (Also Called a Local Flap Phalloplasty)

A pedicle flap phalloplasty serves the needs of a trans man who wants a bulge in the crotch as well as the ability to penetrate a partner by way of an erectile device. In most cases, pedicle flaps are formed by creating a roll of tissue from the abdomen, thigh, or suprapubic area. The tissue roll will be relocated and reshaped over several surgeries, all the while maintaining the connection of the blood vessels at one end. The advantage here is excellent blood flow, and no microvascular surgery is required to connect donor blood vessels to recipient blood vessels. The blood vessels simply travel along in a bridge connected to the tissue.

If you are preparing for a pedicle flap phalloplasty, exercise your whole body, but especially your gluteals, quads, hamstrings, back, and abdomen. This will help you develop collateral (extra) blood vessels. The better your blood supply, the better your pedicle flap will heal.

Although this type of phalloplasty is performed in several stages, each procedure is relatively short. This makes it a reasonable surgical plan for someone who is older or someone who may have more complicated underlying medical conditions and otherwise would not tolerate a lengthier time under anesthesia.

One of the most notable advantages of this technique is that there is no telltale graft scar on the forearm, so your business remains private. There is often significant incisional scarring at the donor sites, but these are easily concealed under clothing.

Let's look at an example of a delayed pedicle flap phalloplasty from the groin. When discussing pedicle flap phalloplasty from the groin, consider the following steps, which are completed over several months.

In each of the first four steps, you will note that the blood supply is maintained at one end of the solid tube created. Step 6 (glansplasty) and Step 7 (placement of erectile device) will occur 8 to 9 months later. Creation of a urethra can be performed, but it is a separate microsurgical procedure done later.

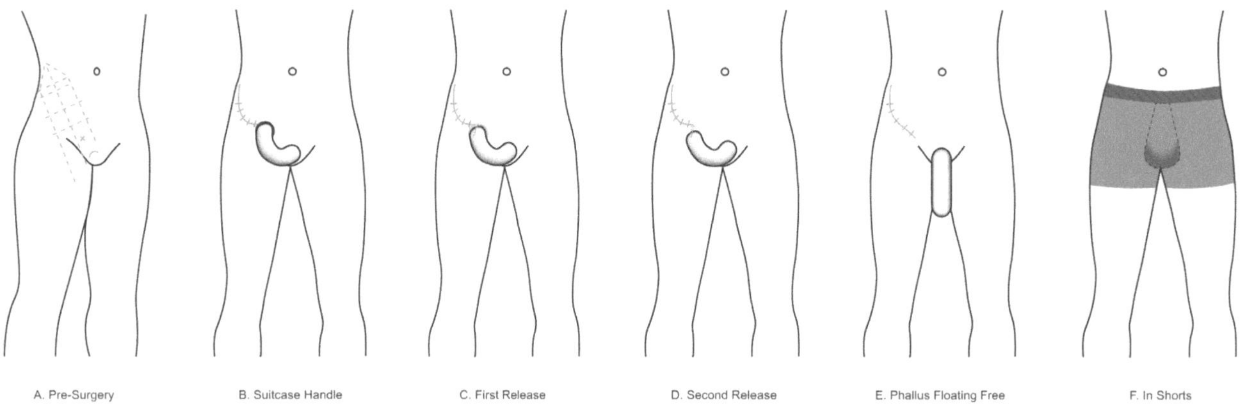

Figure 11.20. Delayed pedicle flap phalloplasty (glansplasty is not shown).

- **Step 1**
  The surgeon draws a template of the pedicle flap on the patient's body. In the groin technique, the flap is outlined with a surgical pen. The outline extends from the groin area all the way to the patient's back above the patient's waist. It is a larger, longer area than the size of the eventual penis.

- **Step 2**
  The surgeon cuts this skin and lifts it apart from the underlying tissue, leaving it attached at the hip end. It is rolled up into a tube, still attached at one end. The loose end (from the patient's back and waist) is rotated and reattached to the patient's midline (see Figure 11.20). When it is reattached, the closed cylinder looks something like an old suitcase handle. The donor site is sutured together, creating a linear scar on the side of the patient's hip and waist area. The patient stays in the hospital for 1 to 2 nights before discharge.

- **Step 3**
  At the next visit, perhaps 2 to 3 weeks later, the outside end of the suitcase handle is surgically narrowed by about 50 percent. The patient recovers with a tourniquet around the side that becomes the tip of the penis; he will gradually tighten this tourniquet per the surgeon's instructions.

  During this first delay, the major blood vessels that feed the flap are divided. The flap survives because of the new blood vessels that have formed at the base of the new penis and the skin that remains attached to the hip. As the phallus is fed by newly established blood vessels in addition to the original pedicle vessels, this tourniquet tightening will not compromise the overall blood supply. This process of delays allows the feeding vessels to be divided while the tourniquet stimulates increased blood supply to the entire flap. If the patient cannot use a tourniquet or cannot execute the process, a secondary additional delay can be done after the first one.

- **Step 4**
  About a month later, the lateral (hip side) attachment of the phallus is surgically narrowed again by another 50 percent. The patient again uses a tourniquet device, gradually tightening it over time according to the surgeon's instructions. As this surgical step is less complicated, the patient has this done as an outpatient procedure, not staying in the hospital overnight. The patient can also elect to have local anesthesia rather than general, if preferred.

- **Step 5**
  Several weeks later, the outer edge of the suitcase handle is completely divided at the hip and sutured closed. The flap is allowed to hang free, still attached with its intact blood supply at the patient's midline. The handle is then flipped upward (vertically) while still joined to the patient at the pubic area. The penis must remain in a vertical position for 3 months, again to maximize blood flow and to prevent swelling. The patient wears briefs or boxer briefs that secure the penis in the upright position.

  At each stage, nitroglycerine ointment is used to dilate surface blood vessels in another measure to ensure robust blood supply and flap survival.

- **Step 6**
  Glansplasty is the creation of a glans penis using a plastic surgery technique. These are done at many phases of a phalloplasty, from the initial surgery of the radial forearm or ALT phalloplasty to several months after the delayed pedicle flap phalloplasty.

  The timing is generally based on what has worked best for the surgeon in their experience. Some surgeons create two circumferential incisions and then "hem" the far incision to create the look of a seam. Others use a silicon cord to create a ridge that won't flatten out over time. Problems with the cord design include erosion and infection. Your surgeon is your best source of information, of course.

- **Step 7**
  If a man wishes to have an erectile device placed, this is done at a minimum of 8 to 9 months after the completion of the phalloplasty. This is to allow sensation to regenerate in the genital area so the man can have an erection and penetrate safely without the device poking through the side of his penis.

  The implantable pump erectile device consists of three parts. First, there is a tube that resembles a single corpora cavernosum, which is implanted in the center of the penis along its length. Then, a saline reservoir is placed in the abdomen to hold the saline to inflate the penile tube. Finally, a pump device is placed on one side of the scrotum (the scrotoplasty having been completed at an earlier surgery).

  The pump activates the saline reservoir to pour saline into the penile tube to make the tube firm. The pump mechanism also has a device to allow the penis to empty or relax after sexual activity by emptying the saline back into the reservoir. The owner pumps the device by squeezing it between the thumb and fingers.

A Surgeon's Advice

Due to its complexity from the sheer number of structures being created, as well as the requirement that they all work together in concert, phalloplasty remains one of the most challenging surgeries done in medicine. Along with this challenge come relatively high complication rates. By far, the most important step in the phalloplasty journey is preparation. Many patients end up with the feeling, "I never knew this could happen."

When considering phalloplasty, it will be important to arm yourself with the facts as best you can, and have those facts inform your expectations so that they are realistic. Speak with your surgeon carefully about all the techniques being used, design your particular surgery carefully depending on your desired functions, get a handle on the anticipated timeline, and make sure to ask not only about complications, but also how they will be managed and how they might change your timeline for recovery.

Just as in so many things with life, the goal in preparing for phalloplasty is to try and have no surprises. Be prepared for the worst and hopeful for the best.

— Dev Gurjala, MD

The following piece was written by UK blogger and vlogger Finlay Games. In this excerpt from May 25, 2019, Mr. Games writes about evaluating his own results.[64]

Managing the Expectations of Phalloplasty

Phalloplasty is all about managing expectations and getting to a place that's "good enough." Otherwise, we could spend our lives changing little bits here and there and never being happy. No penis is perfect. Penises come in all manner of different shapes and sizes and point in funny directions or have bends in them. As for phalloplasty, it's never going to be a cis penis no matter how many advancements the surgeons make. I believe that part of preparing for phalloplasty is acknowledging that fact and working out what "good enough" means for you.

For me, good enough meant being able to have a penis I could pee with and have penetrative sex with a partner. As long as it looked good enough to stand next to other guys at a urinal and make me smile when I looked in the mirror, that was good enough for me.

— Finlay Games

64 Finlay Games, "Phalloplasty Final Stage | AMS Implant Review," *Finn the InFinncible*, May 25, 2019, http://finlaygames.com/phalloplasty-final-stage-ams-implant-review.

Nonbinary (or Less Binary) Genital Surgeries

Penile Preservation Vaginoplasty with Peritoneal Pull-Through: Something New

You will notice that I'm using the terms "penis" and "phallus" quite interchangeably. Embryologically, they are the same structure. Many nonbinary individuals prefer to use the more gender-neutral term "phallus" over the more male term "penis." Does it matter? It certainly can, so check with an individual as to what term they use.

The Penis/Phallus-Preserving Vaginoplasty with Peritoneal Pull-Through

Many transgender females who have both the funds and the opportunity choose not to have vaginoplasty at all. While many trans females are intensely dysphoric about even looking at their genitals, others prefer to keep the phallus.

I've begun to hear about a newer option for AMAB individuals who wish to preserve the phallus but create a vagina suitable for penetration—an adaptation of the vaginoplasty with peritoneal pull-through. (Refer to Dr. Wittenberg's information on peritoneal pull-through vaginoplasty on page 217.)

In this procedure or series of procedures, an individual first has an orchiectomy (removal of the testicles). A vaginal vault or cavity is developed starting from the perineum. A portion of the *peritoneum* is brought into the new cavity to line the walls of the neovagina. This *peritoneal* tissue is brought down from the abdomen by way of robotic-assisted laparoscopy.

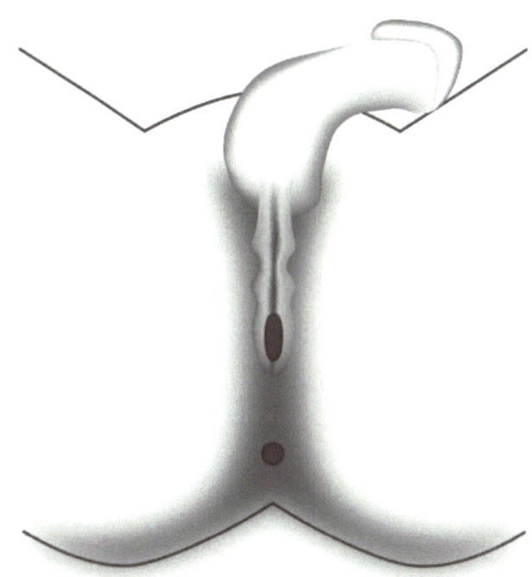

Figure 11.21. The penis/phallus-preserving vaginoplasty with peritoneal pull-through.

(Refer to the "Perineum versus Peritoneum: Big Difference!" on page 217 to review the differences between the perineum and the peritoneum.)

After a person has a phallus preservation vaginoplasty with peritoneal pull-through, the phallus remains above the opening of the neovagina. The phallus continues to serve as the main center for sexual pleasure and the conduit for urination.

The Penis/Phallus-Preserving Vaginoplasty with Full-Thickness Skin Graft

In the peritoneal pull-through procedure or series of procedures, the vaginal vault is developed in the perineum and lined with a portion of the *peritoneal* membrane that encloses the abdominal organs. This tissue is brought down from the abdomen by way of robotic-assisted laparoscopy. Here, the peritoneal membrane becomes the lining of the neovagina.

Alternatively, in the full-thickness skin graft technique, a graft is typically taken from the abdomen and is used as the lining for the vaginal canal. The skin graft is harvested using an abdominoplasty incision (a horizontal incision like you would see with a tummy tuck). The advantage of this approach, of course, is that you can get a tummy tuck at the same time. The disadvantage, when compared to the peritoneal-pull through, is the presence of a potentially long horizontal scar on the abdomen. Scrotal tissue is used to construct the labia.

The phallus remains above the opening of the neovagina. The phallus continues to serve as the main center for sexual pleasure and as the conduit for urination.

Seen on a social media site discussing penis preservation vaginoplasty:

Comment: "Yeah, but do you have a penis or a vagina?"

Response: "Yes."

Gender Nullification Surgery: "The Smoothie"

This procedure includes the removal of the penis and testicles and the reduction of the scrotal sac. It may also be referred to as the "Nullo." The urethra is shortened, so you pee through a urethral opening centered on the perineum but without a penis. The goal is to leave the area as a smooth, unbroken transition from the abdomen to the groin. Tissue from the tip of the penis can be buried under the mons (the lower part of the abdomen just under and above the pubic hair) for orgasmic response.

This surgery may be requested by people who identify as eunuchs and by others who wish an anatomically agender appearance. (See Davis Plastic Surgery's website at davisplasticsurgery.com. See also the information on eunuchs in Chapter 2.)

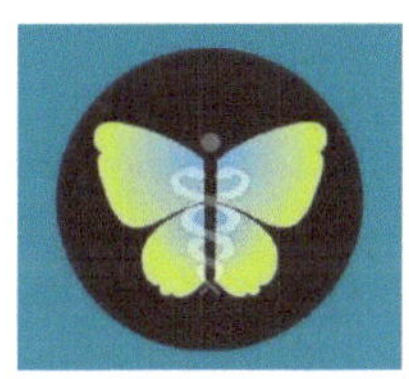

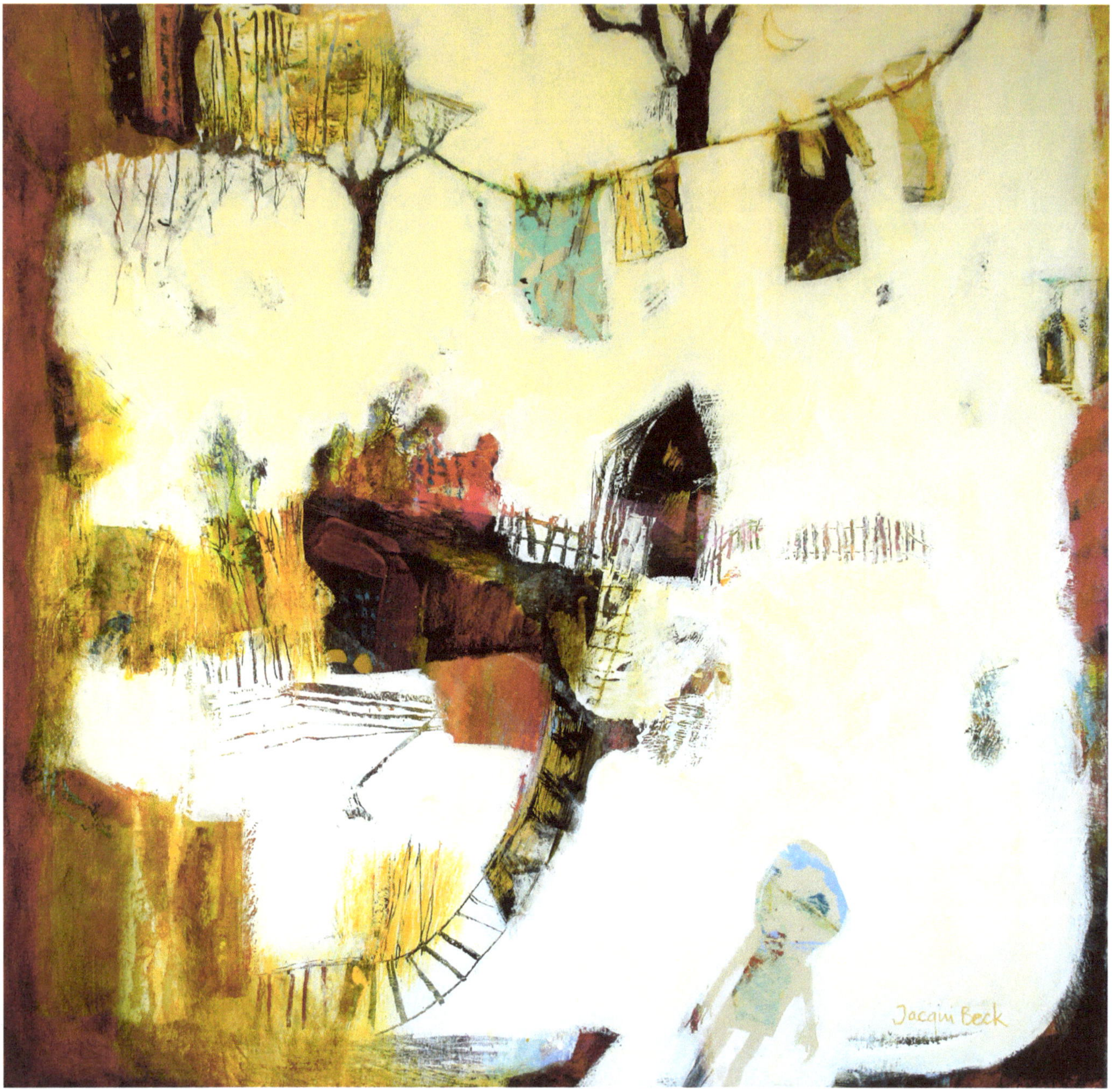

Feels Like Home

CHAPTER 12

Taking Care of Yourself after Surgery

This chapter begins with what happens in the hospital and general postoperative principles that apply to all gender-related surgeries, followed by more specific recovery information for specific surgeries. It is important to keep in mind that everyone will have a unique postoperative course; no two people will have the same experiences.

As always, this information is intended to supplement information from your surgeon, not to replace it. If there is any disagreement between my information and that of your surgeon, go with your surgeon's recommendations.

What to Expect in the Hospital

Having a surgery of any kind can be intimidating, even overwhelming. I remember my family physician used to joke,

> **Q** **What's the difference between a major surgery and a minor surgery?**
>
> **A** **A major surgery is any surgery done on my body. A minor surgery is any surgery done on someone else's body.**

This probably rings true for all of us.

Let's begin by reviewing some concepts about surgery in general, regardless of which surgery a person is having. Most people undergoing a gender-related surgery are having an elective surgery. Does *elective* mean you don't really need it? Not in the least.

An elective surgery is *scheduled in advance* because it doesn't involve a medical emergency. (You could have an emergency gender-related surgery, of course, but that would likely involve an unexpected, rare complication that had to be handled urgently.)

A gender-related surgery usually has a time and a date planned ahead and is listed on a surgery schedule. It is usually performed during the day when the surgeon and crew are awake and everyone is fed and appropriately caffeinated.

You Will Likely Follow the Standard Routine

- Due to the coronavirus pandemic, you will be required to have a COVID-19 test to ensure that you are not infected before being admitted to the hospital. You must isolate yourself until the results confirm that your test is negative.
- You will enter the presurgery intake area, where your name and identity are confirmed. You'll be asked what surgery you are having and the name of your surgeon. A name band stating your name, birthdate, and likely your surgeon's name is fastened around your wrist.
- You will then go to a preanesthesia area where you dress privately in a patient gown, a paper shower cap, and nonskid slipper socks. A nurse or assistant again confirms who you are and what surgery you're having. They double-check that you signed your surgical consent (your permission to have the surgery performed) and that all of the required lab tests have been done.
- Next, you meet the anesthesiologist—a physician or a CRNA (certified registered nurse anesthetist). Expect to answer all the questions you've already been asked and to discuss more about your overall health, the medications you take, whether you've had anesthesia before, and whether you've had adverse reactions to anesthetics or allergic reactions to any medications. (If you find yourself annoyed by the repetitious questioning, remember that it is done as a double-check for your safety.)
- The anesthesia provider may examine your heart and lungs, and they may do an electrocardiogram (EKG). They assess your mouth, teeth, and airway to prepare to place an airway tube. (Even if they are not planning to insert an endotracheal tube, they assess your airway in case an emergency arises.) The anesthesia provider starts an IV to give you intravenous fluids and medications during your surgery.
- The anesthesia provider may give you a medication by IV to relax you before you're wheeled into the operating room (OR) on a gurney (stretcher).

If you're still awake as you are wheeled into the OR, you'll see many expensive machines all over the room. There'll be a scrub nurse dressed in a surgical gown, cap, gloves, and mask. The scrub nurse responds to directions from the surgeon and anticipates their needs, such as handing the surgeon instruments and suctioning blood away from the surgical site so the surgeon can see well. Also present is a circulating nurse, who wears scrubs, a mask, cap, and gloves. Because this nurse is not "sterile" like the gowned scrub nurse, they provide general support for the patient and everything that occurs in the OR, but they don't touch the site of the operation. ("Scrubs" refer to the loose-fitting clothing worn by many hospital staff. A scrub nurse is so named because they scrub their arms, hands, and fingernails prior to gowning up and having their gowns placed and tied.)

Your anesthesia provider stands or sits by your head, which will be at the head of the OR table; they monitor your heart rate and rhythm, your breathing rate, and your levels of oxygen and carbon dioxide as measured through a skin sensor. An anesthetic mask may be placed over your nose and mouth. If you're having general anesthesia through an endotracheal tube (ET) going down the throat, the ET is placed after you have been sedated by the IV medication. Your vital signs (blood pressure, pulse, oxygen level, and so on) are recorded continuously. If you're having a regional anesthetic, an epidural or spinal catheter is placed appropriately by the anesthesia provider. (The type of anesthesia given will have been discussed with you preoperatively.)

> In the OR, everything moves like a choreographed dance; everyone knows exactly what they are supposed to do. As a patient, gain reassurance from the fact that while this operation is new for you, it is very routine for your surgeon and the OR staff.

During your surgery, the surgeon, the surgical assistant, and all of the OR staff work together to accomplish the surgery that you have planned. If unexpected events occur, know that your team has seen such events before or have practiced ahead of time for nearly all possibilities.

After Surgery, You Will Be Moved into the Recovery Room or the Postanesthesia Recovery Area

In the recovery room, you will likely have one-on-one care by the recovery nurse until you are conscious and able to speak and swallow. Unless otherwise planned, your airway tube is removed, and you'll be breathing on your own without mechanical assistance.

Sometimes people go directly to their hospital room after surgery. In some cases (such as phalloplasties with microsurgical procedures), you may go directly to the special care or intensive care unit (ICU) for monitoring of your blood circulation at the microsurgical anastomoses of blood vessels.

If you end up being in the ICU but hadn't expected to go there, remember that the ICU affords you the most meticulous one-on-one care available. Sometimes a patient has experienced an unexpected event during surgery, such as an unpredicted fall in blood pressure, excessive bleeding, or an allergic reaction. In these cases, your surgical team has assessed that you need closer monitoring than the average patient and is moving you to the ICU for your safety.

When You Are Awake and Breathing without Assistance, You Usually Go to Your Regular Hospital Room

If you're having outpatient surgery (sometimes called a "day surgery" since you will be discharged home on the same day and not stay overnight in the hospital), you'll be observed in a recovery area until you're stable enough to have someone take you home. In general, your driver must be a partner, parent, or friend—not a driver for hire.

In your hospital room, your care is likely to be shared by several nurses and assistants. Depending on the size of the hospital, you will meet other personnel, such as laboratory technicians, physical and occupational therapists, social workers, dietary staff, cleaning personnel, pharmacy staff, and members of your surgical team, of course. Someone from the team (often a nurse practitioner or physician's assistant) will "round on you"—meaning evaluate you—at least daily.

In the hospital, expect to get out of bed with help and move around on the day of your surgery, or certainly by the next morning if your surgery is done late in the day. (This would not apply to patients who go to the ICU right after surgery.) Expect to be busy with wound care, bathing, resting, sleeping, eating, getting up to walk, discovering how to pee again if your surgery involved your urinary tract, and spending time with visitors. You may have to wait for various bodily processes (like bowel movements) to become automatic again. Some postoperative days will require more emotional energy than others.

You will likely have pain. Your surgical team expects this and will have provided orders for pain medication to keep you reasonably comfortable. Take your medications regularly; it's often easier to *keep up* with pain rather than try to *catch up* with it.

You may have a patient-controlled analgesia (PCA) device that allows you to get a safe dose of IV pain medication when you push a button. This allows you to get your medication without waiting for someone to administer it. However, the PCA device protects you from getting too much medication by having controlled dose parameters.

It's much more reasonable to anticipate having pain rather than expecting no pain at all. As you recover, your pain medication will come in pill form rather than via injection or through your IV. Many people require at least a limited supply of narcotics when they leave the hospital, although it is becoming increasingly common not to prescribe narcotics postoperatively. (Refer to the part on gabapentin and ibuprofen on pages 261–262.) Narcotics can constipate you, so drink fluids and take the fiber supplements and stool softeners offered.

The length of your hospital stay depends on the type of surgery you have had and the pace of your recovery. When you are ready for discharge to your home or a recovery facility, you will be given medications to take with you (and prescriptions if needed), written instructions on how to care for yourself, and information on where to call if you have questions or need immediate care. You will also be given information on when to follow up with your surgeon and your primary care provider (PCP).

General Postoperative Home Care Guidelines for *All* Surgeries

While every person and every surgical case is different, here are some general principles that apply to all surgeries.

You'll hear this qualifier repeatedly: If I present anything that conflicts with your surgeons' advice, listen to your surgeon and surgical team.

Your healing requires time, restorative rest, more protein than you might imagine, a healthy fluid intake, proper wound care, and gentle attention to your mental health. It also requires you to detect problems that do occur and respond appropriately so that you get the help you need. We will examine each of these areas and then go on to discuss considerations for specific surgeries in the parts that follow.

It Can Take a Village: Your Team of Support

Ideally, everyone undergoing any surgery would have a loving, nonintrusive guardian angel to welcome them home and then prepare food, help them bathe, fluff their pillows, change their surgical dressings, help them take their medications on schedule, drive them to appointments, and massage their shoulders. Sometimes, mothers who have just delivered a baby will hire a postpartum doula (a nonmedical support person) to help them when they first come home. I think everyone coming home from a gender-related surgery could use a doula and maybe such services will develop.

In fact, in researching this, I discovered a company of care providers who can be hired to assist folks after masculinizing surgeries when they stayed at the Quest House in Pacifica, California; visit t4tcaregiving.org for more information. See also the interview with the manager of Quest House on pages 293–296 on aftercare for masculinizing surgeries.

Shortly before going to press, I learned that Quest House was closed due to lease- and pandemic-related problems. Then when making my final checks, I found that Quest House had reopened on a limited scale with expansion plans. Do check the website periodically to follow the progress of Quest House as the story develops (questhouseservices.wordpress.com).

— Linda Gromko, MD

Care for patients undergoing both masculinizing and feminizing operations is also provided at the TransHeartline House in Marin, California (transheartline.org/services).

Perhaps you are fortunate enough to have a spouse or partner, a parent, a close friend, or a sibling to fill this role (or parts of it). Maybe you have the resources to hire a home health aide; if so, arrange this in advance and be certain that your assistant is trans-friendly and familiar with postoperative care.

Perhaps you want *nobody* around you as you recover. If that's the case, identify (and confirm) a few backup people you can contact if you do run into difficulties. If you live in an area where rideshare services are readily available and you can set up delivery services as needed, you will likely do fine for one of the less involved surgeries. But help can be wonderful, particularly in the postoperative period when you may feel more vulnerable than usual.

No matter what your circumstances are, you may find it helpful to go back and read "Planning for Your Surgery" in Chapter 10. Also, review the checklists of helpful items to have on hand.

If you have a network of people like coworkers, friends, or a sports team, look at **Lotsa Helping Hands** (lotsahelpinghands.com) and **Meal Train** (mealtrain.com).

- **Lotsa Helping Hands** can help you or your point person organize people who want to be involved but don't know how to help you most effectively. If you anticipate needing extended support for making or providing meals, doing grocery runs, giving rides to doctor appointments, and so on, you can set up a free temporary website in advance to help coordinate the help you need.

- **Meal Train** is another web platform that helps you organize meals from your community of voluntary donors. Donors who couldn't (or shouldn't) spend time in the kitchen could opt to send a **GrubHub** gift card through Meal Train. Again, Meal Train is a free service, although coordinating additional services on Meal Train costs a small fee.

- **SignUpGenius** (signupgenius.com) is another group-organizing web platform you may like. It's free for friends and family to use.

- **Caring Bridge** (caringbridge.org) offers a different type of support. After you have a surgery, people will want to inquire on your well-being. You might find yourself facing a barrage of calls and messages at times when you're exhausted or simply need your privacy. Caring Bridge gives you a free web platform so you can issue bulletins to friends and welcome their support while maintaining personal boundaries. Caring Bridge asks for donations from readers, but it is quite unobtrusive.

Planning the Length of Your Recovery Time

For planning purposes, it's better to allow for a longer recovery period and be happily surprised than to imagine you'll be back in a few days and then find yourself tanking!

If you're having a major genital surgery, it is fully appropriate to plan for 6 to 8 weeks off work. Longer is certainly fine, depending on your situation. Some people plan for 12 weeks. You may be able to return earlier, particularly if you have the ability to start with part-time or to work from home. If you're having a less involved surgery, less recovery time will be needed. For example, breast augmentation would require less recovery time than a vaginoplasty. But add a few days of recovery time if you have *both* surgeries together. If you're able to return to work on a Thursday or Friday, or even go in every other day, do this to conserve your mental and physical energy.

Remember that recovery is not a linear process. I tell my patients to look at recovery as a spiral that gradually goes up: You progress a little, dip down a little, and spiral up again with the *net* direction in an upward progression. (But talk to your healthcare providers if your spiral moves perpetually downward!)

If you have to travel to a different city or country, allow additional time to recover from the travel itself. Often, the day you go home may take more physical and emotional energy than other days. Remember that the responsibilities that were shouldered by the hospital staff are now borne by you and your personal team.

Resting Effectively after Surgery

Your body needs rest and good sleep to heal. But surgery, anesthesia, pain, varying urinary signals, travel, and even your own excitement may disrupt your sleep patterns. Here are some considerations that may help you:

- **Relax your expectations.**
  It's understandable if you don't sleep perfectly after surgery. Most people don't! Try not to worry about not getting enough sleep. Set the stage to allow yourself to drift off to sleep. If you do sleep, fine. If you don't, just concentrate on resting and know that your body will still heal.

- **Create the most comfortable sleep environment possible.**
  If you can, clean your living space ahead of time so you come home to a reasonably orderly environment. Buy or borrow some extra sheets and pillows with pillowcases before your surgery. Use your extra pillows to help position your body to get yourself comfortable. For example, when you rest on your side, bolster your body with a pillow tucked behind your back, one between your elbows, and one between your knees, as shown in Figure 12.1. Or, get a body pillow.

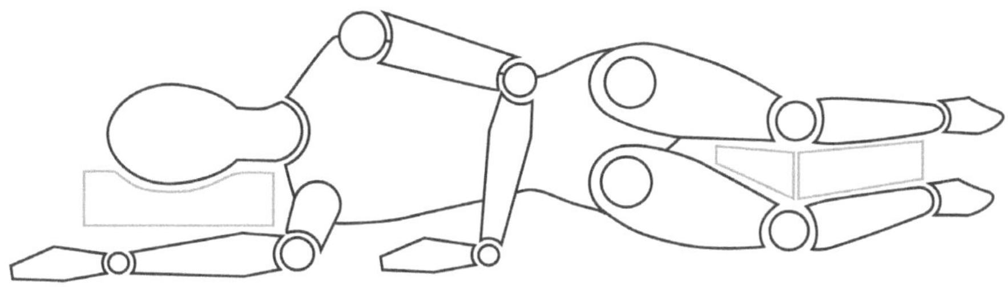

Figure 12.1. Resting on your side with extra pillow support.

If you have been advised to elevate your legs, it probably means elevating them above the level of your heart to help postsurgical swelling subside. A recliner helps, but you'll still need more elevation.

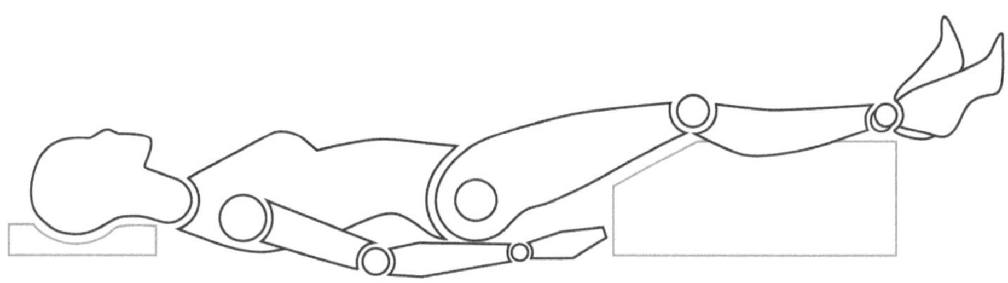

Figure 12.2. Elevation of the legs.

- **Stay clean and dry.**
  If you've had genital surgery, have some Chux pads, a waterproof crib liner, or even puppy training pads to place under your butt. These will keep your bed cleaner and drier and will be much more comfortable for you. You'll find a variety of sanitary pads to tuck into underpants or pajamas in the feminine hygiene or incontinence aisle of your grocery store, drugstore, or online retailer. (See the shopping list at the end of Chapter 10.)

  You may also appreciate having facial wipes and dry shampoo on hand if you cannot shower as often as you'd like. A hairbrush, a hand mirror, a tube of lip balm, and a container of simple lotion or moisturizer may help you feel better too.

- **Take a break from sleeping with your pets.**
  If you're in the habit of sleeping with your pets, take a break for 2 weeks to decrease your risk of post-op infections.

- **Keep some basic cleaning supplies near your bed.**
  You will appreciate having a box of facial tissue, a small wastebasket lined with a kitchen garbage bag, hand sanitizer, and a container of disinfectant wipes close at hand.

- **Set up your phone and charger.**
  For your comfort and safety, set up your phone and charger so you can reach them easily; buy an extra-long cord to make this convenient. It's never a bad idea to have a flashlight with you in case of a power outage. And you may need it for wound care anyway.

- **Create a relaxing environment.**
  A diffuser with essential oils provides relaxing ambience and makes your environment smell nicer. This may sound more like a frivolous luxury than a medical need, but feeling calm and breathing pleasant scents really can facilitate recovery. Unless you're allergic to essential oils, a small diffuser can bubble in the background, misting lavender or peppermint scents throughout your room.

- **Use white noise, ocean sounds, or quiet music to relax you.**
  If you have an electronic smart speaker, ask Alexa (or your Google friend) to play soothing sounds or music that you like, or wear noise-canceling headphones. Adjust your room temperature and lighting to make your environment more conducive to sleep. Consider getting a sleep mask to tune out ambient light. And then finally, just do the best you can. Even if you get sleep that's interrupted by pain, noise, or your bladder, it's better than no sleep at all!

- **Find a meditation app.**
  I first learned about the meditation-relaxation app Headspace from a client: **headspace.com/headspace-meditation-app**. She said that she never makes it to the end of a guided meditation—she's asleep by then! Headspace also tells you bedtime stories. (After a free trial, there is a yearly fee. But it's more cost-effective than a sleeping medication.) There are many similar apps. Here's a post that you may find useful: **appsdose.com/2015/09/10-best-meditation-relaxation-apps-for-ipad-iphone.html**.

Managing Postoperative Pain

Pain is expected after a surgery, although individual experiences vary greatly. Your surgical team expects that you will have pain and will give you prescriptions for medications to help you. Your medications may include any combination of the following:

- **Narcotics or opiates (although these have slightly different definitions, we will use the terms interchangeably here):**
  - Vicodin (hydrocodone + acetaminophen)
  - Percodan (oxycodone + aspirin)
  - Percocet (oxycodone + acetaminophen)
  - Dilaudid (hydromorphone)
  - Codeine
- **As you see from the list above, individual opiates may be prescribed by themselves or combined in a single tablet or capsule with ibuprofen (Motrin) or acetaminophen (Tylenol). These medications—**
  - Are *potentially addictive* but excellent for providing pain relief.
  - Are mind-altering—that is, they can make you "loopy"—and, if you combine them with anxiety medications or alcohol, you may get even loopier. It's best not to combine these without professional advice.
  - Have side effects such as nausea, vomiting, constipation, itching, and so on. *And you can be allergic to virtually any medication.*

- Are regulated with strict laws that govern the prescribing of such medications; we cannot phone these prescriptions into a pharmacy. Other people may steal your narcotics to use or sell. In our practice, we say, "If your cat eats it, your cat gets high." (No refills for meds that go down the sink, either.)

- Contain warnings like, "Do not drive or operate a forklift under the influence of these medications."

- Along those lines, make no truly important decisions while on narcotics. (As one physician friend advised, "Don't buy a grand piano while you're taking these drugs.")

- The effects of opiates can be immediately reversed by using the prescription medication Narcan (naloxone). If someone is living in your environment who is at risk for an opiate overdose, you may even want to consider having Narcan on-site.

Some surgeons are trying to eliminate the use of potentially addictive opiates in the post-op setting and are moving toward nonsteroidal anti-inflammatory medications and gabapentin.

- **Nonsteroidal anti-inflammatories (NSAIDs) (such as ibuprofen, naproxen, and aspirin)—**
  - Are available without a prescription; there are more potent ones that are prescription-only, such as ketorolac (Toradol). Do not combine prescription NSAIDs with over-the-counter NSAIDs as you can easily take too much.
  - Are not advised if you have an ulcer or kidney disease.
  - Have side effects, including gastrointestinal symptoms such as abdominal pain, heartburn, nausea, and vomiting. *And you can be allergic to virtually any medication.*
- **Acetaminophen (such as Tylenol)—**
  - Is generally well-tolerated and available without a prescription, but *you can be allergic to anything.*
  - Comes in a variety of over-the-counter mixtures designed to treat upper respiratory and sinus symptoms. If you are taking acetaminophen from several sources, be aware that it is possible to take too much! Add up the total amount of acetaminophen you are taking; generally, this should never exceed a total of 4 grams per day.
  - *Can cause liver failure with doses over a safe limit or intentional overdoses.* Check with your healthcare provider, your pharmacist, or even your local Poison Control Center if you're concerned.
- **Gabapentin (Neurontin)—**
  - Originally, gabapentin was used as an antiseizure medication; now it is mainly used for peripheral neuropathy and fibromyalgia, but it has been found to help with pain and anxiety. Dosages vary greatly; I start with low doses and increase gradually.

- Gabapentin is sedating at first before one adjusts to it; starting this medication at bedtime can help. If a person takes gabapentin for an extended time, tapering off it is done gradually to avoid precipitating a seizure or discontinuation symptoms (I hear patients complaining about "brain zaps" and anxiety if it is stopped abruptly).

- **Tramadol (Ultram)***
    - Long described as a narcotic-like drug, tramadol is now considered a narcotic. This drug poses addiction risks and all the side effects seen with narcotics, such as constipation, sedation, and nausea.

  ***Note: Tramadol and Toradol sound a lot alike but are totally different medications with different side effect profiles. Know what you are taking!**

Postoperative Nutrition: Getting Enough Protein for Wound Healing

You may not think of your surgical site as a wound. However, it *is* a surgically created wound and you must give your body enough protein to allow your tissues to knit together and heal. (When I see patients in my practice who are not healing quickly, we stress a jump in protein and fluid intake to accelerate a person's progress—and get some great results.)

Our primary nutrients consist of protein, carbohydrates, and fats. All are needed in the diet and all play important roles in tissue growth, maintenance, and repair. Most of us know about carbohydrates, which provide fuel for metabolic processes: sugar, flour, alcohol, and the complex carbohydrates found in starchy vegetables. Fats and oils (like butter, margarine, olive oil, lard, salad dressings) provide highly concentrated sources of calories, enhance the taste of foods, and are necessary for the integrity of cell membranes. Protein is made of amino acids that come from both animal and plant sources. Amino acids can combine to form the "complete" proteins that we do not make in our bodies.

Under normal circumstances, a person needs 0.8 grams of protein per kilogram of body weight. ***But it is estimated that a person healing from surgery needs 1.2 to 2 grams of protein per kilogram of body weight to heal well.***[65] But protein needs vary; a person with kidney disease may tolerate much less protein, while a person with a burn injury may require far *more* protein than usual after a surgery. If you have any doubt about your own situation, contact your healthcare provider and discuss this with them.

Here's how to do the math:

1. Figure out your weight: Take your weight in pounds and divide it by 2.2 to find your weight in kilograms.

2. Then, calculate how much protein you would need per day for postoperative healing (assuming that you do not require adjustments for kidney disease or burn injuries). Take your weight in kilograms and multiply by 1.2 grams of protein for the low end and 2.0 grams for the high end of the range of grams of protein needed per day.

Suppose you weigh 150 pounds (68 kilograms). You would need 54 grams of protein under normal circumstances (0.8 gram per kilogram of body weight) but you could need as much as 136 grams of protein per day for adequate wound healing. Tea and toast aren't going to cut it!

65 Chelsia Gillis and Paul E. Wischmeyer, "Preoperative Nutrition and the Elective Surgical Patient: Why, How and What?," *Anaesthesia* 74, Supplement 1 (January 2019): 27–35, https://doi.org/10.1111/anae.14506.

The point is clear: In most cases, you need more protein to heal well. Ask your surgical team or your primary care physician (PCP), or consult a dietitian if you have questions.

Protein Content of Various Foods from Animal and Plant Sources[66]			
Food (Animal Sources)	**Grams of Protein per Serving**	**Food (Plant Sources)**	**Grams of Protein per Serving**
Beef jerky (4 oz)	44 g	Soy protein powder (1 scoop)	20 g
Salmon (4 oz)	40 g	Veggie burger (1 patty)	12 g
Tuna (6-oz can)	39 g	Lentils or split peas (0.5 cup)	9 g
Steak (4 oz)	27 g	Edamame (0.5 cup)	8 g
Shrimp or prawns (4 oz)	24 g	Beans (kidney, garbanzo, navy, black, white, lima) (0.5 cup)	7 g
Chicken breast (4 oz)	23 g	Soy milk (1 cup)	7 g
Ground beef (4 oz)	20 g	Peanut butter (2 tablespoons)	7 g
Greek yogurt (8 oz)	22 g	Almond butter (2 tablespoons)	6 g
Cottage cheese (0.5 cup)	12 g	Whole-grain bread (1 slice)	4 g
Bacon (4 slices)	10 g	Steel-cut oatmeal, uncooked (0.25 cup)	4 g
Milk, whole (1 cup)	8 g	Hummus (0.25 cup)	4 g
Milk, nonfat (1 cup)	8 g	Brown rice (0.5 cup)	2 g
Milk, 2 percent (1 cup)	8 g	White rice (0.5 cup)	2 g
Egg (1 whole)	6 g	Almond milk (1 cup)	1 g

Table 12.1. Protein content of various foods from animal and plant sources.

If you are using prepared foods, read the nutrition labels to find out how much protein is contained in the food you eat. Pay attention to serving sizes so your calculations are correct.

66 Adapted from *Myfitnesspal*, v. 20.7.0.29453 (Under Armour, 2020).

Drink Your Protein

Protein Smoothie Recipe

1 banana, peeled
1 scoop protein powder of your choice (whey, soy, or pea protein)
¼ cup frozen fruit or frozen kale or spinach
5 to 6 ice cubes
2 cups water, milk, or milk substitute (almond, soy, cashew)

1. Combine the banana, protein powder, fruit or greens, and ice cubes in a blender capable of handling ice cubes (like a NutriBullet or Vitamix).
2. Pour in the liquid and blend away!

Iced Espresso Protein Drink

I wish I could take credit for this protein drink for coffee lovers. I've found it on multiple Pinterest and YouTube sites.

1. Buy a single or double espresso in a venti-size (24-ounce) cup filled with ice.
2. Pour an 11-ounce Premier Protein drink (try chocolate or caramel) over the ice.

This yields 30 grams of protein. Enjoy!

Getting Enough Fluid

How much fluid we need depends on our weight, our metabolic rate (the speed at which we use energy), our activity level, and the amount of fluid we lose through urine, blood, breathing, and so on. Tissue injury and wound healing also increase our fluid requirements. So does fever: We need more fluid to support the elevated heart rate and energy utilization we experience with fever.

At a minimum, plan on consuming at least 2 quarts of fluid per day as a baseline. A good rule of thumb is to drink until you have to pee every hour or two.

Volume Depletion and Dehydration: Not the Same Thing

Note that there is a difference between volume depletion and dehydration.

Volume depletion means that there is not enough fluid (blood) in the blood vessels, and **dehydration** refers to a lack of total body water.

For our purposes, we'll use the terms interchangeably, but it's not entirely correct.

While you're in the hospital, your surgeon and surgical staff keep track of your fluid balance. When you go home, you have to manage this yourself. Fortunately, our body gives us clues as to how much fluid we need. Here are some you may notice:

- **You're thirsty.**
  Thirst can be an indicator of decreased fluid volume; increase your fluid intake if you feel thirsty. Some people, particularly older people, may not be as sensitive to this indicator.[67]

- **Your urine is more concentrated.**
  Our urine gets more concentrated (darker yellow) when our bodies are trying to hold onto every drop of fluid volume. So, drink more fluid when you notice your urine looks more concentrated. If your urine is mixed with blood, it may be harder to see the color differences but do your best. (Brown urine that looks like cola can be a warning sign of an acute kidney injury; call your healthcare provider.)

- **Your urine volume is decreased.**
  If you are peeing very little, you may need more fluid. (This is different than not being *able* to pee—that is, having a full bladder but not being able to pass the urine out of your body. Contact your surgical team, especially if your surgery has involved reconstructing your urethra. You may have a blockage or narrowing of the urethra and need help quickly.)

- **You get dizzy and your heart beats faster when you first stand up.**
  When you first get up after a surgery, sit at the edge of the bed for a few moments before you stand. Then, get up carefully and make sure your body is steady before you walk. If you feel unsteady, sit or lie back down.

  Dizziness or rapid heart rate may signal low fluid volume. You can also get a low red-blood-cell count from blood loss, and you can have a rapid heart rate from fever. I might tell a patient, "Drink a glass of water or have a cup of soup. See if you feel any improvement over the next hour. If you don't, call your surgeon's office." (Call them regardless if you are worried.)

- **You are constipated.**
  Constipation can be a stressful problem after surgery. Opiate pain medications often slow bowel motility to a crawl. Then, if you have fluid depletion, your body tries to conserve every drop of fluid it can, even from the liquid stool moving through the large intestine. That makes the stool dryer and harder. Additionally, if you've had a genital surgery, you may not really *want* to push out a bowel movement because you fear that it may hurt. Make it easier on yourself by increasing your fluid and fiber intake and use laxatives, a laxative herbal tea (such as Smooth Move Tea), and the stool softeners that your surgical team recommends.

67 William Larry Kenney, and Percy Chiu, "Influence of Age on Thirst and Fluid Intake," *Medicine and Science in Sports and Exercise* 33, no. 9 (October 2001): 1524–32, https://doi.org/10.1097/00005768-200109000-00016.

Caring for Your Wounds

If you have a vaginoplasty, you will likely *not* have a postoperative bandage or dressing to go home with at all. You'll be wearing a sanitary pad in your underpants, and you'll change your pads, of course. But that's quite different from wound care after top surgery or donor site care after phalloplasty!

Caring for a postsurgical wound can be intimidating if wound care isn't in your skill set. It's all manageable, but it does take some attention to detail.

Surgical instructions are not "guidelines" or "suggestions." They used to be called "orders." And they are there for your safety.

Before you leave the hospital, your surgical team will give you instructions on how to care for your surgical sites. They will show you how to change your dressings (bandages). Be sure you take any written instructions home with you, along with information on how to contact the surgeon's office for further troubleshooting. Follow your surgeon's instructions ***to the letter***! Their instructions are provided for your safety.

Most surgical wounds *will* heal well provided that they are kept clean and dry and monitored carefully. Serious wound complications are rare, but they do happen. They can be treated, but occasionally some require a surgical revision. As stated earlier, you must support your body with plenty of rest, fluids, and excellent nutrition. Take the medications your surgical team has prescribed. Don't stop taking medications, particularly antibiotics, without your surgical team's okay.

Our bodies are programmed to heal. When I was learning to deliver babies, one of my instructors said, "If you leave both halves of the vagina in the same room, it will heal."

— Linda Gromko, MD

Changing Your Dressings: The Very Basics

STOP! Read this carefully.

Your surgeon will likely change your dressings the first time, whether that is in the hospital or in their office. Ask if you aren't certain.

If my comments are different than those of your surgical team, follow their advice over mine!

The first few times you change a dressing, try to have another human with you for moral support and for more direct assistance. Put your animals in another room.

Review the following general principles ***before you begin:***

1. Wash your hands with soap and water or rub your hands with hand sanitizer as instructed by your surgical team.

2. Assemble all of your wound care and dressing supplies before you take off the old bandages. Put your assembled supplies on an inexpensive flat tray that can be wiped down easily with an antiseptic wipe.

3. Set up your assembled supply tray in a clean area and on a clean surface. Be sure you set up the tray within your reach or within reach of the patient if you are the care partner.[68]

4. For wound care, you will likely use a mix of aseptic (very clean) techniques and a sterile technique. Your surgical team will help you figure out what parts of the dressing change can be aseptic and what *must* be sterile.

   - **Aseptic** (very clean) means devoid of bacteria, viruses, or fungi *that can cause disease*.

   - **Sterile** means devoid of *all* bacteria, virus particles, or fungi. This is the environment you want in an operating room. Do not touch anything that is supposed to remain sterile unless you are wearing sterile gloves and you understand sterile technique.

5. Tear or cut any tape you will need to secure the new dressing *before* you begin the dressing change. Many people place cut tape strips on the edge of their tray or table. The point is to have

68 "Care partner" is the term that was liberally used in the kidney dialysis community in reference to the person who assisted a patient on home dialysis. I learned it from Dori Schatell, the executive director of Medical Education Institute, Inc.

your prepared tape ready and fastened to a place where you can reach it easily with a minimum of handling.

6. Set up a designated "dirty" wastebasket where you will dispose of the old dressings or other contaminated supplies. Line this wastebasket with a plastic kitchen garbage bag so it can be safely discarded separately from regular household garbage. You don't want kids or animals to get into this.

7. If you have Jackson-Pratt bulb drains to empty (the ones that look like small hand grenades), you may want to do this before removing the actual wound dressings. Write down the amount of drainage in each bulb. (This will help the surgical team estimate the proper time for them to remove the drains.) Wearing nonsterile exam gloves, carefully open the tab at the bottom of the bulb and empty the drainage into a designated "dirty" container. Recap the bulb. Cover the container and discard it in your "dirty" wastebasket.

8. Wearing nonsterile exam gloves, gently remove the old dressings. Discard the old dressings and the gloves you are wearing in the "dirty" wastebasket.

9. Take a careful look at the wound to assess the following:

   - **Redness:** Look for red streaks extending from the wound; notice any color you don't expect to see on a wound like gray or black.
   - **Swelling** of the wound and surrounding tissue.
   - **Pus or other drainage:** Clear serous fluid is straw-colored, while pus is white or yellow and has a thick consistency.
   - **Odor:** Notice if the wound has an odor, which can sometimes signify infection.

   If you see something that alarms you, have your care partner or assistant take a photo on a smartphone so you can share it with the surgical team.

10. Cleanse the wound as you've been instructed by your surgical team. Sometimes, you will do this in the shower right before you apply a new dressing; you may be advised to use a gentle soap and to allow water to run over the wound to rinse it. Or, you'll clean a wound using Betadine, provided that you are not allergic to iodine. You may be instructed to use normal saline to rinse the wound. (Saline is medically prepared, sterile saltwater.) Allow the wound to air-dry or gently pat dry with a sterile gauze square (which may be called a "four by four" because they measure 4 x 4 inches).

11. Wash your hands again or rub them with hand sanitizer. Put on the gloves as you've been instructed. These may be nonsterile exam gloves that come in a box or sterile, individually wrapped gloves like those used in surgery. Do what your surgical team has told you to do.

12. If you have been directed to apply any antiseptic or antibiotic ointment, gently spread it over the wound using a sterile swab or a sterile tongue blade. Start applying this at the area that must be kept cleanest (that is, the incision line) and work outward to the perimeter of the wound. This prevents moving bacteria into the area that must be kept the cleanest.

13. Gently cover the wound using sterile technique. Your team will tell you how to do this and what dressing material to use. If a wound is oozing, a layer of nonstick Telfa dressing may prevent the

wound from sticking to the bandages. Cover this with one or two layers of sterile dressings as you've been instructed. Cover this dressing with an outer dressing layer and secure this with the tape you have prepared. If you are using OPSITE (a clear transparent dressing that resembles a window), you won't need tape.

14. Discard used wound supplies safely in the "dirty" container, which is kept away from clean supplies, people and animals, and general household garbage. Any fluid or other material that drains from a wound is considered a biohazard and could potentially spread disease to another person. It is your responsibility to protect other people who could come into contact with biohazardous waste, so be sure to ask questions of your surgical team so you are comfortable with responsible biohazard disposal.
15. Recycle the clean wrappers from your dressing supplies. Use a recycle bin that is clearly distinguishable from your lined biohazard or "dirty" wastebasket.

If you require more complex wound care that requires assessment of other drains, or changing a wound VAC (vacuum-assisted closure) system, you will need more specific help. In some cases, you may be directed to go to a wound care clinic or your primary care provider's office. Or you may have a visiting nurse assigned to you. More information on wound VACs is on page 291.

Gentle Attention to Your Mental Health

The postoperative period can pose a significant disruption to a person's mental comfort. And why wouldn't it? You've just been through a major physical event that required years of planning and periods of logistical uncertainty. You may be under additional stress with travel, fatigue, medication side effects, and the need for more vigilance about your own health.

You undoubtedly have extra expenses, some of which you hadn't anticipated. You may feel isolated from people who ordinarily support you, such as coworkers and friends. You may have experienced worry or fear that you would not *survive* your surgery even though there was never any thought that your risks were excessive.

If you have a partner or spouse, you may find that your relationship with them has weathered stress too; some fundamental aspects of your life and relationship may have shifted. And if you do not have a significant other or supportive family members, you may feel more loneliness and vulnerability than you'd imagined.

If you've had a genital surgery, the world cannot possibly acknowledge what you've experienced. You have no cast or crutches that signal to others, "Please hold the door open," or "I could use help with this grocery bag." In fact, you may have just undergone one of the most significant events of your life and nobody really notices anything at all.

Answer this therapy question: **"If your best friend in the world felt exactly like you do now, what would you do for them?"** Have compassion for yourself and try to support yourself in the same way you'd imagine supporting a best friend.

Are You Depressed?

If you have experienced depression before, you may recognize some the following common symptoms:

- Sadness
- Feeling a sense of being let down or disappointed
- Fatigue
- Sleeping too much or too little; not feeling rested
- Crying more than you ordinarily cry, or not being able to cry
- Difficulty with focusing, concentrating, or reading
- Feeling irritable, cranky, or angry
- Feeling a lack of interest in things that ordinarily interest you or that you usually find pleasurable
- Feeling apathetic and not really caring about anything
- Eating "therapeutically"—that is, eating unhealthy junk food rather than healthy food that helps you heal
- Gaining or losing weight
- Experiencing excessive worry
- Feeling guilty
- Feeling isolated or that nobody really cares or understands

You may recognize that many of the above symptoms of depression actually overlap common postsurgical recovery experiences. If these symptoms are prolonged or severe, tell someone and get help. You may benefit from therapy or medications. Don't allow this to worsen. (Refer to Chapter 17 for more information on depression.)

As stated earlier in the pre-op part, if I know that a patient of mine struggles with depression, we may talk about starting medications *before* the surgery. Most antidepressants take 2 to 4 weeks to kick in.

Be aware that you may be depressed and at serious risk if you're having passive thoughts about dying such as, "It wouldn't matter if I died," or if you're formulating a plan to die on purpose or by "accident."

Recognize That You Are at Risk

Tell someone right away so you can get help. You can also go back and reread Chapter 1 or go on to read Chapter 17 for more information about depression.

Get evaluated promptly. Call 911, your local crisis clinic, or the Trans Lifeline—or go directly to your nearest hospital emergency room for a mental health assessment.

Recognizing When You Are in Trouble: Emergency Warnings That Apply to All Surgeries

We will address specific concerns relating to the individual surgeries later, but the following emergency information applies to all surgeries.

Post and Keep This Emergency Information on Your Phone

- Your surgeon's emergency contact number
- The address **where you are now**—that is, your own home address or the address of the place where you are staying
- Any personal emergency phone numbers, such as family and primary care physician numbers

Chances are excellent that you will get through your surgery and recovery with no major difficulties. But problems do happen, so it is important for you to know when to call for serious emergency help.

When to Call 911

- Call 911 if you are not getting enough air to breathe.
- Call 911 if you are having a severe allergic reaction (anaphylaxis).
- Your care partner calls 911 if you have passed out and cannot be revived.
- Your care partner calls 911 if you are not breathing and have no pulse.
- Call 911 if you are bleeding very heavily and cannot stop it.
- Call 911 for severe chest pain, "the worst headache of your life," seizure, severe injury, etc. If you think of calling, call.

Let's examine these in more detail. But stop reading right now if you are in the middle of any of these situations! **Call 911 and read later.**

- **Call 911 if you are not getting enough air to breathe.**
  - If you know you have asthma and are wheezing or coughing severely, use the asthma inhaler you have brought with you as you wait for the paramedics.
  - A pulmonary embolism (blood clot in the lung) can occur after a surgery. Symptoms can include shortness of breath, pain at the peak of each breath, upper abdominal pain, rapid or irregular heartbeat, coughing up blood, a swelling or lump in the leg, or dizziness, agitation, and loss of consciousness. If this is happening, you will need medical care in the ER.
  - There are other problems, such as panic attacks, heart rhythm problems, or even a heart attack, which can impair your breathing. Call for help.
- **Call 911 if you are having a severe allergic reaction (anaphylaxis).**
  - If you know you have severe, life-threatening allergic reactions called anaphylaxis, you will likely have your EpiPen with you. Use it according to the directions you've been given as you wait for the paramedics (remember that there are directions on the package). The paramedics usually carry EpiPens also.
  - Warning signs can include the throat tightness that comes from narrowing of the airway, hives, flushing, severe itching, and passing out.
- **Your care partner calls 911 if you have passed out and cannot be revived.**
  - Sit down, then lie down if you feel you are going to faint. It is always best to prevent fainting if you can.
  - If you have fainted quickly and without warning, you will likely regain consciousness rapidly as you are guided to a safe horizontal position. If you don't revive, your care partner must call 911 and follow the steps below.
- **Your care partner calls 911 if you are not breathing and have no pulse.**
  - If you are not breathing and have no pulse, your care partner must call 911 and start CPR (cardiopulmonary resuscitation).
  - The 911 dispatcher can talk a caller through CPR if they don't know how to perform it.
  - Continue CPR until the paramedics arrive and take over.
- **Call 911 if you are bleeding very heavily and cannot stop it.**
  - Apply firm pressure to the area of heavy bleeding.
  - As you wait for the paramedics to arrive, lie down with your legs elevated above the level of your heart (nipple level).
  - Call your surgeon as you are waiting for the paramedics. Your surgeon will help assess you and guide you further.

- **Call 911 for severe chest pain, "the worst headache of your life," seizure, severe injury, and other serious symptoms. If you think of calling, call.**
    - The paramedics evaluate a situation and provide emergency care. Many provide emergency-room– or intensive-care-unit–caliber treatment in the field. They will transfer a patient to the ER—or wait with the patient until a transport ambulance arrives.

Having an emergency like any of these by yourself emphasizes the need to have someone with you. But what if you are totally by yourself? In larger communities, dialing 911 (or even 9) will summon help. When you call 911, even if you cannot speak, dispatchers will see your address if you call from a landline. If you're using a cell phone, GPS tracks where you are located, but it can take additional time to locate you unless you've registered your address to connect it to your cell number. You also need to register your address to your phone number if you are using a voice-over-IP (VoIP) phone. Do the best you can in a situation like this.

What Happens If You Call 911 and It Turns Out to Be a False Alarm?

If the paramedics do not need to transfer you directly to a hospital, they will either call an ambulance for you or help you figure out what to do next (follow up with your surgeon, your PCP, and so on). They would much prefer to be called for a false alarm than to be called too late. If your situation improves markedly while the first responders are on the way, you can call again and cancel your request.

Other Urgent Situations You Might Encounter

The following situations require urgent attention but ***may*** not necessitate a 911 call:

You Are Suicidal

If you feel that you are unable to continue living and are thinking about ending your life right now, you must seek urgent help. This is a life-threatening emergency; the life that is threatened is yours! Depending on your circumstances, you must get yourself to someone who can evaluate and treat you. Naturally, you may certainly need to call 911.

You Are Having Pain

Surprisingly—and as callous as this may sound—pain may not represent an emergency. But it does need to be managed.

Important exceptions, of course, are chest pain or "the worst headache of your life," which may signal a heart attack or stroke, respectively. These circumstances definitely warrant a 911 call.

If you are having pain that is suddenly much more severe or different in character than the pain you have experienced, it is very reasonable to contact your surgical team and follow their guidance.

Remember also that regulations dealing with opiates have become quite strict. We cannot, for example, call prescriptions for narcotics into a pharmacy. Plan ahead and contact your surgeon's office before you run out of medications.

You Have a Fever

Take your temperature with the thermometer you were advised to buy before your surgery. A fever is technically defined as 100.4 degrees Fahrenheit, but use the guidelines your surgical team has given you. A fever may signal an infection, and you may need further care. (Sometimes, your temperature is elevated from atalectasis, which occurs when a person is not expanding their lungs enough with each breath. Many postoperative patients have to be reminded to take deep breaths or to use an incentive spirometer device from the hospital. But this problem is generally easy to solve.) Contact your surgeon's office and follow their guidance.

You Are Having Nausea, Vomiting, and Diarrhea and Are Feeling Progressively Weaker

While the reason for your symptoms may not be clear, you may need help to prevent further fluid loss. Of course, it is important to address the underlying cause of your symptoms. Contact your surgeon's office and follow their guidance.

You Are Having Urinary Symptoms

A burning sensation when you pee, peeing more frequently than normal, feeling the urgent need to pee and then peeing only a tiny amount, or peeing blood may signal infection. Or, if your urethra has been revised or built during your surgery and you cannot pee but your bladder is filling fast, you may have a blockage or narrowing (stenosis or stricture). No matter which problem you have, contact your surgeon's office and follow their guidance.

Lists like the one above cannot consider each and every problem that can occur after a surgery. Use your good judgment. Always remember that a call that turns out to be unnecessary is far better than a call that does not get made in a situation that turns out to be serious.

What happens if you cannot reach your surgical team? Contact your PCP, the emergency room, or the nearest urgent care center. It is fair to state that many ERs and urgent care centers may not have a great deal of experience with gender-affirming surgeries.

But do not delay the care that you need ***now*** based on prior experiences or fear.

Specific Postoperative Circumstances Dealing with Specific Surgeries

We'll address specific surgeries or categories of surgeries one by one and in the order in which they were originally presented. As always, your surgical team is your best source of information. Listen to them first!

Feminizing Surgeries

Facial Feminization Surgery: Post-Op Considerations

You may recall that facial feminization surgery (FFS) was referred to as a collection of surgeries done on the same operative day. The fact that it is a collection of several procedures may help to explain why most of *my* patients have found the immediate recovery period to be more difficult than with other surgeries they have had. That said, I know women who would disagree.

Here Are Some Pointers to Help You after Facial Feminization Surgery

- **Control swelling and pain with cooling and medication.**
  Swelling is intense, particularly in the early postoperative period. People may describe "bone pain" from incisions in the skull or jaw. Pain medication is prescribed, but ice packs may help also reduce both swelling and pain. The Facialteam (a facial reconstruction surgery group in Spain) uses "controlled cooling therapy" for the first 24 to 48 hours.

- **Eat well but gently.**
  Many surgeries are done through the mouth; in this case, you may feel like you have had a lot of dental work. Because you will need to eat plenty of protein to help your tissues knit together and heal, look for soft, protein-containing foods that don't require a lot of biting and chewing. You will be able to "gum" foods such as scrambled eggs, macaroni and cheese, and Greek yogurt. Liquid or semiliquid foods like protein smoothies and split pea or bean soups will be comfortable to sip.

  While not high in protein, Popsicles, frozen juice bars, or ice cream can soothe the inside of your mouth like an ice pack. Additionally, anything that is liquid at body temperature counts as a fluid. Fluid helps remove inflammatory debris and swelling.

- **Rest your eyes.**
  If your eyelids or the under-eye area are being modified, you may have swelling to the extent that it is difficult to see for a while. (Your eyes still function, of course, but it is impossible to see through eyelids that are swollen shut.) You may have extensive bruising and swelling. Here's where podcasts or audiobooks may help you get through!

> **A 40-year-old woman told me after she healed from her FFS, "I looked in the mirror and said, '*There* you are!'" It was like she finally found the best friend she'd been looking for all her life.**
>
> *— Linda Gromko, MD*

- **You may spit or vomit *some* blood.**
If you have had a rhinoplasty (nose job), you may vomit some swallowed blood. This can panic you if you haven't heard of this before. Naturally, you should contact your surgeon if you're concerned.

- **Reassure yourself about your breathing.**
Any swelling in the mouth, nose, or neck may make you feel like your airway isn't working properly. This may trigger feelings of anxiety or panic, such as feeling like you are not getting enough air to breathe. Sadly, we were all reminded during the George Floyd tragedy that a person may be able to utter sentences using very small amounts of air. So do not fall back on the old adage that "If you are talking, you are breathing." Try not to take on extra anxiety, which may only make everything worse, including pain.

- **Wear the compression garments that your surgical team advises.**
Your surgeon is likely to have given you a snug facial or neck garment to wear as you heal. Follow your surgeon's instructions on how to use this correctly—that is, how often and for how many hours per day.

- **Gentle massage or manual lymphatic drainage reduces swelling.**
You may be advised to massage parts of your face or neck. This is generally done to help mobilize the fluid that collects in tissues after surgery. Doing massage carefully will help the swelling go down more rapidly and you'll feel more comfortable faster. Your surgeon may advise you about manual lymphatic drainage (MLD). This is a very light-touch massage done to gently coax the lymphatic system to remove extra fluid and debris. Unless your surgeon advises otherwise, search the Internet for MLD therapists in your area.

- **Follow your surgical team's directions about physical activity.**
The Facialteam notes, "Between 6 and 10 days after surgery, when acute inflammation and other symptoms are under control, the patient enters a 2- to 3-week period of progressive recovery, during which time we recommend minimal exertion. After this period, the patient can return to her usual routine. Moderate physical exercise can begin 3 to 6 months after surgery."[69] (Be sure your surgeon knows what kind of "moderate" physical exercise you do.)

Patience Is Critical!

It typically takes between 6 and 12 months to really appreciate the changes created by FFS. I usually tell my patients not to pass judgment until at least a year, but this is your face and it's visible to everyone!

As mentioned earlier, FFS is a surgery (or more accurately, a collection of surgeries) that can make the most impact reducing the effects of testosterone on your outward appearance.

69 The Facialteam has a full playlist of videos that describe the process and many other aspects of facial feminization surgery on its YouTube channel: youtube.com/c/FacialteamEu/playlists.

A gentle reminder: ***Do not start smoking again after any surgery.*** **It's especially hard when you aren't feeling great and the full surgical results aren't visible. Do anything safe and legal to keep yourself from restarting.**

Breast Augmentation Surgery

Follow your surgeon's advice to the letter. Read my guidelines about general surgical recovery. You will likely be able to go home on the day of your surgery unless the breast augmentation is combined with other surgeries such as vaginoplasty.

Be certain not to drive or use alcohol or other substances that make you drowsy while taking your pain medications. If you get into a crash, you could be cited as an impaired driver. Plus, you could hurt yourself or someone else.

In addition, you will want to clarify the following with your surgeon:

- When can you lie or sleep on your front or sides?
- What restrictions do you have on your body's movements? You may be advised not to raise your arms above the level of your shoulders for at least 2 weeks.
- When can you resume exercise? Be sure your surgeon knows exactly what type of exercise you are talking about!
- When can you buy new bras? Following surgery, you'll be required to wear a special postoperative bra except when bathing. (You will not wear new bras until your swelling decreases, likely at least 1 month postoperatively.)
- Will your surgeon (or their assistant) instruct you on how to perform breast massage to help the tissues heal (if that is required after your surgery)?

Orchiectomy

Orchiectomy, or the removal of the testicles from the scrotum, is generally an outpatient surgery (day surgery). It is helpful to rest, elevate the lower half of the body, and apply ice packs.

All postoperative guidelines apply here, but be sure to ask your surgeon and your PCP about stopping spironolactone or other testosterone blockers. Once the testes have been removed, these medications are generally stopped.

Vaginoplasty

Does My Vagina Look Normal?

One of the most common questions I hear from postoperative trans women is, *"Does my vagina look normal?"* And given the enormous variety among the genitals of all women, the answer is almost without exception, *"Yes!"*

The best illustration of this I know is a magnificent art piece titled *The Great Wall of Vagina*. British artist Jamie McCartney asked female volunteers to participate by making plaster casts of their labia! These casts were assembled in a collection of panels. In fact, it was one of my post-op trans women patients who first showed me this piece, which is Panel 4. The Great Wall can be seen in its entirety at **jamiemccartney.com/portfolio/the-great-wall-of-vagina**.

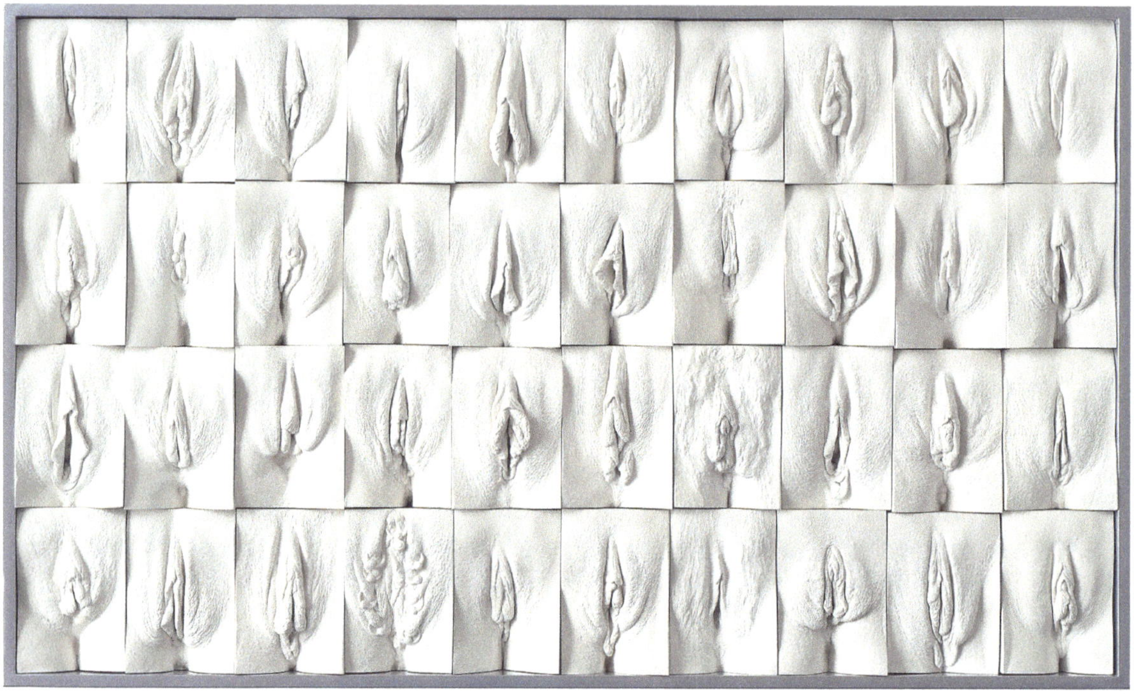

Figure 12.3. **The Great Wall of Vagina** ***by Jamie McCartney.***

Another resource is *I'll Show You Mine*. This book, a photo collection edited by Wrenna Robertson, shows mostly cis women and some trans vulvas—each one unique. Reassuring and educational, many women don't have opportunities to view a lot of vulvas.

As you are examining your postoperative genitalia, remember that you will "remodel" over time—even up to a year. Don't compare your early results with those of women on the Internet who have fully healed.

Dilation Is Critical

If you have a one-step or two-step vaginoplasty and you do not dilate, your new vagina can close!

I have seen this happen several times. It can occur in the span of only a few days, and it can be heartbreaking. It is possible that the neovagina can be revised and reopened, but this may require another surgery and such revisions are technically more difficult to perform. (It isn't known at this writing whether vaginal vaults created using peritoneal tissue require the same diligence in dilating. For now, follow your surgeon's instructions, of course.)

(This is where your pre-op planning is so important. If you really want to have only the phallus and scrotum removed but do not need to have a vagina that can be penetrated, consider a zero-depth vaginoplasty instead. The zero-depth vaginoplasty will take less surgical time to perform and require considerably less maintenance for you.)

Follow Your Surgeon's Dilation Instructions Precisely

You will have a dilation schedule to follow, as provided by your surgical team. As one example, you may be instructed to dilate three times a day for the first 6 months, twice a day for the next 3 months, once a day until the 1-year milestone, and weekly thereafter. But do not follow my schedule! Do what your surgical team has instructed. (Be sure to talk to your surgical team if you have had peritoneal pull-through surgery; those guidelines may be different.)

Surgical instructions are not "guidelines" or "suggestions"; they used to be called "orders" because the instructions are given to ensure that you have the best possible results and to keep you safe. So, follow these instructions even when you're tired and even if you don't want to!

Styles of dilation will vary from surgeon to surgeon. Some will have you insert your dilator to "depth" and stay there for 10 minutes or so; others feel that a rotatory or "dynamic" dilation is preferable.

Helpful Pointers for Dilation after Vaginoplasty

Dilating can be annoying and time-consuming. Many women feel that they've acquired a new part-time job after surgery. Here are some general guidelines for performing vaginal dilation:

- Wash and dry your dilator.
- Get all your dilation materials together before you start:
    - A towel or under-pad for under your butt
    - Surgical lubricant (water-based sterile lubricant like Surgilube, Slippery Stuff, McKesson)
    - A hand mirror and adequate lighting to see what you're doing (you won't need these for long)
    - Baby wipes, facial tissue, or a washcloth to wipe lubricant off your hands and clean up after dilating
    - Pillows and a blanket for comfort
    - Reading materials, TV, audiobooks, or podcasts at the ready
    - Any food or fluids you need for comfort and nutrition
    - Your smartphone to keep you sane, of course. But, if you see something that worries you about your healing perineum, take a picture with your phone and send it to the surgical team.

- Start with the smallest dilator to dilate, or the smallest dilator you used at your last dilation.
- Lubricate the dilator with sterile lubricant. In some situations, you may be advised to put about a teaspoon of medication on the tip of the dilator, so follow those directions if they apply.
    - Enter the vagina with the lubricated dilator, taking care not to touch or enter the urethra above or the rectum below the vaginal opening (women have dilated the urethra or the rectum by mistake).
- Apply slight pressure downward in the direction of the rectum as you enter the vagina; pushing up against the urethra may be painful.
- Take it slowly; don't force the dilator inside.
- Note the number of dots on your dilator once you have gradually reached "depth"—that is, the maximum depth you can comfortably reach or other depth measures you've been told about.
- Leave the dilator at depth for 10 minutes or the amount of time instructed by your surgeon. Some surgeons recommend a dynamic or rotatory process, so do this if instructed. Again, no freelancing.
- After completing dilation, clean yourself up with baby wipes or a warm soapy washcloth. Be sure to move front to back so as not to push rectal bacteria into your urethra, just as you wipe after peeing. Place a new sanitary pad or liner into the crotch of your underpants. At home, some women go without underwear in loose pants or a flowy skirt; tuck a washcloth in the crotch area in case you leak.
- Wash your dilator with soap and water. Then dry or air-dry it in a clean place so it's ready for the next dilation.

Dilation Q & A

Q Does having sex "count" for a dilation?

A No. Penetrative intercourse or penetrative sex toys should not be placed in the vagina by someone else for 3 months after surgery. For that matter, no internal speculum exams should be done for 3 months after surgery, unless approved by your surgeon.

Q So why can I dilate but can't have sex?

A When you are dilating, you know how deep you're going or if it is hurting or otherwise feeling different than usual. Somebody else cannot know this. Anal sex should not be practiced for the first 3 months also; the separation between the rectum and neovagina may be only millimeters in thickness, and anal penetration can cause injury.

Learning to Pee after Vaginoplasty

After vaginoplasty, you will have to get used to urination. Of course, you used to be able to aim your urine stream. After vaginoplasty, your urethra is much shorter, and the surrounding tissue will have varying degrees of swelling that will change from day to day. Your urine stream will run one way on one day and another way on the next! It may even spray like a shower head.

Here are some pointers to help you learn to pee again:

- This stream variation is temporary, but if it bothers you, consider buying a GoGirl, a Shewee, or other stand-to-pee (STP) device to guide the direction of your urine flow (for more information on STPs, see Chapter 9). Or try peeing through the core of an empty toilet paper roll or use a folded paper plate to deflect your urine stream.
- Gently wipe or pat yourself dry from front to back (from the urethra toward the rectum).
- If it is okay with the surgical team, you may use a peri bottle to gently rinse the perineum with warm water. Rinse from front to back and blot the area with toilet paper. A peri bottle is not to be inserted into the vagina.
- If you have been instructed to douche (that is, to rinse the inside of the vagina), follow the instructions from your surgical team. A douche has a rounded blunt tip, whereas a peri bottle has more of a point.
- Place a new sanitary pad or liner into the crotch of your underpants.
- Be aware of the signs and symptoms of urinary tract infections (UTIs); women get them more frequently because of the shorter length of the urethra and its proximity to the rectum.

Watch for the Following UTI Warnings

- Pain when you pee (during or as you finish); one of my patients described this as like "peeing pins."
- Frequency: peeing more often.
- Urgency: feeling the need to go to the bathroom right now.
- Peeing in very tiny amounts.
- Blood in the urine: This may represent a UTI, but it can also be associated with kidney infections, kidney stones, and so on.

- Fever may be associated with kidney infections and severe pain may occur with kidney stones; call your provider.

Swelling in the Perineum

Immediately after surgery, you may not be swollen at all. As you heal, the many incisions and tissue layers will draw fluid from your body into the surgical site. It is possible to have an accumulation of over a quart of fluid—although that is quite rare! Here are some tips to help you if swelling is a problem:

- **Moderate your activity.**
  Although you will want to be up and moving after surgery, too much walking may trap fluid in the perineal area. The same occurs if you are sitting in a "dependent position"—that is, your butt and feet are lower than your upper body and for too long a time. How long? Sadly, you must learn this from your own body; notice when your own swelling gets worse.

- **Elevate.**
  When you are resting, reading, or watching TV, try to keep your butt and legs elevated. Elevating above your heart level (nipple line) can be accomplished with pillows or foam wedges you can buy online.

- **Drink a lot of fluids.**
  This is so you mobilize the fluids retained in the perineal area. Watch your salt intake, as salt and water link together to hold excess fluid in your body.

- **Use ice.**
  An ice pack placed gently over the perineum may feel soothing and help reduce your swelling. You'll find a generous variety by searching "perineal" or "postpartum ice packs" online. A moldable bag of frozen peas is an old and less expensive stand-by that is flexible enough to fit the contours of your body. Wrap the bag first in a clean cloth or paper towel.

Constipation in the Postoperative Period

Narcotic (opiate) pain relievers slow the motility of your bowel. Take pain medications as directed but reduce your use when you can. Hydrocodone, oxycodone, and codeine can all constipate you—that is, make your bowel movements harder in consistency and more difficult to pass. You may not be eager to push anything out of your rectum since everything is tender. So, keep ahead of constipation by doing the following:

- Drinking a lot of fluid.

- Eating high-fiber foods.

- Trying a cup of Smooth Move tea or other laxative herbal tea. (Read the label, follow the directions, and don't try it if you're allergic.)

- Taking stool softeners and gentle laxatives (like Miralax) as directed.

If you go for more than a day or two without a bowel movement, increase your efforts to limit constipation. Call your healthcare provider if these measures don't work, especially if you've gone for 3 or 4 days without a bowel movement.

Common Worries

If Your Sutures Are Coming Out or the Incision Is Opening

It is normal for some sutures to dissolve and come out as you heal. Some sutures are engineered to dissolve while others must be removed; postvaginoplasty sutures are generally self-dissolving, for instance. Let these sutures come out on their own. Don't tug or pull on them.

Some wound separation is common with healing and usually requires no treatment. Talk to your surgical team and be prepared to send a photo taken with your smartphone if necessary.

If granulation tissue is identified (the pebbly, bright cherry-red tissue that you may see at an open incision line), your surgical team or other provider may treat this with silver nitrate. Silver nitrate sticks look something like long matchsticks. Once it is applied to granulation tissue, the silver nitrate helps heal the area and stops bleeding if it occurs. Expect a silver-gray discharge for a day or two after using.

Most of my patients have told me that silver nitrate is not particularly painful, although it is possible to have some temporary burning sensations with it.

If You Experience Vaginal Bleeding or See a Streak of Blood on your Dilator

Unless bleeding is profuse—in which case, call your surgical team right away—a small amount of persistent blood or a streak of blood on the dilator may indicate that you have an area of granulation tissue deep in the vagina or on a side wall. This can be treated with silver nitrate applications by your provider. As above, the silver nitrate chemically cauterizes the granulation tissue, reducing its size and tendency to bleed. It may take treatments on a weekly basis for a while (months in some cases), but it does heal. (No speculums for 90 days except by the surgeon!)

If you have not begun pelvic floor physical therapy, make these arrangements and begin now to maximize your urinary and sexual function.

Peritoneal Pull-Through Vaginoplasty and Phallus-Preserving Peritoneal Pull-Through

Many of the vaginoplasty guidelines—with the possible exception of the specifics of dilation—will apply. You will receive specific dilation information from your surgeon.

Have I forgotten anything? Quite possibly; everyone is different. Please call your surgical team if you experience anything that causes alarm.

Masculinizing Surgeries

We'll now address postoperative considerations in specific masculinizing surgeries or categories of surgeries one by one and in the order in which they were originally presented. As always, your surgical team is your best source of information. Listen to them first!

Remember that all of the same general postoperative information and warnings about dealing with emergent and serious problems apply.

Facial Masculinization Surgery

Facial masculinization surgery is a collection of surgeries that involve the bones and soft tissues of the face, scalp, and neck. Please refer to the postoperative recovery part for facial feminization surgery on pages 275–276. All of the concepts are the same or similar, although you may have an additional recovery area, such as the chest where the rib cartilage has been harvested. If you have had a rib harvested (or for that matter, any surgery involving the upper chest or collarbone area), it is possible—although unlikely—to experience the collapse of a lung due to even a tiny tear of the pleural membrane. This is treatable. Your surgeon will direct you to go to the emergency room if you are having difficulty breathing after your surgery.

After Gender-Affirming Chest Reconstruction (Top Surgery)

Nothing seems to impact the overall life experience of trans men like top surgery does. It is getting to be a commonly performed surgery that allows trans men to stop using the binders that have been so uncomfortable. It is frequently covered by insurance (sometimes even in adolescents). Nonetheless, it is a surgery.

Here are some points to consider to help in your recovery.

- ***Do not start smoking again now* if you stopped smoking before your top surgery!**
  Naturally, this would apply to any surgery. But it is critical in top surgery because the nipple is placed on the chest *as a graft*. Whether a graft "takes" or not depends on the blood supply at the surgical site. More specifically, this relies on the amount of blood delivered, the diameter of blood vessels, and the oxygen content of the blood. Smoking impacts all of these healing factors directly. You could actually lose a nipple graft if you start smoking.

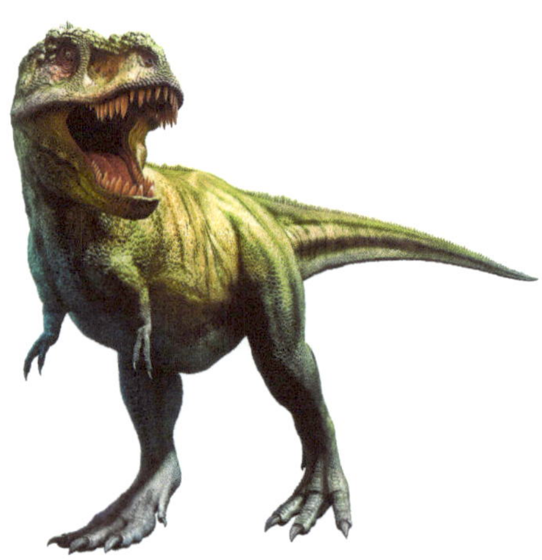

- **Understand how much upper body movement is okay after your surgery.**
  I hear trans male patients referring to the "T-rex position" as a guideline for mobility after top surgery. The Tyrannosaurus rex was a dinosaur with tiny upper limbs that couldn't be raised even to shoulder level. Overhead stretching can disrupt your incision lines and increase your scarring, so move like a T-rex!

- **Expect to wear a postsurgical chest binder.**
  This binder is issued by your surgeon and may be even more restrictive than the binders you have worn in the past. It may zip together in the front or fasten together with hooks and eyes. Use this according to your surgical team's directions. This binder is temporary, though.

- **Sleep on your back.**
  Ask your surgical team about when you may sleep on your sides or front. Pillows or body pillows can help you.

- **Ask your surgical team about scar care.**
  Scars are raised and red for about a year, at which point they tend to become less visible. You may also notice a numbness around the periphery of the scars; this is also normal and will resolve in about a year also.

- **Consider using Pink Pockets to help you if you have post-op drains.**
  The mother of one of our patients is a nurse practitioner in the breast oncology department of a major medical center. She told us about Pink Pockets, a remarkable and inexpensive invention that allows you to secure post-op drains to your shirt, thereby reducing the amount of tug on the drains. They are pink out of respect for folks after breast cancer surgery, but they work for anyone who has a bulb drain after surgery. Search for **pink-pockets.com.**

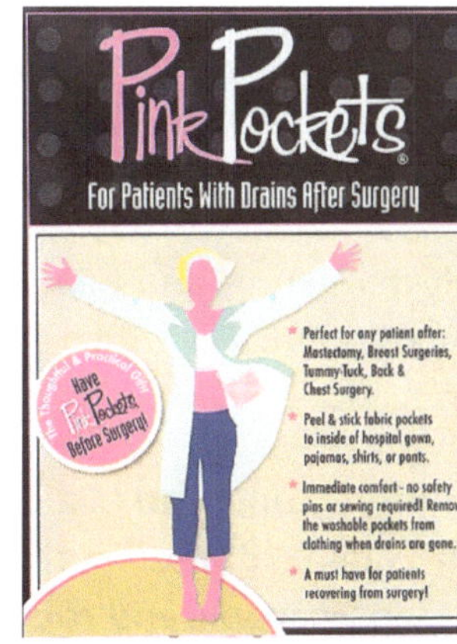

- **Talk with your surgical team about nipple tattooing if, after about a year, you are still having hypopigmentation (reduced pigmentation) over the areolas.**
  The Vinnie Myers Team creates 3D areolar and nipple tattoos that are extremely realistic. One of the cisgender breast cancer patients in my practice had their tattoos by the Team after breast reconstruction. She was ecstatic about her incredible results, and I was simply astonished. I spoke with a representative of the Team, and they do nipple and areolar tattoos on trans men as well. This could include 3D tattooing if your nipple graft didn't "take" well. Contact their office via the website at **vinniemyersteam.com** to get an appointment in the Maryland studio and to learn the Team's travel itinerary.

  If you search the Internet for "nipple tattoos for trans men," you will find others across the country. (Refer also to the phallus tattoos on page 292.)

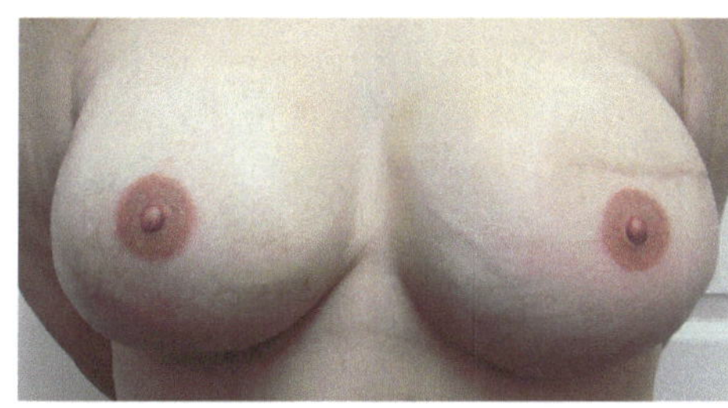

Figure 12.4. A 3D nipple tattoo done on a woman after a breast reconstruction surgery. While these nipples look like they protrude, they are absolutely flat to the touch. The Vinnie Myers Team, who did this tattoo, also does 3D tattoos for individuals after top surgery as well as penile tattoos.

- **Don't burn your binders. Launder and donate them!**
  Imagine how much another transmasculine individual might appreciate inheriting your gently used chest binders! If you don't have a personal friend who would benefit, consider donating them to one of the many organizations that distribute used binders to trans men coming along the path. Point of Pride is one such organization; research them at **pointofpride.org/donate-a-binder.**

After Hysterectomy and Bilateral Salpingo-Oophorectomy

Many—but not all trans men—have their uterus, fallopian tubes, and ovaries removed. Certainly, it is done in preparation for phalloplasty. Removal accomplishes the following:

- It essentially eliminates the possibility of cancer of the uterus, cervix, ovaries, or fallopian tubes. (Fallopian tube cancer is quite rare, but it can occur in people who have BRCA1, BRCA2, or other gene mutations that also increase the risk of a person getting breast, ovarian, peritoneal, fallopian, or pancreatic cancer.) Typically, cancers of the ovary, fallopian tubes, or peritoneum have subtle symptoms that are recognized late in the disease process. Particularly for trans men who are reluctant to seek out gynecological care, removing these organs can be smart.

As a reminder, top surgery does *not* eliminate the possibility of breast cancer, so chest exams done by a man and his healthcare provider are important. The evaluation of any lump is critical, as is special attention to those men with cancer-provoking gene mutations as mentioned above.

- Removal essentially eliminates the possibility of vaginal bleeding that comes from the uterus, which may occur when people run out of their testosterone, forget to take it, or are prescribed a dose that is too low. Bleeding can also occur because of a disease state, such as cancer. That's why bleeding that *doesn't* correct with hormone adjustments must be evaluated further.

Hysterectomy and bilateral salpingo-oophorectomy can be combined with procedures that reduce incontinence of urine or stool. This can be an issue for trans men who have had vaginal deliveries before transition.

Hysterectomy and bilateral salpingo-oophorectomy can be accomplished through the abdomen or through the vagina. But today, these procedures are often done using minimally invasive surgical techniques, such as laparoscopic and robot-assisted procedures. These enable the surgeon to make much smaller incisions. The organs are clearly seen when a camera (the laparoscope) is placed through the belly button, and photographs are projected on large screens opposite the surgeon and assistant. In robotic surgeries, the surgeon actually manipulates the "hands" of the robot and the camera remotely via a computer.

If you have a laparoscopic surgery performed, carbon dioxide gas will flow into your abdomen through the camera port to distend or raise your abdominal wall and make your organs more visible. Visibility is critical for precision! The CO_2 gas floats upward toward your diaphragm (the muscle that separates the abdomen from the chest). This in turn may cause you to experience "referred pain"—in this case, pain that originates below the waist but registers in the upper back or shoulders. Pain in these locations can understandably worry a patient who has had a pelvic surgery, but it is common and it resolves as the body eventually absorbs the gas.

A hysterectomy used to require 6 days in the hospital and 6 weeks off work, but minimally invasive techniques have generally changed all that. Today, it is usually an outpatient surgery (also called day surgery or ambulatory surgery), although some people stay for overnight or for a day or two.

After Monsplasty

Again, your recovery will depend on what technique was used. I had one patient who required a drain with a lengthy horizontal incision across the lower abdomen (although this is rarely needed). This foot-long plastic ribbon sat at the base of the surgical wound, exiting from one side. The ribbon had holes along it to collect fluid and worked something like a drain. Your surgical team or primary care provider can remove this under the surgeon's direction. (I appreciate that many people worry about how it will feel to have a drain removed, but most people don't have these drains at all.)

To remove a drain, I snip the sutures that are securing it. Then I ask the patient if they're ready and then instruct them to breathe in as I count to three and to blow out when I reach "3." When the patient is exhaling, I pull the drain out. The whole thing takes 30 seconds, the patient is distracted, and we're done, with "no trauma, no drama."

After Vaginectomy

In vaginectomy, the walls of the vagina are essentially closed together, which eliminates what some people refer to as the "front hole." It is frequently done in combination with other surgeries, and the postoperative vaginoplasty course may be dictated more by what else has been done as opposed to the vaginectomy alone. Expect pain and swelling, both of which can be managed by following the surgical team's directions.

If you have a urinary catheter, your surgical team will teach you how to manage it. Although you will not have to *change* your own catheter, you will have to empty the urine bag. Sometimes patients are told to remove their own urinary catheters when they no longer need them. (You don't just tug or pull on it; you must first deflate a small balloon that holds the catheter in your bladder. If you need to do this, your surgical team will instruct you.) You should also know how to flush (irrigate) the tubing with normal saline to keep the urine flowing freely into the bag.

After Metoidioplasty

As with vaginectomy, metoidioplasty may be combined with other surgeries; your recovery course may be dictated by the associated surgeries. If you have had a metoidioplasty by itself, your recovery will be limited to the area of what used to be called the clitoris, which now becomes the neophallus. You will not be able to pee through the neophallus unless you have had a urethral extension.

Expect swelling in the area. The swelling may change from day to day, and it may be significant enough to impact your urination, but you should still be able to pee. While it sounds counterintuitive, drink more fluids so you make more urine. This will accomplish a couple of things:

- It will make you feel the need to pee more clearly, and the urine will typically come out faster with more volume and pressure behind it.
- It will make your urine less concentrated. Concentrated urine might irritate the sutures and sensitive surrounding tissues.

Although the swelling will go down in time, you can help reduce it and relieve pain by using ice packs. You can find form-fitting ones online (try searching "perineal surgery ice packs," but I found a much better selection by shopping under "postpartum ice packs"). I know that this reference may trigger dysphoria, but you may appreciate anything that works if you truly need this product.

After Metoidioplasty with Urethral Extension (Lengthening)

Metoidioplasty with urethral extension is naturally more complicated than metoidioplasty alone. Any time that you have your urethra lengthened, there is a risk for narrowing at the connection, which can slow or even stop your urine flow. Your surgical team will tell you what to look for, but here are some things to know:

- You will likely get donor tissue for your urethral extension from the buccal mucosa (the inside of your cheek), from the inside of your lower lip, or from the vaginal labia. These areas may hurt also. Your surgical team will give you tips on how to manage this pain.
- You will have a catheter in the neourethra for several weeks as it is healing. But your urine will actually be emptied through a suprapubic catheter in your bladder; it protrudes from your lower abdomen above your pubic bone.

After Scrotoplasty with Prosthetic Testes Placed

Like all tissue in the perineum, the new scrotum can accumulate fluid after surgery. Expect swelling. A scrotum can easily accommodate a liter of fluid. Reread the part on general postoperative care. For scrotoplasty, you will want to keep your perineum elevated when you are resting. This helps to reduce the amount of fluid the scrotum collects.

You may notice that the testicles are uneven in their location, or that one "rides up." Your surgical team will instruct you on how to massage your testicles so they stay down in the scrotum more easily.

If you have tissue expanders, you will be given special instructions on how to care for them. They will need to be filled periodically with normal saline; like many medical procedures, it isn't that difficult but requires careful attention to what you are doing.

After Phalloplasty (Free Forearm Flap and Anterior Lateral Thigh Flap)

As the most complicated of all gender-affirming surgeries, phalloplasty must be regarded as a combination of surgeries done at different times and with different purposes. Remember that the overarching goals of phalloplasty are to create the following:

- A phallus that can be used for urination, with the man standing up and urinating through his phallus.
- A phallus that can be used for the sexual penetration of a partner.
- Intact orgasmic function.
- Intact urinary function.
- Removal of the uterus, fallopian tubes, and ovaries (hysterectomy and bilateral salpingo-oophorectomy) is usually done early in the sequence. A vaginectomy is also recommended as it is associated with less fistula formation. A fistula is a hole that forms where it doesn't belong; it this case, it can cause leakage from the phallus in phalloplasty. They often heal on their own, but it's better not to get one!

The following information is designed to assist you in your surgeries and recoveries. Since there cannot be a single document suitable for each person going though these surgeries, do read widely, talk to your friends who have had similar surgeries, trust your surgical team, and ask a lot of questions.

This website also has some good information: healthcare.utah.edu/transgender-health/gender-affirmation-surgery/phalloplasty-recovery.php. **If there is a single matter of primary importance in phalloplasty, it has to be the blood flow to the neophallus.**

If you have had a microsurgical connection of a graft or grafts, you may spend your first few days in the intensive care unit or in a special care unit where you are monitored every 1 to 2 hours. This will vary from surgeon to surgeon and facility to facility. If you do go to a special unit, here's what you can expect:

- Your vascular connections where blood flows between a flap or graft and the neophallus will be monitored using a Doppler ultrasound device that attaches near the blood vessel connections in the penis. Other factors like color, warmth, and capillary refill will also be frequently assessed.
- You will be on at bed rest for most of the initial recovery and likely will have SCDs (sequential compression devices) that are wrapped around your legs to periodically squeeze them to move your blood along. This reduces the risk of blood clot formation, as does the use of anticoagulants.
- You will have a urinary catheter in your bladder, but it is inserted in the lower abdomen above your pubic bone. Your urine will empty through the suprapubic catheter (not through your penis) for the first few weeks. You will be trained in how to empty your urine bag and take care of the catheter. You will have another catheter in your penis to keep the neourethra open. This catheter will be removed around your fifth postoperative day, before you leave the hospital. And sometimes, men will leave the hospital with the urinary catheter in place and have it removed in the clinic later.
- You will have a PCA (patient-controlled analgesia) device during the first day or two after your phalloplasty to help you manage pain. You will also receive antinausea medication to keep you from vomiting, thereby keeping your body more stationary.
- You can expect to hear monitors and see LED indicators of various vital signs and body functions if you are in the intensive care unit (ICU). Your sleep will be interrupted, and you may require medications to help you relax and sleep. The sensory overload that occurs in the ICU can make you feel disoriented and you may appreciate medication for anxiety during this time.

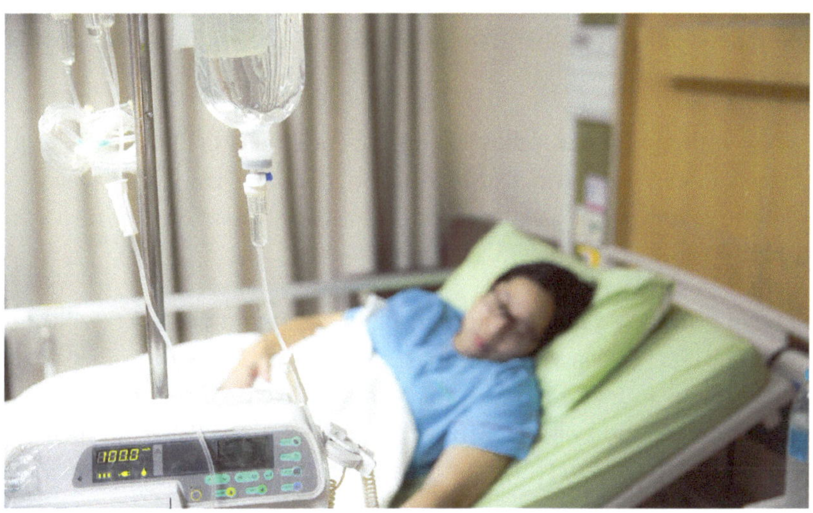

- You will receive fluids and some calories through your IV during your first 24 hours. You may not take anything by mouth in case you have to go back to the operating room quickly (usually to correct a blood flow problem).
- You will likely be moved to a less intensively monitored hospital room on or about the second or third postoperative day.

- Your penis will be elevated in a specialized dressing, and you will continue to be monitored closely.
- You will likely be up and walking and taking all your food, fluids, and pain medications by mouth on about the fifth day. You may be ready to be discharged.
- You will be given detailed instructions on how to take care of your skin graft site.
- You may expect to do physical therapy to keep your wrist, hands, and fingers supple if the donor site was your forearm. You may require a hand therapist, who is a physical therapist who specializes in hand rehabilitation.
- You may receive a specialized burn bandage to help your forearm heal.
- You will be taught how to take care of your penis and how to change your dressings.
- You will be taught by your surgical team how to elevate the penis and how to move your hips, legs, and the rest of your body to ensure adequate blood flow to your penis.
- You and your home caregiver must know how to care for any surgical drains you have. This will not be difficult, but it can feel that way at first.

You will be ready to leave the hospital on or around the fifth day postphalloplasty, provided that you are eating, taking oral fluids and pain medications, and that you do not have obvious problems that need to be addressed.

Problems at this stage include infection, bleeding, inadequate blood supply to the penis or graft sites, the inability to walk without assistance, or the inability to eat and take pain medications by mouth.

Before you leave the hospital, review with your surgical team the care of your penis, your donor graft site, your urinary catheter, your drains, and your surgical dressings. Make certain that your care partner has also received all their instructions. Also make certain that you have the surgical team's contact information available so that the team can "talk you down from the tower"—that is, help you problem-solve a difficult or puzzling situation if needed.

You will be required to stay within a 3-hour radius of your hospital for a couple weeks to a month after the surgery. If you live nearby, you can go home. But if you don't live nearby, you may stay with family in the area. Or you will have made reservations at a hotel or a recovery house well before your surgery. (See the information on Quest House on pages 293–296.)

After phalloplasty, you will be **expected and required** to have a care partner who will help you when you are discharged from the hospital. This can be a life partner, friend, family member, or someone you hire specifically for this purpose. This individual need not be a medical professional, but they must be precise in following directions, as they will be helping you with your dressings, your medications, and your general care. They must see *you* as their priority. (They cannot see you as their ticket for a vacation.)

If you are interested in hiring someone for this purpose, ask your surgical team for recommendations or search online. *Get references.*

Review your postoperative care supplies and make sure that you have everything that was recommended. You can still order things online if needed. A comprehensive list from Meiko Xavier is found at this website: **myphalloplasty.wordpress.com/2016/09/28/medical-supplies-packing-list.**

With the bulk of your surgery completed, don't let down your guard about your good self-care.

Follow postoperative pointers that are both general and specific to your surgery. Review the importance of getting sleep, consuming good nutrition, and keeping your mind sane. **Whatever you do, do not start smoking. The health of your blood vessels is critical to your healing.**

What Is a Wound VAC?

You've already read that having a wound VAC (vacuum-assisted closure) would elevate you to a more sophisticated level of wound care (see page 241). A wound VAC is an ingenious device that allows you to place a spongy material over the wound and cover this with a special plastic wrap and a dressing that attaches to a portable suction. This facilitates the continual removal of debris and drainage and greatly decreases the amount of time required for healing.

Urinary Leakage after Phalloplasty

> The best product I've found for leaking at the tip of the penis is the Male Urine Guard by Jackson Medical. They say it holds up to 2 ounces of urine—so it works great for "dribbling."
>
> — *Trans man, age 62*

After a Delayed Pedicle Flap Phalloplasty

The pedicle flap phalloplasty is done in several stages, and each part of the procedure requires its own specific recovery time. Your surgeon may have different requirements for each step.

Remember that the blood flow to the developing phallus requires the utmost protection. Check the temperature of the skin of the phallus. If it feels cool (as in cold) or appears dusky or pale, this may mean that the blood supply has been compromised. Contact your surgeon. They will have instructions for you and may require you to be evaluated in person.

Report any signs of infection (pus, inflammation, tenderness, fever, or general worsening) to your surgical team.

I had had a metoidioplasty and urethral extension before. I've just had a pedicle flap phalloplasty. I'm so glad I did this. Now I look down and see my penis. There's nothing to put on and I don't have to worry about anything falling off. As far as urinating goes, I pee through the metoidioplasty below the penis. My wife says that the meta is the "workhorse." But now I have a "show horse" too.

— *Trans man in his 60s*

Phallus Tattoos: A Game Changer

Tattoo art can provide a postphalloplasty appearance that better approximates the neighboring skin tone. Subtle color variegations bring the appearance of texture, and nearly hidden blue veins bring greater detail than ever possible. Shane Wallin of Garnet Tattoo in San Diego is one of a number of artists who does decorative tattooing, 3D nipple areolar pigmentation, and phallus tattoo art.

These photos show pre- and posttattoo results in an individual who had free flap phalloplasty by Jens Berli, MD, of Oregon Health and Science University Hospital in Portland, Oregon.

For more information on Wallin's services, search garnettattoo.com, or ftmtattoo.com/phalloplasty. Check with your surgeon as to when it is safe to tattoo after phalloplasty.

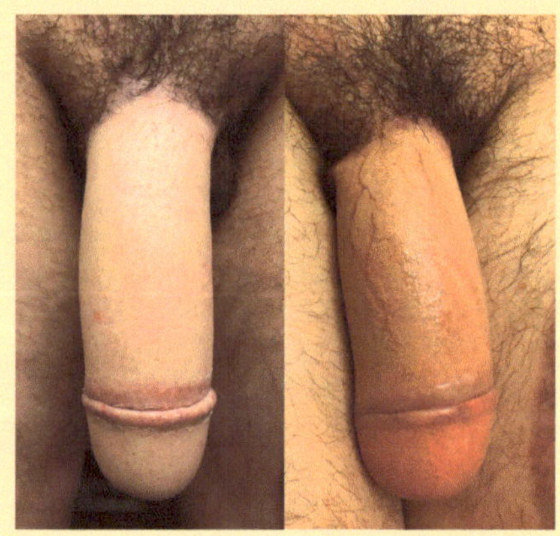

Figure 12.5. A phallus tattoo.

Quest House: A Post-Op Home for Transmasculine and Nonbinary Individuals Recovering from Phalloplasty and Other Gender-Affirming Surgeries near San Francisco

Meiko Xavier is the manager of Quest House in Pacifica, California. He writes an informative blog at myphalloplasty.wordpress.com, and he answered my questions about Quest House here on these next few pages. This email interview was conducted in October 2019. Learn more about Quest House at questhouseservices.wordpress.com.

After this interview was completed, Quest House closed in May 2020 as a result of lease and COVID-19 complications. Meiko and I decided to leave this information in the book, partly because it beautifully describes the functions of a postsurgery recovery house and partly because it emphasizes the importance of such services.

Then, as I was making my final review in July 2021, I learned that Quest House had reopened on a limited scale with expansion plans for the future. Check their website for information on their current situation: questhouseservices.wordpress.com. Hopefully, Quest House will have expanded capacity in the future and they will need our donations.

— Linda Gromko, MD

Linda: I understand you just moved your location.

Meiko: Yes! We have been in our new location in Pacifica since May 1, 2019. We moved from a two-bedroom apartment in Sausalito to a five-bedroom, three-and-a-half-bathroom home.

Linda: Who stays at Quest House?

Meiko: About 70 percent of our guests are having Stage 1 phalloplasty, which is the construction of the phallus. (This varies from surgeon to surgeon.) For most, a Stage 1 phalloplasty is the biggest and most intense of the surgeries. Our guests usually stay for about 1 month and have a caregiver for at least 2 weeks. The other 30 percent are returning for future surgery stages or repairs or are having metoidioplasty. But all our guests are having gender-affirming lower surgeries.

Linda: What are your room rates?

Meiko: Our sliding scale is $75 to $125 per night. It is a self-selected sliding scale and we do not require any proof of income. We ask that people pay what they feel they are able to. We're hoping to be able to reduce the lower end of our sliding scale in the future. In the meantime, we're aiming to create an official scholarship fund sometime this year that we'd like to continue to grow.

Linda: How do you book rooms, and how many people can stay at one time?

Meiko: We book online, first-come, first-serve. We have four guest rooms, each with two beds, plus another room for our house host, who is always managing, supporting, and living in the space. We also have a sofa sleeper and a cot. We try not to overload the house since that makes navigating the bathrooms more challenging. We have three full bathrooms and one half-bath. The half-bath will be getting a shower added to it soon.

Linda: Do most guests have caregivers with them?

Meiko: People who are here for the microsurgery portion of phalloplasty need to plan to have someone care for them for a minimum of their first 2 weeks out of the hospital. This is a firm policy that our house has developed after trying a variety of ways of working with and supporting our guests.

In order to keep the house safe, each person having that big surgery just has to have someone there whose main priority is to help with their needs one-on-one. While not everyone needs around-the-clock support for the 2 full weeks (some need more and some need less), the average person ends up being very grateful that they had a dedicated support person during this time.

Each one of our bedrooms has two beds, and the caregiver stays in the same room. It's not unusual to have mothers come and support their sons. In fact, two of our four surgical guests staying with us right now are here with their mothers!

If a guest is not able to identify someone to help them during their recovery, we refer folks to a project with are in collaboration with called T4T (**t4tcaregiving.org**).

Linda: Are the T4T caregivers or other hired caregivers medical or nursing folks?

Meiko: T4T has caregivers who have been working as caregivers for many, many years—some for well over a decade. While they have some medical training, they are not nurses or CNAs (certified nurse assistants). There's a lot of transparency about this.

Linda: What trans health or medical training do they have?

Meiko: Oliver, the fellow that manages T4T, has more than 16 years of direct caregiving experience, ranging from adults and children with special needs and adults with dementia to end-of-life, HIV, and cancer care patients. He has 9 cumulative years of providing care for trans folks who are undergoing a range of gender-affirming procedures.

Linda: What is T4T's rate?

Meiko: $150 per day if someone wants an around-the-clock advocate during their hospital stay and $100 per day thereafter.

Linda: Is a staff person at Quest House all the time?

Meiko: Most of the time. Our host (which is usually me) spends probably 2 to 4 hours per day cleaning and turning over bedrooms for next guests, emailing with upcoming guests and helping them to prepare for their stay and surgery, and about 3 to 4 hours per day supporting the guests in the house and helping or teaching the caregivers how to support their people.

The host often takes guests to medical appointments and to the ER when emergencies arise. We also spend a fair amount of time providing emotional support; this is actually the largest task of the house host. (A guest's personal and medical needs are generally taken care of by their caregiver.)

Linda: Are caregivers able to administer antibiotics or provide more advanced home care?

Meiko: As someone who has worked in the mental health field in residential settings, I know that there is a subtle but important distinction between "administering a medication" and "assisting someone with their medications." We are definitely not "administering" medications at Quest House. We are simply providing the support that any family member, friend, or partner of a person having surgery would be doing for their loved one. We do suggest that people document their medications by using a medication log and writing down the times they last took a medication to reduce the likelihood of forgetting a med or taking one too frequently.

Linda: What medical supplies do people need to bring?

Meiko: There is a list on our website under the "Your Stay" tab. One of the benefits of our community space is that we have a lot of unopened supplies that end up being donated by previous guests. There is also a supplies list I created for my blog, *My Phalloplasty*, at **myphalloplasty.wordpress.com/2016/09/28/medical-supplies-packing-list.**

Linda: What kind of food is available?

Meiko: People prefer to purchase their own food for the most part. But sometimes folks will use Instacart to order groceries if they don't have a rental car. Uber Eats is a popular choice as well. There is also a fair amount of free food that gets donated when people check out.

Linda: How do you screen your guests?

Meiko: We screen 100 percent of our guests over the phone to make sure that we are a good fit for their needs and that we can meet their expectations. Quest House is a very intentional space. We are creating, protecting, and fostering a sacred healing environment. We hope to be accessible to a wide spectrum of folks who are arriving at this surgical process having gone through a variety of different life experiences or access to resources. We ultimately make decisions by relying on a deep sense of intuition and past experience with what has and hasn't worked for the house.

Linda: Are you supported at all by the surgeons whose patients you see?

Meiko: We have received donations from three different surgical teams as we were fundraising and getting ready to move. We'd love to secure sustaining donations for the future of this project from the surgical teams whose patients we continuously serve.

Linda: And does insurance cover Quest House for your guests?

Meiko: As far as insurance goes, we are not able to bill insurance companies directly since we are a community space and not a medical facility. However, many insurance companies (sometimes easily and sometimes with a lot of pressure) will reimburse folks for travel and lodging costs associated with accessing care when the circumstances require traveling a long distance from their home. The tricky thing is that most insurance companies have this benefit listed as specifically for "transplant patients." The irony is that phalloplasty patients technically are having a transplant surgery of sorts. Maybe in time, supportive community healing spaces like Quest House will be covered by insurance.

Linda: It sounds like guests have great experiences at Quest House.

Meiko: A little more than half of our guests return for one or more stays with us and about 25 percent return two or more times. The bonds formed here are strong. I like to call Quest House "the sweetest home you never had." For many (but not all of us), that's the truth. We take care of one another here. Many of our folks report never having experienced true community until staying with us.

I greatly appreciate Meiko Xavier's information. If you are able to support Quest House, donate through their website at questhouse.services/donate.

— Linda Gromko, MD

SECTION 5
SURVIVING AND THRIVING

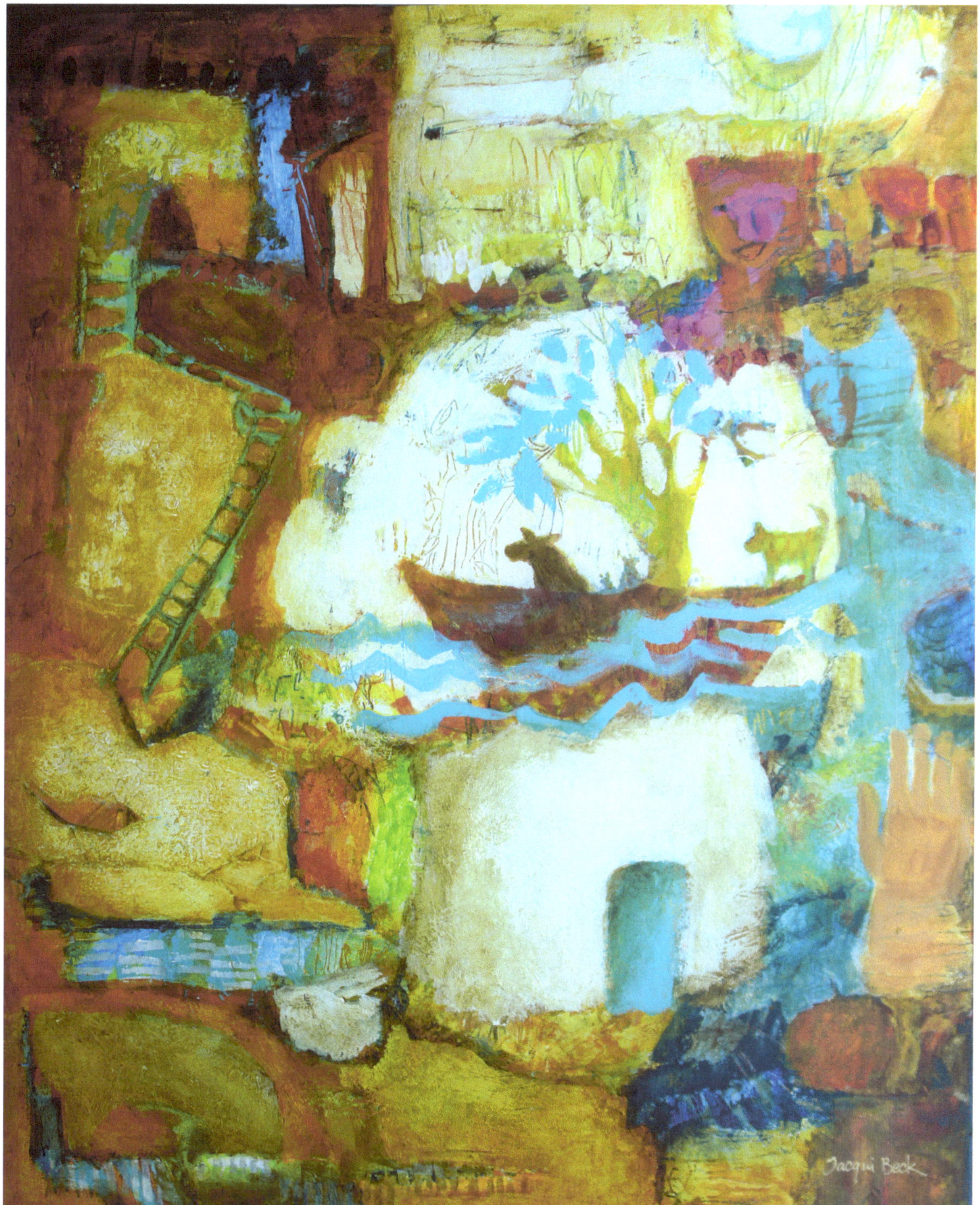

Sueño de Milagros

DAY-TO-DAY INFORMATION THAT GETS YOU THROUGH

Introduction

This section provides a "grab bag" of information. Too diverse to classify, this information is intended to supplement the information in the first portions of this book. You'll find some repetition, of course, and you'll notice that *whole categories* of information are not represented at all. If you're disturbed about any omissions, consider this my respectful invitation to write *your* book.

When I wrote *Where's MY Book?* for trans youth in 2015, I felt an urgency to get it published as soon as possible because of the high suicide rate among trans adolescents. I wanted there to be a good resource for transgender and gender-nonconforming youth. I wanted kids to be able to listen to at least one other voice, perhaps finding a lifeline to sustain them even for a short while. I still feel that urgency, of course, but many more books and services have become available since then.

In compiling this book, I've included suicide intervention resources as well as information on the treatment of depression and the practicalities of getting driver's licenses and passports. But, as I was compiling my outline, I felt it was important to include how to live longer and better, find enjoyment, contribute to your world, and build a legacy. In short, we're moving past essential basics and into areas of contentment, meaning, and joy.

As a result, we're witnessing a community that is rapidly marching up the Maslow's hierarchy—from basic survival into zones of love and enrichment. I didn't always see that in earlier days, but I certainly see it now. Not for everyone, unfortunately, but it is happening more and more.

In spite of the political and social environment that challenges me and so many of my clients, we are experiencing a quiet revolution with too much momentum to be stopped.

— Linda Gromko, MD

You are welcome to send me information that has helped you or is helping you now. If you are a healthcare provider wishing to compare notes or run a case by another doctor in the field, or if you want a speaker for an educational event, I've listed my contact information at the end of this book's preface.

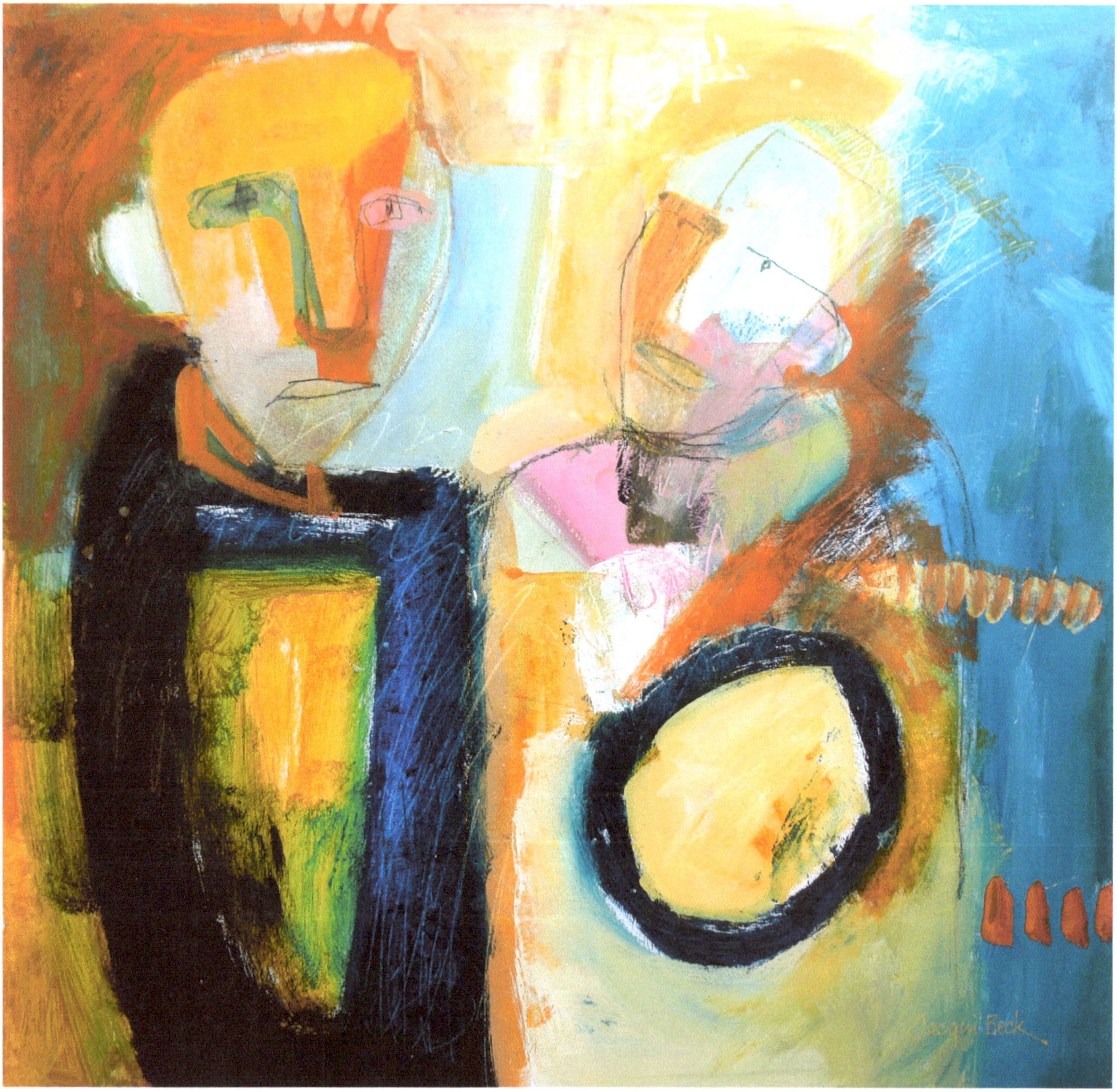

Not the Same

CHAPTER 13
Coming Out

Recognizing Your Gender Identity and Coming Out to Yourself

Whether we are 9 or 90 years old, we find opportunities to get to know ourselves better. We learn what we like and don't like. We learn to define our personal preferences, whether that means what we'll have for breakfast or where we want to live.

Of course, there are people who never bother to get to know themselves much at all. It's likely you aren't one of them. Reading this book implies that you care about yourself and the life you live.

As we grow, we also learn that there are things that are not simply preferences but are rather the fundamental truths of who we are. We learn what we stand for and what we fight for, and we identify the essential things that feed our souls. We learn that we are different from every other being on the planet, and we come to value our strengths and differences.

At some point, we become aware of our gender identity. And like any realization we make about ourselves, we do one of the following:

- We embrace it ("That's me").
- We question it ("I'm not sure; I need more information").
- We reject it ("That is absolutely *not* me!") and we try to put the issue aside—sometimes for the rest of our lives.

Coming out of our own closet (that is, acknowledging our own personal truths) can be complicated. We witness people getting labeled and ridiculed in a world where others' judgments splash over the Internet in a millisecond. We see consequences as real as losing a job, becoming homeless, or being abandoned by our parents and children.

But, *denying* your personal truth comes with a price, too. You get distracted by your own cognitive dissonance, that war inside your head that won't stop. Deny your truth, and you may find yourself connecting with the wrong crowd and with people who don't know how to value, teach, or enhance you. You may be less likely to find the love you want. The struggle with gender spills into other important areas of your life like your education, your career, or your passions. This would seem almost inevitable when you work so hard at denying or hiding who you are.

I've witnessed this struggle many times. It's not uncommon for trans people to say, "I'll just stop" (dressing, getting electrolysis, transitioning, and so on). I've seen trans people throw away one entire wardrobe after another. (People call this "purging.") I've seen people go through multiple marriages while all the while holding onto a deep secret about their gender. (Of course, the children who have come from those marriages can be priceless gifts.)

I've also witnessed that once gender is dealt with, many other things can fall into place. Gender mismatch takes up so much mental and emotional effort that there's little energy left for anything else. But once gender is clarified, other aspects of life become clearer as well. (I also know that this doesn't always happen, and it can be devastating when things don't work out.)

You wouldn't worry so much about what others think of you if you realized how seldom they do.

— Eleanor Roosevelt

I have assisted many individuals with gender transitions at 50, 60, or even 80 years of age. I wonder how much happiness is lost by putting off one's gender transition until later life. And what is the true price of not living as one's true self?

As you come to realize that you aren't like everyone else, you may start to realize that being unique can be wonderful. We aren't *supposed* to be copies of one another! And we find that there are many other amazing individuals who are "different" also.

Be yourself. Everyone else is already taken.

— Oscar Wilde

Recognizing your sexual orientation also takes mental and emotional energy. If you're exploring sexual orientation, read *It Gets Better*, edited by Dan Savage and Terry Miller (itgetsbetter.org); it is a compilation of stories of many famous people who've been down this road—a reassuring and comforting read.

Finding a Support Group

If you are involved in a gender transition for yourself, a friend, or a family member, you may benefit enormously by participating in a support group. Maybe you don't see yourself as a "group" person. Groups may not be for you, but at least take a look at what is available in your area. Search "transgender support groups" or "support for friends and families of transgender adults" in your area.

The Ingersoll Gender Center (ingersollgendercenter.org), which was founded in Seattle by Marsha Botzer, has featured peer-facilitated support groups since its beginning in 1977. Their weekly support group runs regardless of weather, holidays included. When I first attended this group in 1998, they'd have gatherings of maybe a dozen people. Now, their average regular attendance runs over 90 participants each week. On certain meetings of each month, there are breakout groups for special interests like SOFFA ("Significant Others, Friends, Families, and Allies").

There is no fee for participants, and you can come one time or every week without obligation.

Also in the Seattle area, check out Gender Diversity (genderdiversity.org) for support of families and kids of all ages, and PFLAG (pflag.org), originally known as "Parents and Friends of Lesbians and Gays." PFLAG is now the largest of the organizations promoting inclusion of gender diversity in all its forms.

Here's How a Support Group May Help You

- You may learn valuable information (like ongoing research studies and new community resources) that is even more up-to-date than the Internet.
- You learn the language of the transgender community; it changes by the day.
- You meet other people who understand what you're going through more than the general population possibly could.
- You can meet friends without having to hide gender issues. You can be your true self, and that can be a great relief.
- You may find people who have successfully transitioned already. These may become your role models or members to add to your "family of choice."
- You will learn about community events like conferences or TransPride.
- You get other people's feedback about healthcare providers (medical providers and surgeons).
- You learn survival skills that have worked for others.
- You may get relief from the isolation and anxiety felt by many trans people, at least at first. Just telling your story out loud in a supportive environment and hearing the stories of others affirms that you aren't alone. (And you don't have to say a word if you choose not to.)

While many religious groups have not been supportive of the LGBTQIA+ community, there are many who are committed to inclusive support. Search this United Church of Christ website for more information: ucc.org/lgbt_ona.

Defining "Stealth" and "Passing"

The concepts of living stealth, passing, not passing, being able to pass, or having passing privilege make for some animated conversations. It's fair to include these observations if only for the sake of cultural literacy. But it's also fair to say that these concepts can make people uncomfortable, particularly when the terms evoke "good" or "bad" connotations or when the "standard" is seen as only cisgender. (These, by the way, are definitions I've learned in working with the community.)

Living Stealth

In gender-binary terms, living stealth describes a transgender individual who—

- Lives fully in their identified gender in all aspects of life.
- Is recognized by the world as being of the identified gender by their appearance, speech, and social interactions.

- Experiences full binary-gender acceptance (perhaps privilege?) and is never being questioned in a restroom or receiving double takes from others in response to an ambiguous appearance or presentation.

For most purposes, the assigned gender is unknown to anyone but the stealth person's most immediate family, with the possible exception of significant others and maybe limited friends. In some circumstances of family estrangement, the assigned gender is *never* known or recognized by anyone.

The term "stealth" seems to imply that a person is hiding or deceptive. This is unfortunate in the context of gender identity—which is nobody's business—and does not by itself represent ill intent.

Another term for stealth might more accurately be "private." Trans people who live stealth may do so out of personal preference, but it is well recognized that being "out" or being "outed" may have life-and-death consequences.

The term "stealth" carries a connotation of "tricking people." Consider changing that terminology to "nondisclosing" or "undisclosed."

— Johanna Olson-Kennedy, MD, at the WPATH 26th Scientific Symposium Surgeon's Program in November 2020

What Passing Means

An assigned male is said to "pass" (as) female if they look, sound, and "act" female, and more specifically, a cis female. An assigned female "passes" (as) male if they look, sound, and "act" male—that is, a cis male. We hear language like "They pass well." It's easy to see how such language could offend.

It seems that one passes most easily by living in the middle ground of stereotypical physical features (at least without surgery) and by conscientious attention to presentation.

Passing Privilege

The concept of living stealth brings up the uneasy topics of "passing" and "passing privilege."

A trans woman I know says that she "won the genetic lottery." She's not so tall that you'd notice it; she dresses stylishly; she has removed every strand of her facial hair; and she has a peaches-and-cream complexion. She puts obvious effort into her appearance. People look at her because she's attractive and assertive, but not because she sticks out. And not because her appearance evokes questions about her birth or childhood.

Trans males who are taller and have more angular, stereotypically "rugged" features may be said to have won the genetic lotto also. Stealth comes easier for those with specific raw materials (not minimizing the considerable effects of taking hormones, having surgery to masculinize the chest, and being conscious about presentation).

The folks I'm referring to "came with" their passing privilege, in a sense. But I don't mean to imply they haven't put enormous effort into their presentation and haven't had excellent surgical outcomes.

By contrast, another friend identifies as female, but her height of six feet four makes it impossible *not* to be "read" or "clocked." Her low voice makes it hard for her to be recognized as female and she is always "sir'd" on the phone. She dresses with a high-fashion sensibility, but she will inevitably be perceived as a *trans* woman because of her height and voice.

No Cis Counterpart to Passing Privilege

We hear of cis male privilege, white privilege, trust fund privilege (when one is really rich), and youth privilege. And probably everyone is held to annoying standards of physical appearance. I suspect these privileges pile on to other standards that trans and nonbinary people experience. I don't imagine that life comes effortlessly to anyone—even those with various privileges. And I believe most people don't truly know what lies in the heart of another human.

All of this said, passing seems to imply that a person is somehow more authentic. I have talked with so many people who experience considerable pain over passing and its "privileges." It strikes me as ironic that we are judged as "authentic" on the basis of superficial qualities.

We've seen the posters that say, "Trans women are real women." Those of us who are not transgender can only imagine what it must be like to constantly defend one's legitimacy.

These will become important concepts to consider as you read on about adverse childhood experiences, post-traumatic stress disorder, microaggressions, and depression later in this book.

Coming Out to Parents

"Coming out"—the truthful acknowledgment of who you are and what you need to do next—can be intensely liberating, but it can also have its consequences. Let's assume you're operating from the following framework:

- You have made a careful and honest analysis of your situation.
- You are sincerely attempting to be kind to yourself as well as to others who may be impacted.
- Your acknowledgment does not represent a purposeful attempt to harm anyone—yourself or others. You are not trying—
  - To get revenge for anything.
  - To casually step on somebody's heart.
  - To make someone else look bad.
  - To embarrass someone.
  - Or even to inconvenience anyone.

As you weigh the perceived risks, you acknowledge that your disclosure is necessary and that—

- You desire to live your life authentically, embracing your truths rather than sustaining the cognitive dissonance you carry now.

- You may be deeply saddened by some of the consequences that play out, like grief, anger, separations, and accusations, but you cannot sacrifice your real self any longer. All the individuals impacted will have their opportunities to evaluate and restructure their own lives. Granted, this may result in considerable pain all around. But when a kind and honest person says, "**This is my fundamental truth, and it's not simply a 'preference,'**" it calls for some considerable respect. It isn't a casual matter, and you don't approach it casually.

- You are not abdicating responsibilities you have to your parents, partner, children, and family. You are still responsible for supporting your children, for example.

- You are willing to examine behavioral compromises that are based in love and compassion. (For someone to ask you to ignore your fundamental truths forever is not an appropriate request; to ask that you not "dress" for the first time at your kids' graduation could be reasonable.) It's tough and often messy.

How Will Your Parents React to Your Coming Out?

There's a wide range in family responses to a person's coming out. I have seen parents shrug and say, "We only want you to be happy." Or, "I've known that since you were a little kid. I was wondering when we'd be talking about this."

But then, I've also seen college students whose parents abruptly stopped paying for college tuition. One young adult's parents said, "You're dead to me now." Another adult was asked, "How could you do this to your mother?" We've recently read where a father assaulted and attempted to murder his adult son.[70]

Some Suggestions That Might Help You Come Out to Your Parents

- ***You* should be the one to tell your parents, if possible.**
  Tell them in person if you can do so without endangering yourself. This is a courtesy to them that will help you later on.

- **Try not to allow your parents or family to find out from another person or through a public forum like Facebook or other social media.**

What if you've *already* posted every detail on Facebook and your parents have found out in a very public way? Acknowledge to your parents that a Facebook reveal might have been awkward or even painful for them. Apologize if you feel you need to and move on.

You might say something like this: "I was so excited. I didn't take the time to appreciate the impact this might have on you. I'm sorry." (Here, you certainly aren't apologizing for being trans; you're apologizing for the fact that your parents experienced discomfort that you might have prevented. And while your parents may have caused *you* significant discomfort too, that's not the issue at the moment.)

- **Tell your parents in private if you can.**
  This is so they may have the freedom to express their reactions openly. Do not tell your parents by yourself if you believe they will physically harm you. If you do worry about your safety, bring an advocate with you—maybe an adult sibling or another adult they respect.

70 Alex Bollinger, "A Father Slit His Son's Throat for Being Gay in an Attempt to Kill Him," *LGBTQ Nation*, November 12, 2019, https://www.lgbtqnation.com/2019/11/father-slit-sons-throat-gay-attempt-kill/.

- **Consider approaching a grandparent first.**
  Sometimes grandparents respond more positively than parents do. If you think that could be the case in your family, a grandparent may be a good ally and a good buffer.

- **Meet your parents in a discreet but public place like a quiet restaurant if you are worried about a volatile reaction.**
  You'll have other humans around, which may temper your parents' reaction.

- **Try not to come out to your parents at a big event.**
  Your parent's golden anniversary, significant holidays, your mother's birthday, or your grandfather's funeral dinner may not be the best time. While you aren't trying to be insensitive, your announcement may be remembered that way. *Besides, the big event is not about you.*

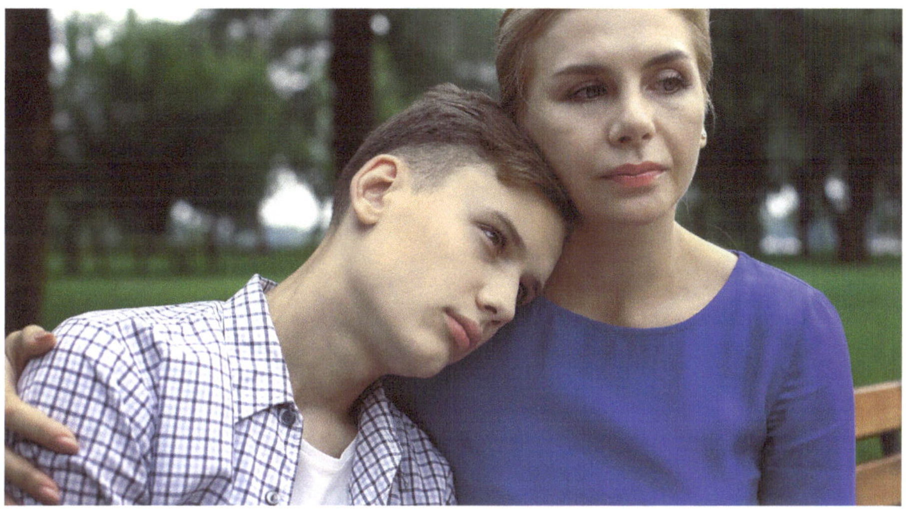

There are rare situations where it may be better if parents are *never* told. In such circumstances, a parent loses the opportunity to fully know and love their child for who they really are. This can be terribly sad, but consider what *would* be best in the following situations (knowing that there may be no right or wrong answer):

- **What would be best if a parent has advanced dementia and no longer knows who you are?**
  In that case, it may be possible to continue to visit and support your parent as a loving presence. There's no point in arguing with them and you don't want them to be alone.

- **What would be best if a healthy parent suddenly falls critically ill?**
  You worry that any shock may literally kill them, but you also know that this could be your only opportunity to come out to them. The imminent death of a parent is not about you, but if you abruptly tell them and they *do* suddenly die, it will become about you in an instant. (You may have missed an opportunity to tell your parent; so be it.)

While there's probably no perfect time to tell your parents, there may be better and worse times. Perhaps you could aim for a Saturday when everyone has a chance to process your information before the regular week begins.

You may want to write a letter to your parents and present it ahead of time or at your meeting with them. This way, there is something thoughtful and concrete for them to read and reread. Do not text this information and do not send this news by email.

Here's an example of how a coming-out letter might read:

Example Coming-Out Letter to Parents

Date ______________________

Dear Mom and Dad,

There is something I have to tell you. I have given this a lot of thought—actually for most of my life. I am transgender. I was born with male body parts, but I have always known that I was female. Maybe this doesn't come as a complete surprise to you.

I didn't talk about this when I was younger because I just didn't know how. But it's becoming more important to live my life as I really am. I am already working with a doctor and have started to take hormones. I know the changes will become more visible in the future and I wanted to be sure you didn't find out from someone else. I won't be quitting my job or anything like that. I need your support and understanding.

I want you to know that you have always been great parents to me. My being transgender isn't because of anything you did or didn't do. I am not doing this to hurt anyone—least of all, you. I love you both very much and hope I can count on your support as I make this change.

Love, ______________________

PS: I can't imagine how it might feel to read this. There is a lot of information and support for families, and I can help you find information if you need it.

When you meet with your parents, go prepared with a copy of a helpful book like this one, or *True Selves* by Chloe Ann Rounsley and Mildred L. Brown, or *Trans Bodies, Trans Selves*, edited by Laura Erickson-Schroth. Know also about support organizations like PFLAG (**pflag.org**) or a SOFFA group (Support of Friends, Families, and Allies).

PFLAG is the major family-support organization available. Ingersoll Gender Center (in Seattle) offers open meetings every week, with certain ones featuring breakout sessions for SOFFA. Search in your area for something similar.

> One of my patients described how her 80-year-old mother reacted to her child's identification as nonbinary: "Well, just as long as you're not a vegan..."
>
> — *Linda Gromko, MD*

- **Plan to meet with a friend or counselor after you've told your folks.**
  This can be a phone meeting. Whether the meeting with your parents goes well or not, it will likely bring up strong emotions for you (such as anger, relief, gratitude, surprise, and sadness). Having a chance to debrief can be helpful for you.

  If coming out to your family went well, great! If it doesn't, give it time. Many families do come around. *Your* family may come around. But if they really don't, remember that you can develop a "family of choice," a network of people who know you and love you just as you are. Hopefully, your biological family will join in down the road.

Coming Out to Your Spouse or Significant Other

Twenty years ago, when I started treating transgender patients, it seemed that most couples just split up. But in more recent years, it hasn't seemed that way at all, at least not in Seattle. I'm sure many couples still separate or divorce, but it isn't a *de facto* answer anymore and it doesn't have to be.

> My spouse transitioned at work years before she had her surgery. I'd just figured she would leave our marriage when she had her sexual reassignment surgery done. But it occurred to me that she didn't have to leave. She didn't want to leave, and our kids are both fine with it. I don't know where I really got that idea. I thought it was just something everybody did.
>
> — *Wife of trans woman who transitioned in her 40s*

Factors to Consider

So many factors enter into whether a couple continues being together after the trans partner comes out. We'll talk more about relationships in Chapter 22. For now, let's get back to coming out. Review the suggestions on telling your parents on pages 305–309. In that part, we recognized that respect and kindness are proper cornerstones of the process. Here, in telling your partner, you recognize that—

- You aren't trying to hurt your significant other, but you realize that your coming out may feel hurtful to them.
- You're aware that coming out will have a life-changing impact on you and your partner, perhaps in both positive and negative ways.

- You appreciate that revealing your gender truth after a long period of hiding can be enormously freeing for you. But you also understand that if your spouse truly hasn't known, it may be very difficult for *them*. Your relief—even elation—may seem insensitive, so give them some time to process the "new" information that you've known for years.
- You both may actually grieve. You may grieve for the relationship you had even though it was based on incomplete information. You may grieve for the things you'll never get to do as a pretransition couple.
    - Review psychiatrist Elisabeth Kübler-Ross's five stages of grief so you can recognize them in your partner and in yourself: (1) denial, (2) anger, (3) bargaining, (4) depression, and (5) acceptance. You may notice that you are traveling through these stages in some order; visit grief.com/the-five-stages-of-grief for more information. (See also "Living with Grief" in Chapter 23.)

Having said all this, remember that *not* coming out may have a devastating impact on you and your relationship as well.

You may have gathered some assumptions and fantasies about what will happen when you have this important coming-out talk. Here are examples of these powerful *assumptions*. For instance, you might assume that—

- Your partner will be horrified, stating indignantly, "You have lied to me for all these years. Our entire marriage is a lie."
- Your partner will take the kids and leave for their grandmother's cabin that very night.
- Your partner will dissolve into tears, sobbing "What did I ever do to deserve this?" or "What did I ever do to *cause* this?"
- Your partner will insist that you leave the house right away and will furthermore press for a divorce where you will have nothing left to your name except for owing child support payments.

But maybe, it goes more like this...

- Your partner shocks you by announcing, "What a coincidence! I can't believe this is happening. I have been doing some reading about transitioning myself."
- Your partner says, "It's not what I was prepared to hear, but our relationship is strong enough to survive anything. Where do we start, and how can I support you?"
- Your partner says, "I just had a feeling that something was going on. We probably both need to talk to a therapist, together and separately."
- "Transitioning?" your partner sighs with relief. "I thought you had cancer or something! Thank goodness you're okay."

If these examples seem unrealistic, know that they are all based on situations I have witnessed.

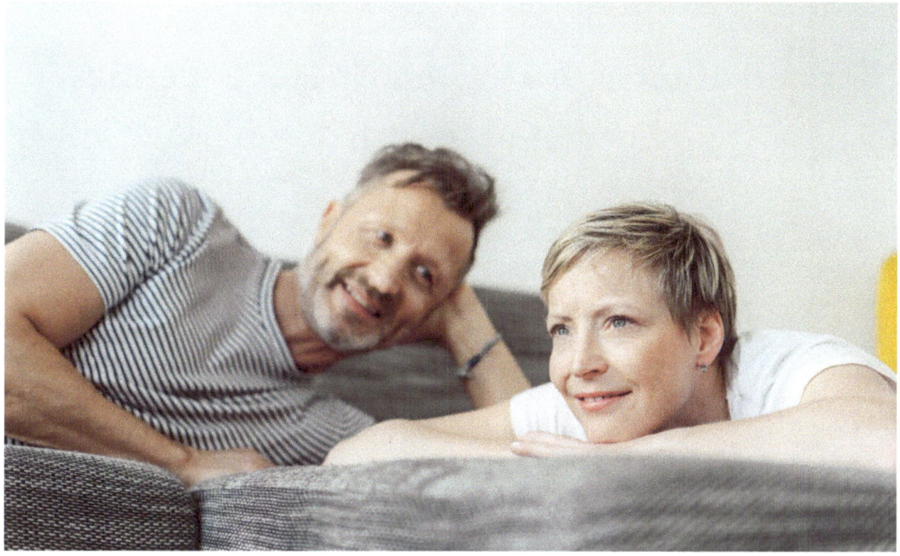

I had to pick up a prescription from my wife's doctor. He had never seen me as Frances so he didn't know who I was. He didn't recognize me. I told him who I was and that I am transgender. There was a funny puzzled look on his face. He called my wife at home to talk to her about her prescription and how to take her medicine. Then he proceeded to ask her questions about me.

My wife was kind enough to tell the doctor that, no, Frances doesn't bother her, that I'm the same person she married, and that I'm a happier person. It really warmed my heart because my wife stood up for me. I truly am in a good place.

— Trans woman in her late 50s

Conversation with a Woman in Her Seventies, Living Stealth

Linda: When did you realize you were female?

I never really thought about it that way, actually. Ask any girl or woman, "When did you first realize that you were a girl and a female?" I'll bet they say they've never thought about it. Neither did I! I just finally knew! I've been asked that question only a few times in my life… way back 40-plus years ago when I was going through my transition as a young adult. When I was very young and self-aware, I just recall always considering myself somehow different… neither a girl nor a boy. It wasn't until I was several years old that I began to feel that I was "different." I felt awkward and confused about how I was expected to fit into the world around me with this alien body!

Linda: Being confused like that, how did you go about expressing yourself to the world?

Early on, I realized that adults and other kids would not handle my thoughts well if I were to tell them about myself. This was the start of what was to be a long time that I felt guilty and ashamed of my body and my thoughts. This type of thinking (about how others around me viewed me and might treat me) started when I was a young preteen. Back then, there wasn't any way for me to learn if there were others who felt like I did. I felt alone and different. So, I did NOT express myself to anyone. I thought that this was the way that I had to be forever. This was the beginning of my life of secrecy.

Linda: How did that work out for you?

I never told anyone about how I felt all through the years of grade school, high school, and into college. I expressed myself to myself in many ways… but always in secret. I was pretty sure that letting anyone know about my feelings would cause chaos in my life and in my family. From the time of my teens, I became more and more sure that I was more female than male. I didn't know what to do with that thought. There was no way for me to change my body and I could never escape my thoughts.

Linda: Did you ever think about ending your life?

Sometimes, when I was in my late teens and as a young adult, but never really seriously. I actually loved my life. I thought of my life as a wonderful gift and I wanted very much to survive these feelings. I always hoped that someday I could change my body somehow and learn more about others who may have the same thoughts that I was having.

Linda: Did you have any social life during the time up to when you were in college?

I felt out of place and awkward. I did not like being among groups of people (and I still don't). Girls were attracted to me, and that was both good and bad; I liked being among girls and had several girlfriends, but I didn't like having them get too close. I was an odd one with the boys. I experienced some bullying at times. I tried my best to fit in as expected in the ways I acted and in the things I did. I didn't want to stand out.

Linda: But you got married. What was that all about?

By the time I was in college, I firmly thought that there was no way out for me. My life would continue on as it had always been. I would try to be the best person I could be. I met a girl in college who liked me, and I liked her. We became very close and I began to think that I could actually play this part alright. I remember standing at the altar in the church, exchanging vows of marriage and thinking to myself, "Are you REALLY sure that you want to do this?" I did it!

Linda: So, what changed?

Time passed. We had a child, a son. But even during those 8 years of marriage, I still had that secret going on in my head. I was with a woman. I loved her as my wife. But at the same time, I envied her for being a woman. I wanted to have a baby myself. I wanted to express myself as a woman. All those thoughts were still with me. It became apparent to me that my wife wanted to have more children and then I would be in a much more complicated and male role, and I was very troubled by that possibility. And I didn't want to go further into our life together and then tell her. I didn't want to spoil her life in that way.

It was at that time in 1973 that I learned about someone else who had been like me and who changed to being a woman. Her name was Jan Morris and she had written a book called *Conundrum*. I wrote to her and asked her for advice and thoughts on my situation. Within the following few months, my mind filled with thoughts of becoming who I really was. Once I learned that there was a path out, I could not deny it. My ex-wife went on to get married, have two more children, and is having a wonderful life. I am still in contact with her from time to time and also with my son.

Linda: Can you fast-forward to today and summarize how your life changed and evolved?

I told my wife about my feelings. We had a peaceful divorce. By that time, we had moved to another state and both had jobs. I underwent my gender confirmation surgery and transitioned on the job in 1974. I met the man who was destined to be my future husband. My doctor advised me that it would be best to just move to another town, state, whatever, and begin my new life. I was proposed to by my, as I call him, "one-in-a-million-man." We moved out West. We got married. Back then, the process was simple: We went to the city hall, got a marriage license, and got married. No big deal. We have been happily married for 42 years and have had a successful life together.

Linda: Okay, but how did you manage to have a "normal" life in this new location?

As I had always done during my life to that point, I maintained my secrecy about my medical and life history. I always considered my issues to be my own medical and private information. I never considered "coming out" to the world since I didn't consider anything that I had gone through to be anyone else's business but mine. By that time, I had gone through all the legal paperwork needed to assume my new identity. And I felt it was also appropriately fair to my husband. I didn't want to put him under some kind of scrutiny because of his marriage to me.

I was fortunate to be employed by a company with strict rules about how the staff treated one another. I wasn't planning on putting any focus on myself to the world. I was not an activist of some sort. I didn't want to be in the public eye. It's not that I was being selfish about my way of life compared with others with my type of history, but I just wanted to be another woman in the world. I didn't want to be defined by any label related to my medical past; I wanted to be free to be myself and to be a good wife.

Linda: Any additional thoughts?

Yes, I do have some thoughts about coming out. There are pros and cons to being silent about this part of my life. The good part is that I am just another woman moving through the world. Most of the people in my life know nothing about my previous life. This approach has meant that my life is peaceful with regard to my interactions with everyone around me. I will not let myself be defined by my medical history!

But, I have learned by my own experiences and watching those of others in my community that no one—NO ONE—can take in this information about someone without it changing how they see you, think about you, and share life with you! I don't care WHAT someone says; when you tell someone about a past such as mine, they are now different toward you. That difference can be either good or bad. The good reaction is a more gentle and caring acceptance of you and a chance for them to learn more about themselves and about you. The bad reaction is one where a friend of decades can shun you entirely (mostly because of religious beliefs and guidance) and lock you out of their lives. In this new place that we live, I have shared my history with only a few select people—for example, my doctor, my lawyer, and just two of my lady friends. I am happy in my role of ordinary citizen, friend, and wife.

Whenever I have an urge about revealing my past to someone, I evaluate that feeling VERY carefully from the perspective of me protecting them. I don't have the right to turn a friendship upside down just because I want to get something off MY mind. I have come to realize that by not outing myself to the world, I am actually protecting people from themselves. There is nothing to gain from this openness in an already wonderful friendship. Do I really want to test a friendship or relationship by bringing this up? If it goes bad (and I have had this happen), both I and my friend could have a much more complicated relationship, or NO relationship going forward. I like just being myself and being seen as just another woman in society.

I am very proud of my life. Not a single day goes by without my realizing how wonderful my life is with me presenting to the world as my true self. I am happy when I look in the mirror. I have no secret shame or guilty thoughts. I can express myself so much better to the world. I accomplished many wonderful things before my transition, and I have accomplished even more afterward. I have had a positive impact on many lives. More than a dozen people close to me would not even be alive if I hadn't been born!

Being Outed by Others: Controlling the Narrative

It's one thing to orchestrate your own coming out, but it's quite another to be outed by somebody else. That takes away the control you should legitimately have about your own self-disclosures. But suppose it happens.

It's a good idea to have some prepared responses at the ready to take back your control. Think of the questions or comments that could derail you, prepare your responses ahead of time, and be able to nail those responses in the moment.

For example, suppose someone says, "I heard you're switching sides, man. You know, turning into a girl."

Who wouldn't want to run? But you might say instead, "Oh, I'm glad you heard. What a relief it is to be finally living an authentic life! How are your kids doing?"

Of course, there's so much that is offensive about the other person's comments: They trivialize what you're going through. You're not "turning into" a girl; if you were "turning into" anything, it would be a woman. By not getting flummoxed by the other person's comments, you take back your own control. And "How are your kids doing?" moves the conversation right along.

Suppose the other person keeps at it: "Have you had the operation?"

That's just nobody's business, and you have every right to react in anger or defensiveness. But you could say something like, "Wow, I had no idea you would be so interested. I'll take that as a compliment. But I do have to be going now. Let's have coffee later."

There's a big difference between people asking honest questions because they care about you and people asking invasive questions because they are simply ignorant and rude. You will probably be able to tell the difference by the feeling in your gut. You don't owe anyone an explanation or justification. You don't owe anyone the most basic of information!

A reasonable response to a question that is really out of bounds is, "Thank you for caring about me. I appreciate your concern." If someone says, "I'll pray for you," just say, "Thank you." Or better yet, "Thank you. I'll pray for you as well."

Watch your tone, of course. Avoid sounding sarcastic or snarky; that would defeat your purpose of an even-handed response.

If you are being called names, ignore the offender and move quickly out of their range. If you are being physically threatened, do what you need to do to keep yourself safe; most importantly, get away. (See more about personal safety in Chapter 16.)

Couples and Families Do Stay Together after Gender Transition

Many factors determine how well your relationship will continue after one person's coming-out. For example, **the age of a couple is one factor**. While much more research must be done on what happens to marriages and families after a spouse declares that he or she is transgender, a 2016 survey of 6,450 trans men and women by the Center for Transgender Equality indicates that more than half of younger couples stay together after a gender transition, but only about a third of those over age 50 do so.[71]

Perhaps this trend reflects greater acceptance of gender fluidity among younger people for themselves, their partners, and in relationships.

> **My husband and I divorced after he joined what I saw as a religious cult. It was as though he announced that all of the rules of our lives were going to be different—and all on his terms. I was terribly hurt and angry. I blamed my husband, and I made no effort to hide this from our 10-year-old son.**
>
> **"Twenty years later, my then-adult son told me how much my comments about his dad had hurt him. I wish I could have been more adult in the way I acted. Looking back, it would have been much kinder to talk to a counselor about my anger—and to have supported my son who was hurting in his own way. I feel regret over this to this day.**
>
> *— Cis woman in her 60s*

Another factor is how sexual the partnership is and how flexible each partner is in their own sexual expression. I would imagine that a couple who is locked into very specific sexual roles and definitions would be less likely to weather a gender transition. Here are comments from folks in my practice:

- "I've never been attracted to men," said a partner in a lesbian couple where the significant other was a transitioning male.
- "I wanted to stay with my husband," said a woman in a 20-year marriage. "But I'm not a lesbian. We are still together, but we live more like sisters now."
- "I'm okay with their transitioning," said a straight woman in her sixties, "and I'm okay being seen by others as a gay couple. I just miss feeling his whiskers in the morning. It's strange the things you miss."
- "We'd been in our feminist, same-sex marriage for over 10 years before my spouse transitioned. At first, it was very different being with a man. We've lost some of our friends over this. But we're doing fine now. I don't think it would have worked out with just anybody. It's worked out because of who *we* are."

71 Gloria Hochman, "When One Spouse Changes Gender, Can the Marriage Be Saved?," *The Philadelphia Inquirer*, December 29, 2016, https://www.inquirer.com/philly/health/When-one-spouse-changes-gender-can-the-marriage-be-saved.html.

If you are the partner of someone who is transitioning, could you be flexible in your own sexual orientation? Some people can, and some simply cannot. Some people view a sexual relationship with a partner as just *one part* of a multifaceted relationship; others see sex as a relationship cornerstone.

If you cannot see yourselves as a same-sex couple, could you go on as sisters, brothers, or best friends in a nonsexual relationship?

Personal Intimacy without Sexual Intimacy

Intimacy, particularly in couples with a rich shared history, may take the form of hand-holding, shoulder-rubbing, cuddling, and even the precious luxury of sharing the most mundane experiences of life. Can trips to Costco be intimate? I think so. From my personal experience, I found that caring for a spouse through a terminal illness can represent *the most intimate*, the most loving actions of the life you share.

Some Couples Transition to a Relationship of Siblings or Best Friends

If you cannot see yourselves as a same-sex couple, could you go on as sisters or brothers or best friends in a nonsexual relationship?

Many people compartmentalize various aspects of a relationship: intellectual pursuits, athletic interests, travel, and so on. It is possible to compartmentalize sexual activity too, although this might not be appropriate for you and your partner.

Exploring this further, have you developed a romantic relationship with yourself? (That is, with gifts of supportive self-care, self-respect, and sexual self-stimulation?) We'll talk more about this in Chapters 22 and 23. Could you develop "friends with benefits" if sexual "benefits" are no longer available in your primary relationship? Might polyamory or separate-but-open relationships be possibilities? Might you relate to someone online and in fantasy? Again, these aren't intended as suggestions for everyone. They may apply to some individuals but be completely devastating and inappropriate for others. It's not a matter of right and wrong; it's a matter of what could work for both of you.

Managing Financially, Apart

If each partner in a couple has financial solvency and can make it financially on their own, people may appreciate more free agency—thus, staying together by choice rather than financial dependency. Many couples are devastated by the enormous costs of divorce and attorney fees, let alone maintaining two separate homes and adding more childcare expenses.

I know of one traditional male-female couple where the wife is in poor health and has no marketable career skills to support herself. She may *not* feel the option to go on alone because she has been so financially dependent on her spouse. Another client, a high-earning professional, anticipates enormous child and spousal support payments to the point where he foresees a life of near-poverty for himself. Both of these folks feel trapped with no great options available. They may benefit from some counseling and from finding other couples who are in similar situations. Both may benefit from a generous division of funds and property if they go their separate ways.

No matter how open or negotiable a relationship is, every couple has more monetary resources together than when they are apart. The ability to enter the workforce or to start over may be more limited than one would think; we even see software engineers finding themselves less marketable in the workplace in their forties and fifties.

And, any major changes in a relationship—gender transitions, an illness of one or both individuals, an illness or death of a child, a natural disaster—will call on each partner to take an honest look at their resources and to explore their own options with clarity and flexibility.

> There's an old saying:
> "Happiness is not having what you want—it's wanting what you have."

Talking to Your Kids: It's a Transition for Them Also

In my experience, small children (maybe through elementary school) seem to weather their parents' transitions more easily than adolescents. Little ones need a few important facts ("Where will we live?" "Who will take me to school?"—in other words, "How will this transition affect *me*?"). Then again, they may shrug off the new information with something as minimal as "Oh, okay."

Adolescents want basic logistical information also. But, as kids move through middle school, it seems that they can find and push *our* buttons with alarming accuracy. If they perceive a flaw or inconsistency coming from us or if they sense that *we* feel guilty in any way, then they may use this as a bargaining tool in future negotiations. So, stand your ground. You as parents have nothing to be defensive about. You will conduct yourselves with courtesy and respect, and it is your expectation that your children will also. If you see your own gender identity as a flaw, they surely will too.

With children of any age, here are some basics to consider:

- **Share the logistical specifics with your kids.**
  Your kids need to know the logistics that impact them, such as where they'll live, what will be new, and what will stay the same. And it's always best if they learn this new information from their parents.

- **Communicate with teachers, school administrators, and counselors on your kids' behalf.**
  You may be able to help your children by talking with their teachers or writing to them. Resource information (even brief pamphlets from PFLAG or Gender Diversity) can impart the basics and give references for helpful websites. Again, controlling the narrative can be a courtesy to your children, and knowing how your kids can share appropriate information with others will be helpful.

  Here's an example:

  Another kid says to your kid, "Who's that?" while pointing at you *en femme* (dressed female). Your kid answers, "Oh, that's my dad. My dad's going through a gender change. He's using the name Anna now, and it would be fine for you to call him that." (Pronouns will shift over time.)

- **Explore together: What should I call you now?**
  Explore with your child what name they'll be using for you and how they'll refer to you. Some parents prefer that their kids use the parent's first name. Many still use "Mom" or "Dad" as before. I've met a few "Maddies" over the years. It's likely that your kids will still call you what they've always called you. It might be confusing to some people, but take it in stride as well as you can.

- **Aim to be matter-of-fact.**
  The more matter-of-fact you are, the more straightforward your kids may be. Develop no-fault language to share with your kids. You may find them using it, too. Here's an example:

  You talking to your kid: "When I was a little kid much younger than you are, I knew that I was a girl. I'm making some changes. The most important thing to me, though, is that I got to have a kid as great as you. No matter what, I will always be your parent."

- **Use opportunities, especially when riding in the car together, to chat about certain details.**
  Even if a child pretends not to hear you, know that they will hear you. These can be important, reassuring times, even if that reassurance isn't obvious at the time.

- **Normalize the process of going to counseling.**
  Tell your child, "Whenever healthy families go through changes, we go to a counselor. Counselors make sure that we are all doing as well as possible. I see my counselor every week."

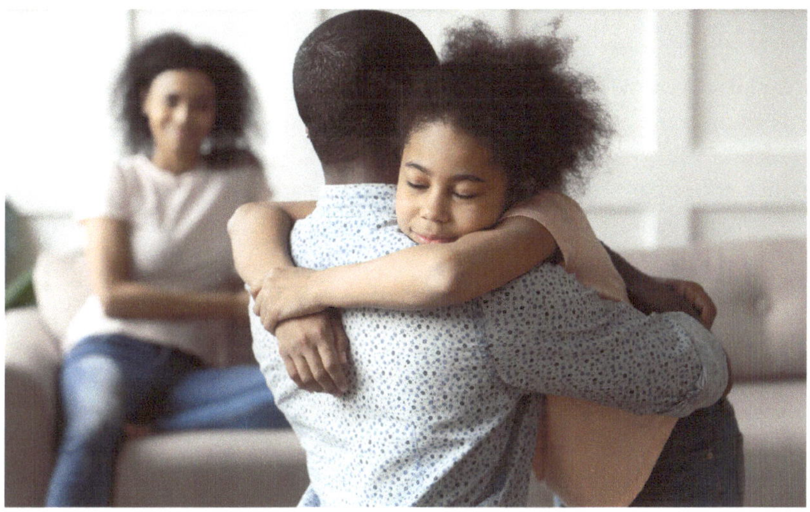

- **Anticipate questions your kids may have.**
  You may want to talk with other trans parents or your counselor about how best to anticipate and answer your kids' questions. What questions might they ask?

  - "Does that mean that I'll be transgender too?"
  - "Couldn't you just go back to the way it was?"
  - "Is Mom (or Dad) transgender?"
  - "Does Grandma know?"
  - "Will you still...?" (play baseball, make cookies, and so on)

For whatever reason, kids in the mid-to-late-elementary-school range seem to think that they are responsible for a lot of what happens in their families. This comes out with the tacit question, "Did I cause it?" or "If I were a better kid, would this have happened?" This applies particularly to situations where parents separate or divorce.

Reassure them to the best of your ability and check in with your kids about these important concerns from time to time. Use the technique of going out to coffee or dinner alone with your kids or taking a "walk-and-talk." When your kids are learning to drive, you'll have hours of "captive-audience" time when you can be with them in the car, and they really want to be with you too.

Aging Together Can Be Better than Aging Alone

As we get older, the simple logistics of our lives may become more burdensome. Particularly if we experience physical limitations or illness, it's a gift to be able to share even the smallest of tasks with someone else. You're going to need someone to take you in for your colonoscopy! It's great to have someone share the responsibility of carrying in the groceries, cooking, doing laundry, traveling, caring for animals, and planning just about anything. Your financial resources are greater together than they are individually. If you respect each other and work through the conflicts that do arise, you may find yourself in a new equilibrium that suits you both well. No matter how things turn out, you as a couple have much shared history and that in itself is a resource for both.

A Few Things to Keep in Mind

First, there's no guarantee that you will stay together in a marriage or relationship after one partner comes out, but there never *has* been a guarantee! (There may have been a promise, but not a guarantee.)

Next, know that all relationships can be modified. To stay grounded as a couple, keep asking, "What is *my* desired outcome?" "What is *our* desired outcome as a couple?" and "What is the desired outcome *for our children*?" Figure out what you want and need. Learn from your partner what they want and need. Don't make assumptions. Brainstorm to expand your options. Include all ideas, even ideas that may seem ridiculous at first glance.

Make it a priority to conduct yourselves respectfully. Resist the impulse to bad-mouth your partner, particularly in front of your kids. If you need to vent, vent to a therapist, not to your kids. If anyone says, "I want it to be just like it used to be," help them understand that is *not* an option. It won't ever be exactly "like it used to be," but, with creative minds and open hearts, it could be even better than it was before. So, find and use the helpful resources you need, like support groups, friends, counselors, and professional advisors.

Work together to find if there are specific compromises that each of you could make and still be true to your own self. If your spouse won't be seen with you dressed in your identified gender, could you start with dressing while traveling, either alone or together? Could you go together to a gender conference in another city? Might you take separate vacations or getaways? Many couples do this.

You and your spouse or partner are assumedly good people with good intentions. Other people have worked through this and you can also. And, if you do not stay together, you'll know that you both gave it a most sincere and honoring try. Remember that you both can learn to survive this too, even if you don't see it now. If you approach the process with love and compassion, everyone involved will have the choice and opportunity to thrive.

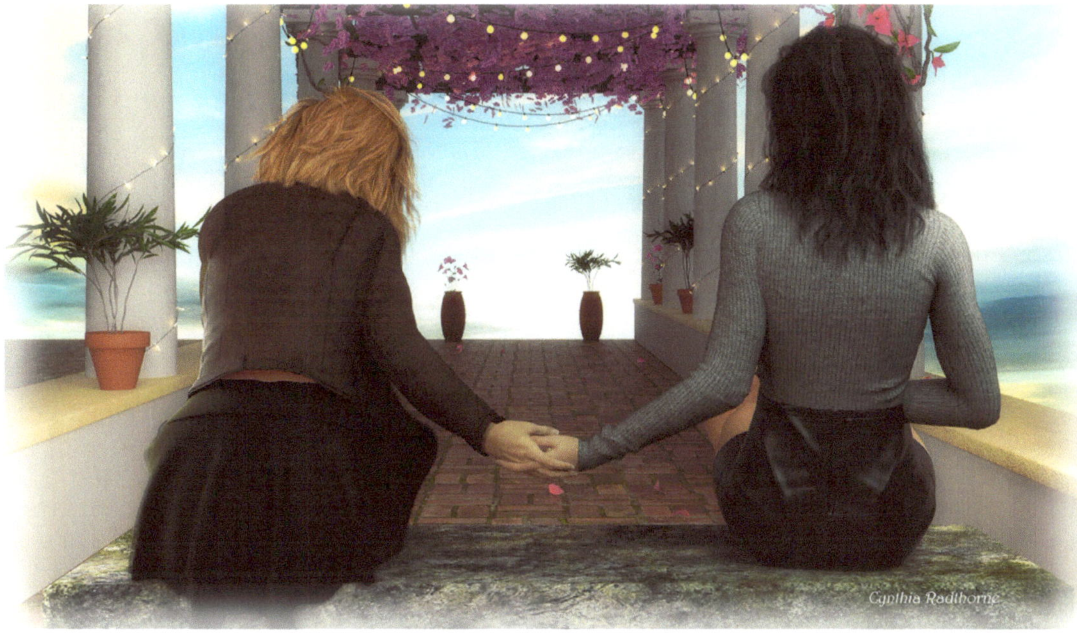

Togetherness after Transition

Written and Illustrated by Cynthia Radthorne

There are many challenges that face a transitioning adult. Things like name changes, gender markers, dealing with bureaucracies, managing workplace expectations, and updating financial and legal records; all of these can be daunting. Yet, of all these, by far the most difficult and most important to your long-term happiness is managing the relationships in your life.

The midlife transitioner typically has many established relationships, some of which may have endured for decades: a spouse or partner, children, siblings, parents, long-term friends, and coworkers. People who mean the world to you and whose ties to you might be impossible to comprehend losing. Yet, the change you are embarking on will test each and every one of those relationships, and each will need to be handled with great care in order to hold on to them.

The first and most obvious one is a spouse or partner. This is the person closest to you, who likely knows more about you than anybody else. Depending on how open you may have been about your gender feelings before deciding you needed to transition, such a change may come like a bolt out of the blue to your partner. Often, we who have held our gender dysphoria in check all the way to middle age or later have made efforts to mask it all from view, even from one as close to us as our partner. This is the person who has the most power to help us, to console us, and to reassure us as we move forward on this path.

Yet, they are also the person with the most to lose from this change. Except in the rare circumstance where one's partner was always aware of your gender feelings from the beginning or might be of a bisexual persuasion themselves, having you be the same gender as they are will most likely not be what they signed up for in the relationship. The odds are that they are comfortably heterosexual in their outlook, and the prospect of you becoming their gay or lesbian partner will shake their foundations.

There is no one-size-fits-all solution to this. It will depend entirely on the dynamics of your particular relationship and in large measure on how adaptable, patient, and understanding your partner is. You must be prepared in case they decide that a changed you is not what they want and that they cannot be happy with that. Will you continue forward or retreat? It is something only you can answer, but think carefully on it so that you know the answer yourself before you first broach the subject with your partner.

Once you do open up about your gender and their initial shock has worn off, it is important to let them know that (a) you are not crazy; (b) you've actually felt this way for some time and no, it's not something that is going away or that you will just get over; and (c) other people in similar circumstances have made this work and managed to hold on to their relationships. It takes work on both sides, it takes patience, and most of all, it takes love. They will be worried that they're going to lose the person they partnered with, that you will change into a completely different person, or that you will want to be with a gay or lesbian person instead of them. But, you need to reassure them that you are still you, with the same personality that they fell in love with. You have a need to live as the gender you feel inside, but the person you are—the things they've always liked about you—are all still there.

Most importantly, communicate. Hopefully, you will have done a lot of research before this point and can provide examples of books or videos to peruse, singly or together. You may know the ins and outs of being transgender, but they may know nothing at all. Start with the key things, such as the difference between gender and sexuality (assuming, for this discussion, that your sexuality has not changed but that we are dealing with just a changed gender recognition). Keep reassuring them that you are not leaving, that you don't want to leave, and that you want to find a path forward together—just with you able to live the gender you feel inside.

Now, to be realistic, while it is entirely possible that your partner might embrace your change 100 percent and love you exactly as they always have, only with you now the same gender as they are, it is not very likely. Your partner's needs, both physical and mental, may not envision a future with someone of the same sex. It does not mean that the relationship must end, but it may have to evolve into something else. For some middle-aged and older couples, the physical things may have lessened already, which makes such a change a little easier to bear. But be very aware and understanding of your partner's needs and be prepared if they cannot give up some of these things.

If they are willing to walk with you and let the partnership grow into something the same but different, a common path to take is to be emotionally connected but in a different way. For example, a male-to-female transitioner may find herself now in a relationship that feels more like close sisters, with much shared history and much affection, but not quite on the same emotional level as before. In place of romance, deeper understanding and acceptance might develop. In place of physical relations, you might have shared experiences in the things that those of same genders do together but which may not have been easily available to you together before.

Explaining things to your children can also be difficult. The good news is that many of the younger generation tend to be more accepting of ideas of gender equality and identity. Even so, on a personal level, children can perceive your transition as "losing" their mother or father. Family interactions can be a little awkward, particularly around what your children will call you (in my case, my son refers to me by my first name). This can be hard for all concerned.

And, as with your spouse or partner, it can feel like some distance has come between you and your children. So, it is crucial to let them know how important they still are in your life and that despite your transition, you care for them as much as you always have. Also, don't assume you can fill the same role as your spouse unless both the children and your spouse are supportive of that. Instead, try to forge a new relationship, blending what you have shared together in raising them with your new experiences as the you that you are meant to be. If your children are older with families of their own, then of course that multiplies the dynamics of change among all their family members, including changes of aunts and uncles. And you thought talking politics at Thanksgiving dinners was complicated!

Siblings can find themselves in a similar situation as children in terms of the potential feelings of loss they may exhibit at "losing" their brother or sister. Help them to see that you are still the same person and that your change does not invalidate all of the memories you have shared with them while growing up. As with all of those close to you, be patient as they adapt to your new name and pronouns. Names tend to be a bit easier for many people; pronouns can take a while. In part, this is due to all those shared memories. When recalling events of the past, it is natural that they "see" you as you were then because that is how the memories were implanted in their brains. So, be patient as they learn to reprocess those memories and layer over them the "new" you.

One of the hardest challenges is your parents. This can be due to any number of things: an older generation unaccustomed to even thinking in terms of other than fixed-gender binaries or religious convictions. But even beyond those fundamentals, your parents have spent your entire life thinking of you one way. They may have decorated your room, bought you toys, and participated in childhood events with a clear idea of what you were. The change you are making may seem to them like a sweeping away of all of that, as either "wrong" or immaterial or unappreciated. It can make them feel as if they have failed at being a parent in not recognizing in you what you may have felt over all those years. And indeed, for those who may have tried to express themselves as they felt they were but were rerouted "back" into what were considered acceptable norms of behavior by their parents, this can be a very fraught situation.

Be gentle with your parents and be aware of their own limits, from their upbringing, their morals, their religion, or their culture. Most of all, understand the things they may feel they are losing—not only their current child but all those memories of a lifetime of rearing you. Focus on the positive memories even if their influences held you back. They are the result of their own times and not your time or the current, more open times about gender. Be the guide for them to show them that you are still their child and, most of all, that you are happy now. For what parent does not want their grown children to be happy in life?

Last, we come to close friends and coworkers. Much like siblings, your friends share many memories with you as you were before. By their nature of not being family, the ties are based more on mutual admiration and respect. They too will have difficulty processing older memories, and you will need to be equally patient with them as they learn how to insert "this" you into the "then." The relationships themselves may also need to change. For example, if you were a male and did male-bonding sorts of activities with your buddy and now you are female, those things may no longer be possible. You both may need to accept that and find a way to bond differently. If they are true friends, they will accept you as you are and see how happy the change has made you. A good friend is more than the shared activities, so with a bit of work on both sides, you can build something new together.

Coworkers are a thing unto themselves, tied as it is into employer policies. Unlike friends who choose to be with you, coworkers often don't have that choice. Some of them may have personal difficulties in dealing with gender transitions. The key here is to involve your employer in this process, clarify their policies, and understand your protections. In a supportive company, your employer will have your back and prevent workplace discrimination. Above all, be professional in dealing with the company and with coworkers. Present yourself as self-assured in your gender, patient but firm in your rights. Coworker reactions will range from "Wow, you are so brave, I admire you so much!" to, well, let's just say, less enthusiasm. Focus on your own work, be thankful for the acceptance you receive, and do your best to deal with any negativity that may arise.

With all of these relationships, remember that the very most important ingredient is time. The longer you are "you" and people see you for who you are and that this change is here to stay, the easier it becomes for everyone. Be patient, kind, and understanding, and be happy that you are now at last able to be the true you.

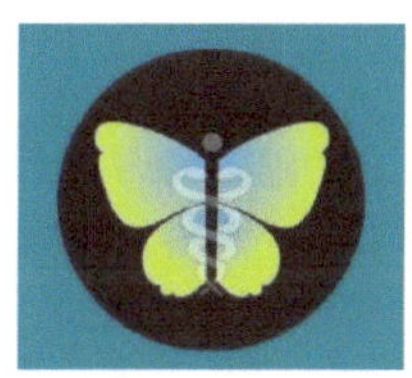

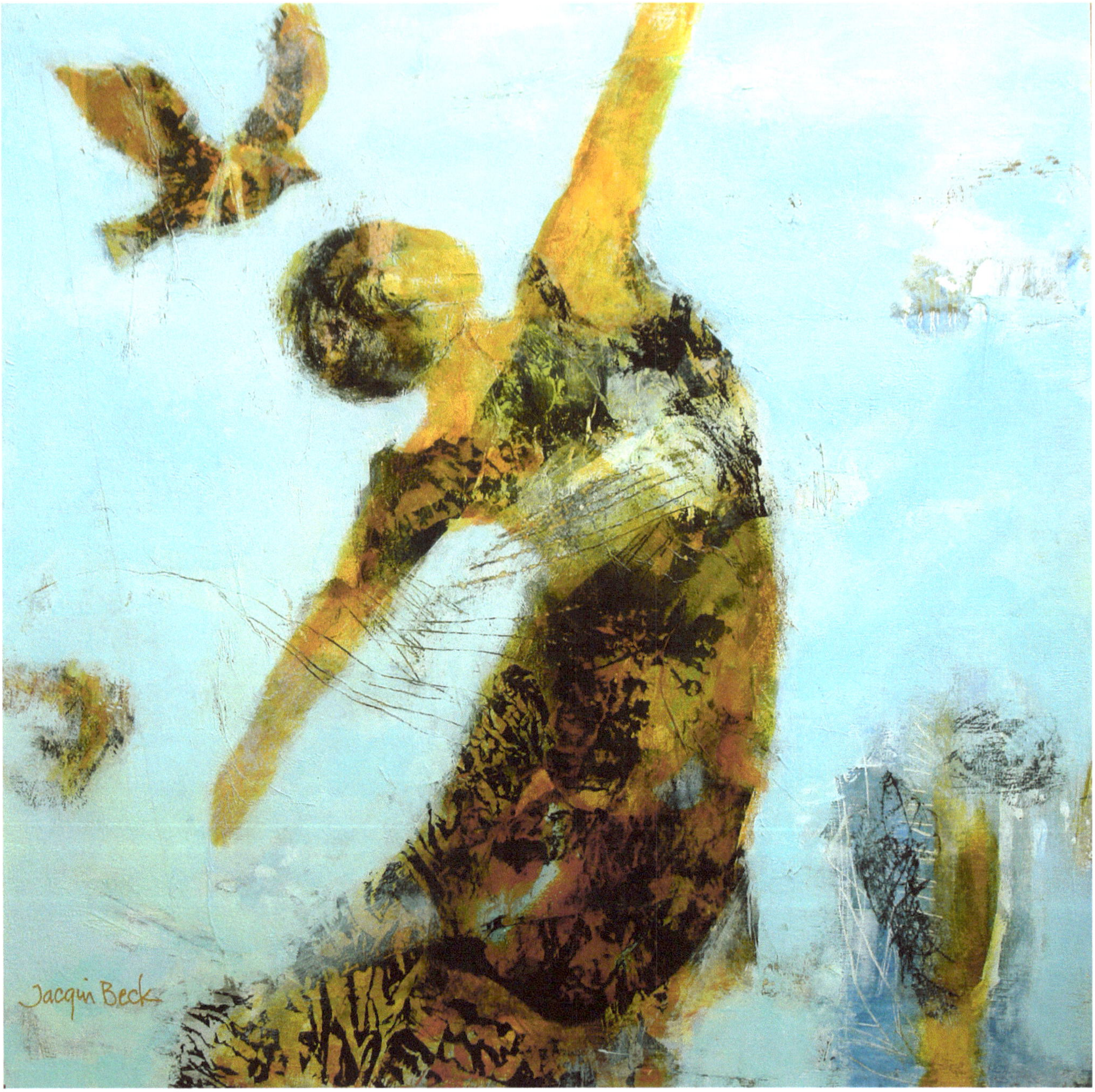

Earth Flying

CHAPTER 14

Finding Gender-Friendly Healthcare and Counseling

To begin a gender transition, you will need the help of a physician or other healthcare provider to prescribe hormones. You will need therapists to write supportive letters if you are considering gender-affirming surgery as well. A psychiatrist friend of mine once said, "It's the healthy people who go to therapy." I'm convinced he was right.

Many transgender folks find that doctors generally know little or nothing about gender transition. Fifty percent of transgender respondents in the National Transgender Discrimination study reported having to educate their healthcare providers.[72]

I think this is inexcusable. But really, why *would* healthcare providers know anything about transgender medicine? I assure you that we didn't learn it in medical or nursing school. Thankfully, this is changing, but not nearly fast enough.

You *can* find providers who are gender-friendly, although they may be more or less accessible depending on where you live. Search "transgender medical care in (your area)" to find your closest resource. WPATH (World Professional Association for Transgender Health) has a list online of their members who are medical and mental health providers at **wpath.org**. In Seattle, search **ingersollgendercenter.org** for local providers.

Talking to Your Own Healthcare Provider and Counselor

Suppose you have a great relationship with a doctor or counselor already. Certainly, you want to maintain these relationships. If these advocates are not experienced in trans healthcare, they may want to consult with providers who are. Many of us who have had more experience are happy to talk with other healthcare providers on the phone or by email.

The first trans woman I treated 20 years ago was someone who called my practice and asked, "Does Dr. Gromko treat transgender women?" I answered, "Not yet," and conveyed that I would be happy to learn if the patient understood that I would be learning as I went. I read the information I could find, spoke with the few doctors who were treating transgender folks in my area, and learned from experience.

You do not have to give up your own doctor or counselor. Sometimes you will want to get your gender-specific care from other providers while continuing to receive primary care from the people you've known longer. Maybe you *will* be the one who helps educate your doctor. Our patients educate us all the time. You shouldn't *have* to be the teacher, but it may be a win-win for both of you. What's important is that you get the care you need.

If you're uncomfortable telling your healthcare provider about your gender issues, put a toe in the water with something like, "I have a friend who is transgender and I'd like to refer them to you. Would you be okay with that?" Their reaction will give you a clue about the provider's comfort level.

72 Jaime M. Grant, Lisa A. Mottet, Justin Tanis, Jack Harrison, Jody L. Herman, and Mara Keisling, *Injustice at Every Turn: A Report of the National Transgender Discrimination Survey*, Washington DC: National Center for Transgender Equality and National Gay and Lesbian Task Force, 2011, https://transequality.org/sites/default/files/docs/resources/NTDS_Report.pdf.

Then, if you see that they are totally okay, say "Oh, thank God. I was talking about me." (Which they probably knew anyway.) If they aren't okay, no personal exposure is needed.

On one level, this seems a bit ridiculous. Your healthcare provider should be comfortable and competent in treating you. But it isn't always the case. I remember a patient who took all of her medical records to an endocrinologist appointment in a small town. She was astonished when the doctor physically tore up her records and said, "We don't treat people like you here."

Of course, that response was absurd, illegal, and highly unethical. There are many of us here to help—healthcare providers who welcome the honor of helping people like you along your journey.

Support Groups for Patients and Professionals

As you proceed through a gender transition, a support group may help you in many ways. Read more about "Finding a Support Group" and "Here's How a Support Group May Help You" in the previous chapter.

If you are a professional working with the transgender and gender-nonconforming community, you might be interested to know that Seattle's Ingersoll Gender Center, founded in 1977, has had a professional group (the Ingersoll Consult Group) since 2012. Founded by Stacy Prince, PhD, and Jana Ekdahl, MA (both gender-friendly therapists), the consult group meets regularly and maintains a listserv for around 400 members. Listserv members can ask open questions to the group via the Internet, and they usually receive answers and opinions within minutes to hours.

Getting Hormones on Your Own: *Not Advised*

Many people do get hormones from friends or from faraway pharmacies online. Is this a good idea? Not in my opinion.

A physician who treats himself has a fool for a patient.

— Sir William Osler

In fairness to people who have self-prescribed, I believe this occurs because of two things. First is a lack of medical care available to trans people. And second is insurance that is a barrier to care and continues to be a barrier in spite of the work of dedicated people who have sought to change this cumbersome system. This is improving, however.

It is fair to say that I have seen many people who have self-prescribed medications without apparent harm. But, if you buy prescription drugs online, it can be a risky choice. I wonder about the sources and the quality control of medications sold on the Internet or on the street.

Self-prescribing is also illegal if you are not a legitimate licensed prescriber.

Transgender Disclosure in a Medical Setting

"Must I disclose that I'm transgender?" I hear this question mostly from people who live completely stealth and also from trans males or trans females who have had gender-affirming surgeries and who never tell anyone about their assigned gender at birth.

But there are some things to consider: Gender, gender-affirming hormones, and surgeries are a legitimate part of a person's medical history. Occasionally, hormones do impact lab values or health conditions. Your primary care provider should know about your medical history and the situation should feel safe enough for you to share it with them.

That said, some concerns are simply far too important to ignore—chest pain, difficulty breathing, or neurological symptoms (such as weakness or numbness on one side). Just get care and sort out the rest later. ***In a life-threatening emergency***, it's probably better for the emergency room healthcare team not to have to puzzle through genital variations as they insert a urinary catheter. ***If your medical problem involves your genitalia, urinary tract, or bowel anatomy***, it's important and to your benefit to find a trans-friendly specialist for routine matters.

But, do you really have to disclose for a mole removal or a sinus infection? I would say no. ***Don't delay care because of gender issues.*** A mole can be a melanoma (a form of skin cancer), and a prompt diagnosis matters in your survival.

If you're pretty certain your genitals won't be involved, just get the care you need and disclose if asked. ("Oh, that's a nonissue for me now; I forgot to mention it.") You also can decline to answer ("I'd prefer not to discuss that"). It would be great, though, to have a doctor or other healthcare provider where you didn't have to "hide."

Find trans-friendly primary care providers and specialists by asking your friends or searching websites like those of WPATH or Ingersoll Gender Center.

Getting Medical Care When You Do Not Have a Doctor

In my observation, medical care is best provided by a physician or an ARNP/PA (advanced registered nurse practitioner/physician assistant) you know and with whom you have established care. This isn't always possible, particularly in an emergency.

A quick Internet search of "transgender-friendly medical care in (my area)" should prompt a listing of appropriate resources. This way, you probably have a better chance of being treated by a provider who knows something about transgender medicine, speaks "the language," and will treat you with respect rather than curiosity or revulsion.

Some Considerations for Emergency Care

You don't have the opportunity to do much screening in a real emergency; you may not even be conscious or able to speak for yourself! But the following tips may help you.

Don't Be a John or Jane Doe (Even *This* Is Binary)!

Carry identification on your person, such as in a wallet or phone carrier. If you're a runner or other outdoor athlete, you can find ID tags that lace into a running shoe (find one of many at **roadid.com**). Carry a cell phone that provides your location by GPS, in case you are able to call 911.

Newer Apple watches will actually check on you if you have a hard fall! According to Apple's website, "If Apple Watch Series 4 or later detects a hard fall while you're wearing your watch, it taps you on the wrist, sounds an alarm, and displays an alert. You can choose to contact emergency services or dismiss the alert by pressing the Digital Crown, tapping Close in the upper-left corner, or tapping "I'm OK."[73] And if you don't respond, your phone will summon 911 and ping your emergency contact people.

Wear a Medic Alert Tag to Identify You and Convey Important Health Information

You may want to order a customized medic alert tag if you have any serious allergies or medical problems. You can also list your name and emergency contact information. Search for customized tags on Amazon or Etsy or pick up brochures at your pharmacy.

Specify conditions like "DIABETES" or "DIALYSIS" OR "BLOOD THINNERS" or any condition that could impact the care you need, especially if you are unable to speak for yourself. If you have had a breast cancer surgery, for example, you may have been advised not to have blood drawn from the arm on the "cancer side." You may specify, "NO BLOOD DRAWS ON LEFT ARM."

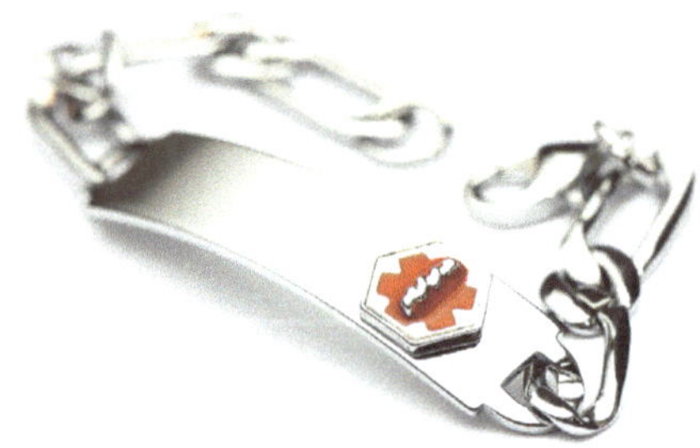

The tags are worn as a bracelet or necklace, and first responders and emergency room personnel look for them first. Some people might want to specify "TRANSGENDER" on a tag, particularly if genital reconstruction has modified the appearance of the urethra.

If you take medications such as anticoagulants or insulin, specify this on your medic alert tag. If you have a condition that could mimic alcohol intoxication, list it. For example, you might list "LOW BLOOD SUGAR" or "SEIZURE."

Don't Allow Insensitive Experiences to Delay the Care You Need

Seeking healthcare, particularly emergency care, has presented barriers for transgender individuals in the past. Many have been treated rudely, and there are even incidents where trans people have experienced violence on the part of ER personnel.[74]

Some patients have found that emergency providers have focused on the transgender piece of their history even when being trans is not critical to their diagnosis. Certainly, the trans part is important in a postvaginoplasty patient having a urinary tract infection; the medical provider must know the surgical background to provide appropriate care.

73 Apple, "Use Fall Detection with Apple Watch," September 17, 2020, https://support.apple.com/en-us/HT208944.

74 Jaime M. Grant, Lisa A. Mottet, Justin Tanis, Jack Harrison, Jody L. Herman, and Mara Keisling, *Injustice at Every Turn: A Report of the National Transgender Discrimination Survey*, Washington DC: National Center for Transgender Equality and National Gay and Lesbian Task Force, 2011, https://transequality.org/sites/default/files/docs/resources/NTDS_Report.pdf.

One woman told me that she had suffered a "transgender broken arm." I asked her what she meant and she explained that it was "a broken arm when the patient is transgender!" The patient went on to clarify that there's really nothing about a broken arm that is specific to being trans. But it was the transgender information that the doctor was most curious about.

You will probably be able to tell when questions are curiosity-driven rather than medically driven. Such questions can help providers help you and other patients get more informed care, but they should come after your arm is casted or the sutures are placed!

But, healthcare is changing, although sometimes slowly. Please do not avoid getting the emergency care you need because you have concerns about how you may be treated. A medical condition may worsen over time, placing you at greater risk and ultimately requiring more complicated care. Don't let this happen to you.

If You Are Diagnosed with a Life-Threatening Illness

No matter how careful we are about our health or how effective medical interventions have become, none of us is getting out of here alive. But even if we confront a life-threatening illness, there are important considerations that make our experiences better or *significantly* worse.

We tend to have better experiences when we know what we want and are able to communicate that information with those around us. Being told about a serious diagnosis, *particularly when it's your diagnosis*, is generally tough. It can be even more difficult if you're estranged from supportive family and lack the advocacy of others.

Read the following suggestions to see if they might make sense for you or someone you know.

- **Learn about your diagnosis.**
  Learn the exact name of your condition and do some Internet research. Some suggest that you avoid "Dr. Google," but I'd suggest that you read what you can find. Just remember that Dr. Google's information may already be out of date or somewhat conflicting.

  Learn the general prognosis and the usual course of your ailment. Is the disease likely to progress to the extent that you will need specialized care or an assisted living facility? Is the disease likely to shorten your life, and if so, over what time period?

  Research the treatment that is available. For instance, if it's a malignancy, what surgery, chemotherapy, radiation, and other options are offered? If you get frightened or anxious when reading about the condition, use my mantra, "What are the *facts* of my situation?" Remember, too, that statistics and predictions may not represent your experience.

- **Appoint a durable power of attorney for healthcare and for financial decisions.**
  This person or persons must agree to serve in this capacity. The designation of "DPOA" allows them to make important decisions on your behalf if you should become incapacitated.

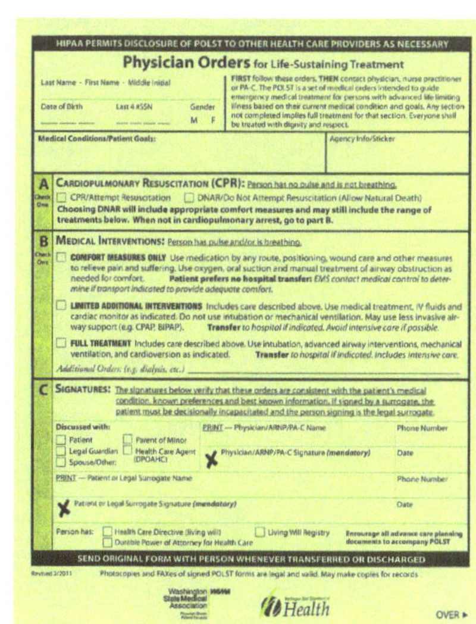

HIPAA PERMITS DISCLOSURE OF POLST TO OTHER HEALTH CARE PROVIDERS AS NECESSARY

Physician Orders for Life-Sustaining Treatment

Last Name - First Name - Middle Initial

Date of Birth | Last 4 #SSN | Gender M F

FIRST follow these orders. **THEN** contact physician, nurse practitioner or PA-C. The POLST is a set of medical orders intended to guide emergency medical treatment for persons with advanced life limiting illness based on their current medical condition and goals. Any section not completed implies full treatment for that section. Everyone shall be treated with dignity and respect.

Medical Conditions/Patient Goals: | Agency Info/Sticker

A Check One — **CARDIOPULMONARY RESUSCITATION (CPR):** Person has no pulse and is not breathing.
☐ CPR/Attempt Resuscitation ☐ DNAR/Do Not Attempt Resuscitation (Allow Natural Death)
Choosing DNAR will include appropriate comfort measures and may still include the range of treatments below. When not in cardiopulmonary arrest, go to part B.

B Check One — **MEDICAL INTERVENTIONS:** Person has pulse and/or is breathing.
☐ **COMFORT MEASURES ONLY** Use medication by any route, positioning, wound care and other measures to relieve pain and suffering. Use oxygen, oral suction and manual treatment of airway obstruction as needed for comfort. **Patient prefers no hospital transfer:** *EMS contact medical control to determine if transport indicated to provide adequate comfort.*
☐ **LIMITED ADDITIONAL INTERVENTIONS** Includes care described above. Use medical treatment, IV fluids and cardiac monitor as indicated. Do not use intubation or mechanical ventilation. May use less invasive airway support (e.g. CPAP, BiPAP). **Transfer** *to hospital if indicated. Avoid intensive care if possible.*
☐ **FULL TREATMENT** Includes care described above. Use intubation, advanced airway interventions, mechanical ventilation, and cardioversion as indicated. **Transfer** *to hospital if indicated. Includes intensive care.*
Additional Orders: (e.g. dialysis, etc.)

C **SIGNATURES:** The signatures below verify that these orders are consistent with the patient's medical condition, known preferences and best known information. If signed by a surrogate, the patient must be decisionally incapacitated and the person signing is the legal surrogate.

Discussed with: ☐ Patient ☐ Legal Guardian ☐ Spouse/Other: ☐ Parent of Minor ☐ Health Care Agent (DPOAHC)
PRINT — Physician/ARNP/PA-C Name | Phone Number
Physician/ARNP/PA-C Signature *(mandatory)* | Date
PRINT — Patient or Legal Surrogate Name | Phone Number
Patient or Legal Surrogate Signature *(mandatory)* | Date

Person has: ☐ Health Care Directive (living will) ☐ Durable Power of Attorney for Health Care ☐ Living Will Registry — **Encourage all advance care planning documents to accompany POLST**

SEND ORIGINAL FORM WITH PERSON WHENEVER TRANSFERRED OR DISCHARGED

Revised 3/2011 — Photocopies and FAXes of signed POLST forms are legal and valid. May make copies for records

Washington State Medical Association — Health

OVER ▸

Figure 14.1. Washington State POLST form.

- **Think about your end-of-life choices well ahead of time.**
  At the end of your life, do you want those around you to let you die in peace with the bulk of medical treatment directed at "comfort care" only? If so, you would want to be designated as a "No Code" or "DNR (do not resuscitate)."

  If it is likely that you will die from your illness, have a POLST form (Physician Orders for Life-Sustaining Treatment) signed by your healthcare provider and posted on the refrigerator—the designated spot where first responders look for it. Find more info at polst.org.

  Or, would you prefer to have everything that's medically possible done to prolong your life? Resuscitative efforts are carried out by default unless an individual has indicated otherwise ahead of time, as in a form. (In the words of one of my 80-year-old trans women patients, "Give it a shot!")

  Make out an advance directive to indicate your wishes for the type of end-of-life care you would want. This form, also called a living will, should be discussed with your physician and DPOA as well as friends and appropriate family members. A state-by-state guide to advance directive forms is available from Everplans: everplans.com/articles/state-by-state-advance-directive-forms.

  Finally, would you prefer to have your physician prescribe a lethal dose of a medication to end your life at the time and place of your choosing? In Washington State, voters have approved physician aid-in-dying, or PAD, which makes this option available in certain circumstances and with very specific requirements. You may find that such requirements require that a person plan well in advance; it cannot be a snap decision.

- **Think about making your own cremation or burial arrangements ahead of time so that your gender and your wishes are respected.**
  There have been some heartbreaking stories where a transgender person has died and their final arrangements were executed by estranged, unsympathetic family members. The example below is from author Christine Colby:

  > "Jennifer Gable died in October 2014 at the age of 32, from an unexpected aneurysm. When her friends attended her funeral, they were outraged to see that she was displayed in the casket wearing a man's suit, no makeup, and her hair had been cut. At no point during the service was her female identity even mentioned."[75]

  Laws pertaining to after-death arrangements for funerals and body disposal vary from state to state. An online state-by-state guide called *Who Has the Legal Right to Make Decisions about Your Funeral* can be found at funerals.org/?consumers=legal-right-make-decisions-funeral.

  An advance directive specifies end-of-life care wishes, but it expires at death. It is recommended that instructions for disposing of the body and the funeral arrangements *not* be included in a legal will, as this is usually read *after* a funeral.

  Better yet, complete a form known as "Appointment of Agent to Control Disposition of Remains." This can be added to an advance directive and includes instruction on how the decedent's body is to be dressed and groomed and what name and pronouns are to be used. In addition, it is possible to designate "those who should have no authority."

75 Christine Colby, "Dying Trans: Preserving Identity in Death," *The Order of the Good Death*, January 10, 2017, http://www.orderofthegooddeath.com/dying-trans-preserving-identity-death.

For further information, refer to the Transgender Law Center's article "Remembering Christopher Lee, Achieving Justice for Our Loved Ones" at transgenderlawcenter.org/archives/3292.

Remember, you are best advised to—

- **Consult an attorney.**
  If you do not have one, call Lambda Legal for a reference: lambdalegal.org.
- **Clarify in writing your wishes for your funeral and the disposition of your body.**
  Include the name and gender you use to refer to yourself, how your body is to be dressed and groomed for a viewing, and how your body is to be disposed of (such as cremation or burial).
- **Identify a willing agent to execute your wishes on your behalf—both for your end-of-life choices (advance directive or living will) and for care of your body after death (appointment of agent).**
  The willing agent must agree to serve in this capacity.
- **Sign the written documents and have them witnessed and notarized.**

Please understand that I am not qualified to give legal advice;
use this discussion to help you find the answers to your own questions.

— Linda Gromko, MD

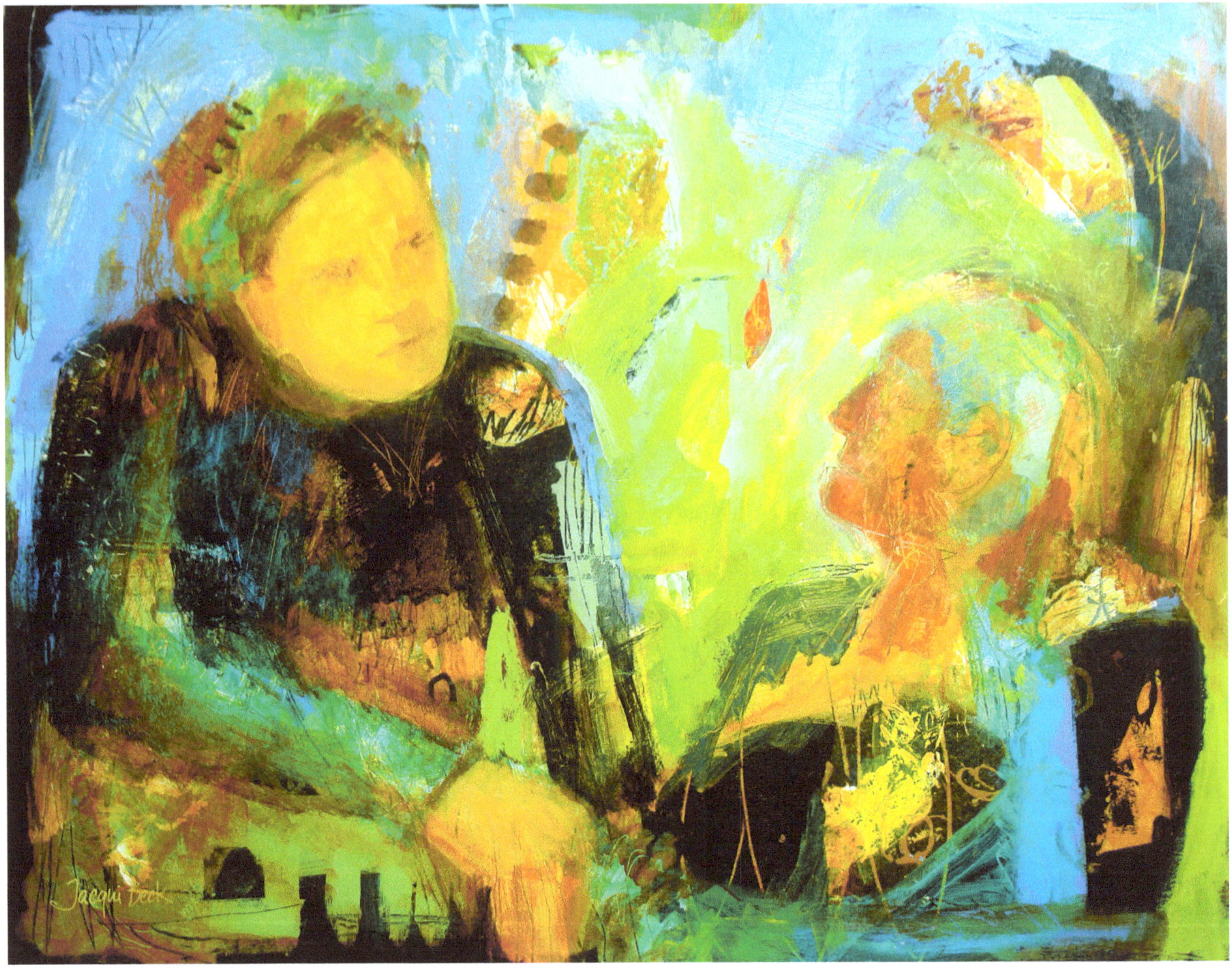

Time Enough

CHAPTER 15
Education and Career Planning

Finishing Up High School and Moving Ahead

Graduating from high school and going on to college or vocational school is important to our personal development. People who finish high school and college generally earn higher incomes. A higher income likely means better housing, healthier living, and less physical risk to you. Plus, if you get to do work that you really enjoy (like I do), you will probably be happier overall.

> Find a job you love and you'll never work a day in your life.
>
> — *Confucius*

Transgender and gender-nonconforming people may have experienced challenges in school, particularly if gender dysphoria has occupied such a large mindshare that it crowded out other things like learning and education. It's not terribly unusual to see such teenagers drop out of high school. But I've seen some impressive options that have equalized opportunities and given people a chance to regroup and catch up. See if any of the following ideas will help if they apply to you.

Assess Your Own Strengths, Weaknesses, and Basic Skills

Take an honest look at your own skills. Do you have difficulty reading or writing? Were you born before computers existed? Have you made assumptions about what you can or cannot do (like "I can't do math")?

- **You really *can* learn new things at any age or brush up on skills that are barriers for you.**
  Two-year colleges often have catch-up courses or human volunteers to help you.
- **Search online for an aptitude assessment or career counseling center.**
  Try to find one associated with a public college or university; search "aptitude testing and counseling in (your state)."
- **You can also learn just about anything on YouTube.**
  Pick a topic and search it on **youtube.com**.

Address Learning and Focusing Difficulties That May Need Attention

I encounter this scenario fairly often in family medicine: An adult has a child who is diagnosed with ADHD (attention deficit and hyperactivity disorder). As the child is successfully treated, the parent realizes that they too have had similar difficulties, but they were never recognized (ADHD can run in families). Common symptoms may include difficulty in reading, difficulty with organization, and the tendency to get more easily distracted than most people do. Medications can truly help, but they aren't the only answers for learning problems.

Some people simply need help in study skills or organization. People also have differences in learning styles. Search online for treating learning differences or read *Driven to Distraction: Recognizing and Coping with Attention Deficit Disorder from Childhood through Adulthood* by Edward M. Hallowell and John J. Retay. Difficulty concentrating can also be a symptom of depression; read more about this in Chapter 17.

A School's Culture Can Hinder a Transgender Student

If you were in the midst of transitioning in middle school or high school, your school culture may not have supported your growth. Of course, the most basic school courtesies should include the following:

- Being addressed by your appropriate name (that is, not being "deadnamed") and referred to by your identified gender pronouns
- Having your appropriate name and gender listed on your student ID card
- Having a safe and appropriate restroom to use
- Having accommodations for gym class like gender-friendly showers and dressing areas
- Having a culture of inclusion demonstrated by a supportive counseling staff and perhaps an LGBTQIA+ support group, as well as institutional protection from bullying by students and staff

If not having these factors negatively affected your education, it's time to build your own educational program. Think, "What would it be like to learn in a supportive environment and in my appropriate gender?" If you haven't transitioned your name or ID, school can be a natural place to begin.

Graduate from High School Officially or Get Your GED

Today, you need a high school diploma or general equivalency diploma (GED) for just about any job or higher educational program. You can get your GED by taking the GED exam, which consists of four separate tests: language arts, mathematical reasoning, social studies, and science. They can be taken together or separately, with each test costing about $30 or about $120 for the entire exam. You can take a preparatory class at a 2-year college to get you ready for the test, or you can even find a 2-year-college program that enables to you get your high school diploma *and* complete an associate degree. You may then be able to transfer directly to a university. Search "GED in (your area)" for more details and for free online practice tests.

Making Your Plans for College or Vocational School: Finding What You Really Want to Do

In the best of all worlds, you will discover your passion and be able to make a living doing it. But if your passion is philosophy or sociology, nail down an alternative that pays the rent. Remember, you can do personal reading in the fields of your passion, but you've got to eat.

Go Where the Jobs Are!

Look into jobs that are likely to be in demand in the decades to come.

The Baby Boom generation will undoubtedly drive a need for more healthcare providers and allied health professionals. Think also about technical positions within healthcare (such as X-ray, ultrasound, surgical, and dialysis technicians).

Culinary skills, cosmetology, and aesthetic laser professionals are always in demand. So are business professionals like accountants, bookkeepers, and financial planners. We're unlikely to run out of the need for electricians, welders, plumbers, and auto mechanics, and we've seen subsidized training available for LGBTQIA+ applicants.

The transgender youth I treat tend to be "digital natives"—that is, they're extremely fluent in computer technology, and many are avid video gamers. Some of the largest software and technology companies have also been leaders in trans health benefits. The computer industry may turn out to be a great career fit for you.

Scholarships and Innovative Educational Programs

One example of a scholarship program that serves the LGBTQIA+ community is the Greater Seattle Business Association (GSBA) Scholarship Fund (**thegsba.org/scholarship-home**). GSBA has awarded over $4 million in assistance to more than 700 qualified applicants since its foundation in 1991. Applicants must qualify by area of residence (Washington, Oregon, Idaho, Montana, or Alaska), academic achievement, community activity, and goals. If you don't qualify by residential requirements, search the Internet on "LGBTQIA+ scholarship information" for many more opportunities.

Here are a couple of alternative learning programs that are reputed to be trans-welcoming and financially supportive:

- **Year Up** (**yearup.org**) is an innovative nationwide program that allows adults between the ages of 18 and 24 to get 6 months of free training followed by a 6-month internship in a technology company; it also provides a stipend for living expenses.
- **ADA Developers Academy** (**adadevelopersacademy.org/organization**) is a tuition-free software coding school for women and gender-diverse adults. It combines classroom and internship opportunities with a focus on serving low-income people, underrepresented minorities, and members of the LGBTQIA+ community.

Where You Work Matters

Microsoft, Google, Amazon, Facebook, and Starbucks have led the employer pack in providing trans-inclusive health insurance coverage. Many employers will help pay for gender transition expenses. Health benefits vary widely, but many companies do cover sexual-reassignment (gender-affirming) surgeries. When genital surgeries are covered, genital hair removal is usually covered also. Some employers cover breast augmentation and facial feminization for trans women, and others are beginning to cover the cost of facial hair removal. In our practice, we have seen some employers cover the cost of our "Nose-to-Toes" laser hair-removal treatments.

You can learn more about a company by seeing if it is listed in the Corporate Equality Index on the website of the Human Rights Campaign (**hrc.org/resources/workplace**). If all things are equal, why *not* look into companies that support you in such significant ways?

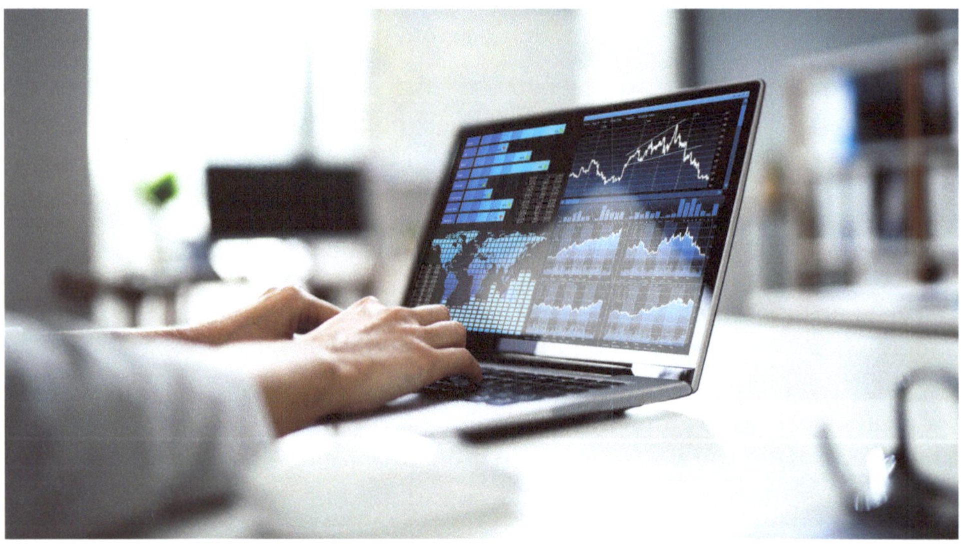

"To all the transgender Americans watching at home, especially the young people who are so brave, I want you to know that your president has your back," President Joseph Biden said on April 28, 2021, urging Congress to pass the Equality Act, which offers expanded protections to LGBTQ Americans from workplace, housing, and healthcare discrimination.[76]

76 Brittany Shepherd, "Biden Tells Transgender Americans, 'Your President Has Your Back,'" *Yahoo News*, April 28, 2021, https://news.yahoo.com/biden-tells-transgender-americans-your-president-has-your-back-023259977.html?guccounter=1&guce_.

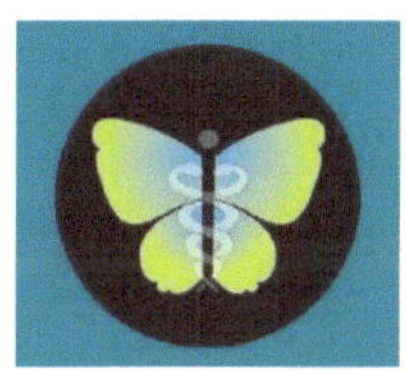

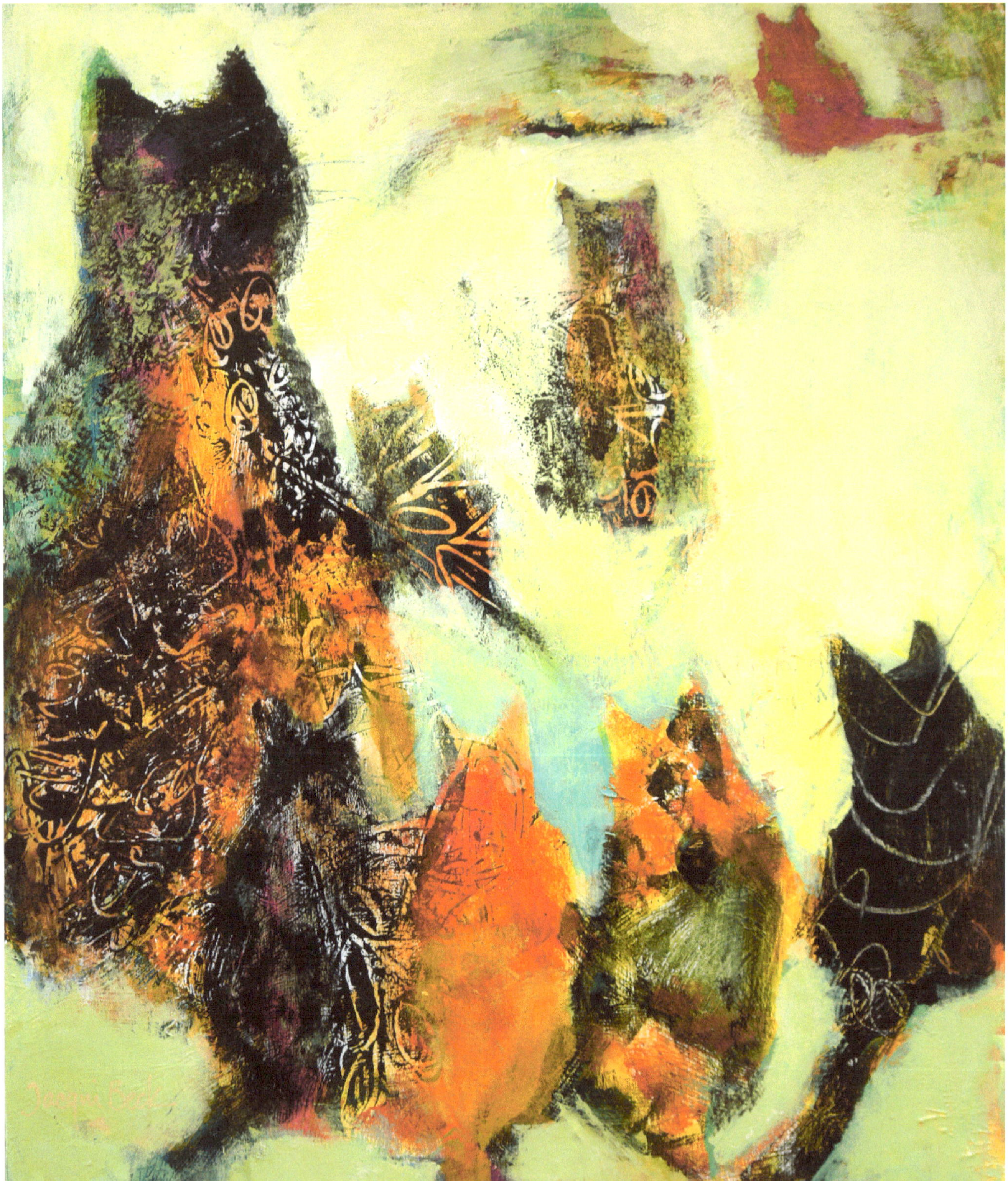

Catwatch

CHAPTER 16
Microaggressions, Personal Safety, and Bullying

As much as I don't want to add to anyone's anxiety, we all have to be careful out there in the world. In this chapter, we begin by discussing microaggressions and move on to bullying and physical violence. Hate crimes, particularly physical assaults based on race or ethnicity, recently hit a 16-year high.[77] Sadly, transgender and gender-nonconfirming individuals are targeted more often than their gender-conforming counterparts.

Identifying Microaggressions

According to Columbia University professor Derald Wing Sue's work, *Microaggressions in Everyday Life: Race, Gender, and Sexual Orientation*, microaggressions are the "everyday slights, indignities, put-downs, and insults that members of marginalized groups experience in their day-to-day interactions with individuals who are often unaware that they have engaged in an offensive or demeaning way."[78]

Transgender and gender-nonconfirming individuals may be the targets of microaggressions. Verbal microaggressions are problematic in that they may sound innocent, are delivered in a friendly manner, and may even be presented as compliments. But because such comments reinforce stereotypes and misconceptions, they tend to distance one group from another. They foster discrimination.

Microaggressions reflect implicit biases "with serious material consequences beyond hurt feelings, from discriminatory hiring to racial inequities in policing and the broader US criminal justice system. In other words, microaggressions matter because they seem to be both symptoms and causes of larger structural problems."[79]

Let's examine some examples of verbal comments and why they may be problematic.

77 Adeel Hassan, "Hate-Crime Violence Hits 16-Year High, F.B.I. Reports," *New York Times*, December 11, 2019, https://www.nytimes.com/2019/11/12/us/hate-crimes-fbi-report.html.

78 Hahna Yoon, "How to Respond to Microaggressions," *New York Times*, March 3, 2020, https://www.nytimes.com/2020/03/03/smarter-living/how-to-respond-to-microaggressions.html.

79 Simba Runyowa, "Microaggressions Matter," *Atlantic*, September 18, 2015, https://www.theatlantic.com/politics/archive/2015/09/microaggressions-matter/406090/.

Microaggressions and Their Implications	
What Is Said	**Why This Might Be a Problem**
"You're trans? Have you had the surgery?"	May assume that all trans people have surgery. This remark is also invasive; it's nobody's business. If I invade your privacy, I assume I am entitled to the information and therefore I'm somehow more important than you are.
"He's gay? What a waste!"	Implies that a desirable individual should be in a "more legitimate" and possibly straight relationship.
"You're so lucky!"	Attributes accomplishments to luck rather than skill, effort, talent, and other variables.
On an invitation to a hospital fundraiser: "Dr. and Mrs. Linda Gromko"	Implies that the doctor, who has to be male, has a wife. My mentor Dr. Barbara Schneidman once said, "When we grew up, you married a doctor; you didn't become one."
To a trans person: "What is your real name?"	Implies that the name the person uses may not be as legitimate as the name or gender they were assigned at birth.
To a trans person: "You don't look trans."	What does this mean? What does it mean to "look trans"? Is this a compliment or a slight? Either way, this comment catches a person off-guard and feels like a judgment.

Table 16.1. Microaggressions and their implications.

Safety comes first. Humor helps you cope. Having someone laugh at me makes me think that they're less likely to start chasing me with a stick. Helping yourself and others laugh makes the world a happier place. Use humor to educate.

Transitioning is a serious process, but don't take yourself too seriously. Take safety seriously. Plan ahead if possible. Go places with a friend. Take a phone. Trust your gut.

— Steve, trans woman, age 61

In a *New York Times* article titled "How to Respond to Microaggressions," Hahna Yoon writes that microaggressions are so commonplace that it seems impossible to tackle them one at a time. Psychologists often compare them to a death by a thousand cuts. Yoon expands that concept, saying that microaggressions imply that the person who receives the message is an "outsider in their own land."[80]

Given the commonality and frequency of microaggressions, choosing one's battles can be impractical and exhausting. Psychology professor Dr. Kevin Nadal created a tool kit called *A Guide to Responding to Microaggression*, which is cited in Yoon's article. Nadal offers five questions to help individuals decide whether or not to respond:

- If I respond, could my physical safety be in danger?
- If I respond, will the person become defensive and will this lead to an argument?
- If I respond, how will this affect my relationship with this person?
- If I don't respond, will I regret not saying something?
- If I don't respond, does that convey that I accept the behavior or statement?

These are difficult choices. Here's an example of microaggression:

- **Person A:** "When are you going to make me a grandparent?"
- **Person B:** "I realize you probably didn't mean this, but when you ask when I'm going to have a baby, I feel pressured and inadequate."
- **Person A:** "Oh, that's ridiculous. You're being much too sensitive."

Now Person B has a new problem. In addition to not measuring up to Person A's expectations, Person B is now "ridiculous" and overreacting. This discussion probably won't end well. It's best for Person A to apologize and move on. So, let's change the script:

- **Person A:** "When are you going to make me a grandparent?"
- **Person B:** "I realize you probably didn't mean this, but when you ask when I'm going to have a baby, I feel pressured and inadequate."
- **Person A:** "Oh, dear. That was terribly insensitive of me! I am truly sorry. Please accept my apology."

In my opinion, recognizing what may be microaggressions is a first step in eliminating them.

Here's another example: Thirty years ago when I joined the medical staff at Swedish Medical Center, there was only one restroom in the medical staff lounge, and it had a sign on the door that read "MEN." Was this a microaggression? Certainly. It wasn't personal, but it reflected the reality of the day: Most physicians were men. It didn't address the underlying stereotype, and it didn't address *my* need to pee! Would it happen in a Seattle hospital today? Not likely. We learn, we apologize, and we don't repeat the microaggressions.

When we misgender another person, a microaggression occurs; it's another insidious put-down. If you are the one who has committed the microaggression, apologize sincerely, move on, and try not to repeat it.

80 Hahna Yoon, "How to Respond to Microaggressions," *New York Times*, March 3, 2020, https://www.nytimes.com/2020/03/03/smarter-living/how-to-respond-to-microaggressions.html.

Other Ways People Can Harm You—and Ways to Survive

Here are some of the ways people can hurt you or make you feel vulnerable. Some would be considered microaggressions, but some become even more serious. In addition to pointing out examples, we discuss ways we can manage difficult situations and protect ourselves from further hurt:

- **People stare at you.**
  This is awkward at the very least. You can stare back. You can ignore them. You can say, "Hi, I'm sorry—I don't remember your name." They will likely be embarrassed and back off.

- **People call you an "it."**
  Ignore this awful comment if you possibly can.

- **People ask you rude direct questions. "Hey, are you a dude?"**
  You owe nobody any information, and it's probably best to walk on. I do remember a patient who was a former hockey player, had had sexual reassignment surgery, facial feminization surgery, and looked fully female. But people would ask if she was "a guy." She would just smile and say, "Oh, I get that all the time. I'm a girl with guy shoulders. Let's go to the restroom and I'll show you." She certainly didn't have to prove a thing, but it was her way of responding and it seemed to work for her.

- **People misgender you (call you by the wrong pronouns) on purpose.**
  I appreciate that people sometimes misgender others by accident. (Even trans people misgender themselves and one another occasionally.) It's probably best to state simply, "I use the pronouns she and her" (or whatever fits for you). This is very different from misgendering somebody on purpose. And it's very different from doing it repeatedly, or after being corrected.

> **I call purposeful misgendering "attack misgendering." The most egregious example I heard was one of my trans women clients being called "son" and "my boy" by an impatient healthcare provider!**
>
> *— Linda Gromko, MD*

- **People "out" you without your consent.**
  If this happens, you might quietly say, "This is an area of my life that still feels new and I'm not totally comfortable being public yet. I'd appreciate it if you would try to keep this information private for now."

  If you're outed by someone you've met in a gender support group, that's very different. Most groups have a rule that what happens in the group stays in the group. Remind the offender of the rule and talk to a group facilitator if it continues to be a problem.

- **People post private information about you on the Internet without your consent or knowledge.**
  See "Cyberbullying and the Upstander Pledge" on pages 346–347.

- **People harm you by sedating you without your knowledge.**
  Slipping something into someone's drink isn't a new phenomenon. If you get "roofied" (have the sedative flunitrazepam, marketed as Rohypnol, slipped into a drink), you are at the mercy of an assailant.

  This happened to a trans woman I know. She was talking to a man at a bar, and it was not during a date—she didn't know him. The man slipped a sedative into her drink and took her to his apartment right afterwards. The man tried to have sex with his then-unconscious victim but apparently panicked when he discovered her male genitalia.

  The police took the trans woman to jail on assault charges and she was bailed out by her father. During her exam at a rape crisis center, the woman was found to have 42 bruises on her body. She appeared in court 3 weeks later and the charges—that *she* had been the assailant—were dropped.

> He beat the crap out of me before he called the police and said that I had attacked *him*. He even said that I had a knife and that he was defending himself. I was the one with bruises, and the police didn't find any knife in the apartment.
>
> — *Adult trans woman*

- **People ambush or attack you with or without the intent of sexually assaulting you.**
  Transgender people are at greater risk of violent attacks.[81] What should you do if you think this is happening to you?
  - Trust your instincts. In his book, *The Gift of Fear*, Gavin de Becker intimates that if you're afraid, there's probably a legitimate reason. Trust your gut instinct to get out of there.
  - Get out of the situation if you can (that is, run or walk fast).
  - Slip into a convenience store or gas station if you see one.
  - Do not let anyone enter your living space or climb into your car.
  - Do not get into anyone else's car.
  - Be aware that if you carry a weapon, it may be used against you!
  - Do carry a smartphone. You can dial or text 911.
  - Do not dress like a target. This is always such a controversial recommendation; the assailant is responsible for their inexcusable behavior, of course. But 5-inch platform shoes won't allow you to run effectively!

81 Linda Gromko, *Where's MY Book?: A Guide for Transgender and Gender-Nonconforming Youth, Their Parents, & Everyone Else* (Seattle: Bainbridge Books, 2015), 201.

Cyberbullying and the Upstander Pledge

In the Internet age, people can post information about you on the Internet (also known as cyberbullying). The most heartbreaking example of this is the Tyler Clementi story (**tylerclementi.org/tylers-story**).

Tyler was an 18-year-old student at Rutgers University in New Jersey. Musically gifted and brimming with potential, Tyler was just coming into his own and adapting to his new university environment. But Tyler's roommate set up a webcam and, without Tyler's knowledge, livestreamed him having a sexual encounter with a man. The roommate Tweeted about the encounter and invited other students to watch online. Soon, Tyler's private time became fodder for an insensitive Twitter feed among the people who were his new dormitory housemates.

Sadly, Tyler died by suicide a few days later by jumping off the George Washington Bridge.

To their enormous credit, the Clementi family took this tragedy and began the Tyler Clementi Foundation to end all bullying in schools, workplaces, and faith communities. The foundation works to prevent online and offline bullying and promotes legislation to protect all vulnerable youth in their schools, especially LGBTQIA+ youth like Tyler. Donate to the Tyler Clementi Foundation and take the Foundation's Upstander Pledge.

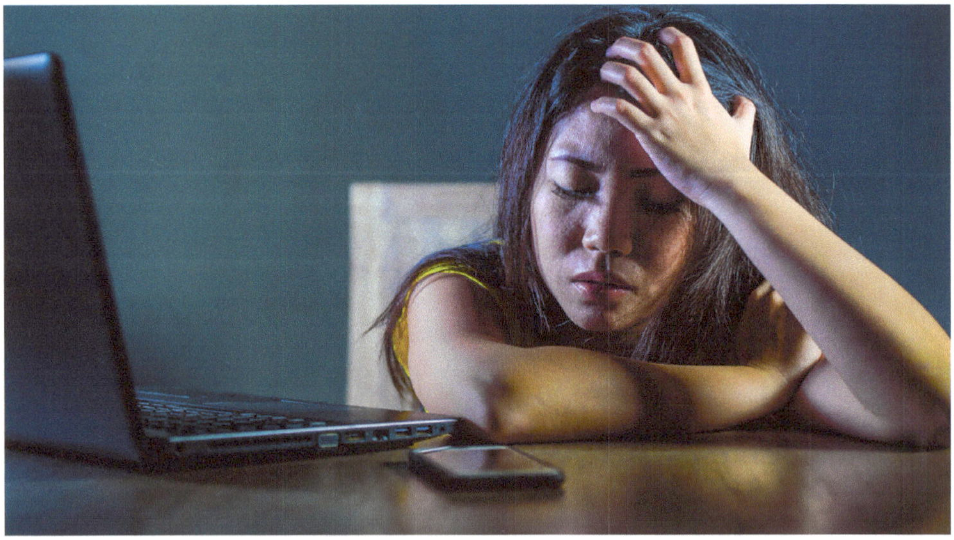

The Upstander Pledge

I Pledge to Be an Upstander.

- I will stand up to bullying whether I'm at school, at home, at work, or in my house of worship; whether I am speaking in the digital cyber world or out in the real world with friends, family, colleagues, or teammates.
- I will work to make others feel safe and included by treating them with kindness, respect, and compassion.
- I will not use insulting or demeaning language, slurs, gestures, facial expressions, or jokes about anyone's sexuality, size, gender, race, any kind of disability, religion, class, politics, or other differences, in person or while using technology.
- If I realized I have hurt someone, I will apologize.
- I will remain vigilant and not be a passive audience or "bystander" to abusive actions or words.

If I See or Hear Behavior That Perpetuates Prejudice:

- I will speak up! I will let others know that bullying, cruelty, and prejudice are abusive and not acceptable.
- If I do not feel safe or if my intervention does not change the poor behaviors, I will tell a trusted adult or person of authority.
- I will reach out to someone I know who has been the target of abusive actions or words and let this person know that this is not okay with me and ask how I can help.

If I Learn in Person or Online That Someone Is Seriously Depressed or Potentially Suicidal:

- I will reach out and tell this person, "Your life has value and is important, no matter how you feel at the moment, and no matter what others say or think."
- I will strongly encourage this person to get professional help.

I Am an Upstander!

Tyler Clementi Foundation

Safety Tips from the Gender Sensei

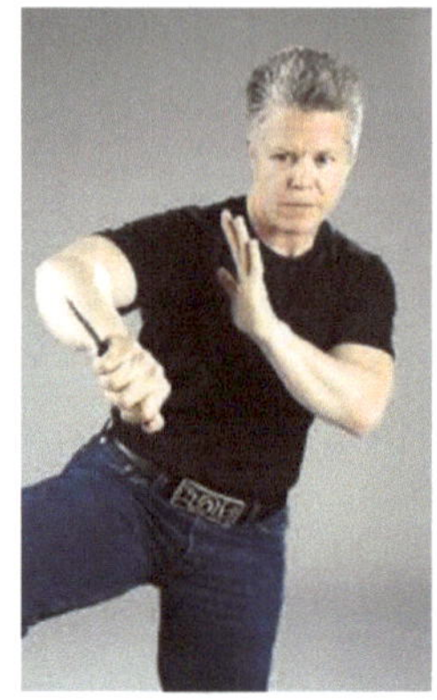

Mac Scotty McGregor, also known as "the Gender Sensei," is a former women's world martial arts champion. He has coached 58 champions and 29 junior Olympic champions. Since his transition, Mac has taught "anything gender": LGBTQIA+ inclusivity, sexuality, and diversity. Mac serves as a contributing writer in The Good Men Project, a media company that explores manhood (goodmenproject.com).

He is also the cofounder and executive director of Positive Masculinity—a nonprofit educational organization aimed at dismantling toxic masculinity and creating a healthier definition of positive masculinity for all. Mac is a frequent lecturer and panelist for healthcare professionals nationwide and hosts his own radio show, *The You Can Make a Difference Show*.

Fitness and self-defense have been priorities for Mac throughout his life. He has taught self-protection in his work with transgender and gender-nonconforming individuals and their advocates. He states, "Safety is even more important when one is transgender or gender-nonconforming. This incites some people, making those of us in the transgender community more likely to be targeted."

Taken from his many workshops on self-defense, Mac offers the following:

Safety Guidelines from the Gender Sensei		
Be Aware		
• Of your surroundings • Of your inner voice • Of things that are out of place • Of your own body language • Of where your keys are	• Of anything that does not feel right • Of anyone that makes you feel uncomfortable • Of where you park	• Of where you are looking • Of exits in any building you are in • Of commonly used manipulation tools

Safety Guidelines from the Gender Sensei	
Do	**Don't**
• Walk with others	• Walk through alleys and secluded areas or close to bushes or shrubbery
• Rideshare with friends	• Walk home alone
• Have keys out and ready	• Walk home alone drunk
• Listen to your inner voice	• Give personal information to a stranger
• Lock doors and windows	• Go home or into a vehicle with someone you don't know
• Put valuables in the vehicle trunk	• Walk with headphones on or earbuds in your ears
• Report suspicious behavior	• Walk around distracted
• Park under lights	• Be hesitant to ask for help
• Walk with your head up and shoulders back	• Listen to unsolicited promises
• Look at people and smile	• Negotiate the word "NO"
• Walk in well-lit, busier areas	• Walk with head down texting or looking at your phone
• Ask for someone to walk you out of meetings and other situations	• Wear your hood up when walking outside (this closes off peripheral vision and hearing)
• If someone makes you feel uncomfortable, call someone and ask them to stay on the phone with you until you feel you are in a safe place; state where you are and describe the person to them if you can	• Feel uncomfortable about asking for an escort to a parking lot at work or school
• Let someone know where you are going	

Table 16.2. Safety guidelines from the Gender Sensei.

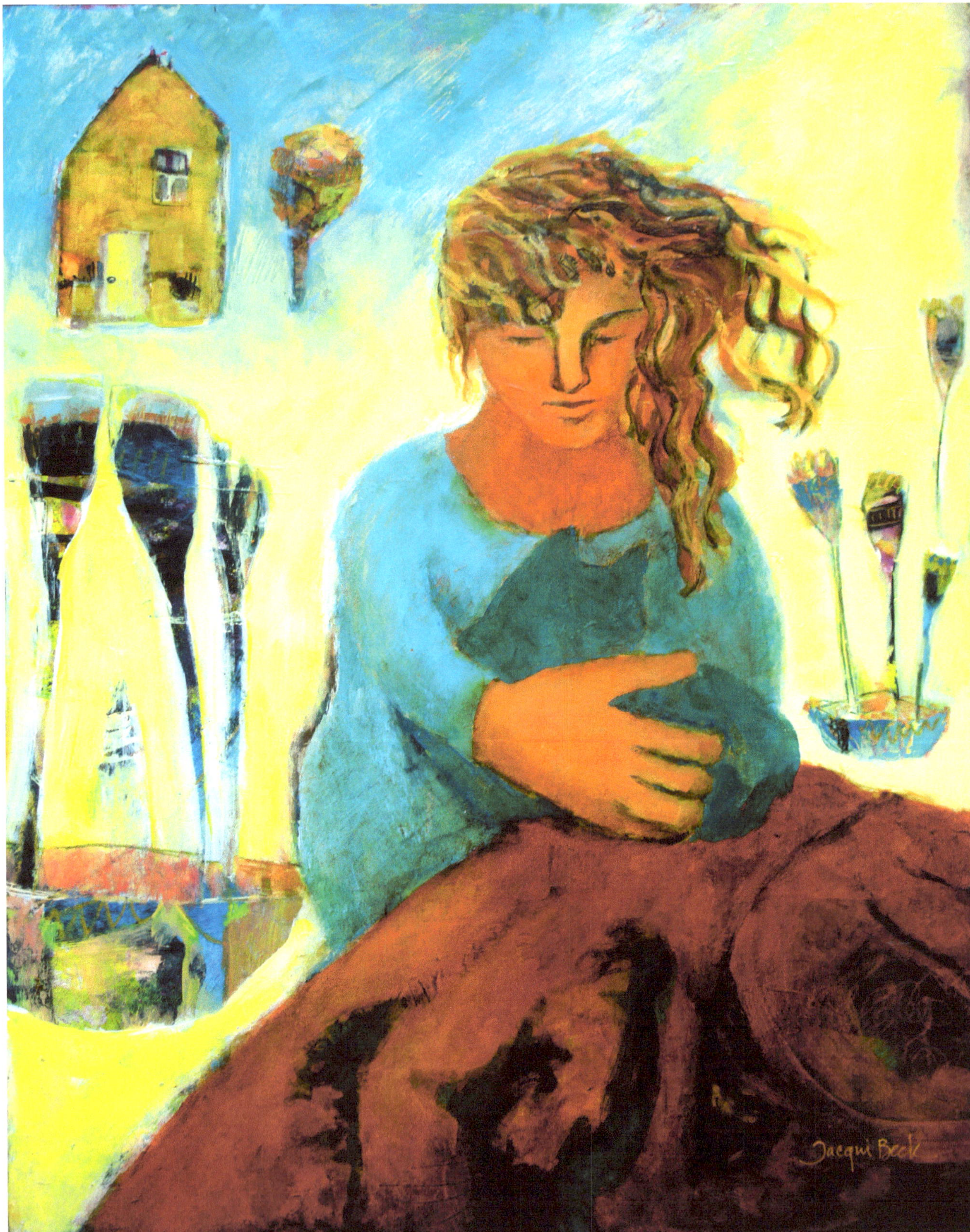

Comfort Found

CHAPTER 17

Recognizing and Treating Depression

Depression is very common, and it impacts the transgender and gender-nonconforming community in greater numbers than their cisgender counterparts.

In this chapter, we will examine the following:

- Symptoms of depression.
- Passive and active suicidal ideation.
- Self-care.
- Treating depression with talk therapy, exercise, and antidepressants. We'll talk about how antidepressants are selected, how they are thought to work, when they begin to work, and how to stop medications.
- Other mental health issues: bipolar disorder, schizophrenia, and borderline personality disorder, as well as their treatment approaches.

> I was talking with one of my young transgender clients and asked if they'd had any problems with depression. Their answer, *Well, I'm trans!*
>
> *— Linda Gromko, MD*

Recognizing Your Own Depression

Most people feel down sometimes. We all have good days and bad days, but having a few bad days is usually not the same as depression.

Depression occurs when a down mood lasts for 2 weeks or more. It may feel like things will never get better. Suicidal thinking, passive or active, can occur. If suicidal thoughts are acted upon, depression can be lethal. (See pages 353–354 for more information on passive and active suicidal ideation.)

Common Symptoms of Depression

- Feeling sad or hopeless, like things will never get better. Seeing the world through this perspective is like looking "through depression glasses."
- Experiencing a sense of emptiness.
- Feeling like a failure even when there's plenty of evidence that you aren't failing at all.

- "Globalizing" things that impact you. For example, rather than saying, "My tire is flat," it's "The whole *world* is flat."
- Feeling personally targeted by general events that impact everyone. For example, during an earthquake, a person might say, "How can this be happening to *me*?" (When, of course, the earthquake is happening to everyone—and more specifically, the earth.) Many people felt extreme anxiety during the 2020 COVID-19 pandemic, while others felt *personally* targeted or *personally* responsible for the illnesses of others.
- Feeling immobilized, like your feet are stuck in glue, and you cannot get moving even to do things that you generally like to do.
- Moving differently—that is, moving or speaking slowly, or being so restless that you fidget or cannot sit still.
- Experiencing a loss of interest in things that normally interest you. You just don't care about playing video games or shopping or doing other things you usually enjoy.

> **I sometimes ask when evaluating a depressed person, "If I could give you a week off and a thousand-dollar bill right now (which I can't), would you feel better?" For people who are truly depressed, it might help for a minute. But overall, it wouldn't seem to matter.**
>
> *— Linda Gromko, MD*

- Dropping out of classes or quitting an "okay" job out of lack of interest or motivation, even though quitting classes or work may not be in one's best interest.
- Feeling a lack of energy.
- Experiencing a disturbance in your sleep—either not being able to sleep or sleeping all the time.
- Awakening early in the morning and not being able to get back to sleep.
- Feeling guilty, often over things that are not within your control.
- Worrying more and often worrying about things that are not in your control.
- Having difficulty concentrating; you find that it is more difficult to read or to remember what you've read.
- Noticing a change in appetite; you eat too much even when you're not hungry or you lose interest in eating altogether. (This may be accompanied by a weight gain or loss even though you aren't trying to gain or lose.)
- Becoming more aware of physical symptoms like aches and pains, headaches, and constipation.
- Isolating or withdrawing from other people.

- Noting a decrease in your libido (sexual appetite).
- Struggling with making routine decisions. Things that are normally easy become difficult for you.
- Feeling more crabby, angrier, or irritable than usual—having a "short fuse."
- Feeling preoccupied about your body's flaws or your appearance with the assumption that nothing will improve. For example, "I cannot ever look female with these hands. Why bother?"
- Becoming preoccupied about death.
- Engaging in risky behaviors.
- Having passive or active suicidal thinking.

Risky Behaviors

Risky behaviors can escalate during depression. These behaviors can "soothe" a person temporarily but often have long-term negative consequences:

- Taking risks with driving, such as driving too fast or driving under the influence of alcohol or other substances
- Making poor sexual decisions
- Cutting and engaging in other self-harm behaviors
- Engaging in eating disorders like anorexia or bulimia
- Using alcohol, tobacco, and other substances more than usual
- Hanging around people who reinforce risky behaviors

A person does not have to have *all of the symptoms* listed to be depressed. But if you have even one or two, *get expert help*, especially if you are thinking of harming yourself. Go back to Chapter 1 and review the emergency resources to use if you are feeling suicidal, and read on for more information about managing depression.

Passive and Active Suicidal Ideation

Passive suicidal ideation occurs when a person imagines, "I wouldn't care if I got cancer or had a serious car wreck," or "It wouldn't matter if I died." But while this person would be "okay" with their own death, they are not currently planning a method of dying or a time to actively end their life.

Active suicidal ideation occurs when a person is thinking of suicide and is orchestrating a way to end their life. When contemplating suicide, an individual may exhibit clues, sometimes called "cries for help." These behaviors may include the following:

- Collecting potentially lethal medications to take in an overdose.
- Researching information about suicide methods.
- Obtaining a firearm with the intent to use it on themselves.
- Composing a suicide note.
- Posting messages on social media platforms about wanting to die.
- Saying goodbye to people who have been important in their life.
- Giving away things like prized possessions or valuables.
- Asking a friend to take care of a pet.
- Becoming more isolated, even secretive ("I won't tell you because you would have to do something to intervene").
- Increasing the use of alcohol or other drugs.
- Taking personal risks, perhaps taking risks with driving.
- Antagonizing or becoming aggressive toward police officers to instigate "suicide by cop." This refers to a situation where an officer shoots a person who is threatening them; the person succumbs in a suicidal act although someone else (the officer) pulled the trigger.

Active suicidal ideation and planning are true life-and-death emergencies. If you notice an individual exhibiting "cries for help," understand that talking with them will not prompt them into suicidal thinking; most likely, they've already thought of it. It's fine to express your concern about their well-being. Give them hotline information or go with them to their counselor or to an emergency room. They need expert help, and you may be the one to help them find it.

Practical Self-Care Measures That Help in Depression and Crisis

Before we discuss the formal diagnosis and treatment of depression, let's examine self-care measures that can help you or someone else going through a difficult time. (Sadly, these measures may be less available in the COVID-19 pandemic.)

- **Structure your time.**
  - Have something to do on the calendar every day. Go to the movies, even by yourself. Watch a TV show you have enjoyed in the past or get hooked on binge-watching something new to you. You aren't trying to have fun necessarily; you're just trying to get yourself through to the next day.
  - Make and keep a routine, including regular calls to a friend or a crisis hotline.
  - Get out of the house. Many venues like public libraries, bookstores, museums, or zoos have free afternoon or evening classes or lectures. Go simply to spend the time; don't worry too much about the subject matter.
- **Try to get some order in your life, even a part of it.**

- Make your bed.
- Put your dishes in the dishwasher, or at least in the kitchen sink.
- Do some laundry so you'll have something clean to wear.
- Take a shower, comb your hair, and get dressed.
- Keep an eye on expenses and bills; late fees or missed payments will make you feel worse.

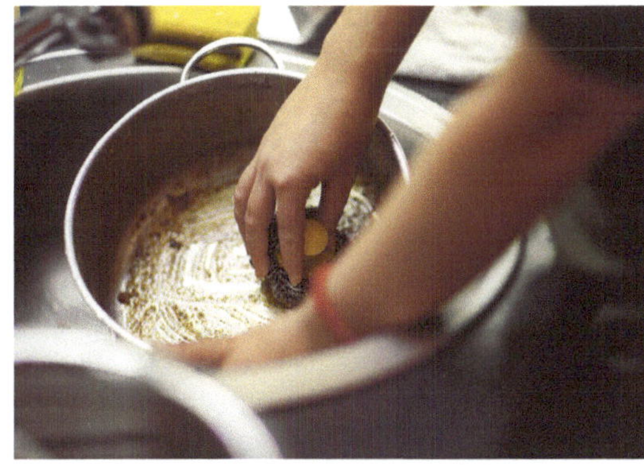

- **Move your body.**
  - Any exercise is fine, particularly activities with a clear start-and-stop time—that is, a walk around a small lake or a YouTube yoga class.
  - Do aerobic exercise like biking, running, dancing, or walking fast if you are trying to defuse anger or frustration.
- **If anything seems appetizing or comforting, do it as long as it's safe and legal.**
  - This might apply to listening to music, reading something that's not too demanding, drinking tea, taking a relaxing bath, eating chocolate, or another pleasurable activity.
- **Be with people.**
  - Depression, sadness, and loss are better managed when not in isolation. Despair or suicidal thinking are enormous secrets that are far too important to keep to yourself. Give yourself or the person you are concerned about the chance to share this information with people who can help.

Do Not Promise to Keep the Secret of Suicidal Thinking for Yourself or Someone Else

If a patient asks me if I will keep a secret, I say, "That depends on the secret. If you are actively suicidal, homicidal, or a danger to yourself or others, I am legally obliged to share this information with people who can help you."

Anyone can say this to a friend, although your obligation may not be a legal one as it is with a healthcare provider.

If You Recognize That You Are Depressed or in Crisis, Seek Help

- Find a therapist if you don't have one. (Ask your healthcare provider, or call a community service agency, your health insurance company, a transgender resource, or—if your city has one—a 211 line.)
- See your therapist more often than usual; some people go every day if they're in crisis.
- Ask your mental health provider about a voluntary admission to a psychiatric facility if you're concerned about keeping yourself safe.
- Use the suicide hotline numbers: Trans Lifeline: 1-877-565-8860; Crisis Connections (formerly Crisis Clinic): 1-866-427-4747; National Suicide Prevention Lifeline: 1-800-273-8255; or call 911. Add them to your phone to keep them available.

- Go to an emergency room and tell the ER personal that you are depressed, particularly if you aren't sure you can keep yourself safe.

Would You Like to Take a Depression Test Online?

Search the Internet for the PHQ-9 (a patient health questionnaire self-test for depression) or the Beck Depression Inventory (BDI). These tools are not substitutions for a visit with a medical provider, but they can give you more information:

ismanet.org/doctoryourspirit/pdfs/Beck-Depression-Inventory-BDI.pdf

Treating Depression

In 1989, a classic study examined the question of how depression is best treated. The investigators took a group of depressed individuals and divided them into four subgroups: One group received interpersonal therapy, another group received cognitive behavioral therapy, a third group was given the antidepressant imipramine, and a fourth group received no treatment (a placebo group). "Patients in all treatments showed a significant reduction in depressive symptoms and improvement in functioning over the course of treatment." That is to say, talk therapy and medications all worked while the placebo group did not improve.[82]

Later studies verified the theory that physical exercise in a variety of forms reduces depressive symptoms.[83]

The "Trifecta" Treatment

My personal preference is to bring out the "trifecta" when patients are depressed. So I may recommend counseling, antidepressant medications, and exercise.

Talk therapy (cognitive therapy or counseling) for people on the gender spectrum is often best done by a therapist who is familiar with gender dysphoria and its many related issues and interventions. If you live in Seattle, look up the Ingersoll Gender Center website (**ingersollgendercenter.org/ingersoll-directory/**) for a list of mental health professionals who are familiar with gender issues.

Exercise can be any form of physical activity (but preferably aerobic) that a person is willing to do. Any sort of movement can help, even simple walking. (I don't think it makes much sense to champion exercise activities that people don't like. If a person is willing to walk regularly in a shopping mall, that can work.) Exercise is also helpful in managing anxiety.

Many people express concern about taking antidepressants, fearing that they will develop a dependency or that it's "putting a bandage on a problem."

---

82 Irene Elkin et al., "National Institute of Mental Health Treatment of Depression Collaborative Research Program: General Effectiveness of Treatments," *Archives of General Psychiatry* 46, no. 11 (December 1989): 971–82, https://doi.org/10.1001/archpsyc.1989.01810110013002.

83 Lynette L. Craft, and Frank M. Perna, "The Benefits of Exercise for the Clinically Depressed," *The Primary Care Companion to the Journal of Clinical Psychiatry* 6, no. 3 (February 2004): 104–11, doi: 10.4088/pcc.v06n0301.

In my opinion, antidepressants are not habit-forming, although people may experience uncomfortable symptoms when they stop antidepressants abruptly. I've personally seen these medications save lives. They help people survive the most desperate of times and simply get to the other side. You cannot solve any of your problems if you die by suicide.

— Linda Gromko, MD

Remember that cognitive therapy and exercise *are* available and effective in treating depression if a person truly wants to avoid medications. But read the next part to see how medications may be appropriately selected and used in lifesaving treatment.

If you or someone in your family is depressed, make sure that potentially harmful medications (all prescription drugs, painkillers, and even Tylenol and Motrin) are locked up and out of reach of the person who's at risk. Consider having Narcan at home to reverse an intentional overdose of opiates. And if you have firearms or other weapons at home, take care to store them properly, locked and separate from ammunition. If you cannot trust yourself to handle firearms, ask a trusted friend or family member to take care of this.

Using Antidepressants

While they are not for everyone, antidepressants do have a role in helping many people. Let's look at some basic information on how they work.

You have roughly 86 billion neurons (nerve cells) in your brain. These neurons communicate with one another. When your brain's messages are not connecting optimally, you may become depressed.

Neurons communicate by sending electrical impulses from one to another. Each electrical impulse originates in the neuron's cell body (see Figure 17.1), travels down the length of a long cablelike structure called an "axon," and jumps across the synapse (the space between neurons) to fire off the next nerve cell.

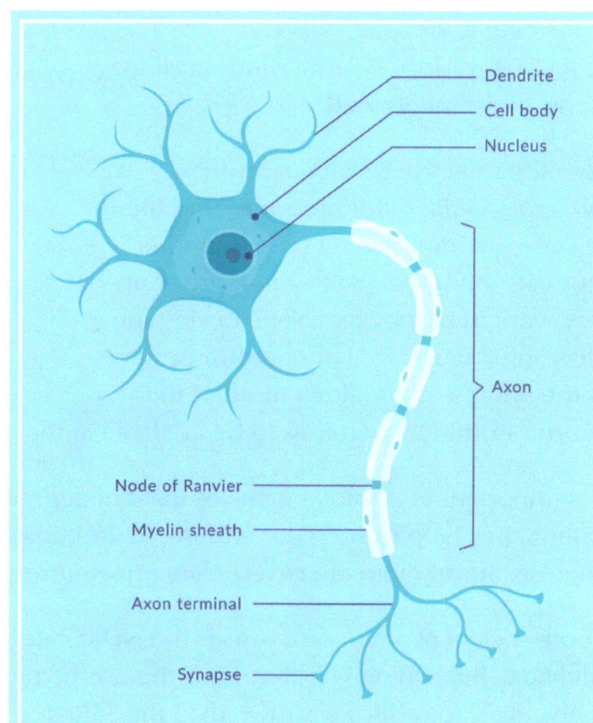

Figure 17.1. Anatomy of a neuron.

Located in the synapse are neurotransmitter chemicals that help the nerve impulses travel from one neuron to another. You've probably heard about the neurotransmitters serotonin and norepinephrine. We also have dopamine, gamma aminobutyric acid (GABA), and probably many more neurotransmitters that are yet to be discovered.

Let's focus on serotonin and norepinephrine. These neurotransmitters are released by the presynaptic neuron, travel across the synapse, and then combine with receptor areas on the postsynaptic neuron in order for the nerve signal to continue on down the chain of neurons in the brain.

Think of it this way: If a nerve conduction is traveling from north to south, the northern neuron is the presynapse neuron and the southern neuron would be the postsynapse neuron.

Neurotransmitters are recycled by being reabsorbed by the presynaptic neuron. It is believed that people with depression may not have as many neurotransmitters available in their synapses, or their postsynaptic receptors are not as sensitive to the neurotransmitters. Therefore, people with depression have neuronal messages that are transmitted less effectively.

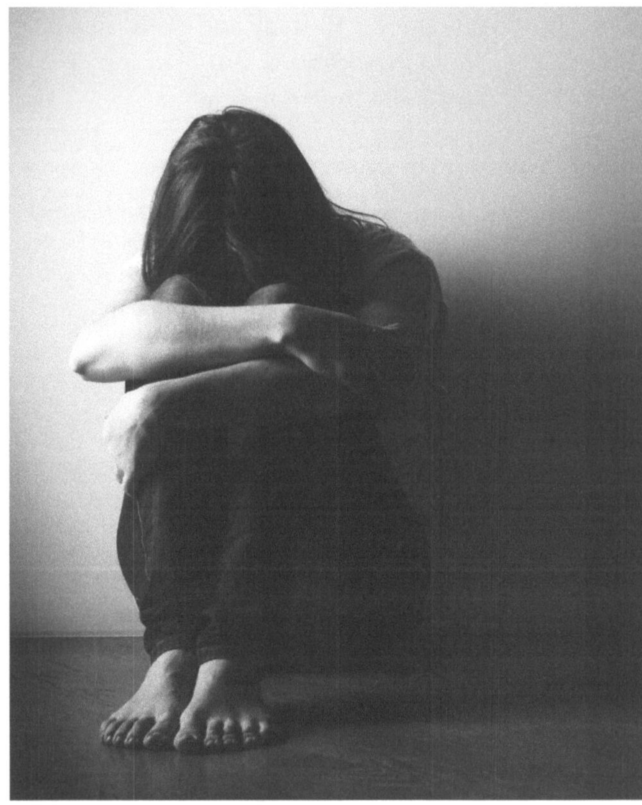

You have undoubtedly heard about the **SSRI (selective serotonin reuptake inhibitors)** with the prototype fluoxetine (Prozac). Others in the SSRI class include paroxetine (Paxil), sertraline (Zoloft), citalopram (Celexa), and escitalopram (Lexapro).

The SNRI class (serotonin and norepinephrine reuptake inhibitors) with the prototype venlafaxine (Effexor) are sometimes known as "combination" antidepressants. Others in this class include desvenlafaxine (Pristiq) and duloxetine (Cymbalta). Refer to Table 17.1 on page 360 for further clarification on all the medications mentioned.

Both the selective serotonin reuptake inhibitors (SSRI antidepressants) and the selective serotonin and norepinephrine reuptake inhibitors (SNRI antidepressants) may work in part by partially blocking the recycling ("reuptake") of neurotransmitters in the synapse. This allows more of the neurotransmitter chemicals to be available in the synaptic cleft to assist with nerve conduction.

It is important to remind ourselves that antidepressants do not *make* more neurotransmitter chemicals. Rather, they help to keep our existing neurotransmitters in the synapse where they can help the nerve impulses travel more effectively from one neuron to the next.

Another class of antidepressants is the **NDRI category, or the norepinephrine and dopamine reuptake inhibitors.** Bupropion (Wellbutrin) is the prototype of this category. Bupropion is well known because it is less likely to reduce sex drive than the SSRI and SNRI antidepressants. It is more likely to be weight-"neutral"—that is, it does not contribute to weight gain or loss. Interestingly, bupropion is also marketed under the name Zyban and promoted to help people lose their craving for cigarette smoking.

The antidepressants listed here are also used to treat panic disorder, generalized anxiety disorder, post-traumatic stress disorder, obsessive-compulsive disorder, and other disorders. SSRIs may be used in premenstrual dysphoric disorder and fibromyalgia. The SNRI duloxetine (Cymbalta) may help reduce symptoms of peripheral neuropathy.

Atypical antidepressants are less likely to fall into the other categories above, and they include the following:

- Mirtazapine (Remeron): known for sedation and weight gain
- Trazodone (Desyrel): used today primarily for insomnia
- Vortioxetine (Trintellix)
- Vilazodone (Viibryd)
- Bupropion: considered "atypical" but is also classified as a NDRI

Tricyclic antidepressants are older medications that were found to have more side effects and greater lethality than the medications commonly used today. Less likely to be first-line medications in treating depression, the tricyclics are sometimes used in smaller doses for treating chronic pain. Examples include imipramine (Tofranil), nortriptyline (Pamelor), amitriptyline (Elavil), doxepin (Sinequan), and desipramine (Norpramin).

The class of **monoamine oxidase inhibitors, or MAOIs**, is generally reserved for specific situations where other antidepressants have not helped. Monoamine oxidase is an enzyme that breaks down serotonin, norepinephrine, and dopamine; thus, *inhibiting* monoamine oxidase makes more of these neurotransmitters available. Examples include tranylcypromine (Parnate), phenelzine (Nardil), and isocarboxazid (Marplan). MAOIs may interact with other medications such as pain medications and decongestants, as well as a number of foods, causing severe blood pressure elevations. The most recent MAOI is Emsam, which is used as a patch. The patch contains selegiline, a reversible MAOI. Emsam has fewer side effects than other MAOIs.

How Healthcare Providers Choose an Antidepressant for a Patient

First of all, it is important to clarify the diagnosis. Is the person suffering from a depressive disorder? Or does an individual have bipolar disorder or another mental health disturbance that may require a different type of medication altogether? (Refer to "Other Common Psychiatric Conditions" on page 363.)

Assuming the diagnosis is correct, here are some guide questions used by healthcare providers in selecting an appropriate antidepressant:

- Has the patient used a specific antidepressant before that worked well? If so, I will often start with the same medication.
- What antidepressants have worked well or poorly with the patient's immediate family members?[84] If I know that a medication worked particularly well in a first-degree family member (parent, sibling, or child), I will often prescribe this first.

84 Richard L. O'Reilly, Lisa Bogue, and Shiva M. Singh, "Pharmacogenetic Response to Antidepressants in a Multicase Family with Affective Disorder," *Biological Psychiatry* 36, no. 7 (October 1994): 467–71, https://doi.org/10.1016/0006-3223(94)90642-4.

Common Antidepressant Medications				
Antidepressant Category	**Neurotransmitters Impacted**	**Generic Names**	**Brand Names**	**Comments**
SSRI (selective serotonin reuptake inhibitors)	Serotonin	Fluoxetine Paroxetine Sertraline Citalopram Escitalopram	Prozac Paxil Zoloft Celexa Lexapro	Caution regarding suicidality applies to all antidepressants
SNRI (serotonin and norepinephrine reuptake inhibitors)	Serotonin and norepinephrine	Venlafaxine Desvenlafaxine Duloxetine Levomilnacipran	Effexor XR Pristiq Cymbalta Fetzima	Cymbalta has FDA indication for peripheral neuropathy; all meds in class help
NDRI (norepinephrine and dopamine reuptake inhibitors)	Norepinephrine and dopamine	Bupropion	Wellbutrin WellbutrinXL Aplenzin Forfivo XL	Weight and sex drive remain neutral; marketed as Zyban to help with smoking cessation
Atypical Antidepressants	Serotonin and norepinephrine	Mirtazapine Trazodone Vortioxetine Vilazodone Bupropion	Remeron Desyrel Trintellix Viibryd Wellbutrin and others	Mirtazapine is sedating and is associated with weight gain; trazodone is used mostly for sleep
Tricyclic Antidepressants (serotonin and norepinephrine reuptake inhibitors)	Serotonin and norepinephrine	Imipramine Nortriptyline Amitriptyline Doxepin Desipramine	Tofranil Pamelor Elavil Sinequan Norpramin	Older meds with more side effects and greater lethality; usually not "first-line" antidepressants
MAOIs (monoamine oxidase inhibitors)	Monoamine oxidase, which breaks down serotonin, norepinephrine, and dopamine	Tranylcypromine Phenelzine Isocarboxazid Selegiline	Parnate Nardil Marplan Emsam	Drug and food interactions may lead to high blood pressure

Table 17.1. Common antidepressant medications.

- Are there any typical side effects that may actually serve the patient? For example, bupropion can help reduce cravings for smoking. It is also "weight neutral" (doesn't impact a person's weight) and doesn't tend to reduce libido (sexual appetite). Remeron may make people quite sedated, but if taken before bed, it can be helpful if insomnia is a problem. Remeron is also associated with weight gain, which can be a desired effect in *some* people.

> **If you look at people who have had one episode of depression, the risk of relapsing into depression is 50 percent in the next 5 years. If you have been depressed twice, the risk is 70 percent in the next 5 years. And if you have been depressed three times, the risk of relapse in the next 5 years is 90 percent.**
>
> **Because of this data, if you have been depressed three times, or if you have been depressed twice and the depression was very severe, the current guidelines suggest staying on the medication or combination of medications that have successfully treated depression because doing so reduces the risk of relapse to approximately 25 percent of what it would be if someone goes off antidepressant medication.**
>
> *— Steven R. Mitchell, MD, PhD*

Antidepressants' Therapeutic Dose: When They Begin to Work

I usually tell patients that it takes about 4 to 6 weeks for antidepressants to reach a plateau. The onset of relief of symptoms may be very variable. During the first week or two, you may feel mild side effects like nausea, fatigue, jitteriness, or yawning, but you really may not feel much different otherwise. That is why it is so important to get help when you feel yourself beginning to sink into depression. *Don't wait until you can barely go on before you try to get an appointment.*

I often start with small doses of an antidepressant and work up to a therapeutic dose. This way, a patient has the opportunity to get used to the new medication. After all, most antidepressants do work. It's important that people aren't derailed by temporary side effects.

You may not experience the full antidepressant effect before 6 to 8 weeks on an antidepressant, and even then, the effects may be subtle. *Other* people may notice improvement before you do. People may say that you "look rested," or they may ask if you've been on vacation or changed your hair. But, little by little, you will start to feel better.

Remember that alcohol is a depressant. Even though it may make you feel more relaxed temporarily, it tends to contribute to depression, and in fact, *it is like taking a depressant.* So cut back on alcohol if this applies to you.

In the meantime, while your medication is starting to work, you will hopefully be involved in counseling and exercising as best as you can. These aspects of treatment can make an enormous difference in your recovery.

The "Black Box Warning" Regarding Suicide and Antidepressants

The FDA requires that all antidepressants carry "black box warnings"—the strictest warnings for prescriptions.[85]

Some people, particularly teenagers and young adults under the age of 25, experience an increase in suicidal thinking or behavior when they begin antidepressants or when a dose is increased. Some physicians have postulated that the medications may make people more "activated," and they may become more likely to *act* on their thoughts—including suicidal thoughts.

Does this mean we shouldn't use antidepressants? Not at all. But it does mean that a person should get emergency help if symptoms of depression worsen, particularly when a medication is started or a dose is increased. Remember that *the greatest risk of depression is suicide*, and antidepressants can be life-saving.

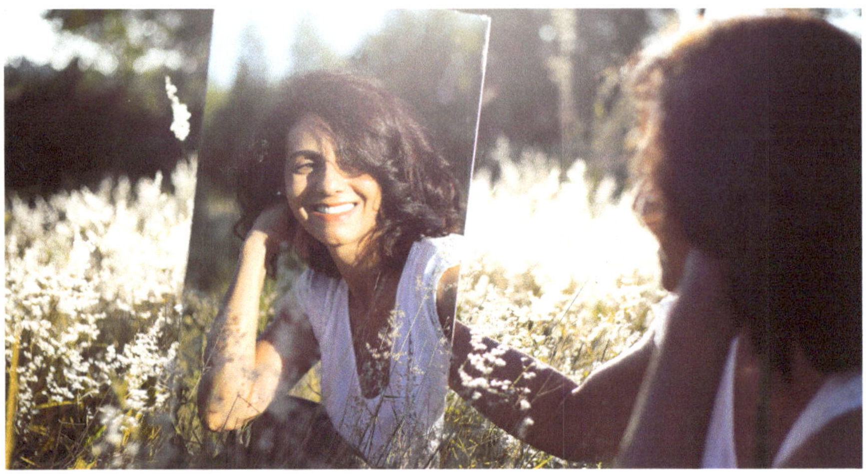

How and When to Stop Antidepressants

Antidepressants are frequently used for a period of about 1 year. They are not physically addictive in the sense that a person does not get a high from them, and increasing doses are not needed to produce the same effect over time.

We often start antidepressants in gradually increasing doses. When I help a patient stop them, I suggest that they taper off the medication gradually rather than stopping them abruptly. People who stop antidepressants too quickly may experience discontinuation symptoms, such as "brain zaps," dizziness, or an unusual sensation of moving your eyes and "having your vision follow behind."

I advise my patients to set themselves up for success when selecting the best time to stop their antidepressants. For instance, don't stop when daylight savings time "turns to winter." And do not stop on the anniversary of a significant date in your life, like the death of a loved one. It may be helpful to take advantage of increased sunlight by stopping antidepressants in the spring or summer, but only if that is a good time as negotiated by you and your healthcare provider.

85 Mayo Clinic, "Antidepressants: Selecting One That's Right for You," *Mayo Clinic*, December 31, 2019, https://www.mayoclinic.org/diseases-conditions/depression/in-depth/antidepressants/art-20046273.

If you strongly oppose the use of antidepressants for any reason, do start treatment for depression by using therapy and exercise. These work! Other methods of treatment, such as transcranial nerve stimulation, light boxes or dawn simulators, dietary supplements, ketamine or esketamine, or even electroconvulsive therapy, can be used in selected patients. Get expert help.

When Hospitalization Is Recommended for Depression

Psychiatric admission is required when a person is actively suicidal and cannot guarantee their personal safety. We may ask patients to agree to a "No-Harm Pact." If they cannot promise *not* to harm themselves, they may require admission or at least an evaluation in the emergency room.

In Washington State, a person cannot be committed to a psychiatric facility without their consent unless they are suicidal, homicidal, dangerous to property due to mental illness, or "gravely disabled." The latter refers to an extreme lack of self-care. In Seattle, these conditions are assessed by a trained designated mental health professional (DMHP)—only recently referred to as the designated crisis responder (DCR)—who may be dispatched by a local crisis clinic. If detained, a person may be kept on a 72-hour hold, but they cannot be held longer unless mandated in a court hearing. Legislation that defines this process protects people from being committed inappropriately by family members or even healthcare professionals.

Sometimes a psychiatric hospitalization is helpful in the process of diagnosing a person's illness. Some conditions can be difficult to diagnose, such as depression versus bipolar disorder. A period of observation can help psychiatrists diagnose and appropriately treat the patient while keeping them in a safe environment.

Other Common Psychiatric Conditions

While a full discussion of psychiatric diagnoses is well beyond the scope of this book, let's look briefly at some common problems that may mimic depressive disorder. Be aware that mental illness is more prevalent in the transgender and gender-nonconforming community—and that there may be considerable overlap between conditions.

Bipolar Disorder

Bipolar disorder (also called manic depressive disorder) is a condition characterized by swings in mood (highs and lows). It is easy to spot someone with bipolar I disorder (BP1) who is experiencing an acute manic "high." They talk too fast ("pressured speech"), move too quickly, have racing thoughts, spend money liberally, and become more sexual than usual. While initially creative and engaging, a manic individual may become "out of control," agitated, and sometimes threatening or violent to those around them.

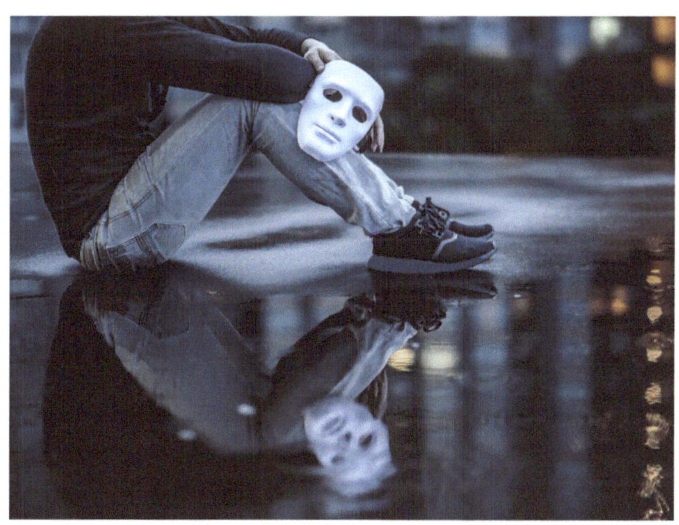

Manic individuals may experience delusions of grandeur and an absolute belief in their own special powers. They may lose touch with reality and sometimes experience hallucinations. Manic individuals may go for several days without needing sleep. Mania may be followed by periods of hypomania (an elevated but more normal mood), or by a normal mood, or by periods of deep depression. Due to the extreme and unpredictable nature of mania, it is not uncommon to see manic individuals detained involuntarily in psychiatric emergency facilities.

While symptoms of bipolar disorder can be quite dramatic, there is often a long delay in accurately diagnosing this disease. One reason is that patients with bipolar disorder have no mood symptoms about half of the time. For one third of the time, they have some symptoms of depression and only one sixth of the time do they have any manic or hypomanic symptoms. When they do have manic symptoms, these are usually mild.

Patients with bipolar disorder, on average, spend only 14 hours a year in full-blown mania. For the vast majority of the time, they do not show the classic symptoms of mania. Bipolar patients are very often misdiagnosed as depressed, and it may take years before they are correctly diagnosed.[86]

Individuals with BP1 are treated with "mood stabilizers," including the following:

- Lithium (Lithobid or Eskalith)
- Lamotrigine (Lamictal)
- Ziprasidone (Geodon)
- Lurasidone (Latuda)
- Valproic acid (Depakote)
- Aripiprazole (Abilify)
- Olanzapine (Zyprexa)
- Quetiapine (Seroquel)
- Carbamazepine (Tegretol) and others

Some of the mood stabilizers have antipsychotic properties; some are also anticonvulsants.

Things to Watch for with Antidepressants

Antidepressants like SSRIs that are used without mood stabilizers may actually worsen mania. It is critical that people taking medications for bipolar disorder have expert advice. Transgender women taking estradiol should be aware that estradiol and lamotrigine can interact. Estradiol increases the clearing of lamotrigine and may result in lower levels of lamotrigine and decreased therapeutic effects.

See drugs.com/ppa/estrogens-progestins-transdermal-combination-products.html.

86 Judd, Lewis L. et al., "The Long-term Natural History of the Weekly Symptomatic Status of Bipolar 1 Disorder," *Archives of General Psychiatry* 59, no. 6 (July 2002): 530–37, https://doi.org/10.1001/archpsyc.59.6.530.

Individuals who experience bipolar II disorder (BP2) experience periods of depression interspersed with normal mood or hypomania, but not full-blown mania. Hypomania may be described as an individual feeling upbeat or confident rather than invincible. Psychiatrists use mood stabilizers to treat BP2.

Bipolar disorder can be hereditary. The disorder generally begins in the teens or in young adulthood and lasts lifelong in varying degrees. Manic or hypomanic individuals may attempt to decrease agitation by using alcohol, and it is not uncommon to see alcohol dependency become a separate problem or comorbidity.

Schizophrenia

Schizophrenia is a serious and often disabling mental illness involving distortions of reality. As with bipolar disorder, it frequently begins in young adulthood and lasts lifelong. People who are schizophrenic have delusions (false beliefs) or hallucinations (experiencing visions or voices that aren't real). They may experience depression or paranoia; they interact with others in ways that isolate them or prevent them functioning in society. As in bipolar disorder, there is a genetic predisposition. Depression and suicide are prevalent, and it is common to see people trying to manage their symptoms with substances such as alcohol.

Medications for schizophrenia are typically antipsychotics that help to give order to and organize an individual's thoughts. A psychiatrist I knew used to refer to antipsychotic medications as "mind glue." You will notice some overlap between the following medications used in schizophrenia and those used to treat bipolar disorder:

- Aripiprazole (Abilify)
- Brexpiprazole (Rexulti)
- Cariprazine (Vraylar)
- Clozapine (Clozaril, Versacloz)
- Lurasidone (Latuda)
- Olanzapine (Zyprexa)
- Quetiapine (Seroquel)
- Risperidone (Risperdal)
- Ziprasidone (Geodon)

Borderline Personality Disorder

It is important to mention borderline personality disorder, if only for clarity. Borderline personality disorder is often referred to as "BPD," so it is understandably confused with bipolar disorder. The two conditions are not the same, although there may be some overlap. As with any diagnosis—or any label for that matter—be certain which condition you are describing!

Borderline personality disorder is classified as a *personality* disorder, whereas bipolar disorder is considered a *mood* disorder. With a personality disorder, the symptoms are more pervasive over time whereas bipolar symptoms occur when a patient is activated or depressed. Borderline individuals have frequent shifts in opinion ("I love you/I hate you"), and they tend to see things in a black and white, concrete way (for instance, they may view a person as being 100 percent right or 100 percent wrong with no middle ground). They frequently experience conflict in relationships. (A patient of mine swears by the book, *I Hate You—Don't Leave Me*, by Jerold J. Kreisman and Hal Straus; the title alone is an apt description of BPD.)

Use the following table to identify some important differences and similarities between the conditions.

Bipolar Disorder and Borderline Personality Disorder Comparisons

Features of the Condition	Bipolar Disorder: Bipolar I And II	Borderline Personality Disorder
Classified as a mood or a personality disorder?	Mood disorder	Personality disorder
Can medications help?	Mood stabilizers, antipsychotics, and anticonvulsants Caution: If antidepressants are used without mood stabilizers, they may activate mania.	Frequently uses the same meds as with bipolar disorder but is often medication-resistant; dialectical behavioral therapy (DBT), developed by Marsha M. Linehan, PhD, focuses on mindfulness and is a mainstay of treatment
Symptoms	The individual is essentially normal* between episodes of highs (mania) and lows (depression) and likely to be functioning at work and in relationships	Pervasive features of personality, such as fear of abandonment, unstable relationships, frequent suicidal ideation, dissociative symptoms, and difficulty interacting with others
Type of therapy	Individual or group cognitive behavioral therapy, medications	Dialectical behavioral therapy (DBT) focuses on mindfulness; also transference-focused therapy
Thought patterns	Essentially normal* between episodes of mania and depression	Black-and-white thinking: all good or all bad
Impulsivity	Essentially normal* between episodes	Frequent suicidal ideation and threats of self-harm
Genetic role?	Yes	Yes

*Variability may be influenced by rapidity of cycling of highs and lows.

Table 17.2. Bipolar disorder and borderline personality disorder comparisons.

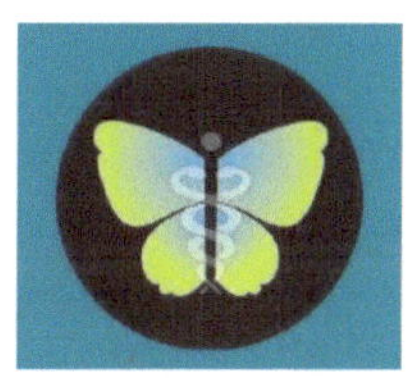

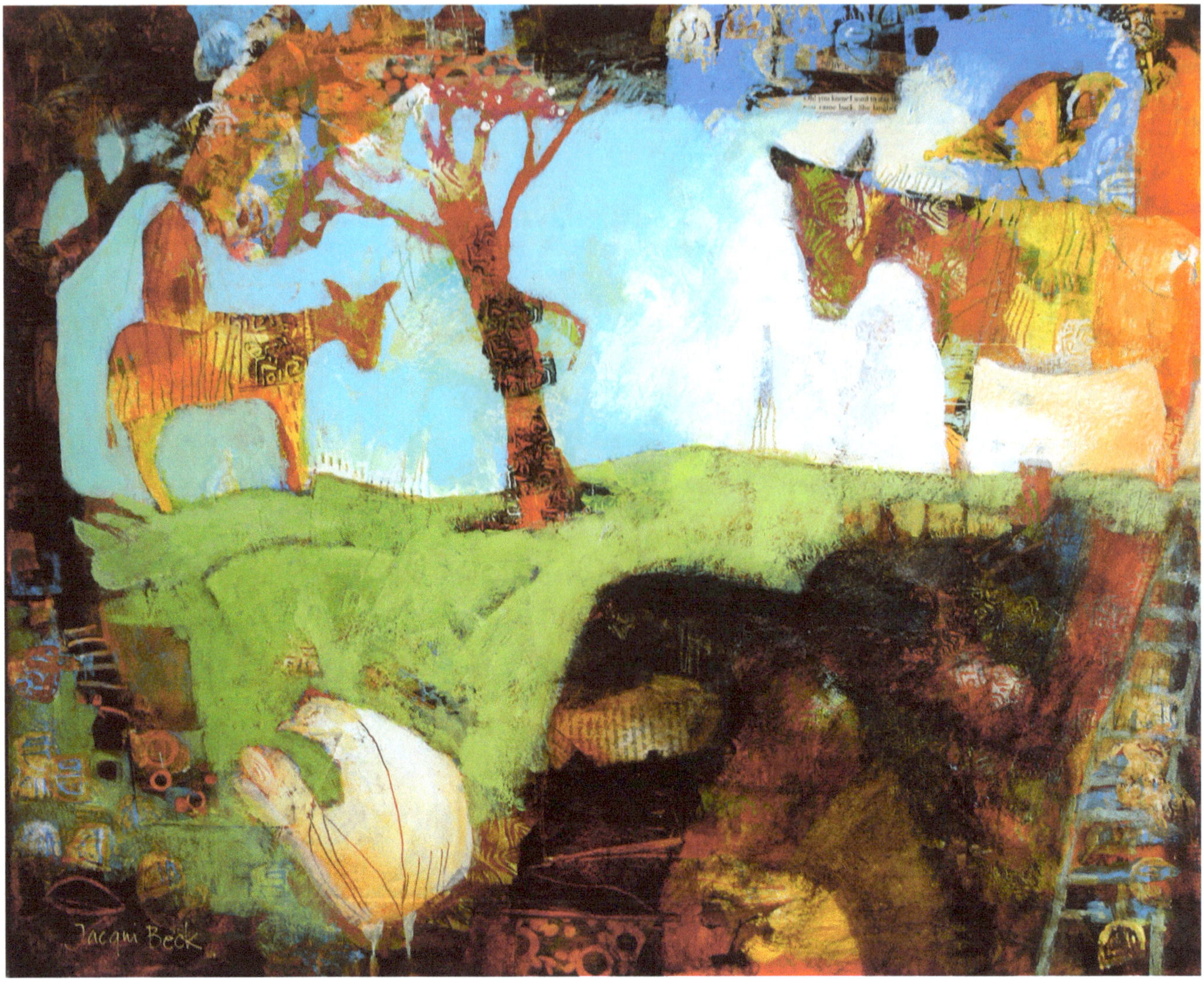

Hidden Underneath

CHAPTER 18

Trauma-Informed Care and Resilience: Adverse Childhood Experiences and PTSD

Like many healthcare providers, I've been learning about trauma-informed care, adverse childhood experiences, and PTSD. I know I can't possibly do justice to these topics, but I feel compelled to include some of the basics.

Trauma and resilience are topics of extreme importance in the transgender and gender-nonconforming community. In this chapter, we will take a *very* brief look at the following topics:

- **What we have learned about the inequities experienced by transgender individuals through national surveys**
- **Adverse childhood experiences (ACE)**
  - How are these experiences quantified through the ACE questionnaire?
  - What outcome differences are observed in people with high ACE scores?
  - How can we help people with high ACE scores develop resilience?
- **Post-traumatic stress disorder (PTSD)**
  - What is post-traumatic stress disorder? What are the symptoms of PTSD?
  - What are some forms of treatment for PTSD?
  - What is complex PTSD?
- **How an individual with PTSD or a high ACE score can protect themselves in vulnerable healthcare circumstances**
- **How healthcare providers can support patients in vulnerable clinical experiences**

What We Have Learned about the Inequities Experienced by Transgender Individuals

The National Transgender Discrimination Study (NTDS) and the US Transgender Survey (USTS) uncovered volumes about the traumas and inequities experienced by transgender individuals. (The NTDS surveyed more than 6,400 transgender and gender-nonconforming people, and the data were reported in 2011 (**transequality.org/issues/resources/national-transgender-discrimination-survey-full-report**). The USTS surveyed 28,000 respondents in 2015 and data were reported in 2016 (**ustranssurvey.org/reports**).

For many of us serving the community, the data confirm various inequities we had observed in our clients for years. Most importantly, the data validated the experiences of members of the transgender and gender-nonconforming communities.

Through these studies, we know that "transgender and gender-nonconforming people face injustice at every turn: in childhood homes, in school systems that promise to shelter and educate, in harsh and exclusionary workplaces, at the grocery store, the hotel front desk, in doctors' offices and emergency rooms, before judges and at the hands of landlords, police officers, healthcare workers, and other service providers."[87]

The differences were so all-encompassing that the first survey was nicknamed "Injustice at Every Turn." Rather than cite the surveys more broadly, let me present a small sample of findings from the 2016 main report:[88]

- Nearly one-third (29 percent) of respondents were living in poverty compared to 12 percent in the US population.
- The unemployment rate was 15 percent among respondents, 3 times higher than the unemployment rate in the US population at the time of the survey (5 percent).
- Of respondents, 40 percent had attempted suicide in their lifetime, nearly 9 times the rate in the US population (4.6 percent).
- Of respondents, 7 percent attempted suicide in the prior year—nearly 12 times the rate in the US population (0.6 percent).
- Of respondents, 10 percent of those who were out (as transgender) to their immediate family reported that a family member was violent toward them because they were transgender, and 8 percent were kicked out of the house because they were transgender.
- In the year prior to completing the survey, 46 percent of respondents were verbally harassed and 9 percent were physically attacked because of being transgender.
- People of color, particularly African Americans, fared far worse than study participants in general:[89]
    - Of Black respondents, 42 percent had experienced homelessness at some point in their lives, compared to 30 percent in the USTS sample overall, and 22 percent experienced homelessness in the prior year because of being transgender.
    - Of Black respondents, 34 percent who saw a healthcare provider in the prior year reported having at least one negative experience related to being transgender, such as being refused treatment, being verbally harassed, being physically or sexually assaulted, or having to teach the provider about transgender people in order to get appropriate care.
    - Of Black respondents, 6.7 percent were living with HIV, nearly 5 times the rate in the USTS sample overall (1.4 percent) and more than 20 times the rate in the US population (0.3 percent).

---

87 Jaime M. Grant, Lisa A. Mottet, Justin Tanis, Jack Harrison, Jody L. Herman, and Mara Keisling, *Injustice at Every Turn: A Report of the National Transgender Discrimination Survey*, Washington DC: National Center for Transgender Equality and National Gay and Lesbian Task Force, 2011, https://transequality.org/sites/default/files/docs/resources/NTDS_Report.pdf.

88 Sandy E. James et al., *The Report of the 2015 U.S. Transgender Survey* (Washington, DC: National Center for Transgender Equality, 2016), 24, transequality.org/sites/default/files/docs/usts/USTS-Full-Report-Dec17.pdf.

89 Sandy E. James, Carter Brown, and Isaiah Wilson, *2015 U.S. Transgender Survey: Report on the Experiences of Black Respondents*, Washington, DC and Dallas, TX: National Center for Transgender Equality, Black Trans Advocacy, and National Black Justice Coalition, 2017, https://transequality.org/sites/default/files/docs/usts/USTS-Black-Respondents-Report.pdf.

The research demonstrated some hope in that when transgender individuals were supported by family, their outcomes improved. But there was no doubt that enormous discrepancies exist between the experiences of trans-identified versus nontrans individuals.

Now, hold on to that information as we turn to another important study.

Adverse Childhood Experiences

In the fall of 2019, the national media released a number of reports linking certain adverse childhood experiences with negative health outcomes in adults. The data came from The Adverse Childhood Experiences Study done by Kaiser Permanente in collaboration with the Centers for Disease Control and Prevention.

In the mid-1990s, Kaiser Permanente asked 144,000 clients in 25 states to participate in a ten-question survey. The researchers gathered information about adverse events experienced when the participants were under 18 years of age and correlated them with physical examinations and outcomes data in later life.[90]

This information was not specific to trans or LGBTQIA+ folks at all, but rather to the general, reasonably affluent, employed, and educated patients of Kaiser Permanente. We can reasonably assume that transgender participants would have worse outcomes than the general group studied.

The ten-question survey measured categories of adverse experiences. "Five are personal—physical abuse, verbal abuse, sexual abuse, physical neglect, and emotional neglect. Five are related to other family members: a parent who's an alcoholic, a mother who's a victim of domestic violence, a family member in jail, a family member diagnosed with a mental illness, and the disappearance of a parent through divorce, death, or abandonment. Each type of trauma counts as one. So, a person who's been physically abused, with one alcoholic parent, and a mother who was beaten up has an ACE score of 3."[91]

> **When I first heard about the ACE report on NPR, I immediately thought of one of my gender-variant patients. That patient's mother literally drove off and abandoned her at a truck stop when she was only 12 years old. When I told my patient about the ACE test, she was eager to take it. She scored an 8 out of 10. A transgender male I've followed for nearly a decade took the test during one of our visits and scored a 10 out of 10.**
>
> *— Linda Gromko, MD*

90 Centers for Disease Control and Prevention, "Preventing Adverse Childhood Experiences (ACEs) to Improve US Health," last reviewed April 6, 2021, https://www.cdc.gov/media/releases/2019/p1105-prevent-aces.html.

91 ACES Too High, "What ACEs/PCEs Do You Have?," *ACES Too High News*, accessed July 30, 2021, https://acestoohigh.com/got-your-ace-score/.

Important Information from the ACE Study

It turned out that the number of certain types of adverse events experienced reliably predicted health outcomes in later life. It was not the total number of events, but rather the total number of *different types* of events that counted. Additionally, one type of stress didn't count more than another.

Study participants with four or more of the adverse experiences had significantly more physical illnesses as adults; they were often chronic conditions like heart disease, diabetes, depression, and cancer.

Quantifying Adverse Childhood Experiences

The original ACE questionnaire was devised in 1985 by Dr. Vincent Felitti, who wondered why some of the patients in his obesity clinic had dropped out in spite of satisfactory weight loss. Felitti postulated that obesity was related to adverse experiences in childhood, particularly sexual assault, physical abuse, neglect, domestic violence, and drug or alcohol issues.[92] Over the years, the survey has been modified for different target groups.

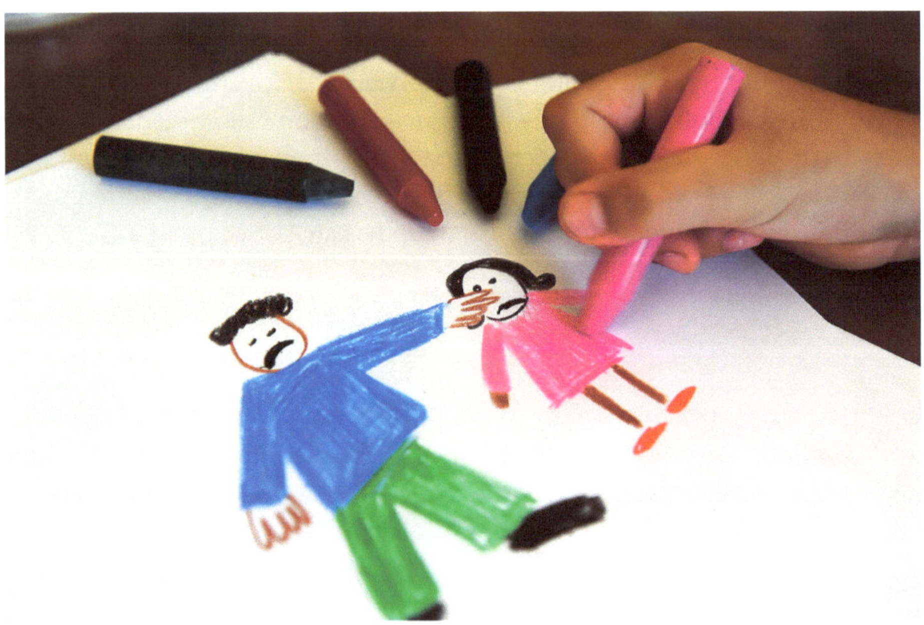

92 Jane Ellen, "The Adverse Childhood Experiences Study—the Largest, Most Important Public Health Study You Never Heard of—Began in an Obesity Clinic," *ACES Too High News*, October 3, 2012, https://acestoohigh.com/2012/10/03/the-adverse-childhood-experiences-study-the-largest-most-important-public-health-study-you-never-heard-of-began-in-an-obesity-clinic/.

Finding Your ACE Score

Prior to your 18th birthday:

1. Did a parent or other adult in the household often or very often…Swear at you, insult you, put you down, or humiliate you? or Act in a way that made you afraid that you might be physically hurt?

   No ______ If Yes, enter 1 ______

2. Did a parent or other adult in the household often or very often…Push, grab, slap, or throw something at you? or Ever hit you so hard that you had marks or were injured?

   No ______ If Yes, enter 1 ______

3. Did an adult or person at least 5 years older than you ever…Touch or fondle you or have you touch their body in a sexual way? or Attempt or actually have oral, anal, or vaginal intercourse with you?

   No ______ If Yes, enter 1 ______

4. Did you often or very often feel that…No one in your family loved you or thought you were important or special? or Your family didn't look out for each other, feel close to each other, or support each other?

   No ______ If Yes, enter 1 ______

5. Did you often or very often feel that…You didn't have enough to eat, had to wear dirty clothes, and had no one to protect you? or Your parents were too drunk or high to take care of you or take you to the doctor if you needed it?

   No ______ If Yes, enter 1 ______

6. Were your parents ever separated or divorced?

   No ______ If Yes, enter 1 ______

7. Was your mother or stepmother: Often or very often pushed, grabbed, slapped, or had something thrown at her? or Sometimes, often, or very often kicked, bitten, hit with a fist, or hit with something hard? or Ever repeatedly hit over at least a few minutes or threatened with a gun or knife?

   No ______ If Yes, enter 1 ______

8. Did you live with anyone who was a problem drinker or alcoholic, or who used street drugs?

   No ______ If Yes, enter 1 ______

9. Was a household member depressed or mentally ill, or did a household member attempt suicide?

   No ______ If Yes, enter 1 ______

10. Did a household member go to prison?

    No ______ If Yes, enter 1 ______

Now add up your "Yes" answers: ___. This is your ACE Score.

Adapted from acestoohigh.com/got-your-ace-score.

The Adverse Childhood Experience Study demonstrated that many individuals have some ACE events in their background. Nearly two-thirds of respondents had one positive ACE score; 17 percent had four adverse childhood experiences.[93] Higher ACE scores correlated with a range of negative health conditions, risk behaviors, and social and psychological conditions.[94]

Here are some interesting take-home points:[95] [96]

- A person with an ACE of 4 was found to be:
    - Twice as likely to smoke
    - Four times as likely to be an alcoholic
    - Nearly five times (460 percent) as likely to experience depression
    - Over 12 times (1,220 percent) as likely to have attempted suicide
    - Four times as likely to have emphysema or chronic bronchitis
    - Over twice (240 percent) as likely to have hepatitis
- People with an ACE score of 6 statistically shortened their life span by 20 years!

Participants with high ACE scores were more likely to have unplanned pregnancies and to contract sexually transmitted infections (STIs) than their low-scoring counterparts. They had more sex partners and became sexually active earlier as well. They were also more likely to have experienced sexual assault or sex trafficking than low-scoring counterparts.[97] [98] [99] [100]

The initial research, as well as the dozens of spin-off studies that followed, suggested that a person (particularly a younger one) doesn't differentiate between the type of adverse events. Rather, for *any* stress, they experience a physiological response—an increase in their levels of the circulating stress hormones cortisol and epinephrine (adrenaline).

Cortisol and epinephrine are the hormones needed to prime the body for its response to stress, whether that is to fight, flee, or freeze. Toxic stress, extreme stress, or repetitive stress may impact brain development as early as infancy.

---

93 Centers for Disease Control and Prevention, "Preventing Adverse Childhood Experiences (ACEs) to Improve US Health," last reviewed April 6, 2021, https://www.cdc.gov/media/releases/2019/p1105-prevent-aces.html.

94 V. J. Felitti et al, "Relationship of Childhood Abuse and Household Dysfunction to Many of the Leading Causes of Death in Adults: The Adverse Childhood Experiences (ACE) Study," *American Journal of Preventive Medicine* 14, no. 4 (May 1998): 245–58, https://doi.org/10.1016/s0749-3797(98)00017-8.

95 ACES Too High, "What ACEs/PCEs Do You Have?," *ACES Too High News*, accessed July 30, 2021, https://acestoohigh.com/got-your-ace-score/.

96 Vincent J. Felitti, "The Relation between Adverse Childhood Experiences and Adult Health: Turning Gold into Lead," *The Permanente Journal* 6, no. 1 (Winter 2002): 44–7, https://www.ncbi.nlm.nih.gov/pubmed/30313011.

97 Susan D. Hillis, Robert F. Anda, Shanta R. Dube, Vincent J. Felitti, Polly A. Marchbanks, and James S. Marks, "The Association between Adverse Childhood Experiences and Adolescent Pregnancy, Long-Term Psychosocial Consequences, and Fetal Death," *Pediatrics* 113, no. 2 (February 2004): 320–27, doi: 10.1542/peds.113.2.320.

98 Susan D. Hillis, Robert F. Anda, Vincent J. Felitti, and Polly A. Marchbanks, "Adverse Childhood Experiences and Sexual Risk Behaviors in Women: A Retrospective Cohort Study," *Family Planning Perspectives* 33, no. 5 (September 2001): 206–11, doi: 10.2307/2673783.

99 Juliet Bonnay, "How High ACE Scores Can Impact Adult Health," *Juliet Bonnay: Different Perspectives* (blog), November 15, 2019, https://by-julietbonnay.com/2019/11/how-high-ace-scores-can-impact-adult-health/.

100 Centers for Disease Control and Prevention, "Preventing Adverse Childhood Experiences," last reviewed April 6, 2021, https://www.cdc.gov/violenceprevention/aces/fastfact.html.

Toxic stress, in turn, infers a dose-responsive increase in depression, suicide, substance abuse, overweight and obesity, ischemic heart disease, liver disease, traumatic injury, cancers, PTSD, kidney disease, diabetes, asthma, and other chronic medical conditions.

Helping People with High ACE Scores Develop Resilience

It is important to know that a high ACE score does not doom an individual to poor outcomes. Resilience, although it is more subjective than ACE factors, can also be examined; resilience score indicators have been developed.

One such resilience assessment is the Connor-Davidson Resilience Scale developed by Dr. Kathryn M. Connor and Jonathan R. T. Davidson, professor emeritus of psychiatry and behavioral sciences at Duke University School of Medicine.[101]

Davidson stated, "Resilience is the ability to bounce back, pick yourself up from the ground if you've been dealt some blows, to be able to cope well or effectively with adverse conditions. It certainly includes various properties like being optimistic, having confidence in yourself, or belief in yourself to overcome things, to have the skills you need, social support, ability to find some meaning or purpose in life. Probably one of the most important or critical things of all is something called 'hardiness,' which is thought to be a mix of commitment, control, and challenge."[102]

The 2016 documentary film, *The Biology of Stress and the Science of Hope,* discusses the ACE model and various means to enhance resilience. The documentary introduces the "Miss Kendra Program," a tool developed by Dr. David Johnson for creating a trusted (although mythical) ally to listen to kids and help them cope with their stressors. It also features the work of Dr. Nadine Burke Harris, a pediatrician who incorporates a trauma-informed model into her work with high-risk kids. Burke Harris makes the point that medical schools should validly be teaching students about adverse childhood stressors and their prevention as good medicine.

According to Dr. Monique Tello in an article on *Harvard Health Blog* about trauma-informed care, "the first step is to recognize how common trauma is, and to understand that every patient may have experienced serious trauma. We don't necessarily need to question people about their experiences; rather, we should just assume that they may have this history, and act accordingly."[103]

Trauma-informed health and human care shifts the focus from asking clients "What's wrong with you?" to the more insightful "What's happened to you?"[104]

---

101 Kathryn M. Connor and Jonathan R. T. Davidson, "Development of a New Resilience Scale: The Connor-Davidson Resilience Scale (CD-RISC)," *Depression and Anxiety* 18, no. 2 (September 2003): 76–82, http://dx.doi.org/10.1002/da.10113.

102 White, Christine Cissy, "Putting Resilience and Resilience Surveys under the Microscope," *ACES Too High News*, February 5, 2017, https://acestoohigh.com/2017/02/05/__trashed-4/.

103 Monique Tello, "Trauma-Informed Care: What It Is, and Why It's Important," *Harvard Health Blog*, Harvard Health Publishing, October 16, 2018, https://www.health.harvard.edu/blog/trauma-informed-care-what-it-is-and-why-its-important-2018101613562.

104 Family and Youth Services Bureau, US Department of Health and Human Services, "Asking: "What's Happened to You?" A Focus on Trauma-Informed Care, *NCFY Reports, Summer 2011*, July 27, 2012, https://www.acf.hhs.gov/archive/fysb/newsletter/fysbnewsletter/asking-whats-happened-you-focus-trauma-informed-care.

Directing resources toward supporting families socially and economically, strengthening the work of schools and community organizations, reinforcing an individual's ability to connect with others to problem-solve and gain mastery, and promoting self-care are all critical.

Let's shift gears again; let's turn our attention to PTSD.

Post-Traumatic Stress Disorder (PTSD)

Post-traumatic stress disorder is a condition that develops in some people who have experienced a shocking, frightening, or particularly dangerous event at some time. Such traumatic events may include a motor vehicle accident; a natural disaster like a hurricane, fire, flood, tornado, or earthquake; sexual assault or domestic violence; a criminal or terrorist attack; or another potentially life-threatening situation. When related to military service in wartime, PTSD used to be known as "shell shock."

In the *Diagnostic and Statistical Manual of Mental Disorders* (*DSM–5*), PTSD is an anxiety disorder that develops in relation to an event such as those listed above. The exposure must involve directly experiencing the event, witnessing the event in person, learning of an actual or threatened death of a close family member or friend, or repeated firsthand, extreme exposure to the details of the event.

People naturally react during and after a traumatic event with a "fight, flight, or freeze" response mediated by the stress hormones cortisol and epinephrine. These hormonal signals have evolved to prepare our bodies to fight back, to run away from the tiger intending to eat us, or to freeze so we won't attract more tigers. Cortisol increases our body's available glucose to energize our skeletal muscles, while epinephrine makes our hearts beat faster and our lungs work more effectively with wide-open airways and increased oxygen exchange. These changes (more glucose to skeletal muscles and more oxygen from more effective breathing) are normal and adaptive when you're faced with an actual tiger. However, when there is no tiger, the body experiences what amounts to a physiologic "false alarm."

Symptoms of PTSD

According to the *DSM-5*, symptoms of PTSD represent the following categories:

- **Reexperiencing the event**
  Seeing a news report or hearing loud sounds may prompt unwelcome memories of the event. Reliving experiences are often called "flashbacks," and provocateurs are called "triggers." Recurring nightmares are common, as are physical symptoms such as shaking, nausea, and vomiting. A person may experience dissociative reactions and prolonged psychological distress.

- **Alterations in arousal**
  Symptoms can include feeling on-guard, jumpy, irritable, reactive, and ready to fight; using alcohol or other drugs; smoking; and driving aggressively. They may also manifest as sleep disturbances, elevated blood pressure and heart rate, and hyperventilation.

- **Avoidance**
  Another symptom is avoiding certain people, locations, or activities that remind one of the event, or keeping overly busy to avoid thinking of the trauma. Avoidance may also take the form of detachment or isolation.

- **Negative alterations in cognition and mood**

Other PTSD symptoms include feeling more negative or numb than before the traumatic event, experiencing guilt or shame, and losing interest in things one normally enjoyed. Mood swings and anxiety are common. (Doesn't this sound like depression? Depression and suicidal ideation can also be found in decreased mental agility, as can the use of illicit drugs and potential addiction.)

What It Means When a Person Is "Triggered"

"Triggering" has become a contemporary buzzword. Knowing what triggering is can help healthcare providers identify problem areas and help our clients find greater comfort in the world.

According to trauma therapist Elaine Duncan, MA, LMHC: "When a person overreacts with anger, anxiety, or freezing, that is a clue that the person is probably getting triggered. What seemed like just an annoying event, such as getting cut off in traffic, can cause a person who has been triggered to be angry for a couple of days, not able to sleep, and feel anxious for days. Most likely they are reacting not just to the triggering event but also to the memory of a traumatic event. A referral to a trauma counselor would be appropriate in this case, as the traumatic memory can be reprocessed and resolved."

Treatments Available for PTSD

There is considerable overlap between PTSD and other conditions such as anxiety or depression. Trauma-focused psychotherapy is the mainstay of treatment, but treatment must be individualized and may include group support and medications. PTSD therapy may include the following:

- **Trauma-focused psychotherapy**
  This usually takes the form on one-on-one talk therapy that occurs over a period of several months and focuses initially on the traumatic event.

  - **Prolonged exposure therapy**
    Sometimes called "flooding," this therapy exposes patients to intense and sustained images of trauma. It may involve desensitization so that patients may process the trauma without experiencing the feelings or emotions that have accompanied it before.

  - **Cognitive processing therapy**
    Through talk therapy, patients focus on the trauma and feelings they carry with them about the trauma, such as guilt or shame. Over time, they can think about the event without provoking a stress response.

Bessel van der Kolk, MD, in his book, *The Body Keeps the Score*, states, "While trauma keeps us dumbfounded, the path out of it is paved with words, carefully assembled, piece by piece, until the whole story can be revealed."[105]

105 Bessel van der Kolk, *The Body Keeps the Score* (New York: Penguin Books, 2014): 234.

- **Eye movement desensitization and reprocessing (EMDR)**
  Although the mechanism is not fully understood, EMDR allows a person to reprocess their memories and think about their trauma without it triggering a larger reaction. The therapist uses eye movement techniques (having you look back and forth) or a clicker device to produce sounds, first on one side and then the other.

I'll admit that EMDR seemed like an odd technique to me until I noticed that my clients who experienced it were doing better even after serious lifelong traumas.

I asked psychotherapist and certified EMDR specialist Elaine A. Duncan for more information. She explained, "EMDR is an extensively researched, effective psychotherapy method proven to help people recover from trauma and other distressing life experiences, including PTSD, anxiety, depression, and panic disorders. EMDR therapy does not require talking in detail about the distressing events. Conducted by a trained mental health professional using gentle, painless bilateral stimulation, it allows the brain to reprocess the memory and proceed with the natural healing process. Most clients will begin to see definite improvement in symptoms in a few sessions. For more information on EMDR therapy, see **emdria.org**."

- **Medications**
  - **Antidepressants**
    Selective serotonin reuptake inhibitors (sertraline, fluoxetine, and paroxetine are examples) and serotonin and norepinephrine reuptake inhibitors (venlafaxine) make more of the neurotransmitters serotonin or norepinephrine available to facilitate nerve transmission in your brain. Refer to Chapter 17 on treating depression and also see **apa.org/ptsd-guideline/treatments/medications**.

  - **Prazosin (Minipress)**
    This is used specifically for the reduction of nightmares. Prazosin is an older medication used to treat high blood pressure; however, for some patients, it reduces the frequency and intensity of nightmares. While its efficacy is controversial, its use is common.

Complex PTSD

While PTSD is usually connected to a single event such as a fire or motor vehicle accident, complex PTSD is the result of multiple traumatic events occurring over a period of time. Included under this umbrella are "multiple incidents of child abuse, particularly child physical abuse and child sexual abuse, prolonged domestic violence, concentration camp experiences, torture, slavery, and genocide campaigns."[106] A commonality of these various circumstances is the prolonged powerless nature of the individual with no ability to get away. This is also referred to as "complex trauma" or "disorders of extreme stress not otherwise specified" (DESNOS).

In complex trauma, individuals may appear to have features of personality disorders, such as borderline personality, dependent personality, or masochistic personality. As such, the clients may be seen as being "weak" and are often "blamed" for their symptoms, which may include anger, detachment, suicidal ideation, altered perception of a perpetrator, and alterations in states of consciousness. Alcohol use, drug use, and self-harm behaviors are not uncommon comorbidities.[107]

106 Traumadissociation.com, "Complex Posttraumatic Stress Disorder," accessed June 24, 2021, http://traumadissociation.com/complexptsd.

107 National Center for PTSD, US Department of Veterans Affairs, "Complex PTSD," updated January 31, 2020, https://www.ptsd.va.gov/professional/treat/essentials/complex_ptsd.asp.

Dissociation and Complex PTSD

According to Elaine Duncan:

> "Dissociation is another common condition found in those with complex trauma. Dissociation is sometimes evident when a person 'checks out' and they may not remember what has taken place when they were 'checked out.' Dissociation often manifests as multiple personalities. This is not always as dramatic as the popular notion of multiple personality disorder, now called dissociative identity disorder. The more common manifestation we see involves different parts of the personality taking over at different times.
>
> "Much like everyone has various *facets* of their personality (that is, their child part, their professional part, their parent part), a person with dissociative disorder and a history of childhood trauma has parts that are *more strongly separate from one another and from the adult self.* These parts may take turns taking control. This may be seen, for instance, when an angry part gets triggered and dramatically flares. Or the little-girl part might get triggered, and the next thing you know, you see a little girl in an adult body in front of you. All of this reflects the fact that the psyche developed during trauma and provided mechanisms for self-protection."

Connecting the Dots

From the US Transgender Surveys, we learned that transgender individuals experience a range of social, economic, and mental health disparities. The ACE studies clarify that while the majority of people have experienced some trauma, the people who have experienced *multiple* traumas have significant adverse health outcomes. Finally, a review of PTSD reinforces that there *are* things that can be done individually and systemically to help.

Working with Healthcare Providers

Interactions with healthcare providers can raise anxiety levels for anyone. Imagine how it might be for a person with PTSD, complex PTSD, or a high ACE score! Elements of invasion, exposure of one's private parts, and the feeling of being trapped without possibility of escape can all contribute to a difficult clinical experience or an avoidance of healthcare altogether.

Let's look at some ways patients and providers may make these experiences more positive, or at least less traumatic.

How an Individual with PTSD or a High ACE Score Can Self-Protect in Vulnerable Healthcare Circumstances

An individual with PTSD or a high ACE score may experience difficulty in medically vulnerable situations. I recommend that such an individual tell their provider that "these exams are difficult for me" or "I've had bad experiences with exams." Hopefully, the provider will hear that information and be gentler by taking a bit more time or offering more explanations. Or maybe they will ask you how they can help.

Think ahead about what parts of an exam or appointment worry you. Your preferences *may* not be honored, but it is perfectly reasonable to ask for what you need to make the experience less difficult. For example, it is okay to ask the following:

- That you are addressed by your correct name and gender.
- That your body is covered during any exam; if you feel you need a reason, say, "I'm modest."
- That your face and airway are not covered.
- That you may have a friend in the exam room with you to hold your hand or otherwise support you.
- That there not be extra people in the exam room (this is more difficult in a teaching facility, but you can still ask). Or the reverse—that you can have a second healthcare person in the room so that you are not alone with the examiner.
- That the provider tells you what they are doing as they go along.
- That they stop any exam or procedure at your request, even for a small break or to re-collect yourself.
- That they move a bright light that is shining in your eyes or fix other irritants that make your experience worse.

Also remember that you may leave a clinical visit and reschedule if you need to.

Tips for Healthcare Providers to Prevent Patients from Having a Traumatizing Healthcare Experience

- **Assume that *every* patient you see has a history of trauma.**
- **Be polite.**
  Simple courtesy goes a long way, particularly with people who have been harmed by people in power. I remember doing STI exams on 13-year-olds in the youth detention center. These kids had been charged with "O and A" (offering and agreeing, which meant prostitution). They were already regarded as "throwaways"—not even "runaways." Courtesy and kindness were all I had to offer.
- **Use a quiet voice.**
- **Take care to use the patient's correct name and gender pronouns.**
  "What name do you go by? What pronouns do you use?" If the patient asks why, say, "It's very important to many people, and we want to show our respect."
- **Explain what you will be doing.**
  Say, "I'll tell you everything I'm doing as I perform your exam." Then be sure to tell them what you're doing. You can add, "I haven't found the element of surprise to be helpful in medicine."
- **Offer to stop if something is "too difficult, too uncomfortable, or even if you have a question."**
  Then stop when asked.
- **Give the patient a moment to gather their presence of mind, and then say, "Tell me when you're ready to continue."**
  This shifts some control to the patient.
- **Respect if a patient says *not* to do a part of the exam.**
  Transmasculine adults or kids may not want to remove a chest binder or permit a breast exam (out

of respect, I would say "chest exam"). Sometimes I defer that part of the exam, ask the client if they have any concerns about their chest, and remind them to ask me later if they do have concerns one day. I generally do this exam after they've had top surgery, for example; that's when I would take that opportunity to talk to the patient about breast exams and the fact that top surgery doesn't protect one from breast cancer.

- Could I miss something? Yes. Clarify with the patient that you would not be able to find something if you did not examine the area, but that you trust they will notify you with concerns. Document that the patient was asked and that they declined the exam.
- I've said to a number of people, "Did you know that if I examined you when you have specifically told me not to, my exam may be considered an assault?" It's different in an emergency, of course.

- **Tell the patient what to expect and make a plan together before you start the exam.**
  This is especially true when doing an exam or procedure that you know will likely be painful—that is, a pelvic exam in a patient with pelvic inflammatory disease (PID)—or a complication after pregnancy termination).
- **Offer local anesthesia, or more local anesthesia, as long as it is safe.**
  If a procedure is painful and we can reduce that pain, we should try. At the very least, give the patient a choice: "We're just about done, but I have two more stitches to place. We can stop for more anesthesia. Some people would prefer to go ahead without stopping. What would *you* like to do?" It really *is* their decision.

  One of my patients went to an emergency room for evaluation after a suture line opened up (dehisced) following vaginoplasty. She needed a number of sutures, and the ER doctor proceeded to place several stitches in the patient's perineum—without local anesthesia. The patient asked for numbing medication, but the doctor seemed annoyed by the request. Of all the memories this patient has from a rocky postoperative course, this is the one that seemed to stand out the most—that of the ER doctor who didn't even offer anesthesia.
- **Use the "1-2-3" technique if you are doing something quick but painful.**
  Suppose you are removing an IUD, and you know it will likely cause cramping. Ask the patient to breathe in as you count "1-2-3" and blow out hard when you say, "Blow!" As they blow, you remove the IUD. The patient's forceful exhalation distracts them from the cramping that often occurs.
- **Maintain eye contact and keep talking with your patient as a way to keep them from dissociating.**

One of my patients had bleeding after a metoidioplasty and had to be seen in the emergency room. He told me later, "They wanted to catheterize me. I figured if I stayed very still and was very quiet, it wouldn't hurt so much." This comment prompted a referral to an EMDR therapist to discuss the PTSD that had been there for years.

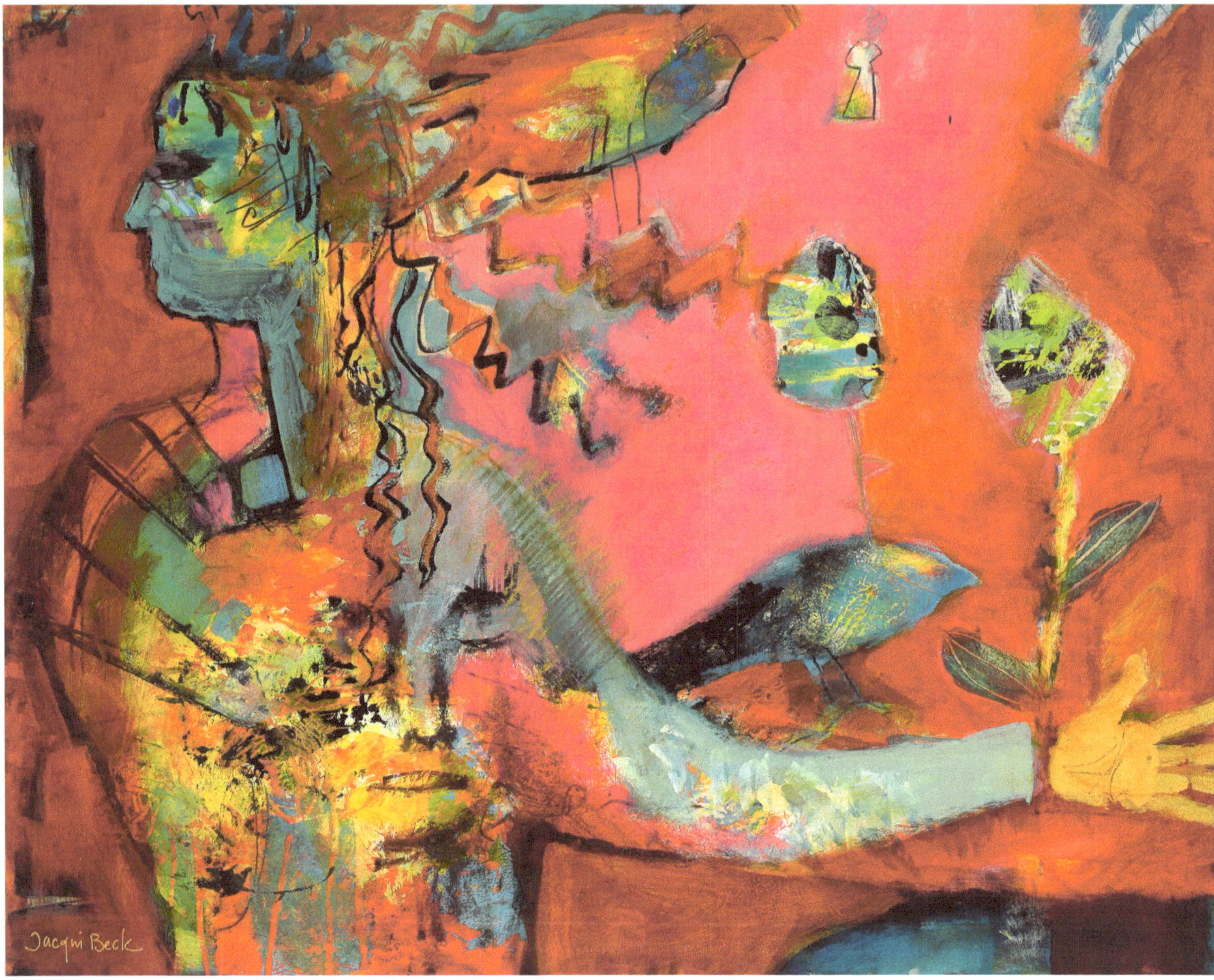

Inattention to Detail

CHAPTER 19
Changing Your Documents

At first glance, changing your legal documents may seem sort of boring or perhaps daunting. But I assure you that this is critical to a smooth gender transition. Paying careful attention to this information will save you enormous difficulties down the road. We'll go through each item separately.

Most people begin the process by changing their name or the gender marker on their driver's license or state identification card. (It can be done in either order.) There may be circumstances in which you will need the help of an attorney (Lambda Legal at **lambdalegal.org** is one reference). But if your situation is reasonably straightforward, you can likely proceed on your own. Minors will need the assistance of parents or legal guardians.

And, to save you time, let me direct you to an extremely helpful web resource from the National Transgender Center for Equality. It's a central hub for information on how to make the document changes you need, and it's easy to use and particularly helpful because regulations vary from state to state: **transequality.org/documents**.

Changing Your Legal Name

When I used to deliver babies, my patients and I would often talk about choosing names for them. I recommend that people pick a name that would work just as well in the boardroom as the day care facility. Something "cute" may not cut it when they're running a company.

Now that you are selecting your own name, here are some considerations:

- Be aware that names that are popular today may seem dated later. My own name, Linda, is a great example of this. Now, when you meet a Linda, you can be reasonably sure that she's over 60 years old. (That said, if you are an older person, you may want to consider a name that was popular when you were born so you can fit in with all the other Lindas!)
- Many trans people continue to use the same initials they started with. Using your initials as an informal nickname works as a good "bridge" name for some people.
- If you have an easily adaptable first name, you might want to take advantage of that: Christine becomes Christopher, Robert becomes Roberta, and so on.
- Some people change their last names too; for example, they sometimes use their mother's maiden name.
- But it is *your* name, the name that represents your true self. Give it careful thought and choose what works for you. You can change your name as often as you like, but it costs money for each change.

The process of completing a legal name change isn't all that difficult. You must do this in the county in which you live.

As an example, here's how it works in Seattle: Go to the website of the King County Courthouse or one of its regional branches and enter the words "legal name change" in its search function. You must complete a Petition for Name Change form and pay a moderate fee (although the cost varies, so check your local reference so as not to be surprised). Then you will be scheduled on the court calendar, often for that day or the following day. Be sure to bring your current photo ID. You will appear in a small courtroom and get sworn in. The judge will ask you to confirm your new name and sign some papers, and then your name change is official. The legal name change will then be recorded by the county.

In my opinion, this is a celebration time. Plan to go out to lunch or do something else to mark this as the important life-changing day that it is!

Changing the Gender Marker on Your Driver's License or State ID

Checking this task off your list can make your life *much* easier, especially if you travel or do something that attracts the attention of law enforcement. You will also need appropriate photo ID when you apply for a job, open a bank account, and engage in countless other day-to-day interactions.

In Washington State, you must provide your name, address, and other identifying information on the form. **As of January 27, 2018, you are no longer required to have a doctor's letter or court order in Washington State.** We used to keep these forms in our office when a doctor's signature was required.

In Washington State, you may designate your gender as M, F, or X. You then sign your name and mail this form to the state department of licensing. In turn, it will send you a document indicating that your gender marker has changed. Then you take *this* document to the vehicle licensing office where you can get a new driver's license or state identification card with a new photo (if you like) and your appropriate gender marker. (Time for another celebration!)

Again, you can check your state's requirements by visiting transequality.org/documents.

Remember to Do These

- To change your name, deal with the county where you live.
- To change your gender marker or change your name on your driver's license or state identification card, deal with the state where you live.
- To change your birth certificate, deal with the state or country in which you were born.
- To change your Social Security and passport documentation, follow federal procedures (covered later in this chapter).

Changing Your Birth Certificate

Changing your birth certificate varies from state to state, according to where you were born. Look this up on transequality.org/documents. **In Washington State, you no longer need a letter from your physician.**

For states that do require a physician's letter, I use the template below and print the letter on our medical office letterhead.

Example Letter to Change Your Birth Certificate

I, (physician's full name and medical license or certificate number), (issuing US State/Foreign Country of medical license/certificate), am the physician of (name of patient), with whom I have a doctor/patient relationship and whom I have treated (or with whom I have a doctor/patient relationship and whose medical history I have reviewed and evaluated).

(Name of patient) has had appropriate clinical treatment for gender transition to the new gender (specify male or female).

I declare under penalty of perjury under the laws of the United States that the foregoing is true and correct.

Signature ______________________

Typed Name ______________________

Date ______________________

Changing Your Social Security Information

Because the Social Security Administration (SSA) is a federal (not a state) agency, the requirements for specifying a gender change are the same nationwide.

Changes you will likely want to make to your SS information include your name and your gender identity. Note that your gender identify is recorded in the SSA's computer records only and *not* on a Social Security card. **Your SS number will not change.**

The easiest way to make this change is to ask your doctor (a licensed physician who can be a primary care doctor or a specialist) to write the appropriate letter to enable you to make the change. This letter must be written using the following template and it must be on your doctor's letterhead. These rules are nonnegotiable.

Here is the template:

Example Letter to Change Your Social Security Information

I, (physician's full name and medical license or certificate number), (issuing US State/Foreign Country of medical license/certificate), am the physician of (name of patient), with whom I have a doctor/patient relationship and whom I have treated (or with whom I have a doctor/patient relationship and whose medical history I have reviewed and evaluated).

(Name of patient) has had appropriate clinical treatment for gender transition to the new gender (specify male or female).

I declare under penalty of perjury under the laws of the United States that the foregoing is true and correct.

Signature ______________________________

Typed Name ____________________________

Date _________________________________

So, what constitutes "appropriate clinical treatment for gender transition?" This may include surgery, but it doesn't have to. It may include therapy, hormone treatments, changes in outward presentation, or any other combination of treatments to support gender transition. But there is no requirement to specify what particular clinical treatment has been received.

For more information on how to change your name on your Social Security card, see the SSA's website at faq.ssa.gov/en-US/Topic/article/KA-01981. For helpful general information regarding transgender people and the Social Security Administration, see this link at the US National Center for Transgender Equality's website: transequality.org/sites/default/files/docs/kyr/SSAResource_June2013.pdf.

Changing Your Passport

At the time of this book's printing, the changes you will likely want to make to your passport information include your name and your gender identity. On June 30, 2021, it was announced that by the end of 2021, a gender marker can be self-identified as "X" on US passports without the need to provide medical documentation.[108]

And you can self-identify even if the gender you select does not match the gender on your supporting documentation such as a birth certificate, previous passport, or state ID, according to the US State Department. It is also working to add a gender marker for nonbinary, intersex, and gender-nonconforming people as soon as possible.

For more information on how to change your gender identity on your passport, see the US State Department's website at **https://travel.state.gov/content/travel/en/passports/need-passport/selecting-your-gender-marker.html**.

Save yourself time: Find the National Transgender Center for Equality at transequality.org/documents. This central hub for information on how to make changes in documents is easy to use and particularly helpful because regulations vary from state to state.

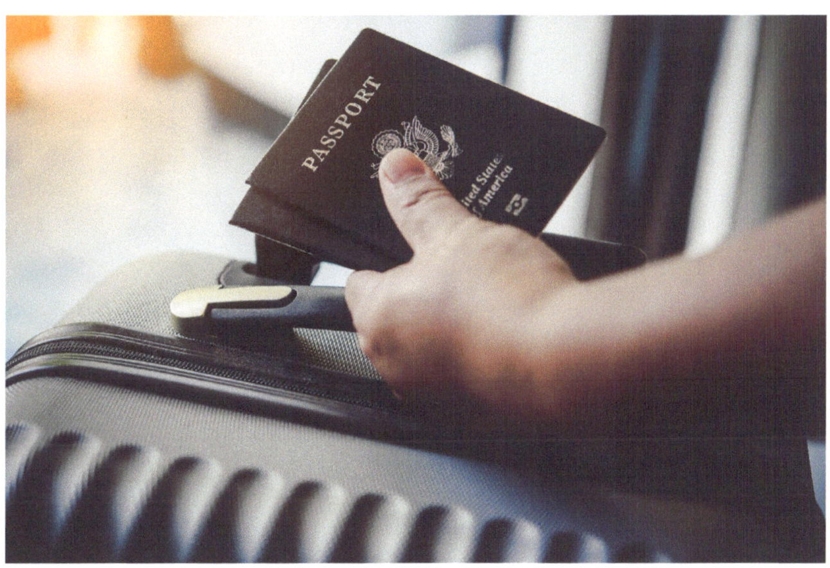

108 Kate Sosin, "U.S. to Add 'X' Gender Marker on Passports," *The 19th*, June 30, 2021, https://19thnews.org/2021/06/u-s-to-add-x-gender-marker-on-passports/.

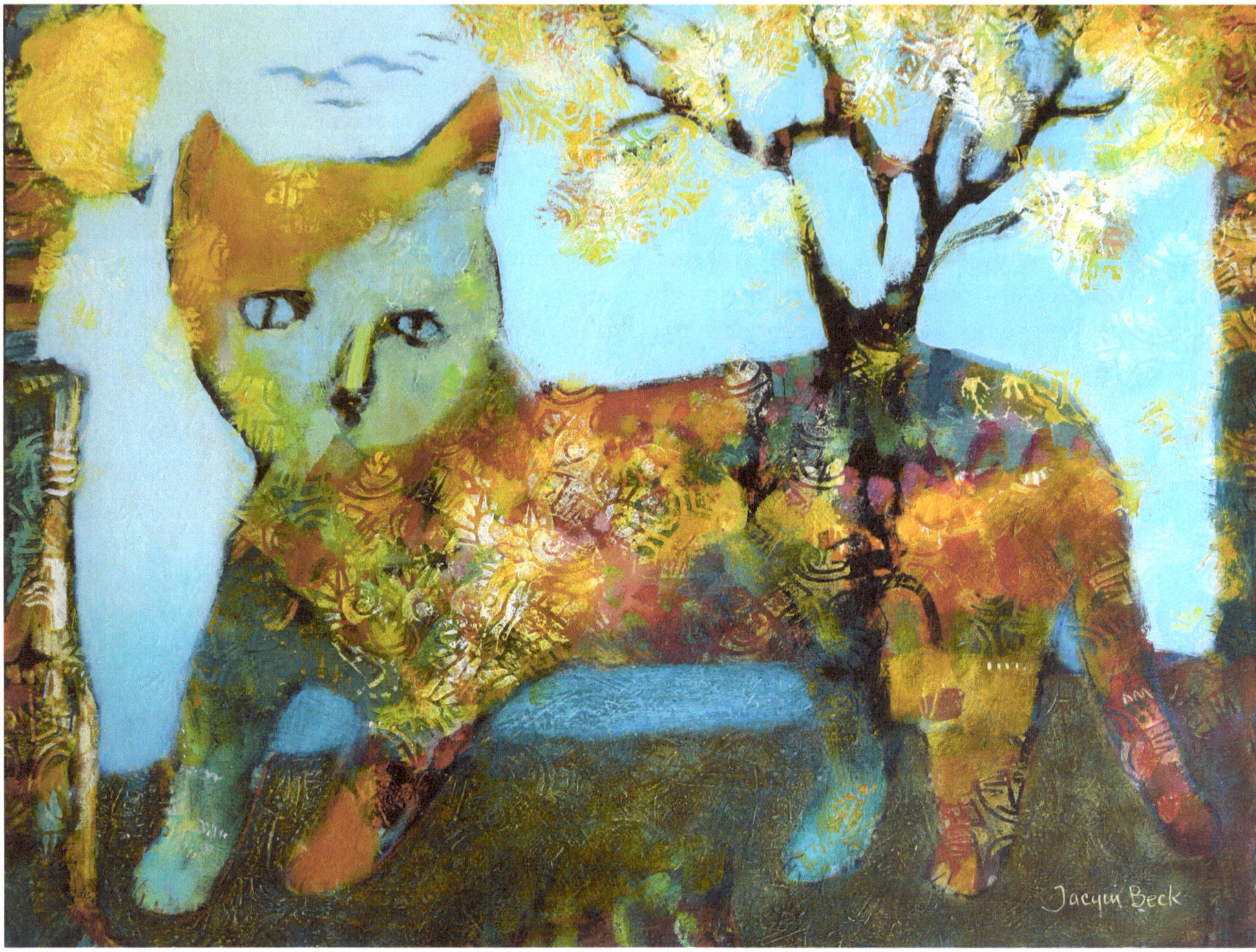

Tree in Cat

CHAPTER 20
Traveling

If you have the opportunity to travel, excellent! But take some time to plan ahead and avoid unexpected hassles. Naturally, consider where you are traveling. Do an Internet search to get an idea of the local culture and how gender-nonconforming people are typically received. (Amsterdam sounds great, for example, while traveling through portions of the United States sounds stressful.)

Here are some pointers to help you:

- **Ensure that your boarding pass matches your identification (with your appropriate gender marker) and your passport or enhanced driver's license.**[109]
  Refer to the previous chapter and get your identification documents completed in plenty of time if you are preparing for a big trip.

- **Check the Transportation Security Administration (TSA) for specific information regarding transgender travelers at tsa.gov.**
  You can also call the TSA Cares Helpline at 855-787-2227.

- **Use the TSA website to prepare yourself with information about going through airport security.**
  The TSA does require that you pass through a scanner. But you can request a search done in private by an individual of the same sex. Needless to say, this experience can vary according to the airport and the TSA personnel who work there. Expect this to take extra time, so plan accordingly. You can ask to speak with a supervisor if you have difficulties.

- **Avoid security hassles by having a "carry letter."**
  A carry letter is typically written by a healthcare provider and indicates that you are transgender, that you have or are receiving appropriate treatment, and that you are to be addressed in your appropriate gender. The letter that is written for your passport or Social Security Administration documents may serve you perfectly, and you may want to take a copy of this when you travel.

- **Know that a "carry letter" may require more specific information if you are using injectable hormones and carrying the necessary needles and syringes.**
  Your doctor may simply write something to this effect on a prescription sheet or on letterhead:

  > *"John Jones is under my medical care for the treatment of gender dysphoria. He is required to travel with appropriate hormones for treatment, along with syringes and needles for administration of this medication." Signed: (doctor's signature)*

---

109 From the TSA website: "When making a reservation or at the security checkpoint, you are encouraged to use the same name, gender, and birth date as indicated on your government-issued ID. All baggage must go through the screening process. If a traveler has any medical equipment or prostheses in a carry-on bag, the items will be allowed through the checkpoint after the traveler completes the screening process. If a bag must be opened by an officer to resolve an alarm, the traveler may ask that bags be screened in private." To find out more info, visit the TSA's Transgender Passengers website page: tsa.gov/transgender-passengers.

Or, alternatively:

"John Jones is under my medical care for a condition that requires the self-injection of medication. He is required to travel with injectable medications along with syringes and needles for administration." Signed: (doctor's signature)

A young trans man wanted a doctor's letter to participate in an out-of-country science program. I signed the paperwork and recommended the following:

- **Have a ready-made explanation for the phalloplasty scar on your leg (for example, a skin graft after a burn or an infection).**
- **In the off-chance that you have a serious injury and have to have a urinary catheter, write in your phone or ID: "I had surgery to correct a birth defect of the urethra. Call Dr. _______________ at ________________."**

— Linda Gromko, MD

- **Take your oral medications in bottles with the original prescription labels from the pharmacy.** The same applies for injectable hormones or transdermal patches.
- **If you have any concerns about gel breast forms, get a note from your healthcare provider indicating that you are being treated for a medical condition and that your breast forms are a medical necessity.** Gel breast forms may be taken in your carry-on luggage without consideration of the 3-ounce rule. (I've never been asked to write a note about breast forms; remember, these are frequently used in cis women postmastectomy.)
- **Take with you a list of all your regular medications for your general health.** If you are a cardiac (heart) patient, a copy of a baseline electrocardiogram (EKG) can be invaluable in the emergency room.
- **Know that you are responsible for the safe disposal of needles and syringes.** Refer to Stealth Brothers for excellent hormone replacement therapy (HRT) travel kits with needle and syringe disposal cases (stealthbrosco.com).
- **One last tip: Packers and vaginal dilators are not metal and will not trigger metal detectors.** Show your doctor's letter if anyone asks.

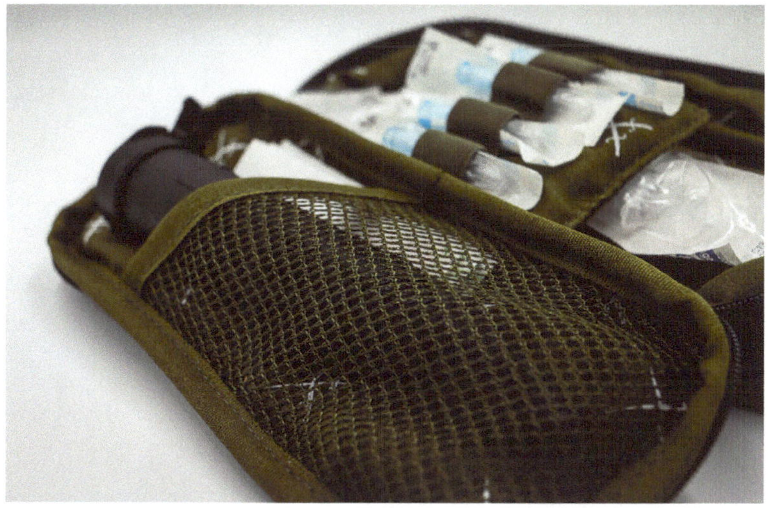

Figure 20.1. Stealth Brothers HRT travel kit.

All of the above aside, do travel if you get the opportunity, learn some of the language out of respect for the people you are visiting, and have an amazing time!

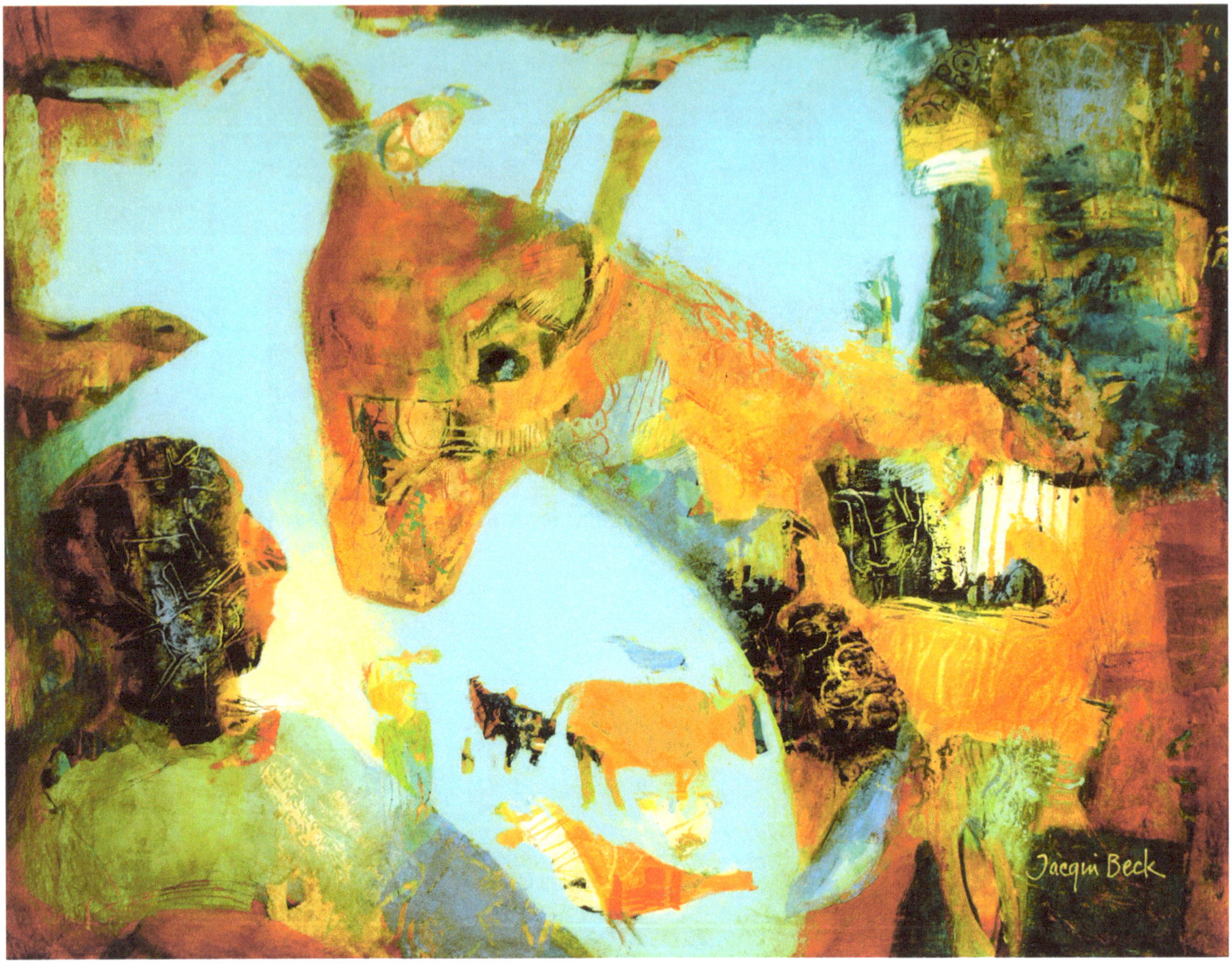

Who I Listen To

CHAPTER 21

Pregnancy Planning—and Avoidance—for Transgender Folks

Pregnancy doesn't come with guarantees for anyone. When I used to deliver babies, I found it remarkable how many things had to go just right for a baby to be conceived, carried in the uterus to full term (38 weeks from conception or 40 weeks from the date of the last menstrual period), and then delivered with both the parent and baby healthy.

Requirements for Having a Healthy Baby

Here are some of the basic requirements that apply to everyone hoping to have a healthy baby:

- **A healthy sperm from someone assigned male at birth must combine with a healthy egg from someone assigned female.**
  Both the egg and the sperm must each have the proper number of chromosomes; each of the gametes (sperm or egg) must have 23 normal chromosomes to combine to form a fertilized egg, or zygote, with 46 chromosomes. The sperm must be normally formed (no two-headed or two-tailed sperm, for example) and swim normally to meet and penetrate the egg.

  The egg must not be too old or it will have a greater likelihood of chromosomal abnormalities. Individuals assigned female have all the eggs they will *ever* have in their ovaries when they are born. They don't make new eggs, like people who are assigned male and make new sperm continually. So, you may have sperm that were produced yesterday from a 90-year-old assigned male and eggs from a 36-year-old assigned female. It's the assigned female who is termed "elderly" in this mating. Chromosomal abnormalities are thought to be the primary factor in pregnancy loss or miscarriage, which can occur in up to half of all pregnancies.

- **The sperm and egg, combined together, must nestle into the fluffy lining of the assigned female uterus at just the right time in the menstrual cycle.**
  If implantation occurs too late, the hormonal environment will not support and nourish the fertilized egg (zygote), and it will be passed out of the body in the menstrual flow.

- **The uterus and its carrier (the assigned female) must be healthy enough to retain the zygote for the duration of the 38 weeks.**

Many Things Can Go Wrong

Here are the most basic problems:

- The sperm or egg may have chromosomal or other abnormalities that do not support proper joining and viability.
- The hormonal environment of the host may not support the healthy implantation and continuation of a pregnancy.
- The uterus may be abnormally shaped. For instance, it might have a heart-shaped configuration or contain a midline septum (wall) that distorts the cavity. Such variations may crowd the pregnancy or interfere with its blood supply—causing pregnancy loss.
- The uterus may contain fibroids, which are benign muscle growths that can distort the shape of the uterus; these are most common in women starting in their 30s. The fibroids often grow during pregnancy under hormonal stimulation. As they grow, they may interfere with the uterine blood supply, crowd the pregnancy, and in some cases, may be related to pregnancy loss.
- The cervix (the mouth of the uterus) must stay closed until the end of a pregnancy. If it begins to dilate in the middle of pregnancy, a baby may be born very early and not survive. If a person knows that they have this condition (incompetent cervix), the cervix may be sutured closed to prevent early dilation.
- The placenta (the organ that looks something like a liver and connects the person with the uterus to the baby via the baby's umbilical cord) must be healthy enough to provide nourishment to the baby and to carry waste products from the baby's system. If the placenta is not up to the task, the baby may not grow as robustly. Placentas are impacted by many factors: maternal age, maternal illnesses (such as diabetes), infection, high blood pressure, smoking, and many others.
- Uterine contractions may begin too early, and if they cannot be stopped, a baby may be born prematurely. Neonatal medicine has made enormous advancements in caring for premature babies and even "micro-preemies" (which are born weighing less than a single pound after fewer than 26 weeks of pregnancy). But these babies do not always survive and are sometimes born with chronic conditions with lifelong impacts.
- The process of labor and delivery generally goes well, but not always. Early separation of the placenta from the uterine wall (placental abruption) may result in hemorrhage for the parent and anoxic (inadequate oxygen) injury to the baby. Cord accidents—such as the umbilical cord being compressed, the cord coming out of the uterus before the baby, or a cord wrapped tightly around a baby's neck—can all endanger a baby's oxygen supply. There are many other factors that can go wrong; surprisingly, though, things generally do go well, and most babies are very resilient.

Contraception: If You Have a Uterus and Ovaries and Don't Want a Pregnancy

Most healthcare providers advocate that their patients have safe sex to protect them from contracting or spreading sexually transmitted infections (STIs). Using latex condoms will reduce STI spread and your chance of becoming pregnant if you have a uterus and have sex with partners who make sperm.

Don't count on the quality of your testosterone effects—your deep voice and heavy beard growth—to prevent pregnancy. Of course, pregnancy is less likely to occur in a heavily testosterone-influenced person. But it isn't impossible.

If you have sex with a "sperm maker," do consider birth control in addition to latex condoms. Some of the more popular options include the following:

- **Progesterone-containing intrauterine devices (IUDs)**
  These include brand-name IUDs such as Mirena, Skyla, and Kyleena. These IUDs must be placed in the uterus by a trained provider; ask your provider if ibuprofen is appropriate for you to take before insertion to lessen discomfort. These IUDs generally are associated with minimal (if any) bleeding, last for 5 years (and now 6 for Mirena), and are simple for your provider to remove. (The Paragard IUD has copper in its stalk; it prevents pregnancy but doesn't reduce bleeding. On testosterone, however, bleeding may be minimal, and the Paragard lasts for 12 years.)

- **Progesterone-containing implants**
  These are easily placed in the upper arm near the elbow and last for 5 years.

- **Depo-Provera**
  This progesterone injection is given every 3 months.

- **Low-dose oral contraceptives**
  These are made of progesterone only, or a low-dose combination of estrogen and progesterone. Trans men may not appreciate the estrogen-related side effects (breast fullness, swelling, nausea), but progesterone-only pills have minimal side effects for most people.

There are many user-friendly contraceptive methods available. If your provider does not feature these options, Planned Parenthood does, and they serve many transgender clients.

Planning for a Pregnancy If You Want One

Many transgender individuals *do* want to reproduce and have their own biologically related children. There are many reasons why trans men do or do not want to have biological children; none of these reasons are necessarily right or wrong. Here are some suggestions to help you.

To Assure the Best Results Possible, Address the Matter of Planning a Pregnancy *Before* Starting Gender-Affirming Hormones

If you were assigned male at birth, bank sperm.

Fertility experts recommend doing this *before* you take estradiol or a testosterone blocker; the quality of sperm may decrease after being on hormones or hormone-blockers.

- **Find a reproductive technology clinic or fertility clinic in your area.**
  You may want to search online using the phrase "fertility clinics that serve transgender individuals" to find the clinicians who truly want to help you and won't seem judgmental. There will be a setup charge and yearly banking (freezing) fees, so get this information before you go. It may be worthwhile to see if your insurance covers this, but it is typically rare.

- **Get a prescription from your primary care practitioner for "semen analysis and sperm banking for fertility preservation" that you will take to the fertility clinic.**

- **Make an appointment to collect a sample. Collecting a semen sample is done like this:**
  1. You are given a labeled specimen cup with a lid and then you're directed to a private enclosed cubicle or office with a door you can lock.
  2. You masturbate until you climax and produce a sperm specimen that goes into the cup. (The clinic usually has sexually explicit magazines; bring your own materials if you prefer.)
  3. You take your labeled and lidded specimen cup to the desk and make your next appointment. The semen analysis report will give you information on the quality and characteristics of the sperm, such as its shape, motility, the number of sperm present in the specimen, concentration, pH and viscosity, and the number of white blood cells present. Most people are advised to collect several specimens on several different days.

If you were assigned female, learn about egg harvesting and cryopreservation from a fertility specialist.

Egg harvesting is a more complicated process. It is a minor gynecologic surgery that is timed with your ovulation (egg release). As such, this process may be problematic if your gender dysphoria is severe. Your hormonal environment may be manipulated by medications to temporarily stop your usual hormonal release, and an ovulation stimulator medication is given to induce the ovulation of a number of eggs. Egg harvesting is done with ultrasound guidance and by inserting a needle deep in the vagina and into the ovarian follicles.

Expect to pay around $10,000, more or less, for egg harvesting and freezing. Check to see if insurance covers it, although it likely will not. Because of potential complications associated with advancing maternal age, egg harvesting and cryopreservation are best done when a person is on their 20s or early 30s. This way, you can be in your 40s and use one of your own 20- or 30-year-old eggs. You can take your time and have a pregnancy when it works best in your life, yet still minimize the risk of chromosomal abnormalities and miscarriage.

If you were assigned female at birth, consider keeping your reproductive organs (uterus, tubes, ovaries, and vagina) intact, and delay any gender-affirming genital surgery until your reproductive decisions are carried out.

You may be able to become pregnant and carry a baby in your uterus. (See the interview with Jack Shephard on pages 399–405.)

You will be required to stop testosterone several months prior to conception. If you want to carry a baby in your uterus, you may also want to consider chestfeeding your infant. If that is your urgent desire, you may even wish to avoid top surgery until after you have your kids. Chest reduction is less conducive to chestfeeding because of the disruption of milk glands and milk duct tissue, but many trans men have done it.

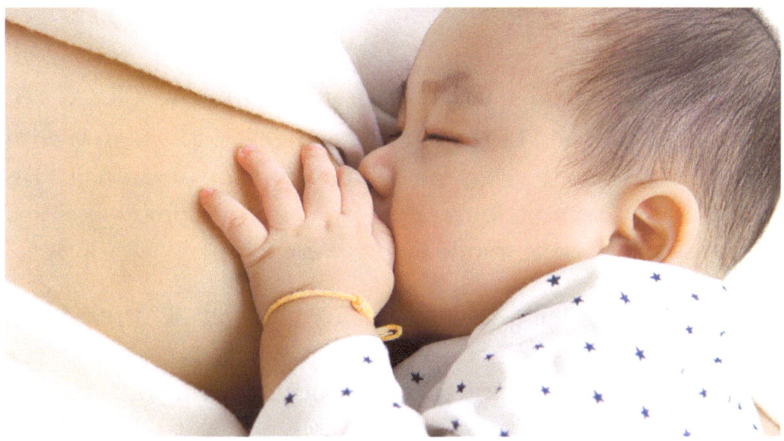

You may need to find sperm, eggs, or a surrogate to carry a pregnancy for you.

Fertility clinics will have information about young, healthy donors of both sperm and eggs.

I have spoken with folks who have arranged less formal sperm donation, such as when a best male friend or a relative donates sperm. You don't have to have sex with this person, but you must get the sperm into the vagina. People have placed the semen without a needle in a syringe, in a diaphragm, or in menstrual cup and then inserted those objects into the vagina of the person hoping to carry a baby. This isn't how it's done in a fertility clinic, of course, but I've seen it work.

A legal contract is encouraged. Remember also that sperm processed through a sperm bank is tested and retested for STIs (particularly HIV). Clients may read extensive information about the potential donors' personal characteristics, professions, and aptitudes—and even inspect handwriting samples—as part of selecting their donor.

Talk with a fertility clinic and later with an attorney if you are considering having a surrogate carry a pregnancy for you. This can be a wonderful solution for many people, but go prepared.

Adoption is another excellent option, but it removes the option of having a child who is genetically related to you or your partner. If you are still looking for a partner and want to parent, consider a partner who already has a child or children.

A Seahorse: Pregnancy in a Transgender Man

When a transgender man carries a pregnancy and delivers a baby, he is sometimes referred to as a "seahorse."

Seahorses (the undersea kind) have a unique reproductive setup: The seahorse who was assigned female deposits the eggs she makes—all 1,000 of them—into the pouch of her partner seahorse who was assigned male. The male fertilizes and carries the eggs in his distending pouch and delivers fully formed baby seahorses in about 45 days. (Seahorse birth is remarkable; take a look at **youtube.com/watch?v=b_nEA3dtOZs**).

For a human experience, consider watching the YouTube movie trailer listed below before you read Jack Shephard's compelling interview in which he details his own experience with transitioning, pregnancy planning, delivery, and child-rearing.

The documentary movie, *Seahorse: The Dad Who Gave Birth*, was directed by Jeanie Finlay (the UK film director best known for *Game of Thrones: The Last Watch* and *Orion: The Man Who Would Be King*) and was released on August 30, 2019. *Seahorse* is the compelling story of journalist Freddy McConnell's pregnancy, labor, and delivery of his son. He found pregnancy troublesome as he describes "moving backward," almost losing himself as male hormone effects were temporarily stopped.

You can find the trailer on YouTube: **youtube.com/watch?v=0MUtJJDaDPk.** There is also an article about Freddy McConnell in *The Guardian* newspaper (**theguardian.com/society/2019/apr/20/the-dad-who-gave-birth-pregnant-trans-freddy-mcconnell**).[110] You can find other accounts on YouTube as well.

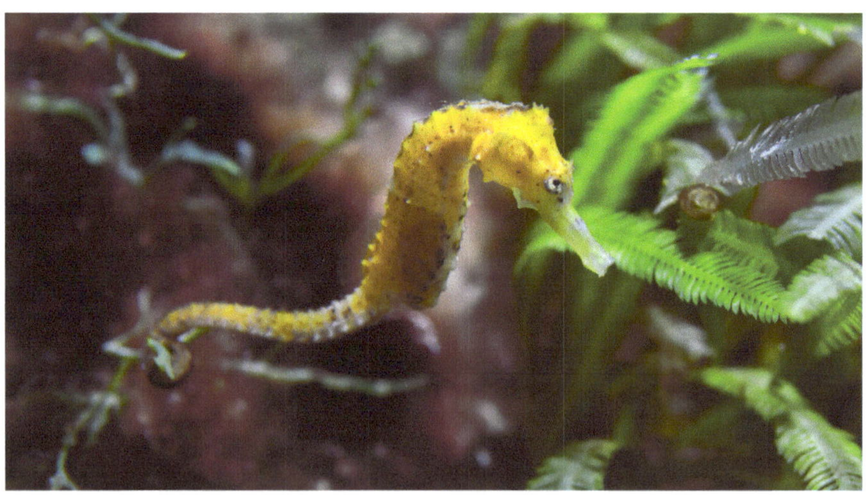

110 Simon Hattenstone, "The Dad Who Gave Birth: 'Being Pregnant Doesn't Change Me Being a Trans Man,'" *Guardian*, April 20, 2019, https://www.theguardian.com/society/2019/apr/20/the-dad-who-gave-birth-pregnant-trans-freddy-mcconnell.

My Interview with Human Seahorse Jack Shephard

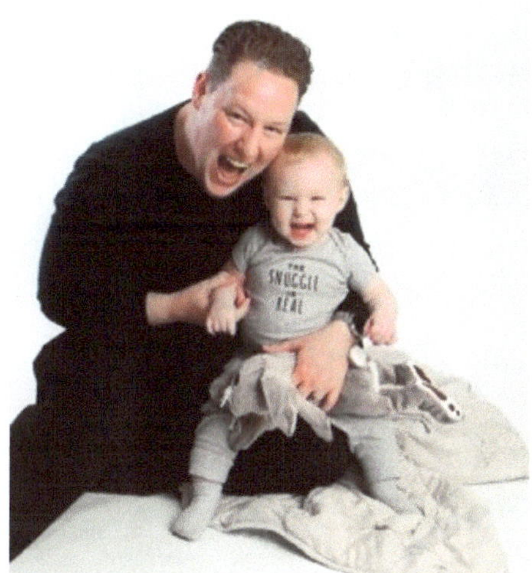

Jack Shephard, RN, BSN, BS, was the first man I had ever met who had given birth to his child. I found the interview to be fascinating and the photos enchanting. Here's our conversation from December 14, 2019.

Linda: Tell us a little about your background: Where did you grow up, what kind of family did you have, and what was your earlier life like?

Jack: I was born in Nuremberg, Germany, because my father was in the military. I don't remember moving around much because my father's time with the military ended when I was still pretty young. We moved to California to live with my grandparents for a while. I have an older brother and a younger brother, so it was difficult being a family of five squished into two rooms in a shared house.

My birth name was unpronounceable to most people until long after I had stopped using it and it became popularized by some television star. So, from the start, I knew I was different from those around me. I learned early to anticipate, though, that others wouldn't understand me, the simplest example being my name. Sometimes a new or substitute teacher would just pause around where my name was supposed to fit in on the attendance roll call, and I would volunteer my name's correct pronunciation.

Being the perceptive kid that I was, I also learned about social roles and what was expected of me. I repeated the favorite colors of my friends, wore the things I was told to wear, and behaved the way other children of my perceived sex behaved. My family was also very strictly religious, so the social programming was intense. I wasn't aware of how intense until I entered high school and college, when I finally had something to compare it to.

Linda: Tell us about your education, your career, and career goals.

Jack: I had to get away from home before I could really go to school in earnest. I was very lucky to have found a relationship with a guy who was very enthusiastic about education. I approached my family about moving out (to move in with him) after I was 18 and did so with the intent of going to school, which they were supportive of.

It took me 7 years to get my first bachelor's degree in general biology, but I did it. During the last year of my initial schooling in 2008, then-President Bush cut funding for biological research in half, which not only meant that I couldn't finish an internship that I was lucky enough to get, but also that my shiny new degree was approximately worthless.

I discovered that I didn't like being alone all day after working several isolating jobs, and I felt that I would be well-suited to work with people, so the next logical step was nursing. I got my nursing-assistant certification through a food-stamps retraining grant, completed other prerequisites, and applied to nursing school at the University of Washington. I graduated from the UW School of Nursing in 2013 and had a whirlwind nursing career where I became a jack-of-all-trades.

I held jobs in psychology, clinical research, orthopedics, medical-surgical nursing, corrections, spinal cord injury, and hepatology. After about 4.5 years after graduating from UW, I began taking a graduate family-nurse-practitioner program primarily online. I had to take a leave of absence after a year due to life changes, including a divorce. I still have plans to return to graduate school, but it may be a while before I am financially able to return. When I finally do go back, I plan to provide gender-affirming care as a primary care provider and hopefully do some research by data mining with existing patient records.

Linda: Please give us some basic information about your transition.

Jack: My transition really began when I started to have the language to describe my feelings. Before having this ability, I still *felt* who I was inside; it wasn't as if the language gave me the feelings. I identified with male characters in film, television, and books, and I imagined myself as those characters as I was doing almost everything. I came by this language when I took a human sexuality course in college. It was there that I learned the difference between sex and gender, as well as the existence of folks who identified as somewhere in between, which was at the time called "genderqueer."

At first, I thought that I must be genderqueer, because how could I not acknowledge that I had female body parts even though I walked around imagining myself as Luke Skywalker? The female parts were kind of staring at me in the mirror every morning. But the things that got me the most excited sexually were when I imagined myself as a man, so how did that factor in? Then I learned about people who were called "transsexual" and how that differed from transgender or other related terms.

During this course, I discovered that there are people who actually choose to make physical changes to their bodies to varying degrees to better align their appearance with who they felt they were inside. This rang pretty strongly inside me as I was frequently (constantly) imagining myself as someone else—someone male.

From there, I learned all I could about transition and what I would have to do to accomplish it. Fortunately, I had resources at the school I was attending. I also wanted social support though, not just counseling, so I started an LGBT group on the campus and became a bit of a microcelebrity in school as I began to transition socially. I changed my preferred name to Jack and most of my teachers caught on easily enough.

I went through counseling through the school, but because there were no counselors at the satellite school I was attending in eastern Washington, I had to drive 2 hours one way to get to appointments. Thankfully the counselor was kind and flexible enough to allow me to have 2-hour counseling sessions every other week to cut down on the driving expenses, but it was still a lot of time and effort.

It wasn't until I had moved back to Seattle that I was able to find a provider who was willing to prescribe testosterone for me.

Several months later, a friend of mine started to see the changes that were happening in me and became excited to start testosterone also. He started shortly thereafter and we basically went through transition together, which was very important to both of us so we could have that support. It took me many years to get to a place where I was hardly ever mistaken for a woman, even in spite of a baritone voice and a decent amount of facial hair.

Linda: When did you first want to be a parent? How did you actively include getting pregnant in your plans to transition? How did you arrange your plans with a sperm donor, and what were your considerations?

Jack: I don't know if it was just something that was always expected of me, but I can remember wanting to be a parent almost from the time I realized that I had that potential. I think that happened at around age 6 or 7. I might have realized that I would one day grow big enough to be like my parents, even though the specifics of this were somewhat unclear. The year before I started taking testosterone, Thomas Beatie had given birth to his first child after being on testosterone for many years and having undergone a bilateral mastectomy. But I thought that it was probably not something I'd be able to do for many reasons. So, I resigned myself to adopting if I wanted to have children in the future, and I started testosterone as quickly as possible.

I arranged with my conceptive partner to not have him named on the birth certificate and to release him from responsibility related to the child. I had a friend draft the legal paperwork for us, and we had them signed and witnessed by a notary. I wanted to make sure that my conceptive partner didn't fear the future—that is, fear the financial or social support of the child. I also found that I didn't necessarily want another person making big decisions about how to raise my child.

Linda: I understand that listing a trans parent on a child's birth certificate can be problematic. How are you listed?

Jack: I am listed as the mother and I am actually listed under my birth name, which I have yet to have changed on my own birth certificate; the law required the names of parents as they were listed on their birth certificates. I do not know if I would be able to have my title changed on my daughter's birth certificate, but I am certain that I can have my name changed on her birth certificate once it has been changed on mine.

Linda: Tell me about your conceptive partner.

Jack: My conceptive partner was someone with whom I had had a previous sexual relationship. We had also lived together, and he was an incredibly supportive person in my life. We had talked about the possibility of having a child together several years before I started to plan seriously. He is part of my daughter's life still but currently lives in another state. I'm Daddy and he's Poppa. I send him pictures of her and keep him updated on her development.

It was ideal for me to have someone that I know and trust as my conceptive partner, but I think I would have eventually compromised with someone I knew less well if it came to it. It is nice being able to look at my daughter and her traits and behaviors as they emerge and see the similarities from both of us. It is also helpful to know some genetic history for her future healthcare.

Linda: What experiences did you have in getting care for your pregnancy confirmation and pregnancy care? How did you find a supportive healthcare team? What experiences were affirming? What experiences were difficult?

Jack: I was very fortunate in that I had a friend in nursing school who was part of our queers-and-allies group and was in school to be a nurse-midwife. I talked to her about what it might look like and she was supportive and gave me as much information as she had. She said that she wanted to specialize in this area of midwifery (mid-husbandry?) and would be happy to help when I was ready.

For me, the symptoms of pregnancy and the shape changes weren't so big of a deal because I had seen myself as a man for so long, but I had also wanted to be a parent for so long that I had read about and written stories about male characters who got pregnant through magical or technological means. So I felt like my identity didn't suffer too much, except when others would misgender me during that time.

The hospital my college friend worked at (Overlake Medical Center) was really great about their approach when I became her patient. They had a meeting with all the hospital birthing managers—labor and delivery, postpartum, social work, outpatient clinic, patient education—and we came up with a plan. I let them know what sorts of things were important to me and they also created a one-on-one birth education class for me to attend so I wouldn't have to have the majority circumstance make me feel awkward or embarrassed. I had pretty much everything I needed in part because I had such an amazing midwife.

Chestfeeding was something I wanted to try, but I knew that because I had had a bilateral mastectomy (top surgery) years earlier that there was no telling what might happen. I ended up not chestfeeding, mostly due to the difficulty in mechanics and concern over my daughter getting enough nutrition, especially when she was born a few weeks early. I tried formula and a nursing kit with tubes, but it was all a bit difficult to manage. With everything else I had to handle, it became less of a priority to chestfeed, and I found other ways of bonding with my daughter, like through skin-to-skin contact.

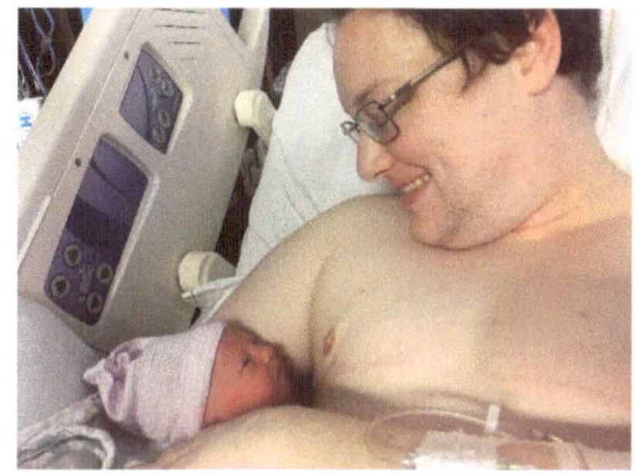

Part of me was honestly a little scared that my parents would show up and kidnap my daughter from the hospital, lest she be doomed to life with an unbeliever, but the hospital was very reassuring about their policies regarding infant security.

Linda: What personal support did you have? What was your experience with community during pregnancy (being welcomed, avoided, and so on)?

Jack: I had support from a few good friends. Those I told about the pregnancy were excited for me, but I was so busy otherwise that I didn't really have a gauge for whether I was being avoided or not. I had a baby shower that a bunch of friends came to, so I don't think I was generally avoided.

Linda: Did you experience depression or anxiety during pregnancy or after childbirth, and if so, how did you manage this?

Jack: I was a little nervous during pregnancy, but it was after my daughter was born and I had to take care of her and do things for her that I became more anxious. It was very useful that my college friend told me that postpartum depression usually manifests as fears of not being an adequate caregiver. Understanding that those thoughts could get out of hand were what helped me to stop and really think about what I was able to do for my daughter and how what I could do was enough.

Linda: What was your labor and delivery like?

Jack: It was kind of like a TV sitcom delivery, short of the baby being born in a car or a barn. My daughter literally punched her way out of me. I woke my partner by asking for a ride to the hospital, and he thought I was joking at first because it was a bit early (both in gestational date and hour of the morning). Then he saw how much pain I was in. When I spoke with my midwife about my symptoms, she said my experience was a bit unique in that I was experiencing blinding period-cramp pain separate from the tight muscle contractions I was experiencing at the fundus (top) of my uterus.

When we got to the hospital, they couldn't check me in because my gender in the medical records didn't allow for it and I hadn't been preregistered. It took what felt like an eternity to get an epidural because it took so long to sort out my registration and because I had had a previous reaction to Demerol, so the staff was concerned about a cross-reaction allergy with another opioid. Once I had the epidural, things went more smoothly. Once my midwife was able to check my cervix, she was able to ascertain why I was in so much cramping pain; my cervix had dilated to 10 centimeters in about 3 hours.

Linda: What were your experiences like in dealing with the medical community during labor and delivery?

Jack: The labor and delivery staff were great, for the most part. There were a few dinosaurs who couldn't refer to me by my desired pronouns no matter how often they were reminded, but they didn't stay for long.

It was actually the obstetrics bosses of my midwife who were more offensive. They set requirements for my care that my testosterone level be monitored several times during my pregnancy so they could make sure I wasn't doping (taking testosterone). This made me indignant for a couple of reasons, the first of which was that they thought that my gender was wrong because they were trying to avoid "virilization of the fetus," which is one of the theories about how trans men come to be. The other was that they thought I would try to harm my child by injecting something with unknown effects into my body during pregnancy. I was also asked to consult with a high-risk obstetrics program at UW and have STI monitoring several times because my conceptive partner was HIV-positive, even though he and I had been on antiretrovirals during the conception process.

Linda: What did you think of that baby when you first saw her?

Jack: I thought she was amazing and the cutest thing I had ever seen. So did everyone else.

Linda: How has it been to raise your daughter? Global question, of course, but what are your greatest challenges in parenting?

Jack: Raising my daughter has been challenging, but it brings frequent joy. She is so happy all the time! I think one of the greatest challenges has been trying to parent by myself. It's a big job, but I find I'm able to get help when I need it.

Linda: What have your experiences been like in interacting with other parents?

Jack: I don't know a lot of other parents. My midwife friend from college has a teenager and she was able to give me some really good insights on parenting—like no matter what, it's expected that you are not going to be perfect as a parent. And that's okay! That was so comforting and took some of the pressure off.

Linda: What advice would you have for other men like yourself who are now considering parenting?

Jack: Go with what your heart says, whether that's to have kids or not. If you feel weird about it, don't force yourself. If it's something you want to do, I encourage you to find out more about your options and make a plan that will work for you.

There will not be a right time to have kids. There are always things you could do to be more prepared or more financially stable or save for the kid's college before they're even born.

There are no guarantees that everything will go smoothly and you may have to sacrifice some things to have this experience, but you shouldn't have to deny yourself fatherhood because of someone else's definition of gender.

Linda: What do you see ahead for you and your daughter?

Jack: I think she's going to be an amazing young person and I will try to give her options and exposure to the different conceptions of gender. From what her teachers tell me, she may also be destined for a career in healthcare.

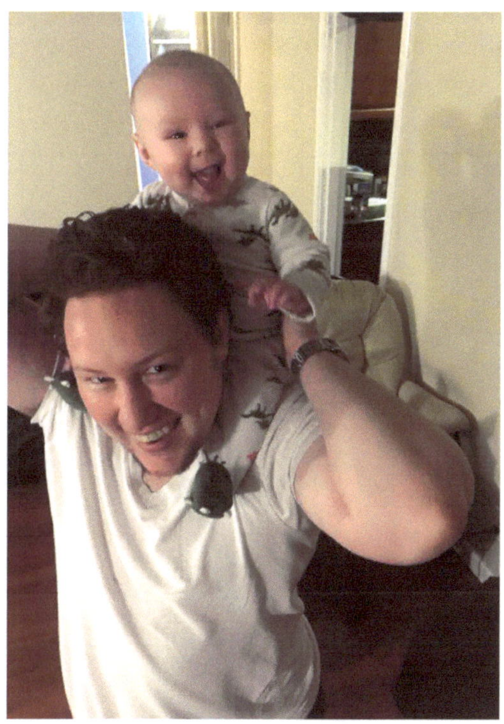

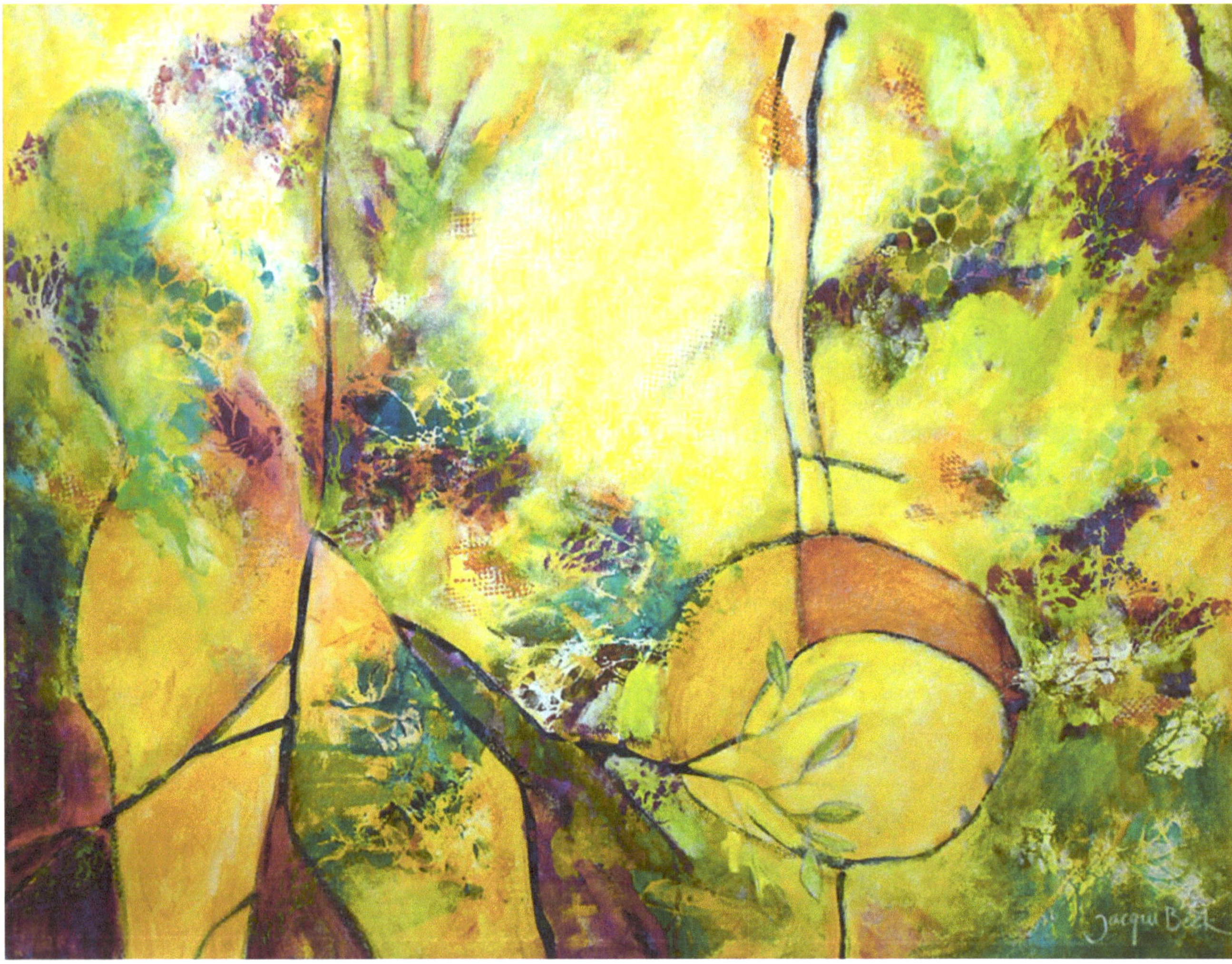

I Belong

CHAPTER 22
Sex and Relationships

I have been working in the areas of family planning, treating sexually transmitted infections (STIs), delivering babies, providing care for gender-nonconforming individuals, and counseling people with respect to issues of sex and sexuality beginning when I was about 20. Decades! Sexuality certainly isn't boring and it's often complex.

At its best, sexuality can represent one of our greatest paths to love, intimacy, comfort, neurobiological emotional healing, and personal growth. At its worst, our sexuality—how it's used by us or others—can seriously demean our own sense of self-worth and lead us into high-risk behaviors with profound consequences like STIs, unplanned pregnancies, physical injury, emotional and psychological trauma, or just an old-fashioned broken heart.

As sexual beings (at least for those who define themselves in this way), I've always imagined that we must have two circulatory systems: one that carries blood "north" to the brain, and one that carries our blood "south"—that is, to the genital region. I also think that the "southern circulatory system" is dominant; it has the capacity to override the northern circulatory system completely. (You appreciate that this is a metaphor only. We do not have northern and southern circulatory systems, of course.)

My point here is that "genital thinking" can be mighty compelling, and it's a smart idea to consider sexual matters with our actual brains first.

In this chapter, I'll present matters of body image, dating in its various forms, sexual response (learning about original-issue bodies and learning what to do with reconfigured parts), toys that help people learn and enhance their sexual response, sexual consent, poly and kink, and safe sex. Then, we'll go briefly into what may be even scarier territory: dealing with personal rejection, handling the death of a long-term partner, and grieving and recovering. This cannot possibly be comprehensive. But buckle up and come along.

Body Image

I have examined thousands and thousands of people's bodies in my career as a nurse, a nurse practitioner, and for decades more, as a physician. I have examined more living bodies than most humans could imagine, and I have probably heard more people express concerns about their bodies than I would ever have expected.

It always startles me when someone who looks stereotypically beautiful complains that their breasts are too big or too small or shaped "wrong," that their bodies are too fat or too skinny, or that their face has features they describe as ugly. I have heard people agonize over "bat-wing arms" or "flawed" skin. I have heard many people question whether their genitals look "normal" or "right." (The answer to this question is almost always a resounding "yes" because of the enormous range of normal in the human body. Go back and look at Jamie McCartney's *Great Wall of Vagina* in Chapter 12.)

All of this body dysphoria doesn't even begin to cover bodily concerns related to gender dysphoria. If you were assigned female at birth (AFAB) but identify as male, you may want your chest reconstructed to appear as a male chest, not out of vanity (whatever that is) but out of a core need to have a synchronous body and mind. If you were assigned male at birth (AMAB) but know yourself to be female, your dysphoria may be so profound that you may not want to use the penis to save sperm for later fertility or even to collect a urine specimen!

Body image is complicated for many of us. Following are some points that may be of help.

There exists an astonishing range of normal in the human body. As in everything else, we will likely find ourselves *somewhere along a bell-shaped curve of normal*. Of course, there are congenital or trauma-induced abnormalities. But, for the most part, we simply vary.

If you find yourself being critical about your body, talk to yourself about this. Try allowing a little positive self-talk into the mix. And then, try to give your positive self-talk at least *equal time* with the negative self-talk. (If you succeed at establishing that balance, apply this to other areas of your life for improved mental health in general.)

Realize that most of the images that we see in the media are heavily altered. The company that makes Dove soap ran a commercial a number of years ago where they took a model who was beautiful to begin with and then digitally "corrected" her bit by bit until she was "perfect."[111] The point is, nobody has a chance by these standards. Has it occurred to you that the media and the advertising industry sell us concepts or products by inviting us to feel badly about ourselves? We don't have to let these messages in, but it's hard not to!

Almost nobody has porn star genitals. We just don't. Genitals can be as varied-looking as our faces. No matter how they look, our genitals function to enhance the pleasure of our lives and perhaps to facilitate reproduction.

If there's something about your body that you really do not like, change it. Take the energy spent in pain and worry and redirect that energy into making the changes you need or want to make. This applies to your weight, the shape of your nose, the color of your hair, and most certainly to the body asynchronies associated with gender dysphoria. Go back and reread the part in this book about choosing a surgeon in Chapter 10 and start doing your research.

If you truly cannot get around this body image dilemma, talk to your therapist. But do not allow these issues to take over and interfere with your mental health and happiness going forward.

Dating

Many people seek connections with others. Whether it is for recreation, companionship, intellectual stimulation, affection, sexual contact, reproduction, or simply to go to a movie, we tend to connect with others. Often, we find one person to spend some or most of our available free time with; some people spend time with several or many people. (Others, of course, do not seek these connections. If that is a person's position—a free choice to be singular rather than to avoid real or imagined pain—so be it.)

111 Unilever, "Dove Evolution," October 6, 2006, YouTube video, https://www.youtube.com/watch?v=iYhCn0jf46U.

Finding Someone You'd Like to Date

When we were in high school or college, the world seemed set up to help us find partners. We were in classes with similar-minded, eager potential friends and lovers. We could "sample" people (with some consequences). In general, it was the perfect time to explore. Looking back, this exploration of people may have been as important to our development as the academics.

When our attention turns more seriously to our work, the selection available for dating and relationships can narrow. We may start looking for activities that recreate the concentration of people we experienced in school; a drama group, volunteer activities, a political campaign, an ultimate Frisbee team, and so on.

Online Dating

Online dating is more private (until you go out with someone), and you can choose from a variety of online sites depending on your interests. Examples include Match.com, POF.com (Plenty of Fish, as in "in the sea"), Bumble.com, Grindr.com (male and more overtly sexual), FarmersOnly.com, OKCupid.com, Tinder.com, eHarmony.com, ChristianMingle.com, It'sJustLunch.com, Zoosk.com, SilverSingles.com, EliteSingles.com, and so on. There are sites for younger and older people, same-sex seekers, and LGBTQIA+ sites. (For a review of LGBTQIA+ sites, go to Mashable.com/roundup/best-gay-dating-apps. As their site says, "The best dating apps for gay users, since meeting people IRL is hellish." IRL means "in real life.")

Dating sites work in a variety of ways, but in general you are expected to provide a profile of yourself. This consists of a current photo or preferably several photos that you download via your computer or smartphone, plus a brief personal statement. You label your post with a title such as, "I'd Like to Meet a Nice Democrat." Then you will be asked to specify various bits of information about yourself. You don't have to provide any details at all, but you're more likely to find someone you like if you volunteer more information. This might include age, weight (or some judgment like "HWP" or "height-weight proportionate"), religious preference, whether or not you are a smoker, political affiliation, your pets, favorite movies, athletic activities, field of work, whether you have a professional degree or not, and on and on.

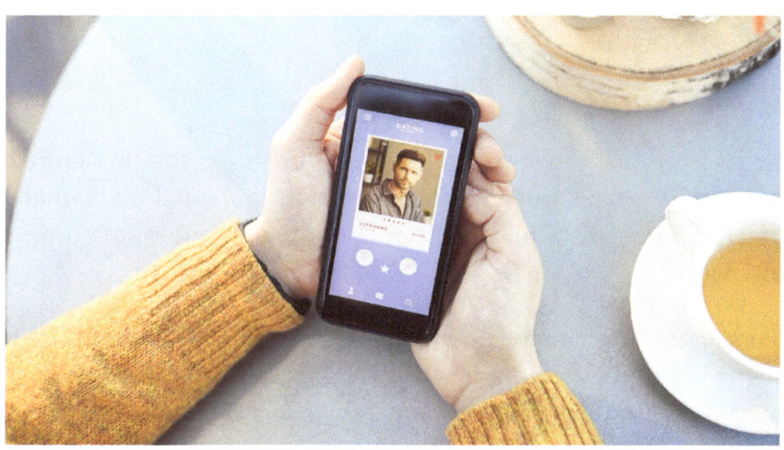

Sites generally have a fee, which ranges from a few dollars per month to much more; some are free. When you want to contact someone, you can signal them (for instance, Match.com has you "wink" at another subscriber). Once you've both made contact, you may begin an online correspondence if you wish.

While online browsing has its drawbacks, it does allow you to express and learn "deal-breaker" information right away. You know immediately who smokes, who drinks, who drives a motorcycle, who has herpes if you ask or volunteer this, and who has a dog or cat.

Some sites allow a way to offer your gender identity and dating preference. But if you are transgender or gender-nonconforming, there are always ways to articulate this information even on the more traditional sites. For example, you could say "originally a boy; exploring my feminine side." Or when they ask if you want children, you could say something like, "I want children so much that I've already frozen the ingredients." *That* could start a dialog!

Write your introductory information carefully. Understand that you do not have to physically meet anyone at all. Remember that you will communicate initially through the online site; your identification and your contact information is hidden. Keep it that way until you trust the new person.

Be careful when you meet someone in person for the first time. Let a friend know where you are going. (I had my office manager page me 30 minutes into my first date with my late husband Steve at a Starbucks with two exits!) Trust your intuition. Don't go anywhere with anyone who makes your stomach uneasy.

What Is a TERF?

TERF is an acronym for trans-exclusionary radical feminist.

According to Dictionary.com, a TERF is defined as "an advocate of radical feminism who believes that a trans woman's gender identity is not legitimate and who is hostile to the inclusion of trans people and gender-diverse people in the feminist movement."

Life is too short to surround yourself with people who discount you from the start.

Sharing Your Gender Information

When you are starting a relationship, gender truths should probably come up before you become intimate. Maybe it's not at the moment you meet, but it is a matter of your personal safety that you do not allow this information to be discovered by surprise. Tell a partner about your gender nonconformity ahead of time if you hope to become intimate.

In an online dating circumstance, you can introduce this as one part of your profile. Be aware that potential dates are hidden by the privacy of their computers. If they disapprove of you and trans people in general, they can insult and offend you with relative anonymity. They can also stand you up (arrange to meet you and not show up), or prepare to meet you in person and drive by with honks and slurs. Worse, there are people who may have an agenda to harm you physically. Be careful; these are people who are not worth your time or feelings. Do the best you can to weed them out as early as possible.

Back to the gender reveal. Let's take an example: Suppose you are a non-op trans woman (you either haven't had gender-affirming vaginoplasty or you don't intend to). You and your potential assigned-male-at-birth partner are becoming sexually aroused, you begin sexual play, and he is surprised to find that you have a penis. Startled, your date may not know how to conduct himself. If his surprise translates into transphobia or homophobia, he may get angry and you may be in physical danger.

It's better to discuss your body and sexual preferences with clothing on and "feet on the ground." Your safety of both body and mind are important.

Over the years, I've spoken with several non-op trans women who make it a practice to conceal their genitals during sexual intimacy, even with a long-term partner or spouse. They may satisfy a partner by oral or anal sex, and they say the partner doesn't know the penis is even there. Again, a surprise reveal may place a woman in jeopardy. I wonder how the trans woman's needs and desires are met?

Be aware also that there's a segment of the population that is intrigued by a transgender woman with a penis as a fetish. A fetishist may require a particular body part for their sexual gratification. Such a person may obsess about the penis of a trans woman. This is to the extent that they are not attracted by the *person,* but rather, the object of their fetishism—that is, the penis. As in anything sexual, if the trans woman is looking for someone to obsess about her penis, that could work, but be aware of "chasers"—meaning cis men who seek out *only* trans women without being completely upfront about their sexual preference or their motivation.

We have to remember that with consenting adults, any practice that is *mutually* desired and not injurious to one party can be fine. Even sexual practices that involve physical pain can be alright as long as both participants agree and can stop any behavior with a single safe word. Clearly this is not the case where one partner is controlled by the other or is being hurt without seeking out rough sexual behavior.

Having Sex

"Having sex" undoubtedly means different things to different people. However, it is never the forced contact of rape or sexual assault; these are acts of power and violence rather than sex.

Sexual intimacy usually starts with a foundation of attraction, affection, and, hopefully, trust. You feel that you want to be with a particular person. Maybe you like the way they look. Maybe you are attracted to their irreverent sense of humor or the fact that they vote the way you do. You like to be close to them, and it feels good when they touch you or hold you.

Hopefully, you trust this individual enough to share private information. If you don't trust them, stop and wait until you find someone you do trust. Get the blood back up into your brain. This is the moment to stop and move on; you'll find someone else.

If you are transgender or gender-nonconforming, you must trust a person with whom you are intimate with your private information. They must understand that you may have body parts that differ from your overall presentation. For example, suppose you were assigned male at birth but identify as female. Your special person understands that your genitals don't include labia, a vagina, or a clitoris unless you've had sexual reassignment surgery. And that's perfectly fine with them. Additionally, you trust that your person will not post this information on social media platforms because you know and trust that they care about you.

As for any couple (or group) becoming intimate, it's very normal to begin to explore each other's bodies. You will find that touching certain parts of the body result in a sensual excitement called arousal. A trans female may prefer the term "aroused" to "having an erection." A trans male may talk about his clitoris as his penis or by some other name. It will likely be arousing to your partner to use the terms they like.

The mouth, the breasts, and the genitals are all erogenous areas, meaning that stimulating these places is likely to produce sexual excitement. You will likely find other areas that feel particularly nice for you or your partner, such as perhaps the thighs, the buttocks, and the rectum. It really doesn't matter as long as those enjoying the journey are consenting adults.

Touching, kissing, using the tongue in ways you both enjoy, hugging, breathing, moving together, and encouraging each other all lead to an increase in sexual arousal, culminating in (or not) the climax of orgasm. Having sex does not require penetration. It all depends on what you and your partner enjoy and what works for all involved.

Sexual Q & A

Q **Do you and your partner have to climax?**

A **Not necessarily.**

Q **Do you and your partner have to orgasm at the same time?**

A **Lord, no! Not required. Can be nice; can be distracting.**

Q **Do you have to have orgasms at all?**

A **It depends on the person, but I'm reminded of the words of Beatrice Kaufmann: "I've been poor and I've been rich, and rich is better."**

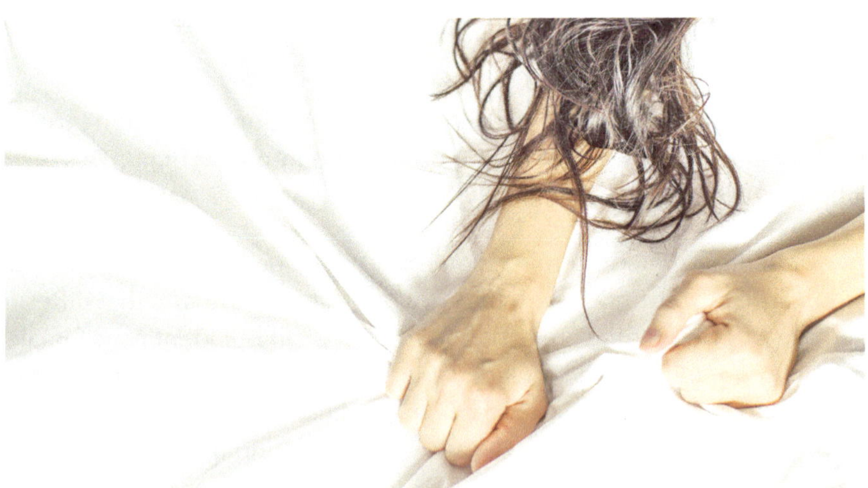

A Surgeon's Notes on Trans Female Ejaculation

As far as female ejaculation goes, I don't know how frequent it is, but I can say that some patients have reported consistent ejaculation with each orgasm, with varying amounts of ejaculate, from minimal to a lot. The post-op trans female ejaculate is not truly semen. It is clear, slippery like lubricant, and much the same as precum. And yes, aroused trans women will secrete precum. At times, precum may be copious and allow for penetration without synthetic lubrication.

I looked up the composition of semen. It is about 65 to 70 percent seminal fluid (which surgeons do not excise), 25 percent prostatic fluid (not removed either), and 5 percent fluid from bulbourethral glands (also left in place). And 2 to 5 percent of semen comes from the actual testicles and epididymis (which are removed). Trans female ejaculate is composed of the first three types of fluid.

— Ellie Zara Ley, MD

Learning What Works to Experience Orgasm

What is orgasm anyway? Here is a Merriam-Webster dictionary definition: "Intense or paroxysmal excitement; especially the rapid pleasurable release of neuromuscular tensions at the height of sexual arousal that is usually accompanied by the ejaculation of semen in the male and vaginal contractions in the female."[112]

Since that definition left me unsatisfied, I turned to Dr. Emily Nagoski's excellent book, *Come as You Are*. Dr. Nagoski says: "When you strip it down to the universal essentials, here's what you get: Orgasm is the sudden, involuntary release of sexual tension."[113]

The experience may be the "humdrum" orgasm or what Nagoski terms the "brain-melting, toe-curling, turn-the-stars-into-rainbows type of orgasm!"[114]

While Nagoski's book is, by her description, "basically a book about cisgender women," I think it has enormous merit for everyone. She covers the obligatory anatomy, but in the context of the embryologic homologues (meaning the fundamental information that male and female embryos are identical until the process of testosterone-driven differentiation begins). She reassures us that our anatomy and sexual response are normal. She walks you through orgasm with her model of accelerators and brakes, simple coaching, and encouragement. Nagoski's book also takes us gently through the basics of self-stimulation.

Other nominees (mine) include these books:

- *For Yourself: The Fulfillment of Female Sexuality*, Lonnie Barback, PhD, 2000.

---

112 Merriam-Webster, s.v. "orgasm," accessed July 14, 2021, https://www.merriam-webster.com/dictionary/orgasm.

113 Emily Nagoski, *Come as You Are: The Surprising New Science That Will Transform Your Sex Life* (New York: Simon & Schuster, 2015), 361.

114 Nagoski, 282.

- *Female Ejaculation and the G-Spot*, Deborah Sundahl, 2014.
- *Sex for One: The Joy of Selfloving*, Betty Dodson, PhD, 1996.

Getting to Gender Euphoria

Lately, I've been feeling different in my transition. It's a feeling that's hard to describe. I think in a lot of ways it's all starting to feel more embodied. I think in the years prior to where I am now, I was distracted by the details in how to get where I wanted to be. I was obviously experiencing transition, but it was just a different space. Also, not to say necessarily that I've arrived at where I want to be, but I'm closer to it than I ever have been.

I feel like I've just now been able to relax a little bit and just experience it in my body, live it in this body. I think part of it has to do with finally socially transitioning, but there are other pieces of the puzzle as well that all seem to be coalescing: where I'm at with electrolysis, being gendered correctly more and more, legally changing my name and gender, and rhinoplasty. Also I'm getting glimpses of my real self when I look into the mirror.

I feel more and more that I am being seen, by myself and by others. I think a side effect of all of that was having that crazy-intense orgasm. I feel like I really am in my body, that there's a sense of alignment taking place.

I recently came across the term "gender euphoria," and I guess I've been having more moments like that. All of those things together are carrying me deeper and deeper into my Self. That orgasm felt like complete and total surrender. In some ways, that feels like where I'm at with transition.

There are obviously things that I'm consciously working toward, but at the same time I feel like I've surrendered to the experience of it. Like I've let go and have allowed myself to just experience it instead of trying to manage it. I tried so hard for so long to be strategic about my transition and make choices that would make it less difficult. The entire time, though, my body had other plans. I felt like my strategies or plans were in constant struggle with how things were playing out in real life (that is, breast growth right out of the gate). I feel like I've gotten to a place where there are no more strategies—just living and experiencing.

— *Trans woman in her 40s*

Sexual Interaction with a Partner

If any area begs for excellent communication, it's the area of sexual interaction. Tell your partner what feels good to you; ask them to tell you what feels good to them. You may begin to develop your own words or phrases to explain what you prefer.

Let's go back briefly to the Netter drawings of embryologic development. Refer to page 209 to remind yourself of the color-coded genital structures. While all of the genital structures are erogenous (that is, responsive to sexual stimulation), the most sensitive areas are the clitoris in an AFAB and the glans penis in an AMAB. These structures are analogous, different only in their size as mediated by testosterone. (Even the shape and structure of both the clitoris and the penis are virtually identical, although it's a little trickier to see the smaller clitoral shaft and there's no urethra passing through the clitoris.) The prostate in an AMAB responds to sexual stimulation and is not removed in vaginoplasty. You may be able to feel it along the front (upper or anterior) wall of the neovagina, much as an AFAB may feel the G-spot in the analogous location. (The G-spot, female ejaculation, the periurethral sponge, and the Skene's glands: All have been such medical mysteries to the traditional, mostly male (back then) medical community!

For a helpful review on the clitoral-versus-Gräfenberg-spot controversy, read the online article "Models of Sexual Response" on the *Our Bodies, Ourselves* website (**ourbodiesourselves.org/book-excerpts/health-article/models-sexual-response**) to learn information from Shere Hite, Harold Lief, Helen Singer Kaplan, Bernie Zilbergeld, Carol Rinkleib Ellison, Beverly Whipple, and Karen Brash-McGreer, which all expand on the work of sexologists William Masters and Virginia Johnson.[115]

When we think of orgasm in an assigned male, we think of the penis becoming erect and ejaculation occurring with seminal fluid pulsing through the urethra to the outside world. (I believe it may have been Lily Tomlin who said, "Nice girls don't use words like 'throb.'") Semen consists of spermatozoa from the testicles and fluids from the prostate, seminal vesicles, and bulbourethral glands at the base of the penis.

> **Most people think ejaculation is synonymous with orgasm in a person who is assigned male at birth. Not necessarily. Assigned males can learn to separate their sexual contractions from the ejaculation itself. This is a tantric practice that allows the individual to "last" longer, delaying orgasm.**
>
> — *Tina Schermer Sellers, PhD, LMFT, founder of the Northwest Institute on Intimacy*

In an assigned female, erectile tissue in the clitoris and its supporting crura (legs) become engorged in response to sexual stimulation. The crura are analogous to the penile corpora cavernosa. With orgasm, contractions may occur in the upper portion of the vagina and in the uterus. Although not all assigned females experience ejaculations during orgasm, many do. Fluid pulses out of the periurethral area, probably originating in the periurethral sponge wrapped around the urethra, much the same as the prostate gland wraps around the assigned male urethra.

The G-spot, located on the anterior vaginal wall, becomes enlarged and more defined with stimulation. In addition to the clitoris, the G-spot in the anterior vaginal wall becomes another "sexual center" for many assigned females.

Learning What to Do with Reconfigured Body Parts

If you or your partner has had genital reconstruction for gender affirmation, you will want to familiarize with the embryologic equivalents.

115 Our Bodies, Ourselves contributors, "Models of Sexual Response," *Our Bodies, Ourselves*, October 15, 2011, https://www.ourbodiesourselves.org/book-excerpts/health-article/models-sexual-response/.

In Vaginoplasty

The glans penis is reconfigured into the neoclitoris. As in the assigned female, it will have a shaft and be protected by the neoclitoral hood. (If a woman has had a two-step surgery with labiaplasty after the initial vaginoplasty, the clitoris will be hooded at the second step. Prior to that, the neoclitoris is more exposed and may even feel too sensitive for stimulation.) The prostate gland is not removed but remains wrapped around the urethra on the front or anterior wall of the neovagina. It too responds to sexual stimulation.

What the neovagina does *not* have is the capacity to "sweat" or self-lubricate. Choose one of the many personal lubricants available (see "Toys to Augment Sexual Response" on page 421) to make vaginal stimulation more pleasurable and to prevent the development of microtears from penetration. (**Note:** Neovaginal lubrication does occur when the neovaginal lining is derived from peritoneal or colonic tissue.)

Advice from Dr. Wittenberg

I discuss with patients having vaginoplasty that the nerves are preserved to the essential area of the clitoris, but their orgasm is going to be different postoperatively than preoperatively. After 3 months, they can start masturbating. I don't give them a road map for this because, just like AFAB adolescents, every woman has to find out what works for them with excitation. It is different for each person, and it can take up to a year for the nerves to heal. In the first year, there can be excessive numbness, excessive sensitivity, or both.

I do discuss that there is a second erogenous zone, the G-spot, where the prostate is. I ask them if they have had vaginal or clitoral orgasm.

— Heidi Wittenberg, MD

Advice from Dr. Ley

For post-op trans women, the majority are able to orgasm by 3 to 9 months, although my patients have ranged from 2 weeks post-op to over 2 years post-op for a first orgasm. Some patients have shared that the mechanism to achieve orgasm are the following (but, as expected, quite variable from one to another): direct clitoral stimulation, vaginal penetration (which could have a relation to or be the equivalent of prostate stimulation), stimulation of the neuromuscular bundle* of the neoclitoris, or most probable, through a combination of these along with their mental and emotional state at the time of sexual intimacy.

**The neurovascular bundle is composed of the superficial penile fascia (dartos), dorsal artery and nerves, deep penile fascia (Buck's fascia), and the tunica albuginea. This strip of tissue is folded onto itself and sutured in place, positioning the clitoris anatomically; it is the folded bundle of nerves over the pubic bone and behind and above the clitoris that can be quite stimulating by bumping, tapping, rubbing, and so on.*

— Ellie Zara Ley, MD

In Metoidioplasty

When an AFAB has a metoidioplasty, the clitoris—already enlarged from the influence of testosterone—is configured to make it protrude more. This continues to function as the primary arousal center.

Refer to pages 422–423 for information about GenderCat's Fascination Sleeve and Buck Angel's Buck Off. Both are pleasure-inducing products that facilitate masturbation; a ribbed cylinder is placed over the hormonally enlarged clitoris—stimulated by suction and repeated in-and-out hand movement.

Advice from Drs. Wittenberg and Ley, Combined

While a person may take up to a year to heal after metoidioplasty, for the most part an earlier response than a year can be expected since the nerves are preserved, and less surgical "organ-gami" (according to Dr. Wittenberg) is involved with the metoidioplasty phallus than other surgeries. Again, finding the right stimulation is an individual adventure.

In Phalloplasty

In any of the phalloplasty types we've talked about, the hormonally enlarged clitoris is either tucked inside the base of the neophallus or it remains exposed at its base. Erection occurs with the use of an implanted pump or malleable rod. Remember that the glans penis portion of the neophallus is constructed from tissue of the forearm, the anterior thigh, or other sites such as the abdomen. While neither of these sites is particularly erogenous to begin with, rely on the powerful override of the brain as well as the sexual response from the testosterone-enhanced original parts.

> Everyone's genitals are made of all the same parts, just organized in different ways. The differences don't necessarily mean anything, they're just varieties of beautiful and healthy. Actually, that could be the most important thing you'll ever learn about human sexuality.[116]
>
> — *Emily Nagoski, PhD*

On the next several pages is a wonderful piece is contributed by NadjaDee. Read, laugh, and learn!

116 Emily Nagoski, *Come as You Are: The Surprising New Science That Will Transform Your Sex Life* (New York: Simon & Schuster, 2015), 282.

Confessions of a Post-Op Trans Girl: Does Anyone Know a Good Electrician?

by NadjaDee

I was asked to write about how it feels to have sexual relations postsurgery, but in order to do that, I must first give a little backstory.

After I transitioned, the only seriously depressing moments were in the morning, when I would shower and get ready for work. I was one of the luckier ones; most people wouldn't know I was trans just by looking at me. This meant that most of my day was good, and I would get the pronouns that matched my identity. Being called "she," "her," or even "Miss" was a win in my book. I was even happy with "Ma'am" even though it implied I was older, but it was still a feminine pronoun. But, in the mornings, I would step into the shower, be faced with male genitals, and feel dysphoric again. I went from undressed to depressed in a matter of seconds.

So I knew I wanted to get gender-affirmation surgery for most of my life. I just never knew how I was going to find a good doctor and pass a therapist's evaluation, let alone save up all the money. It seemed like surgery was a lifetime away, a brass ring that would always remain hopelessly out of reach.

But then I met the man who would later become my husband. He didn't care that I was pre-op—he had the ability to see me simply as me, a woman. When we had sex, he knew that my genitals were off-limits. I didn't want to be reminded of the fact that I didn't have a vagina, and he didn't ever call attention to it. I wished I could be like some non-op trans girls I knew, but I couldn't convince myself that my male organ was just an elongated clitoris. Nope. To me, it was a part that was attached to me, but I was not attached to it.

My partner and I both knew that I wanted surgery, that I *needed* surgery. This was before the days of legal same-sex marriage in any state and he wanted to marry me. For me, it was a matter of mind not matching body and creating a deep sense of body dysmorphia, which led to severe depression.

Finally, we got there. I was able to schedule myself for gender-affirmation surgery. We didn't have a lot of money and couldn't afford the local surgeons in the States. Doing some research, we found that even with added airfare and hotel, the surgeons in Thailand were affordable. They did excellent work and the hospitals were top-notch, complete with an English-speaking nursing staff. Not only could we manage the cost, but we would also get to travel, or at least my other half would be able to sightsee while I was stuck in bed, recovering from major surgery. In addition, for the cost of just lower genital surgery in the States, I could get both vaginoplasty plus breast augmentation if we went to Thailand. I could finally travel abroad while traveling as a "broad." A win-win in my book.

So, the surgery came and went. I was recovering and it was time to travel back home. After surgery, you spend a lot of time healing and even more time spent on the tasks of aftercare—things like dilating, which by the way, is zero fun. I knew that my body needed to heal before I could take it out for a "spin." There's a lot of scar tissue, a lot of blood reflowing, and nerves upon nerves learning how to respark. The doctors tell you to wait several months.

It was quite a while before I felt secure enough to test out my new configuration below. You see, after all the blood has dried up, after all the gauze has been removed, after all the sutures are removed, and purple skin has turned flesh-colored again, it's scary thinking about sex. You feel a little nervous running your new parts into overdrive. But eventually you get braver and braver, your confidence begins to build, and dammit, you deserve some gratification! After all, you didn't go through all that pain and surgery just to park your car in the garage, right? Okay, so maybe using so many car analogies is still the masculine part of me talking. But you must admit that it's rather fitting. After all, you could buy a new car with what you spend on a brand-new vagina.

The problem comes when you can't, well... come. You see, it's easy with a male body. You know exactly where to go to get off. You simply grab the stick shift and put it in gear. But, now your "outie" is an "innie." It's not as convenient to navigate. It's an import and you not only don't have the instruction manual, but you've also lost the key to the ignition. It doesn't help that you're fueled up and ready for a road trip. If you don't have directions on how to get there, you're going to be stuck at home.

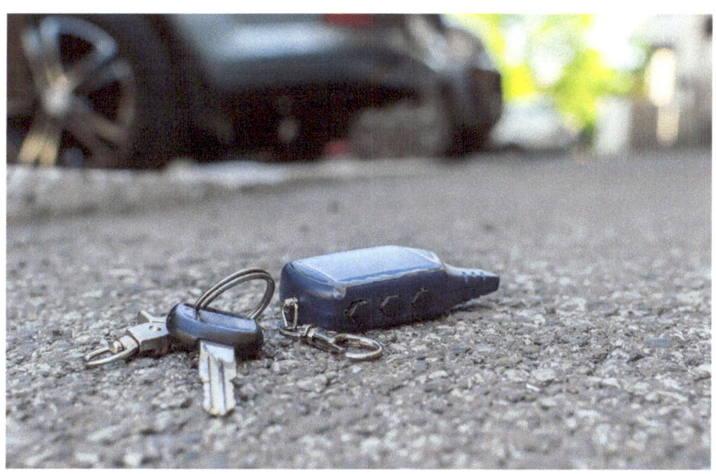

I'll be honest. For a while, I tried and tried to masturbate but couldn't. Everything I tried just didn't seem to work. Like I said earlier, it was easy before. You knew where to grab and what to do. It was obvious when you climaxed and there were no hidden surprises. But now your parts are not only split up and dissected, but they're turned inside out and you don't know what nerves are still working or where they've relocated. Your sensitivity isn't the same.

The same goes for breasts. Sure, your boobs look great, but they feel numb. You have no idea if someone is touching you or not because it feels like you're wearing mittens on your breasts. As far as your vagina is concerned, you might as well have your lover attempt foreplay from the next room because that's as much success as it's having on your arousal center.

Nothing seemed to be working. I faced the very real thought that I would never have another orgasm. The realization hit me like a ton of bricks. Is that it for me? My life isn't even half over, but I had to ask myself if that was the end of my sex life. I began to mourn over the fact that the only pleasure I'd experience from now on would come from a tub of coffee Häagen-Dazs ice cream that I'd eat alone. But I'm not one to easily give up. I'm descended from a science-minded family, and I needed to conduct some experiments.

I spoke to a few cisgendered females who told me that many of them have never been able to climax through vaginal intercourse but instead needed clitoral stimulation. Meanwhile, other women could climax vaginally but had clitorises that were too sensitive to touch. Yet others were a combination of the two. The main thing most of my female friends agreed upon was that the mental stimulation was just as important as knowing what to touch (or not touch) down below.

Armed with this new information, I went to work. Without getting into too much detail, it turned out that I needed a combination of stimulation, both mental and physical. Because my nerves were now literally spread out, I needed to be touched in many areas. Some nerves had been severed and there was little to no feeling in certain zones.

One secret that I'll pass on to other M2F trans women who may be having trouble achieving orgasm is that we still have access to one part that cisgendered women lack—namely a prostate. Cisgendered women don't have a prostate, they have Skene's glands. So that makes us trans women special. If all else fails and your surgeon was more a butcher than an artist, you can always try to take advantage of prostate stimulation. Like many cisgendered women have told me, they have erogenous zones, but they're just spread out. Being a post-op trans woman is no different: You just have to find them ... again.

It's like Kate Bornstein said: "The plumbing works and so does the electricity." Sometimes, you just gotta find the right electrician for the job.

Toys to Augment Sexual Response

Discovering what type of sexual stimulation is most effective has a learning curve, whether it's learning what you like or learning what works for a new partner. Women who have transitioned have told me that their sexual response feels different that it was when they had male parts.

One said, "Masturbation was pretty easy as a male. But I'm getting closer to having orgasms again." (And most do climax, usually within 6 months to a year after vaginoplasty.) Another woman said, "Orgasm as a female is more of a whole-body experience—it goes on longer. It's not penis-oriented."

Postoperatively, sexual satisfaction is reported to be excellent, although there may be a learning curve in adapting after vaginoplasty.[117] There are many products designed to enhance sexual function. I've referred many patients, particularly postoperative folks, to Seattle's Babeland.

Babeland (babeland.com) was founded in Seattle some 30 years ago and is now part of the larger company Good Vibrations (goodvibes.com/s). Combined, the company has a total of 15 stores in New York, Seattle, Boston, and the San Francisco Bay area. They feature sex toys, some lingerie, books, personal lubricants, vibrators (of course), anal plugs, packers, dildos, and a particularly nonthreatening, helpful staff. You can find events and sound advice on their websites.

Committed to pleasure and education, the Babeland and Good Vibrations staff were *the* people I wanted to talk with about serving transgender and gender-nonconforming clients. See my interview on pages 425–428.

A Few of the Many Products from Babeland and Good Vibrations

The products below and on the next few pages can be found in many sex stores and online retailers. However, I recommend Babeland and Good Vibrations because you can get professional assistance and you don't feel like you need a shower after shopping.

- **Lubes and more lubes**

  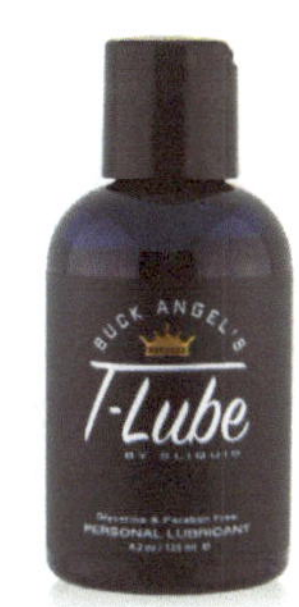

  "Lubes" stands for personal lubricants, of which there is a huge variety. Water-based lubricants are often recommended postoperatively. Examples include Surgilube, Slippery Stuff, Astroglide, and Good Clean Love's water-based formula. Silicone-containing lubricants include Sliquid, Astroglide X, Wet Platinum, and others. Be aware that silicone lubes may erode silicone sex toys over time, making them more difficult to clean effectively. Many companies make both water-based and silicone-containing lubricants, so read the labels. Do not use petroleum jelly as a lube; this oil-based product can erode latex condoms, as can other products containing petroleum. Because products and people vary, you may find that you are sensitive or even allergic to some products. Be aware of the acidity (pH) or fragrances in some products, look up ingredients, and ask the folks at Good Vibrations or Babeland if you have questions.

  Lubes are beneficial because—

  - They're protective. Sexual friction can result in injury or pain; microtears can lead to the spread of STIs through the vaginal, neovaginal, or rectal tissue.

117 Jochen, Hess et al., "Sexuality after Male-to-Female Gender Affirmation Surgery," *BioMed Research International* 2018, no. 36 (May 2018): 1–7, http://dx.doi.org/10.1155/2018/9037979.

- They help with dryness. Trans-masculine individuals taking testosterone may find that they experience dryness, something like a menopausal AFAB may experience. Celebrity trans activist and film star Buck Angel markets "T-Lube," a water-based Sliquid product, to address dryness in trans men who have not had vaginectomy.
- They simulate AFAB vaginal lubrication. The neovagina is constructed with penile or scrotal tissue, which does not produce its own lubricant as occurs in an AFAB.
- They make sex more comfortable.

- **Kiss-X FTM Stroker**
According to the Good Vibrations website: "Based on feedback on Buck Angel's original stroker Buck-Off, this new toy, designed with Buck, offers a snugger fit for trans men whose body parts are smaller, those not in medical transition, or those who are earlier in their hormone replacement therapy. Trans porn superstar and activist Buck Angel's mission to help trans men become comfortable with their bodies is now accessible to more people, thanks to the Kiss-X's smaller-shaped base that allows for a snug, pleasurable fit over bits that are smaller in size."

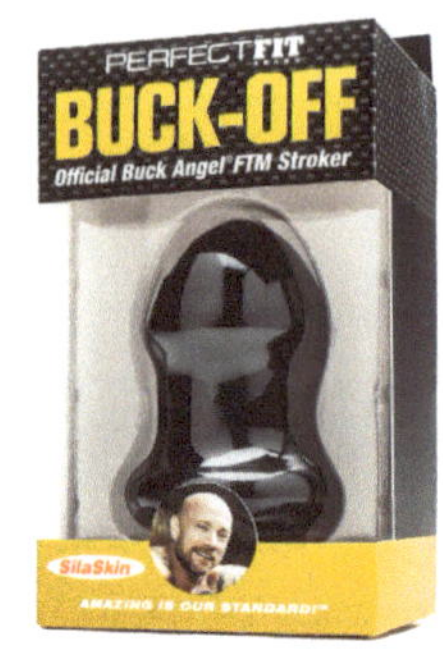

- **Nipple and clitoral pumps**
Similar in concept to the penile pumps used to manage erectile dysfunction, these pumps create stimulation through suction. Many people use the cylindrical pumps in preparation for metoidioplasty.

- **Penis rings**
Like most sex toys, penis rings are available in a wide variety of styles, depending on one's preferences. A penis ring is used to sustain an erection by temporarily trapping blood within the penis. Rings can be applied by stretching a ring over the penis (and testicles) or by snapping it on at the base. New users are advised to avoid rigid rings as they can be more difficult to remove, as well as to remove a ring if the penis becomes numb or discolored (a good tip!). Here's a guide from the mainstream media: **menshealth.com/sex-women/a19532760/cock-rings**.[118]

- **Vibrators**
There are so many vibrators available; just go shopping. Browse the website of Babeland (**babeland.com**) or Good Vibrations (**goodvibes.com/s/**). These really *aren't* back massagers. Find anything from the little rabbit-ear vibrators to the "Titan Waterproof Rocket." A word of caution: Do not insert a vibrator into the rectum unless it is specifically designed as an anal vibrator or plug. Without a flare at the base, a vibrator can travel up into the rectum and colon and may require a visit to the emergency room to remove it.

- **Dildos**
Like vibrators (and many dildos *are* vibrators), dildos are available in many shapes, colors, and sizes. They are basically penis-shaped and are used for penetration. Dildos can be used as strap-ons by securing them to a harness that the stores also sell. Dildos may have suction cups to secure them to a bathtub or other surface. As with any sex toy, use with lubricants, give and get consent, and avoid pain unless mutually agreeable.

118 Carrie Borzillo and Men's Health Editorial, "How Penis Rings Can Help You Have Better Sex," *Men's Health*, July 8, 2020, https://www.menshealth.com/sex-women/a19532760/cock-rings/.

- **Anal plugs**
  Rectal stimulation can be erotic. It's an area rich in nerve endings with easy access to the sensitive prostate gland in a cis male or trans female. Again, just browse the websites for ideas. Here are some important safety tips:
  - Use products that are designed for anal insertion. They must flare at the base so an anal toy does not escape and travel north into the colon.
  - Use lubricants liberally.
  - Do not use numbing cream; pain is a warning that helps you stay safe.
  - Use safe-sex techniques—that is, condoms on penises and sex toys—to avoid sharing bacteria or virus particles.
  - Engage in safe and smart sex practices. Any toy or body part that goes into the anus shouldn't go into any other orifice afterwards.

GenderCat's Fascination Sleeves, Packers, and Play Prostheses

GenderCat is a company that specializes in prosthetic penises and "Fascination Sleeves." Watch its founder Joseph Mudge on YouTube (youtube.com/watch?v=gSVlT-WezVY) or meet him at a trans conference. GenderCat is known for its individually customized products and for its payment plans for purchases over $69. Here's a rundown on GenderCat's products (web links were current at the time of publishing):

- **Fascination Sleeve** (gendercat.com/products/fascination-sleeve-for-pleasure)
  Used as a masturbation device, the Fascination Sleeve is a silicone cylinder with a longitudinal opening. By placing the Sleeve over the "sensitive parts," the user squeezes the sleeve to create suction. Then, by masturbating in the "traditional" style, they are able to climax without direct genital contact, a dysphoria-producing factor for some. The Sleeve's internal diameter is customizable; smaller diameters may be suitable before an individual has taken testosterone. Additionally, the buyer selects the interior texture as bumps or ridges and selects from many different colors.

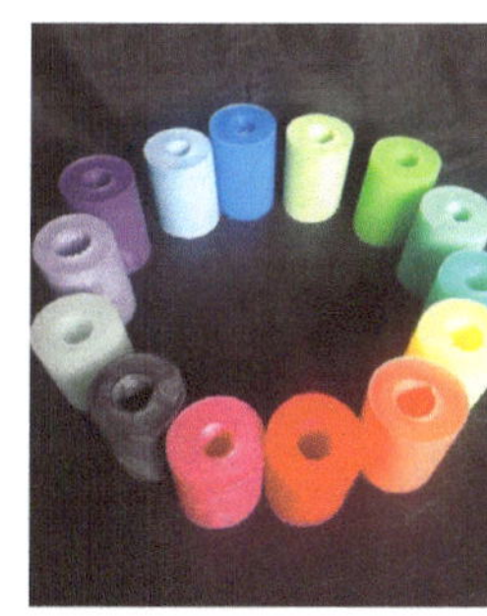

- **4RLZ GenderExtender**
  gendercat.com/collections/fascination-products/products/4rlz-genderextender-a-fascination-sleeve-product
  This is the Fascination Sleeve in an "affirming shape"; it looks like a penis and comes in a variety of customizable skin colors. The buyer chooses from a color sheet with numerous color variations available. Masturbating with the GenderExtender is masturbation with a penis. This minimizes dysphoria and connects the visual and tactile experience with genital pleasure.
- **GenderCat's Packers**
  gendercat.com/collections/gendermender-packers-and-penis-prosthetics/products
  These gender-affirming packers (including the 4RLZ Slim, JR, and Girthy models) are designed for wearing in underwear, which creates a bulge and decreases visual dysphoria when the wearer is naked. The buyer customizes the packer by specifying the following options:
  - Color (numerous colors are available, using a color sample sheet; variegations of color are possible)

- Texture (soft, semi-hard, hard, and superhard, depending on the model)
- Size (these include 3, 4, 5, and 7 inches; uncircumcised options are also available)
- Scrotum with or without Amazeballs (incorporated as two individual and mobile testicular prostheses)

- **GenderCat's Play Prosthesis**
  gendercat.com/collections/gendermender-packers-and-penis-prosthetics/products/dual-texture-hard-prosthesis
  Designed for penetration and masturbation, this device features an internal opening patterned after the Fascination Sleeve. Incorporating the Sleeve minimizes dysphoria and connects the visual and tactile experience with the wearer's genital pleasure. The Play Prosthesis adheres to the wearer with the use of a self-adhesive sheet. The buyer customizes the prosthesis by specifying the following options:
  - Color (same options as above with the packers)
  - Texture (semi-hard, hard, and superhard)
  - Size (these include 4, 6, and 8 inches; a uncircumcised 4-inch option is also available)
  - Fascination Sleeve size
  - Scrotum (customizable as above)

Because there are so many products, textures, sizes, and functions, how does one possibly choose? Here is further clarification from GenderCat founder Joseph Mudge:

> **My personal preference is to have a super-soft for everyday packing and either a hard or super-hard for play. The semi-hard is meant to be soft enough to pack but firm enough for some penetration. So it's great for occasional packing and occasional play. It's a compromise, so it's not *great* at either. What it is great for is the occasion when you're going out and you know you'll have the opportunity to use it in a new and exciting setting. This is when I will choose a semi-hard. If I were to pack with it every day, I would find it distracting and tiring to have a semi-erection all the time. I like to pack with a super-soft daily because it's so comfy and does its job well. I spend most of my time with this prosthesis and so it's my priority.**
>
> **I like to switch to a hard or super-hard for play because then I have the exact length and firmness that I want during play. I do get some dysphoria sometimes when switching, but I've found that if I switch early enough, then the erection feels right once I'm really ready for action.**
>
> *—Joseph Mudge, founder, GenderCat*

GenderCat also makes breast prostheses and other products. See more at GenderCat.com.

Answers from the Sex Educators at Good Vibrations and Babeland

I figured Babeland could answer some of my many questions about sex toys and respectful marketing to transgender and gender-nonconforming individuals. When I first contacted Seattle's Babeland, I was referred to Good Vibrations and learned that it had acquired Babeland in 2013. Together, Good Vibrations (GV) and Babeland have 15 stores in the San Francisco Bay Area, New York, Boston, and Seattle—all women-founded, sex-positive retailers where you can find anything vibratory and erotic but not feel, well, slimy.

Extremely helpful in providing answers to my questions were Andy Duran, the education director of GV and Babeland; Lisa Finn; and Carol Queen, PhD, who also serves as GV's staff sexologist and curator of its Antique Vibrator Museum in San Francisco. For more information, visit **goodvibes.com/s/** and **babeland.com**.

The first batch of questions are answered by GV educators Andy Duran and Lisa Finn.

Linda: Do you recommend any specific books or references for the trans and gender-variant communities?

AD and LF: Absolutely! We carry several books on gender identity both for folks exploring and affirming their own gender, and titles specifically aimed for their loved ones, service providers, and clinicians. I really love the book *Red: A Crayon's Story*! Its simplicity in how it describes the story of a crayon that's labeled red but is able to draw only in blue no matter how hard it tries is an excellent way to help youth and adults alike to understand some of the challenges that trans people may face.

Linda: We are seeing more clients who identify themselves as nonbinary, but on a spectrum of feminizing or masculinizing. What sexual issues are they presenting with and what is your approach to helping them?

AD and LF: Nonbinary identities have always existed. Many of us live and operate in societies where gender "roles" are thrust upon us at infancy and expected to last our whole lives. And for as long as that's been happening, there have always been people who have felt confined by it and not fully seen and accepted for who they are. The rise in nonbinary visibility is what happens when individual whispers are combined to create a loud collective voice of a community. The sexual challenges that ENBY (phonetic for NB or nonbinary) folks might face are ultimately due to the rest of us not doing our part to create a world safe enough for them to exist inclusively.

It's an ongoing practice that can start with simple steps, such as removing antiquated language like "ladies and gentlemen" from our lexicon, respecting pronouns (including "they/them" and so on), and celebrating nonbinary body positivity.

Linda: Many trans women who are on estradiol lose erectile function. Besides medications like sildenafil, what are you recommending for female-identified folks who either want to maintain penetrative sex using the penis or do not want to use the penis at all?

AD and LF: A simple ring at the base of the penis can often assist folks looking to maintain an erection, as long as they don't have other health concerns that would make constriction of the blood flow more dangerous, such as diabetes or blood clotting disorders.

Since gender congruence and connection to our bodies is so individual and personal from trans person to trans person, there is no one way for trans bodies to look or be. Many trans women who have not had bottom surgery will still stimulate their phallus and may refer to it as a clitoris or a penis, since it is homologous tissue that functions similarly for sexual pleasure.

With that said, there are plenty of trans women who experience dysphoria of their genitals or who simply find sexual pleasure in other ways. That's why it's important for us to meet each customer where they're at individually, versus trying to push folks to some place where they're not.

Linda: With transmasculine individuals, what words do you use besides "clitoris," "labia," and so on? One individual I know uses "sensitive parts." Same question for transfeminine folks.

AD and LF: That's easy! Because we never know what's in someone's pants, we simply use the words they feel the most comfortable with. When it comes to our products, we assign no gender. We explain how they work on various parts of the body instead. For example, "This vibrator is great for providing stimulation over the clitoris, head of the penis, and for vaginal and anal use," allowing the customer to determine what might work best for them without having to disclose their anatomy. When we are referring to a body part of that person, we use the name they provide. For example, some trans men might refer to their nonanal orifice as their "front hole" or "bonus hole," as opposed to "vagina," whereas others might actually prefer to call it a vagina.

Linda: How do you help trans women "relearn" orgasm after vaginoplasty?

AD and LF: It depends on how they like to orgasm! For example, if they found orgasm through anal stimulation, then perhaps very little needs to be "relearned." Because orgasms change throughout everyone's lifespan, be it because of hormones, medications, trauma, or surgeries, there is a constant need to relearn how we find it. Many trans women come in after vaginoplasty looking for dilators, as it's recommended to use dilators to help hold the shape, depth, and elasticity of the vagina.

Linda: I've been advised that "strap-on" is an old, offensive term. What terms do you use?

AD and LF: It's not that strap-on is an old or offensive term so much as that it may not apply to the relationship that trans folks may have to their products. A strap-on refers to harnesses and dildos being used as sex toys. However, for many trans folks (particularly trans men), they may think of their harness and dildo less as a sex toy and more of a prosthetic or an extension of their own body. In our stores, we know that someone may come in looking for a strap-on, while others may come in for the same product but for the purpose of gender congruency.

The following questions are answered by Carol Queen, PhD.

Linda: How do hormones impact sexual response and expression?

Carol Queen: As people (of all gender identities) may remember from puberty, hormones can play a significant role in sexual desire and response both in and out of a supplemental, replacement, and gender-affirming context. One thing that's very much worth noting is that the way hormones change the physical body might have an effect on a person's sexuality because they allow that person to begin to inhabit the gendered body with which they identify. This can open up a comfort level for some who have previously been uncomfortable. So while this is essentially psychological, hormonal change has facilitated it.

Those taking testosterone often reference heightened sexual sensitivity and also a higher sex drive. Those taking estrogen often reference feeling more connected to their emotions. I note here, though, that just as male-female and masculine-feminine are not "opposites," there is a lot of variability in sexual feeling and response. So I don't think it would be correct to say that these changes are always going to be noticed (or certainly noticed equally strongly) by all people taking hormones.

Linda: Please give us some information about sexual response after surgery. Let's start with vaginoplasty.

CQ: With vaginoplasty, an especially significant variable in sexual response is the degree to which postsurgical dilation is kept up. Some people let it lapse, especially if they don't have partners at the time (this happens with cis women during postcancer treatments and in similar contexts too). And it can be subsequently more difficult to start or return to dilation.

Another factor is the specific way the vaginoplasty was done and how the surgeon used the especially sexually sensitive glans tissue. This area on the penis is homologous to the clitoral glans, and some surgeons used to use it as a kind of cervix analog when they invert penile tissue in the vaginoplasty. This is an interesting choice, though, as it reinforces that the vagina is for penetration, not just that a woman has a vagina that she may or may not want to engage with sexually. (I am using gendered language on purpose here because I want this to reflect a specifically gendered attitude.)

The more usual way now is to reconfigure this tissue as a clitoris, which gives the person more options for pleasure, including self-pleasure. It can be sensitive to vibration as well as partnered stimulation; of course, genital responsiveness may depend on how well nerves were preserved during surgery.

And I should add that regardless of gender identification and the procedure done, a person may find themselves really rediscovering their body and sexuality, and we may want to remember that almost all of us in the United States have had terrible sex education! So it won't just be the "new" genitals that need to be understood; it's the whole body and its role in arousal. Kissing, touching (including nongenital touching), and all kinds of other stimulation will help optimize turn-on, and this is important for people who have had no medical procedures as well as for those who have.

Linda: And phalloplasty?

CQ: Here too, it partly depends on what kind of procedure was done. Metoidioplasty tends to affect the nerves much less than some phalloplasty variants, reserving clitoral sensation in the neophallus. But lately, phalloplasty more routinely includes a procedure that incorporates the clitoris and allows sexual sensation to be more significantly retained than the old-school techniques allowed.

There's generally a size difference between the two procedures, and that means that toys intended for larger penises or for sex acts like intercourse might not work as well for all guys who have opted for metoidioplasty. The Buck-Off stroker is designed for these folks, and there may be specific kinds of partner play (oral, manual, and so on) that are especially pleasurable. And as for the guys who've opted for phalloplasty, the erotic sensations on the surface of their new penis may be less, and techniques required to optimally stimulate the clitoral tissue that remains might need to be explored. For example, instead of stroking the skin of the penis, try grasping it and moving the whole thing so as to engage the clitoral tissue.

Linda: Tell me about pumping before masculinizing surgery.

CQ: Pumping is often done for pleasure and can be done by people of any gender identity. It supports blood flow into the area being pumped, which is one important component of arousal. It can also temporarily enlarge the area being pumped as well as engage the skin's flexibility while this is happening. So pumping might be a useful strategy premetoidioplasty.

Whenever I talk to any customer about pump use, I warn that it can be overdone, and I'm actually most concerned about those who want to add size. They are the pump users who really wish to (literally!) gain something from pumping. So I think this warning is an important part of any discussion about pump play or use in a surgical context too.

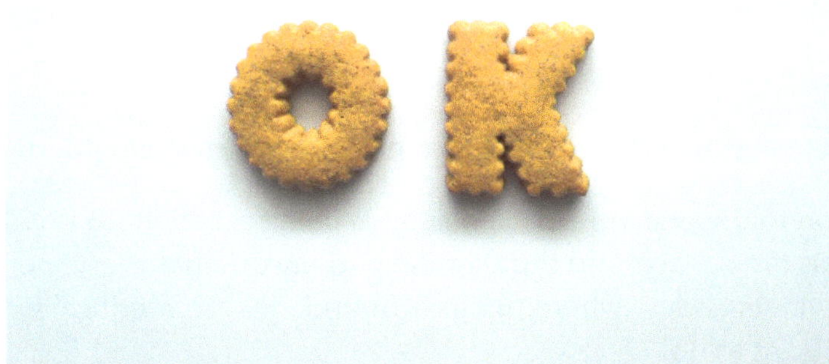

People interact sexually in a kaleidoscope of different ways.

— Andrew M. Faulk, MD, physician and author

Consent: Sexual and Otherwise

This portion was contributed by Rachel Drake of the Consent Academy, an educational collective based in Seattle. Rachel is an educator and consent advocate who helped found the Consent Academy in 2016. She is one of the authors of *The Consent Primer: Foundations for Everyday Life*.

Consent for Sexual Activity

Consent in a sexual context is like consent in any context. Having an understanding of what consent is and how it works is particularly important with sexual activity because it is more intense and more "high-stakes" than many of the interactions we have. Knowing yourself, your own boundaries, and what you want to do with your body, mind, and spirit are paramount in healthy consent practices.

The basics of consent include **capacity**, **information**, **agreement**, and **autonomy**. (An easy way to remember this is the acronym **CIA-A**—that is, be your own intelligence agency.) Consent is really about building on the foundation of autonomy of the self and using the three pillars of capacity, information, and agreement to uphold the autonomy of others. Practicing the tenants of consent in nonsexual areas of your life helps to build those muscles so when there is a highly charged sexual interaction, you are better able to state and hold your boundaries.

Capacity is the level of cognitive ability required to understand what is happening. For instance, are you in a state of mind to understand what is going to be happening? Things that can impact one's capacity include substances (such as alcohol or recreational drugs), a lack of food, sleep deprivation, one's emotional state, and prescription medications. Any of these can either impair or improve capacity. When people communicate and understand their own personal capacity, they can help assess another person's capacity and in turn assess the risk in engagement. We must remember that no one is likely to be at 100 percent capacity all the time. Capacity builds on sharing information. Here are some important considerations:

- Does everybody know and *understand* what is being asked of them?
- Do you have *enough* information to engage?
- Is the information being shared coming from a place of honesty and goodwill?

Having enough information to understand what a person is being asked to do is critical in creating clear agreements. Details such as time, place, and duration help to ensure that everyone is comfortable with what will be happening. Understanding where people's boundaries are is critical in knowing what a person wants to do and does not want to do.

How to Get Consent

Every consent interaction is different and every person is different. The interaction depends on the relationship dynamic and the consent framework that you build over time. Building an understanding of someone's desires, boundaries, and stipulations over time is at the core of a consent framework.

By remembering what people agree to, you can create a shorthand of consent. For example, suppose you know how a friend takes their coffee. You do not have to ask every single time, "What do you want in your coffee?" Rather, you create a shorthand where "Do you want coffee?" means coffee with two sugars and cream. Sometimes these frameworks need to be updated, so if your friend decides to cut out sugar, it would be their responsibility to update the framework.

If you were not aware that your friend had a dietary change and you made the coffee in the usual way, this creates what we call "a consent incident." The consent framework was not updated. You made coffee for your friend the way you thought they liked it, the friend then updates the consent framework (that is, makes it known that they want coffee without sugar), and you make the change to the agreement about coffee.

Now, if you were to continue to put sugar in your friend's coffee even after being told not to, that territory needs to be explored. Is this intentional? Are you a forgetful person? Are you neurodivergent and is it difficult for you to integrate new information? Understanding the reasons for pushed or seemingly ignored boundaries is necessary.

This works the same way in a sexual situation. The amount of information you need to share and the explicitness of a consent agreement varies. For example, are you having a one-night stand or your first sexual interaction? Or is this with somebody you have been with for 5 or 6 years and you have a solid consent framework that you are constantly updating?

Updating a framework is important because people can change and evolve over time. With any sexual encounter, simply asking questions can update the framework and also make the interaction sexier. Using sentences like "Does that feel good?" "Do you like this?" "Do want harder, rougher?" "Do you want it softer?" "Is it okay if I put my hand here?" help you gain clarity. A statement like "I really like it when you do this to me" establishes approval. Getting that verbal agreement early on is helpful. It is also important to follow up by talking about what happened afterwards.

The more you talk, the easier it becomes to build a healthy consent practice. You can also have nonverbal consent, so watch for nonverbal cues as well. The longer you know someone, the more you know their nonverbal cues. If you have a shorter-term relationship (and thus a smaller consent framework), you will have to use your words more.

Types of Sexual Activity That Involve Consent

All types of sexual activity involve consent. Here at the Consent Academy, we have a list of over 250 possible sexual activities that people can talk about to start the conversation. All conversations involve a discussion of safe sex, sexual hygiene, disclosure of any physical issues that may be impacted by sexual interactions, and any emotional triggers that you are comfortable disclosing (or if you are willing to accept any consequences if you do not disclose). We cannot always know if a sex act is going to trigger an emotional or physical response. We encourage people to be prepared and to understand that any interaction has inherent risk.

What to Do When Consent Is Ignored or Violated

The first thing to do is breathe and take time to process what happened. We have minor consent violations every day.

In a sexual situation, this depends on the relationship dynamic. If someone has their consent ignored repeatedly by the same person, they need to make a decision as to whether or not they want that person in their life.

When looking at how we communicate, we have discovered that many consent incidents are not intentional. Rather, they may be a matter of someone either not understanding because of a capacity issue or a lack of clear information. Nevertheless, it causes a communication breakdown.

If you have an ongoing relationship with the person and you know how to communicate with them, you might simply say, "Hey, this wasn't okay" or "I didn't feel good about how this went." Then, follow this up by talking about what happened with the person involved in the incident.

If you feel your consent has been violated and you cannot talk to the other person involved, get help from a trusted person. This would be someone who can engage in active listening and who is not going to label the incident or tell you how you "should" feel. This would be someone who can just let you have your response and constructively help you figure out what you want to do. If it is something very serious, of course, seek professional help.

Introducing the Consent Academy

The Consent Academy is an educational collective based out of Seattle. Our mission is to teach consent in all of its complexity, aspects, and potential. We offer a variety of workshops and other training events, as well as private and business consultations. With over 50 years of collective education experience, our approach incorporates the disciplines of psychology, sociology, public health, psychotherapy, and personal coaching to create a systemic view of how consent impacts everyone from the bedroom to the boardroom. We believe consent is part of everyday life and its practice builds stronger, safer, and more connected communities.

Access the Academy at consent.academy.

Poly and Kink in a Trans-focused Private Therapy Practice

by Paulette de Coriolis, MA, LMHCA

The following information and resources are contributed by Paulette de Coriolis, MA, LMHCA, a mental health therapist and transgender specialist practicing in Redmond, Washington (paulettecounseling.com).

Most of the clients that I see are trans in the umbrella sense of that word. Some of these trans clients are also poly or kink. Additionally, several clients that do not identify as trans have come to me because they feel, correctly, that I will not judge them for being poly or kink. I see trans and poly as identities; I'm not sure kink is an identity or is something some people do.

Poly

Poly in a narrow scope of the term is *polyamory*, which is having multiple long-term, loving relationships with the full knowledge and consent of all parties involved. Polyamory does not mean that all parties have sex with each other. In a "vee" relationship, Person 1 has a romantic relationship with both Persons 2 and 3, but 2 and 3 do not have a romantic relationship. In this example, 2 and 3 are *metamours*. There are many other forms of poly relationships besides the vee.

"Loving relationships" does not always include romantic and sexual relationships. Some relationships may be deep friendships that in heterosexual, monogamous relationships could be seen as suspect—for example, a friendship between a man and a woman.

Poly is also an umbrella term, the breadth of which people disagree on. In the broadest sense, it includes polyamory, ethical nonmonogamy, consensual nonmonogamy, polyfidelity, solo poly, open relationships, swinging, relationship anarchy, and more. Polygamy, polygyny, and polyandry are relationship forms with multiple marriages and are not legal in the United States.

Nesting partners live together and may be married or not and may share finances or not. A *solo poly* person does not nest with any of their partners. A *polyfidelity* relationship is a closed poly relationship.

Children raised in stable, loving poly families do just as well as children raised in stable, loving monogamous families. However, poly families may be at a disadvantage if the family divorces or dissolves, as the legal system in the US generally does not recognize the rights of nonbiological partners.

Selected Books on Polyamory

- *The Ethical Slut, Third Edition: A Practical Guide to Polyamory, Open Relationships, and Other Freedoms in Sex and Love*, Janet W. Hardy and Dossie Easton, 2017.
- *Opening Up: A Guide to Creating and Sustaining Open Relationships*, Tristan Taormino, 2008.
- *More Than Two: A Practical Guide to Ethical Polyamory*, Franklin Veaux and Eve Rickert, 2014.
- *Eight Things I Wish I'd Known About Polyamory Before I Tried It and Frakked It Up*, Cunning Minx, 2014.
- *The Polyamorists Next Door: Inside Multiple-Partner Relationships and Families*, Elisabeth Sheff, 2013. Sheff is academic researcher who has published on both poly and kink, some of which is behind paywalls. Her curriculum vitae is at **elisabethsheff.com/cv**.

Podcasts on Polyamory

- *Loving without Boundaries*: **lovingwithoutboundaries.com**
- *The Multiamory Podcast*: **multiamory.com**
- *Polyamory Weekly*: **polyweekly.com**

Where to Find More

Local poly discussion groups may be found on **meetup.com**. Facebook has poly groups, although many are closed and some are secret. Wikipedia has many articles on poly.

Kink

Kink may refer both to nonconventional sexual practices and also to *BDSM,* which is not necessarily sexual. BDSM is a multiple abbreviation: BD is bondage and discipline, DS or D/s is dominance and submission, and SM is sadism and masochism or sadomasochism. These are broad categories of behaviors that are best practiced with the full, noncoercive consent of the participants.

Some activities are organized as a *scene* or *play session,* which has a discrete beginning and end, often with cool-down period or *aftercare*. Prior to the start of a scene, the participants agree on words or signals such as "green," "yellow," or "red"; or "more," "less," or "stop." A *safe word* may be used by the *bottom* to call a stop to a BDSM scene.

Some people live the lifestyle 24/7, especially in D/s relationships.

The popular book *Fifty Shades of Gray* was *not* a good example of full, noncoercive consent of the participants. A more recent book that explores consent is *The Consent Primer:*

Foundations for Everyday Life by The Consent Academy (2019) and authors Sar Surmick, Rachel Drake, Lara-Ashley Monroe, Kelley O'Hanlon, and Leah Hirsch, along with editor Lessa Lamb.

Major metropolitan areas may have a *BDSM dungeon*, which is a room with BDSM equipment and ideally provides written rules and supervision of activities. The Seattle area had a BDSM dungeon as part of the members-only Center for Sex Positive Culture (CSPC). The space also hosted educational activities by the Foundation for Sex Positive Culture (FSPC). Unfortunately, the CSPC/FSPC lost its space in 2016 to gentrification and CSPC and FSPC split apart. The FSPC rebranded as the Pan Eros Foundation and is housed in Gallery Erato in Seattle's Pioneer Square area. The CSPC has regrouped and rents out the Gallery Erato space for occasional play parties.

Where to Find More

- Center for Sex Positive Culture (CSPC): **thecspc.org**
- Pan Eros Foundation: **pan-eros.org**
- The Consent Academy: **consent.academy**
- Wikipedia has articles on kink and BDSM.

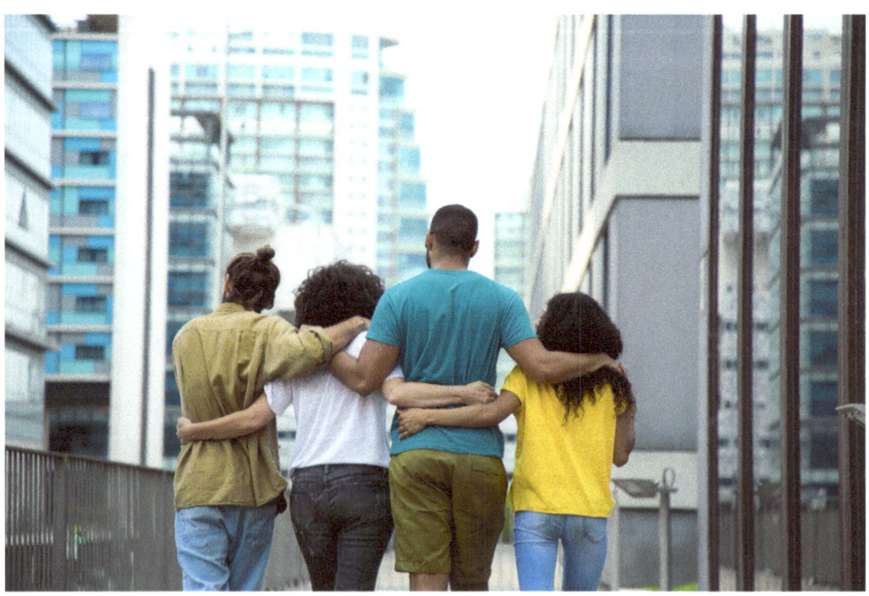

Safe Sex

Having sex with another person has certain risks. In the best of worlds, you would assess your risk *before* you are sexually intimate with someone. For many people, it's a rite of passage to start a sexual relationship with each partner by having STI screens. Included in such screening panels are tests for HIV (the virus that causes AIDs), herpes type 1 (usually oral) and type 2 (usually genital), syphilis, hepatitis B, hepatitis C, gonorrhea, and chlamydia.

Tests for the first five are done by way of a blood draw. Gonorrhea and chlamydia testing can be performed through a urine test or a cervical sample during a pelvic exam. (It used to be commonplace to insert a swab into the penis, but somehow that's "lost favor.") HPV (human papillomavirus) can show up on a Pap test. You may have been immunized against HPV when you were in middle school; you can still be immunized at many pharmacies up to age 45. Without immunizations, your best protection are latex condoms and dental dams.

If the above tests are negative for both you and your partners (meaning that they show no infection), you have a reasonably good chance that you are in the clear. But if you have had a recent exposure to, for instance, HIV or herpes, it may take several months for these to show up on a lab test. Therefore, use latex barriers to protect yourself from transmitting these viruses or HPV. Many people rescreen 3 months after the initial screen, assuming that they're practicing safe sex and haven't had new exposures.

Pre-Exposure Prophylaxis (PrEP) against HIV

Pre-exposure prophylaxis (PrEP) is a single daily pill consisting of two anti-HIV medications, specifically Truvada (emtricitabine and tenofovir disoproxil fumarate) and the newer Descovy (emtricitabine and tenofovir alafenamide).

Be aware that at the present time, Descovy is not for use in people assigned female at birth who are at risk of getting HIV from vaginal sex because its effectiveness has not been studied in this group.

Taking PrEP every day can drastically reduce your risk for contracting HIV. When taken daily, PrEP reduces the risk of contracting HIV through sex by 99 percent and reduces the risk of contracting HIV through injecting drugs by 74 percent.[119] People must be HIV-negative when they start Truvada or Descovy, and they must have a blood test for HIV as well as liver and kidney function tests every 3 months.

Consider taking PrEP if you do the following:

- Have multiple sex partners.
- Have partners who are known to be HIV-positive.
- Don't know the HIV status of your partner(s)—or for that matter, the HIV status of other partners *they* may have.
- Experience penetration as part of your sexual activity. If you are the "receptive" partner (this usually refers to having penetration of the vagina or rectum), you may be at greater risk for contracting HIV because of the surface area of the penetrated vagina or rectum and because of small microtears or tissue injuries that allow the virus to enter your bloodstream.

119 Centers for Disease Control and Prevention, "Pre-Exposure Prophylaxis (PrEP)," last reviewed June 23, 2021, https://www.cdc.gov/hiv/risk/prep/.

- Have anonymous hookups or sex for money.
- Are trying to get pregnant with a partner who is HIV-positive.

For more information on PrEP, go to the Centers for Disease Control (CDC) website at **cdc.gov/hiv/basics/prep.html**.

If you were born after 1990, you may not recall the heartbreak of the AIDs epidemic. Many of us who remember the epidemic at its height are elated to tell our patients about PrEP. One of the best accounts of this time period was captured in the book *My Epidemic: An AIDS Memoir of One Man's Struggle as Doctor, Patient and Survivor* by Andrew M. Faulk, MD. Dr. Faulk was both an HIV patient and an HIV doctor at the time.

PEP (Post-Exposure Prophylaxis) against HIV

PEP is post-exposure prophylaxis. Check the CDC website for details, but at this writing, PEP consists of three antiretroviral medications started within 72 hours after a potential HIV exposure and continued for 28 days. PEP is generally used by an HIV-negative person after any of the following:

- An occupational exposure by a healthcare worker treating an HIV patient (that is, a high-risk needle stick injury or an exposure to amniotic fluid in an HIV-positive mother)
- A sexual exposure where a condom breaks or no precautions are taken
- A sexual assault[120]

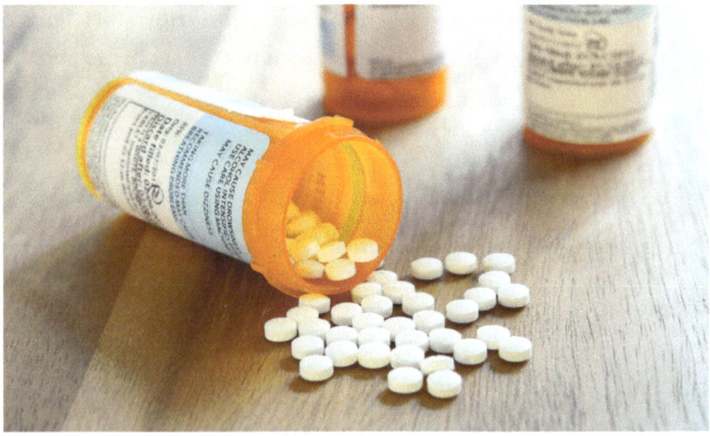

120 David T. Kuhar et al., "Updated US Public Health Service Guidelines for the Management of Occupational Exposures to Human Immunodeficiency Virus and Recommendations for Postexposure Prophylaxis," *Infection Control and Hospital Epidemiology* 34, no. 9 (September 2013): 875–92, https://doi.org/10.1086/672271.

Birth Control

If you were assigned female at birth and are on testosterone for masculinizing, you may become pregnant if you have sexual contact with people who make sperm. (If you are planning a pregnancy, you must stop your testosterone because of masculinizing effects on a developing fetus. Refer to "Planning for a Pregnancy If You Want One" in Chapter 21.)

While unlikely, trans men occasionally do have unintended pregnancies. Here are some important guidelines to consider:

- **Do not miss your testosterone doses.**
  Even taking a dose several days late can make a difference. You could potentially ovulate and have period bleeding again. Do not assume that a "good" testosterone level will protect you.

- **Use birth control if you have sex with partners who make sperm.**
  Barrier methods like condoms and IUDs may be good choices because they have no estrogen in them. (The Mirena, Skyla, and Kyleena IUDs do have the progesterone levonorgestrel in their stalks.) You may also want to consider a progesterone-only birth control pill or an implanted progesterone device. (Look up Nexplanon; it is easily placed by your healthcare provider under the skin on the inner portion of the upper arm and provides 5 years of contraception as of this writing.)

- **Consider permanent sterilization for either you or your partner if you do not want a pregnancy ever.**
  For example, your partner could have a vasectomy. You could consider having a tubal ligation or a hysterectomy with removal of the fallopian tubes and ovaries; you may want to do this if you are considering a phalloplasty anyway.

- **Remember that birth control methods, with the exception of latex condoms, do not protect you from STIs.**

Emergency Contraception

In a moment of panic, you realize you've had a contraceptive emergency. Maybe you had no birth control protection, you took your pills wrong, or a condom broke or fell off during sex.* "Morning After" treatments do not end an existing pregnancy and they do not protect you from STIs. The options include the following:

- **Over-the-counter pills**
  These do not require a prescription and can be taken up to 5 days after the event. All are forms of the progesterone levonorgestrel. They include brands such as Plan B One-Step, My Way, Preventeza, and Take Action.

- **A prescription method called "Ella"**
  This contains the selective progesterone receptor modulator ulipristal and can be taken up to 5 days after sex.

- **A Paraguard (copper) IUD**
  This device is inserted into the uterus by your healthcare provider or a Planned Parenthood clinician and can be placed up to 5 days after the event. The copper IUDs now provide up to 12 years of contraception!

Contact your healthcare provider or Planned Parenthood (**plannedparenthood.org**) for more information.

*If the pregnancy exposure occurred during a sexual assault, you are encouraged to have a medical evaluation ***as soon as possible***. An emergency facility can provide STI evaluation, post-exposure prophylaxis against HIV, and emergency contraception, as well as documentation and treatment of other injuries.

Finding a Long-Term Partner

While not everybody wants a partner to grow old with, it can have its advantages. A real life partner is someone who knows you inside and out, cares enough to give you a kidney if you need one, and at least tries to catch you when you fall. They've got your back and it feels good. Life is better with a partner in many ways, but it can be more complicated too. Of course, you can have a friend or friends who know you very, very well. And I don't think you must be in a partnered relationship to be happy.

In my opinion and experience, good relationships can take an enormous amount of work and time. They also provide an unparalleled framework for personal growth and the opportunity to experience love you'd never imagined. Even having been through the grief of losing a life partner, I'd do it again in a heartbeat.

Dealing with Rejection

Rejection is painful for everyone. In some ways, though, the potential hurt of rejection is the price we pay for the *chance* to find a partner. I once had a therapist who said, "You can't win the lotto if you never buy a ticket." She wasn't suggesting that I start gambling.

Rejection 101

If you are rejected—that is, someone doesn't want to be with you or you get dumped, which will likely happen because it seems to happen to everyone—here are some things that can help you get through it:

- Call or text someone who knows you well.
- Try not to be home alone—that is, get out of the house, go to a movie, or do *something*.
- Get exercise. Spinning or martial arts classes are helpful in working out anger or aggression.
- Protect yourself from risky or self-destructive behaviors (too much alcohol, substance use, and so on).
- Don't settle. Have you ever known people to have sex with anyone to prove to themselves that they are still desirable? Don't be that person.
- Be prepared to hold out for someone who is worth your time. In my 50s, I employed a young medical assistant who would tell me, "Dr. Gromko, *men should be an enhancement!*" She was right. Dr. Tina Schermer Sellers recalls similar advice: "The person you're with should be a partner, not a project!"

If you are thinking of suicide because you've been rejected, treat this as the emergency it is and get some professional help (see Chapters 1 and 17).

Living with Grief: Suppose Your Long-Term Partner Dies

If you manage to find a love worth having, the sad truth is that one of you will likely die before the other. It's sort of a cost of doing business, I guess. But it is a huge cost, probably steep enough to keep many people away from even seeking a relationship.

Whether your partner's death occurs suddenly and without warning, or it is anticipated, grief can feel overwhelming. Nothing in life feels the same, and you wonder how the world manages to go on when you feel so devastated.

My husband Steve died of diabetic kidney failure after more than 3 years of home dialysis and a week after a leg amputation. He wasn't a well man, although his superior intellect and irreverent humor carried us through to the end. At first, I remember grief surrounding me during every waking moment. Occasional thoughts of "life" would interrupt me, but mostly I remember just how achingly sad I felt. For the most part, I soldiered on. I had important work to do being a doctor (the only thing that felt normal) and caring for Steve's daughter. I remember crying literally every day on the way to work.

I took some comfort in knowing that by *my* doing the grieving, Steve didn't have to do it. I don't think he wouldn't have weathered grieving well.

The first year after Steve died was the most difficult with every holiday, Steve's birthday, my birthday, and Father's Day punctuating my loss like a punch to the gut. But those were days that could be anticipated. Far worse were the unexpected times when the color of the sky, the sight of a couple walking comfortably together, or the smell of a restaurant breakfast would claim, "You don't belong here anymore; you're not a part of the normal world."

The next year, everything became more routine, if perhaps boring. Clearly, the rest of the world had moved on from Steve's death. A degree of normality returned, with thoughts of Steve—and missing him—intruding often. During that time, I volunteered at a homeless shelter kitchen; the guests were far worse off than I was. Or perhaps it was just that we were all miserable.

By the third year, I started to notice tears being replaced by smiles. (So did President Joseph Biden after the death of his son, Beau!)

Ten years later, I don't cry. I smile easily at the heady, inclusive memories of being Steve's partner. I have several great friends, I have good work to do, and I enjoy living with the knowledge that I was fully loved.

Tomorrow Will Be Different: Love, Loss, and the Fight for Trans Equality **was written by United States Senator Sarah McBride, our country's first transgender senator. Read her unique—but still universal—story of her first great love and marriage.**

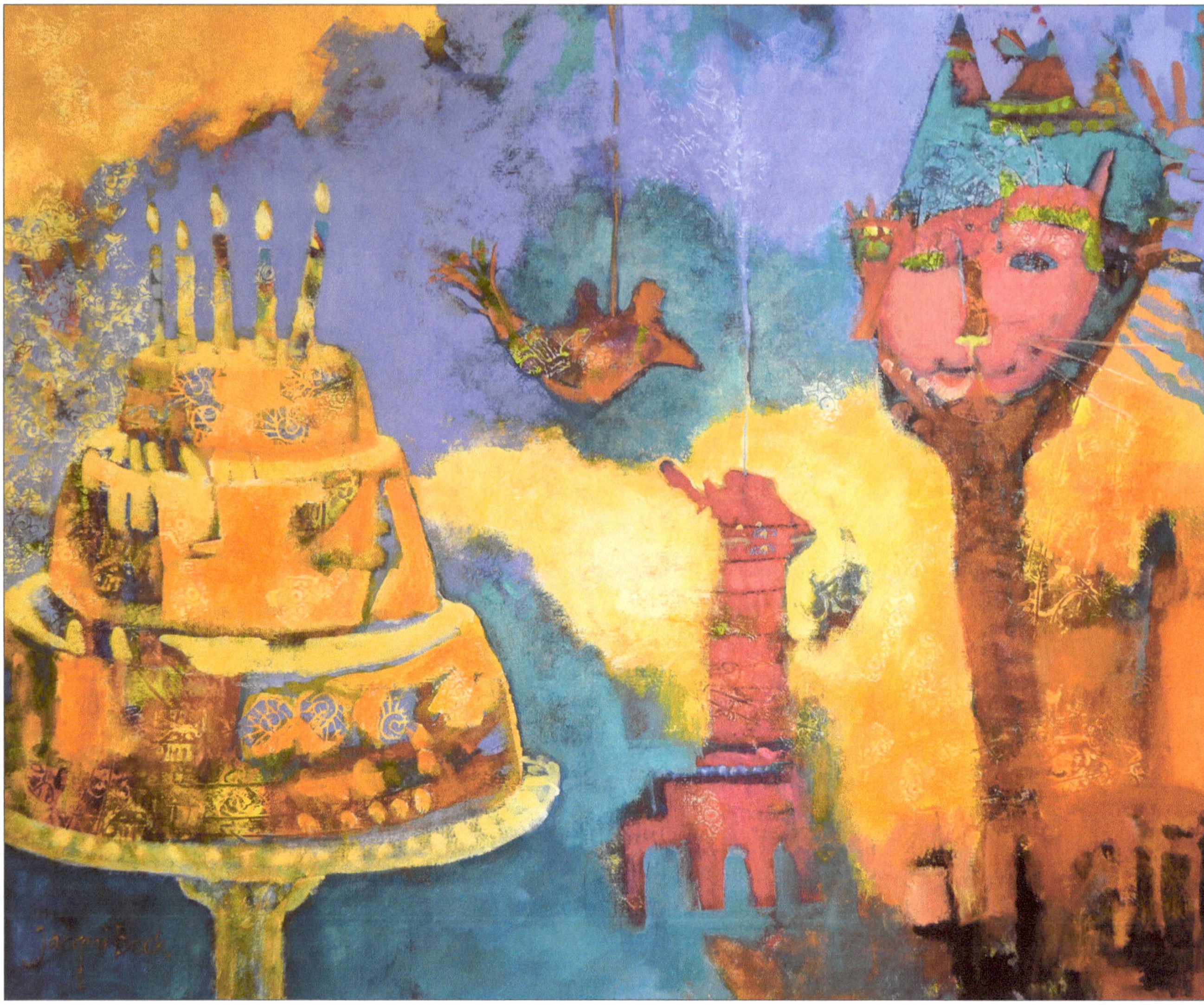

The Birthday Cat and the Giraffe Piñata

CHAPTER 23

How Transgender and Gender-Nonconforming Individuals Can Live Long, Healthy Lives

We've covered a lot of information in this book, mostly dealing with gender dysphoria and many of the ways to begin to manage it. As people find that their gender dysphoria becomes less urgent—perhaps through hormones, surgery, and finding ways to manage it more comfortably—we turn our attention to living long and living well.

We will look at living more fully throughout life. As often happens in the practice of transgender medicine, we're limited by our knowledge. We have to take data about society as a whole and make inferences about the transgender community specifically.

Yet stories like the three I highlight in the next few pages enable me to make those inferences. And I hope they inspire you as well.

Following those stories, we'll look at how Americans die because if we want to live our best lives, we have to understand the risk factors and behaviors that lead to an untimely death.

- What are the leading diagnoses that end the lives of most Americans?
- How can we recognize the risk factors for these disease entities?
- How can we separate the risk factors that are beyond our control and examine the personal risk factors we can control?

Doing so allows us to exert the control we do have to make our lives better.

We recognize that, as I say to my patients, "Nobody's getting out of here alive." But in the time we all have left, how can we live our lives as well and as long as we can? Once we discover how best to live, we assuredly want more life! Can we live with commitment, meaning, and even joy? And what is the legacy we leave for those who come after us?

We now focus our attention on three trans women who have distinguished themselves with their creative excellence and their courage.

Life Stories of Excellence: Women Finding Their Way

Ginger Chien: A Transgender Rock Band Walks into a Rural Bar…

Ginger Chien, who holds a master's degree in engineering from Princeton University, is modest about her many achievements. I heard her storytelling performance on Ignite Seattle in the summer of 2019. Ginger contributed her bio below. This is followed by a transcript of her performance essay, "A Transgender Rock Band Walks into a Rural Olympic Peninsula Bar." Be sure to watch the actual performance on YouTube: **youtube.com/watch?v=6dpqBVCEcKI**.

Ginger Chien: In Her Own Words

I call myself a creatrix at the intersection of intellect and emotion, words and music, and fact and imagination, with communications at the heart of everything I do.

I'm an electrical engineer at a major wireless telecommunications company where I transitioned on the job in 2011 with support from peers and management. After I transitioned, I found myself expanding into speaking roles at national technology conferences on subjects including queer authenticity and emotional intelligence, as well as the latest wireless device technologies.

I am an open-mic storyteller, sharing tales of life, love, and being around the country. I am an advocate for and teacher of diversity and emotional intelligence and the collaborative creativity it fuels. I'm active in a local PFLAG chapter where I advocate, educate, and provide emotional support to families and allies of LGBTQ people. I am a prolific inventor, with over 50 sole and shared patents in areas of business processes, communications, computing, and user interfaces. I am also a musician in a transgender '80s cover band who has seen the power of shared experiences and authenticity open hearts in the most unexpected places.

The following is my story.

A Transgender Rock Band Walks into a Bar…

When I was a little kid, one of my favorite TV shows was *The Partridge Family*. It was about a mom and her kids. They played in a band together. They had all kinds of funny adventures and it was such a neat family. I wished I could have called that one my home.

I also dreamt of someday being Lori. She was the smiling girl behind the keys. But none of this was in the cards for me because I was the only son of a hopeful immigrant family and I had a role to play.

I did well in school, got married, had a great kid, and had a successful career, but everyone's affections were directed to the accomplished facade of the man I had created. And I felt very alone.

So, I came out late in life, and I saw some transgender friends playing in a band and I was absolutely mesmerized. Now I knew nothing about rock music. I hadn't even been to a concert before. All I had to offer to them were my childhood skills as a violin player, but I promised I would work hard, I would study any instrument, and I asked them, "Can I join the band?" And they said yes!

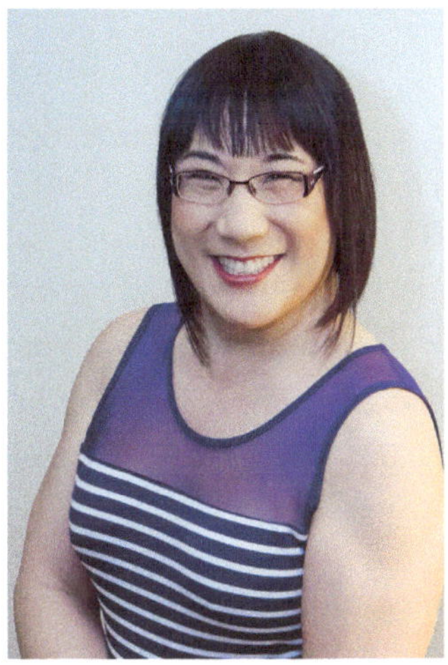 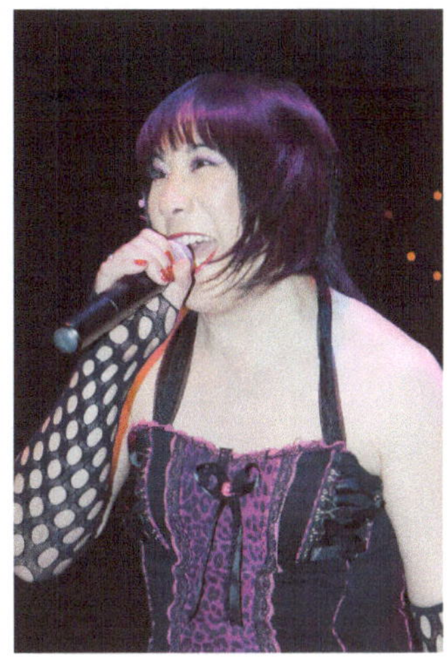

And so I bought a whole bunch of equipment. I learned how to play the keys. We put together hours and hours of music so we could fill an entire night, and we started looking for our first big public shows to play in the town of Port Angeles, Washington. Port Angeles is a pretty rugged coastal town way out on the Olympic Peninsula. It's known mainly for logging and fishing. It's the last place you'd expect to find a trans band playing in a bar.

But we put on our colorful outfits and we strutted into that bar at 9 o'clock. It was already packed because everyone knew that "that" band was coming. And the men... they clutched their beers... and the women... they looked us up and down as we walked toward the stage. And then we started playing. The '80s music drew the women on the floor, and then the men followed. Now we have played there for 15 years to packed houses.

At these shows I met this man. He was a self-described redneck. At first, he was really creeped out by us, but now we have conversations and give each other hugs. He told me a story about a friend of his with whom he'd lost touch. This friend had gotten back in touch with him and said that she had transitioned and was living as a woman and wanted to reconnect.

And much to his credit, because he had come to know us as people, not as fears and assumptions, but at the level of music and connection, he said he was not afraid to meet her and they did meet and they did reconnect.

I had to ask him: "Knowing who you are and where you came from, and you're standing here now talking with me giving me hugs. And knowing your friend, where your friend came from and who she has become, which one of you changed more?" And he thought for a second and this little smile crept across his face and he said, "Me. I've changed more!"

This thing that we do… it is a risky thing. There are people and places who would have nothing to do with us. We stick out everywhere we go. But because we have authenticity, people tell us that they're inspired. I think it's like we lift this suffocating wet blanket of conformity off of everybody by being a little bit bigger than life, and it creates space underneath where people can finally breathe and be themselves.

One of my favorite songs that we play is called "Major Tom." It's an obscure song about an astronaut who gets lost in space and even though he's lost, it ends on this beautiful chorus over and over singing that he's coming home. And I can look across our audience and see young, old, gay, straight, queer, trans, abled, and not… they're all dancing and singing together because we're taking the risk to be ourselves and they can join us. And when that chorus hits, everyone tips their heads back, and they reach their hands for the ceiling, and they're all singing that they too are coming home.

And me? I'm the smiling girl behind the keys. I'm making music and people are dancing and singing with me.

It feels like home.

Linda's note: Learn more about The Nasty Habits at thenastyhabits.com. And while we're on the subject of singing, next is another unique and powerful story about holding on to the essence of who we are no matter what our gender expression is.

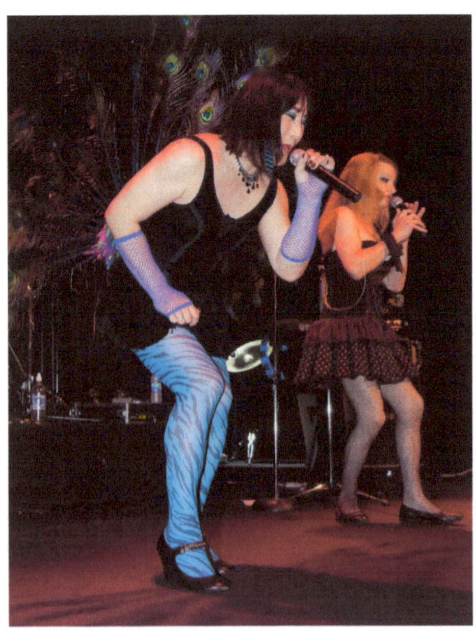

Dr. Stephanie Dykes: A Trans Woman in the Seattle's Men's Chorus

College administrator Dr. Stephanie Dykes has sung since high school.

When she transitioned at age 50, she was concerned about how she would be able to continue singing as a trans woman who sang bass. The consummate researcher, Stephanie discovered GALA choruses (galachoruses.org), an association of LGBTQIA+ choruses.

After moving to Washington State, she auditioned for the Seattle Men's Chorus. Director Paul Caldwell welcomed her into the chorus ranks with the provision that she would wear a tuxedo. She became the first trans woman to sing as a member of the Seattle Men's Chorus in its 40-year history.

Stephanie won the respect of her chorus "brothers" with her solo of "Stars" from *Les Misérables* at a chorus retreat in November 2018. Then in June 2019, she won the hearts of the broader Seattle audience at the Seattle Men's Chorus's "Summer of '69" concerts at Benaroya Hall.

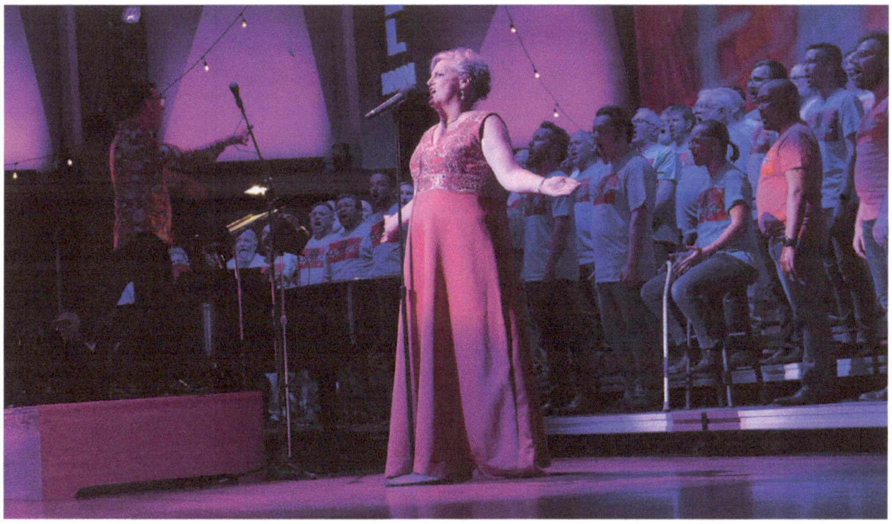

With her hair styled in a princess updo and wearing a floor-length fuchsia gown, Stephanie sang "My Way," becoming the first trans woman to ever solo as a member of the Seattle Men's Chorus. She received a standing ovation at both of the chorus's performances.

In Stephanie's words, "The Seattle Men's Chorus has been the musical highlight of my life. Being a member of this chorus is like having 200 brothers." Stephanie missed singing with her brothers during the pandemic, but music is always in her heart.

Hear Stephanie Dykes's solo on YouTube at youtube.com/watch?v=s64L00qnVMU.
Read more about the Chorus at seattlechoruses.org/learn/seattlemenschorus.

Katherine Johnson: Christmas Eve in Las Cruces

The following is by Katherine Johnson, used with permission from her blog *Una Voce Sola* at unavocesola.wordpress.com.

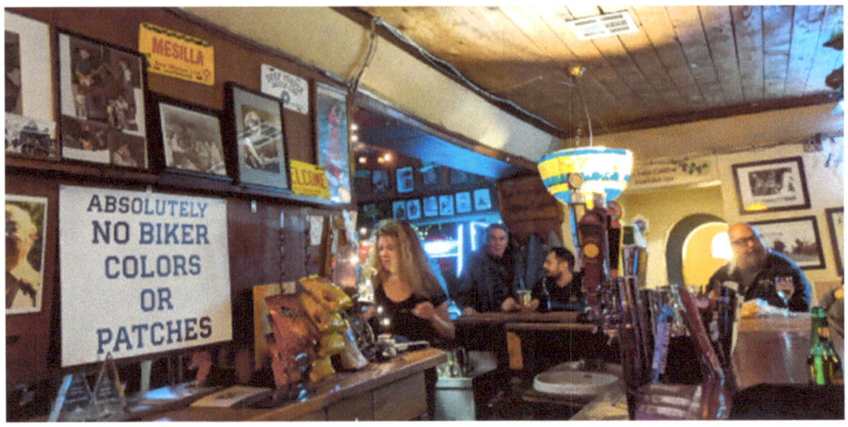

December 24, 2019, El Patio Cantina, Mesilla, New Mexico (the oldest bar in New Mexico)

Tonight I thanked my excellent friends, one by one, at the High Desert Brewery for their sustained generosity that welcomed me to Las Cruces. Later, not settled into this Christmas Eve, I wandered with purpose to the El Patio Cantina in Mesilla, NM. This is where those who are short on places to go over Christmas, be that eve or day, come. Moths to a flame, so to speak.

My wings are burned for better or worse.

Long live the El Patio, the patron saint of the young, the lost, the abandoned, and those like me that are ending up, either by circumstances, luck, or choice, their lives where they can barely be found. I am OK with all this.

Neither bitter or with joy; I live in a solitary place where my end game rectitude is often corrupted by the El Patio. On this Christmas Eve, I find myself at peace here, quite drunk. Here in this bar I am consumed with thoughts about when my young son, beloved, once believed in Christmas and me. There I sat downstairs, far into the night, drunk, making that lie come true.

I wish everyone that reads this on this Christmas Eve to not to be troubled by this place where I find myself tonight. Rather, ground yourself in love, family, or community as you find it.

I am good with what life has brought me. No, actually I feel blessed by everything, good, bad, indifferent. Here in New Mexico I live under clear blue skies that are nothing less than the iris of God.

Merry Christmas to all.

The Leading Causes of Death in the United States

Having shared the richness of three creative life stories, we shift to a more sobering topic: How are we likely to leave this world? Although we cannot apply data to the transgender community, we begin by looking at the population in general.

Examining death rates is only one way of looking at the health of a people. Below, you will find the leading causes of deaths in the United States as tracked by the Centers for Disease Control and Prevention. (This tracks all deaths, not just those in the transgender community.)

This particular list does not track deaths by age. Were we to look at deaths among teenagers and young adults, for example, accidental deaths and deaths by suicide would top the list. The list below does not examine death rates by income levels, race, education, or geographical location. So far, I have not found death rates by age and gender identity. But we can take information we know clinically about the transgender and gender-nonconforming community to make some important inferences.

CDC's Top 10 Causes of Deaths in the US in 2019[121]

1. Heart disease
2. Cancer (lung, colon, and breast are typically cited as the leading all-cancer deaths)
3. Accidental deaths
4. Chronic lower respiratory diseases (such as COPD or emphysema)
5. Stroke
6. Alzheimer's disease
7. Diabetes
8. Kidney disease
9. Influenza and pneumonia
10. Suicide

Note: Statistics for 2020 were not available at the time of this writing, but COVID-19 as a cause of death broke into the US "Top Ten" in March 2020, fluctuated throughout 2020, and peaked in January 2021 when it surpassed all other US causes of death. In January 2021, it was speculated that COVID-19 would rise to third place, behind heart disease and cancer—and ahead of accidental deaths.[122]

Following the resolution of COVID-19, we may expect a return to the prepandemic lists.

121 Centers for Disease Control and Prevention, "Leading Causes of Death," last reviewed March 1, 2021, https://www.cdc.gov/nchs/fastats/leading-causes-of-death.htm.

122 Jacqueline Howard, "Covid-19 Likely Ranks as the Third Leading Cause of Death in the US in 2020, CDC Statisticians Say," *CNN*, January 5, 2021, https://www.cnn.com/2021/01/05/health/covid-third-leading-cause-of-death-cdc-wellness/index.html.

Risk Factors for Premature Death

Looking at each of these causes of death, we can tease out the risk factors that increase our chances of having—and dying of—each condition. For example, high blood pressure and diabetes are the leading risk factors for kidney failure. Influenza and pneumonia are more likely to be lethal in older people and in immunocompromised individuals.

Then we can look at those risk factors that impact the trans community disproportionately, examine whether these risk factors are modifiable, and extrapolate from that whether or not mortality might be reduced. Let's take a couple of examples:

- **Tobacco smoking is significantly more prevalent in the LGBTQIA+ community but particularly high in the transgender community.**[123]
  A higher incidence of smoking could increase the trans community's risk of *every single item* on the Top 10 Causes of Death list.

  Is smoking a modifiable risk factor? Yes. Although highly addictive, smoking can be addressed by the prescription drug Chantix, over-the-counter nicotine replacement products, the antidepressant bupropion (marketed as Wellbutrin and as Zyban to help people stop smoking), hypnotherapy, cognitive therapy, and the time-honored cold-turkey method.

  Is smoking mortality reduceable? Yes. People with a 30-pack-a-year history of smoking are now screened with low-dose CT scans to look for lung cancer. And cancer is only *one* of the causes of death that is increased by smoking.

> **I have more than a dozen individuals in my small family practice who have now lived for a decade beyond their lung cancer diagnoses. Years ago, there would have been no way to foresee such survival accounts.**
>
> *— Linda Gromko, MD*

- **Depression impacts the transgender community disproportionately.**[124]
  Depression increases the risk of death by suicide and accidental death in all LGBTQIA+ subgroups. Is depression treatable? Yes, with antidepressants, cognitive therapy, exercise, and other methods.

---

123 "Transgender adults are 2.1 times more likely than cisgender adults to smoke. Only 11.8 percent of heterosexual young adults indicate that they currently smoke cigarettes, compared to 19 percent of homosexual, 16.9 percent of bisexual and 33.2 percent of transgender young adults." Truth Initiative, "Tobacco Use in LGBT Communities," *Fact Sheet*, February 18, 2018, https://truthinitiative.org/sites/default/files/media/files/2019/03/Truth_LGBT%20FactSheet_FINAL.pdf; US Food and Drug Administration, "Tobacco Use in the LGBT Community: A Public Health Issue," updated June 2, 2021, https://www.fda.gov/tobacco-products/health-information/tobacco-use-lgbt-community-public-health-issue.

124 Virupaksha, H. G., Daliboyina Muralidhar, and Jayashree Ramakrishna, "Suicide and Suicidal Behavior among Transgender Persons," *Indian Journal of Psychological Medicine* 38, no. 6 (November–December 2016): 505–09, http://dx.doi.org/10.4103/0253-7176.194908.

> **My best woman friend from medical school and I have had dinner together once a month since graduation. Continuity enriches an already meaningful friendship, particularly when either of us is experiencing a crisis.**
>
> *— Linda Gromko, MD*

Can death by suicide be prevented? Yes, through early identification, treatment, and ongoing vigilance.

All of the Top 10 causes of death have identifiable risk factors, some of which are preventable and some not. One of the most important ways by which we can alter our health and life span is to recognize risk factors that are within our control and those that are beyond our control. There are many *more* factors that are within our control, which we will detail.

Assessing Your Own Risk: Factors That Are *beyond* Your Control

Here are the factors that are beyond our control:

- **Genetics**
  Most of us have no control over the genes we inherit from our parents. But should we inherit a genetic propensity for a lung disease, we can control our exposure to cofactors like smoking that further increase our risk of dying.

- **Race**
  Our race and ethnicity can influence our exposure to systemic racism and its impact on our economic environment, health, education, and other opportunities.

- **Random accidents**
  While many accidents are preventable, many occur as a strike out of the blue and are, at the time of the incident, beyond our control. Once an accident has happened, it becomes a fact of a person's life; there's nothing to do but to manage the consequences.

> **It's not what you get, it's how you cope.**
>
> *— Linda's mom at age 96*

- **The parenting we received and other advantages or disadvantages we had growing up**
  These all occurred in the past. We can't change our upbringing, although we can change how we deal with it. (Refer to adverse childhood experiences in Chapter 18.)

- **Our financial status at birth**
  The financial advantages or disadvantages we were born into are beyond our control. They may have been beyond our parents' control also.

- **Adverse events we have experienced in the past**
  These include sexual assaults, injuries, and mental illness of those around us, which can impact our health.

Finding Contentment, Meaning, and Joy: Lifestyle Factors We *Can* Control

Here are the factors that we *can* control and that can impact the quality and length of our lives:

- **Nutrition**
  We can choose healthier or less healthy foods within our means, and we can prepare our own food ahead of time to maximize our own nutrition. We may have more or less healthy food options depending on our resources, but a fast-food diet is a relatively costly one both in terms of initial and long-term financial outlay for future medical issues.

- **Weight maintenance**
  While a propensity to obesity is arguably related to genetics and environment, we can avoid extremes of weight through modifiable factors like body movement and food habits.

- **Exercise**
  A great stress reliever, exercise prevents diabetes and helps us manage our weight. It can be part of a treatment program to deal with depression. Walking is the exercise most often used by long-term weight managers in the National Weight Control Registry (**nwcr.ws/research**).

- **Restorative sleep**
  If we are not sleeping effectively, we can be evaluated by a doctor that specializes in sleep problems. Obstructive sleep apnea is related to hypertension, diabetes, and cardiac arrythmias and is often manageable through weight control and CPAP devices (continuous positive airway pressure masks that extend the length of time we oxygenate our blood during sleep). We can examine our "sleep hygiene" and manage our sleep environment more effectively. Sanjay Gupta, MD recently explained in his excellent book *Keep Sharp: Build a Better Brain at Any Age* that sleep quality is critical in repairing and "organizing" our thoughts.

- **Positive contact with others; loneliness impacts longevity**
  While there's a difference between being alone and being lonely, contact with other people helps. Even contacts that may seem trivial help.[125]

- **Regular contacts with friends**
  We need friends and longer friendships as well as new ones. Having friends of different age ranges is interesting, and we're more likely to have some friends that outlive us (a practical matter). The quality of friendships surpasses quantity; a shared history can be the best.

- **A feeling that we have purpose in life and that our lives matter**
  If our purpose is watering a plant or feeding a pet, it *is* purpose. Of course, there are many examples that can be tailored to individuals. We can find activities that give us purpose: rocking hospitalized infants, walking shelter dogs, advancing political causes, or just being kind to people.

125 Harvard Health Publishing, "Can Relationships Boost Longevity and Well-Being?," Harvard Medical School, June 1, 2017, https://www.health.harvard.edu/mental-health/can-relationships-boost-longevity-and-well-being.

- **Recreation**
  Whatever we see as fun or gives us pleasure, such as movies, art, music, traveling, reading, and sex.

- **Conscious appreciation of quality (gratitude)**
  Are we consciously recognizing the excellence of food, art, sunsets, and music? Do we notice and recognize these life-enriching entities and experience gratitude? Do we record it, as Dr. Gupta suggests, in a gratitude journal?

- **Lifelong learning**
  We can keep our minds sharp and curious since learning is available to all of us. Are we using our libraries, YouTube, and low-cost or free apps that teach us to relax, to speak French, and to nurture our interests?

- **Financial management**
  This allows us to live securely and within our resources and manage our future with less fear.

- **Spiritual practices of our choice**
  More than going to a church, a spiritual practice may be walking near a lake, keeping a journal, meditating, engaging in prayer, listening to or writing music, giving to the local food bank, and so on. Spiritual practices may be anything that connects us to a greater power—whether we identify that as God in whatever name, peace, nature, light, or love—or anything that connects us to a greater whole and a greater good.

- **Provision of a personal legacy that honors our lives and helps those beyond ourselves**
  Our personal resources vary greatly, but we may have more than we think.
  - Provide for friends or family members as you can through a will, even if your assets are modest. You may have a retirement account at work or life insurance through an employer.
  - Make a simple will and have it witnessed and notarized. Designate beneficiaries on retirement accounts or insurance policies.
  - Think about who or what organization might be your beneficiary through an inexpensive term life-insurance policy, making you a philanthropist (on your death anyway). Online resources such as Mama Bear or FreeWill can help you construct your own will for a small fee or no fee, respectively. If it's notarized, it's supposed to "count," but consult an attorney to be safe: **freewill.com** and **mamabearlegalforms.com**.

A life-changing experience for me came when a penniless man in public housing deliberately left all of the items in his subsidized apartment *to me* many years after he had been my patient. His flamboyant shopping brought him floor-to-ceiling Le Creuset cookware, Asian art pieces, and angora scarves in all colors from the catalog. My unexpected windfall enabled me to donate a gymnasium-size space full of pricey items to the Lambert House trans youth fundraiser. It shook my own priorities and prompted my search for Steve, my very best husband, now deceased.

— Linda Gromko, MD

- **Involvement in modifying things we care about**
  These include politics, causes, and charitable giving. Give in honor of someone you remember, honoring their life and contributions.

- **Humor**
  Medicine is a field rich in humor that keeps us going and gives power to its generators. Look for it. When a patient makes me laugh, my life and their life both expand.

> **I know I may look like an old-timer to many of you. It's true, I'm 72 years old! But my vagina is only 30, which makes me a millennial!**
>
> *— Barbara Sehr, age 72, trans woman and comedienne*

- **Careful respect for our own medical needs**
  We must seek and get the healthcare we require:
  - Do we get our personal immunizations? (preventing pneumonia, influenza, and more recently, COVID-19)
  - Do we get dental care? (Which can prevent heart disease.)
  - Have we figured out our medical maintenance regimen? Do we have a system like a Mediset weekly pill organizer, or online pharmacy delivery, or other methods to minimize errors or avoid running out of the medications we need?
  - Are we being screened for breast cancer, cervical cancer, colon cancer, or prostate cancer—in other words, are we being appropriately screened considering the organs we have?
- Awareness of our own mental health needs and the willingness to seek help as we need it:
  - Do we have a maintenance plan if we have depression or anxiety?
  - Do we have an emergency plan for when we go off the rails or decompensate?
  - Are we controlling our post-traumatic stress disorder (PTSD) if we have it? Have we talked to providers about medications or therapies? Have we read the book *The Body Keeps the Score: Brain, Mind, and Body in the Healing of Trauma*? Or the more recent book by Oprah Winfrey and Bruce Perry, *What Happened to You: Conversations on Trauma, Resilience, and Healing*?
  - Are other mental illnesses (like bipolar disorder, dysthymia, and panic disorder) optimally managed?

- **Intimacy**
  Both physically and emotionally, intimacy can decrease our isolation and shore up our resilience.

- **Minimizing sexual risks**
  If PrEP (preexposure prophylaxis) is appropriate, have we arranged to have that prescribed, and do we follow up with maintenance lab work every 3 months? Are we knowingly taking sexual risks that might be modified?

- **Respectful use or avoidance of alcohol**
  Approximately five drinks in a week will cancel the effect of an antidepressant medication and increase our risk of suicide, accidental death, and injury to others.

- **Avoidance of smoking and other tobacco products**
  Have we supported our quitting, or can we not start at all?

- **Support for substance management**
  If opiates are risks for us or those around us, have we sought treatment? Have we purchased Narcan (naloxone) to have on hand to help manage an accidental or purposeful overdose?

- **Self-imposed exposures**
  Do we have firearms in the home? Are we trained in firearm safety if we own weapons?

- **Cleanliness and order**
  Doing your laundry may "spark joy" for Marie Kondo and you, but not me. However, starting the day with a clean sink and an ordered mind can help me, so I work at that.

Finally, we need to have respect for ourselves and the use of our time because our time is our life. This list above is a lot to consider, but it is hardly an exhaustive one; add your own categories to personalize it.

Your Minimum Daily Requirements

If you need clarification about what *you need* on a daily basis, fill out my Minimum Daily Requirements table on pages 454–455.

The point of the exercise is to outline what you need on a daily basis: how much food, how much water, how much touch, how much humor, how much intellectual stimulation, and so on. Be as specific about your requirements as you can be.

You may meet more of your requirements on some days than on other days. As always, the more we know what it is we want and need, the more likely we are to have our needs met. Meeting our minimum daily requirements—or at the very least knowing what they are—is fundamental to good self-care.

Minimum Daily Requirements (May be daily, weekly, monthly, or as needed. List as many other categories as apply to you.)			
Category	**What exactly do you need?**	**Obstacles**	**Plan**
Work			
Exercise			
Being on water			
Sunlight			
Sex			
Contact with friends			
Body care (basic)			
Spa care			
Massage			
Music			
Art			
Motion pictures			
Shopping			
Water			
Travel			

Category	What exactly do you need?	Obstacles	Plan
Sleep			
Crying			
Therapy			
Chocolate			
Conversations			
Life theater/music			
Study			
Finding a bargain			
Volunteering			
Giving money			
Teaching			

Table 23.1. Minimum daily requirements.

Words to Live By: A Few Verbal Self-Care Tools

Throughout my years in healthcare, I've found a few simple verbal tools that seem to help people. None of them is original; a couple come from 12-step group models like Alcoholics Anonymous. These self-care tools are useful in many situations—direct, memorable, and cutting quickly to the essence of many of our problems.

When you're grappling with a problem, examine where you are meeting or failing to meet the Four Agreements. I've tried this with patient problems and staff challenges. It's enlightening, clarifying, and fast.

The Four Agreements by Don Manuel Ruiz[126]

Be impeccable with your word.
Don't make assumptions.
Don't take anything personally.
Always do your best.

I've had many occasions to use the HALT acronym with patients—particularly those who are overwhelmed with life's stressors or an ongoing crisis. Isn't this, after all, the essence of self care?

The HALT Acronym from Alcoholics Anonymous

Don't let yourself get too Hungry, too Angry, too Lonely, or too Tired.

A question asked by my own Queen Anne Medical's office manager, Barb Boni, this tool cuts to the essence of any problem.

What is your desired outcome?

126 Don Miguel Ruiz, *The Four Agreements: A Practical Guide to Personal Freedom*, San Francisco: Amber-Allen, 2018.

Here is the Serenity Prayer from Alcoholics Anonymous.

The Serenity Prayer

Grant me the serenity to accept
the things I cannot change,
the courage to change the things I can,
and the wisdom to know the difference.

This abbreviated version of the Serenity Prayer above was adopted by Bill Watson, the founder of Alcoholics Anonymous. It is repeated at the beginning of every AA meeting and in many types of 12-step meetings that modeled themselves on AA.

However, the full text of the prayer, below, was written by theologian Reinhold Niebuhr and contributed by author and editor Barbara Mulvey Little. It's worth reading and reflecting upon, although from a Christian perspective.

God, give me grace to accept with serenity
the things that cannot be changed,
Courage to change the things
which should be changed,
and the Wisdom to distinguish
the one from the other.

Living one day at a time,
Enjoying one moment at a time,
Accepting hardship as a pathway to peace,
Taking, as Jesus did,
This sinful world as it is,
Not as I would have it,
Trusting that You will make all things right,
If I surrender to Your will,
So that I may be reasonably happy in this life,
And supremely happy with You forever in the next.

Amen.

Linda's tool for navigating in a sexist world:

How would a man do it? (Or how would a woman do it?)

This quote is from Barbara Mulvey Little, who has written several books dealing with spirituality. How many spiritual practices focus on "the now"!

The past is gone, the future is yet unknown.
The only moment we have is the present.
Unwrap it and enjoy it.

I've worked with many individuals in crisis over the years. Sometimes, I try to help them discover what kind of support they need. The real question, of course, is what do you need to do to support *yourself*? Sometimes you have to step aside a little to see it.

If your best friend were in exactly your situation,
what would you do for them?

As a physician, mom, and business owner, I've heard and used the advice "Choose your battles" many times. Our practice uses a variation of this advice that I think I heard from a hospital orderly years ago.

Don't poke a skunk.

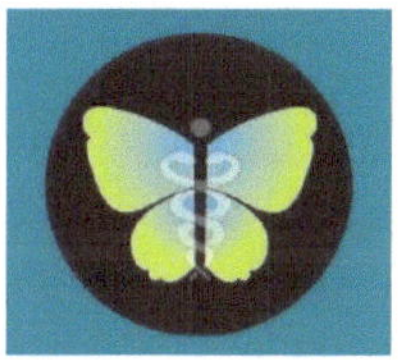

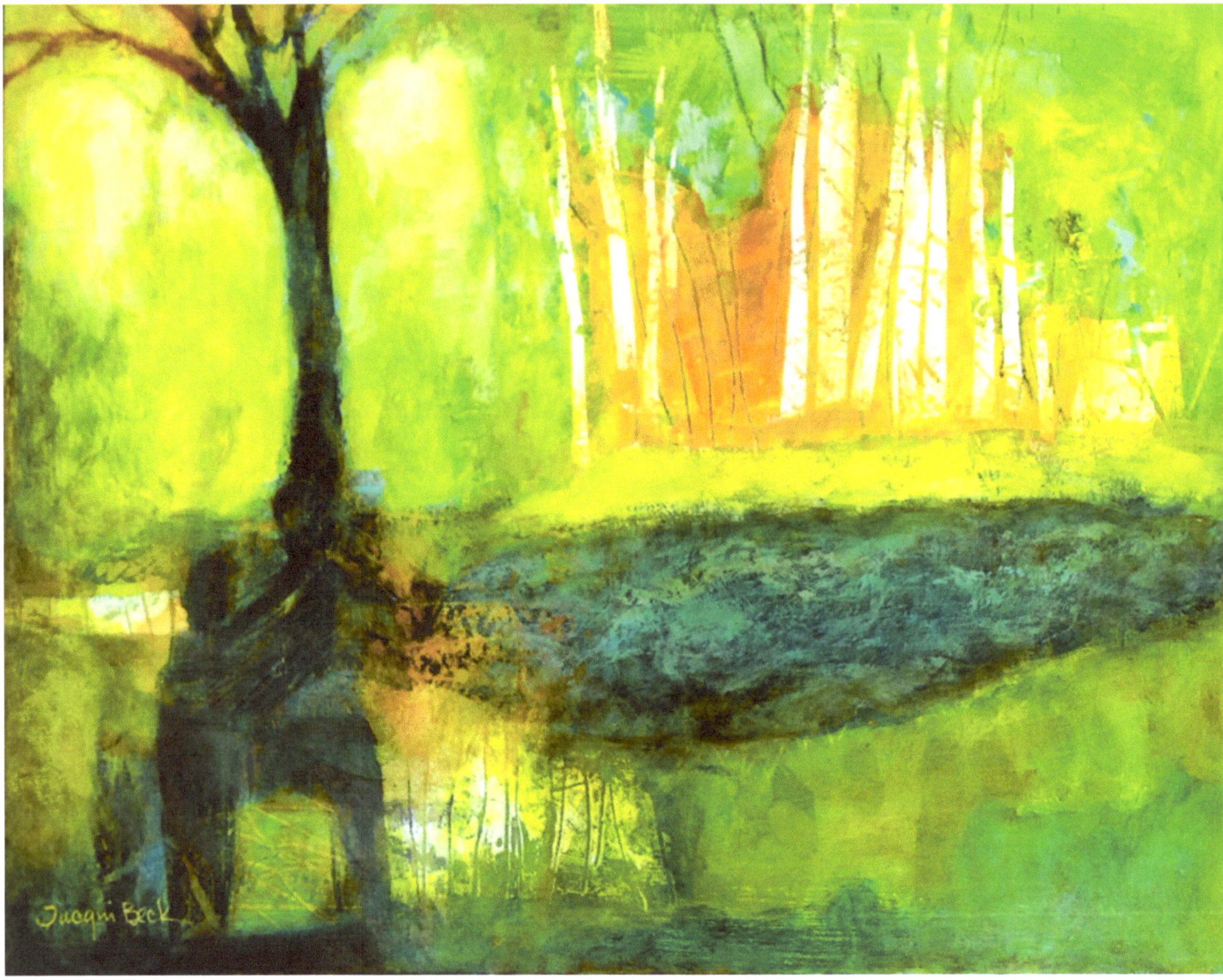

Still Forest

CONCLUSION

I finished writing *A Practical Reference for Transgender and Gender-Nonconforming Adults* in early 2021—amidst the COVID-19 pandemic and between impeachments of Donald Trump.

We have all shared these potent experiences, but each of us gathered our own unique insights. No matter what experiences we have had, it is good to be breathing air—most especially without a mechanical ventilator.

I recognized again how little control I have in the world at large and in the immediate world around me. I learned that good medicine can be practiced remotely, reaching more people. I reminded myself that the practice of medicine is fundamentally a practice of teaching—teaching not only patients, but also professional colleagues. (I have recently released an online course, *Transgender Medicine for Healthcare Professionals*.)

I was reminded of the precarious financial balance of a tiny independent medical practice. My staff and I struggled from one Payroll Protection loan to the next, not knowing if the practice would even survive. This book survived on the good graces of numerous content providers and GoFundMe angels who pitched in to help.

I hope that I have many more years to live, to practice medicine, and to gather more stories to tell. But I can truly say that if I died tomorrow, I have had an amazing life! Never boring, often challenging, and usually hopeful.

I have been honored to occupy a position of privileged intimacy in the lives of so many people who have come to my medical practice: clients and staff alike. They are all my teachers; I bring their wisdom to you. I sincerely hope this book helps you or someone you know.

— Linda Gromko, MD
July 2021
Seattle, Washington

EPILOGUE TO THE DEDICATION

David—to whom this book is dedicated—died on March 6, 2021—15 months after his horrible paralyzing fall (refer to the Dedication on page v). I arrived a few minutes after he died, helped the caregivers bathe him, and stood witness as the mortuary person zipped him into the blanket body bag. It was important to me that David's body was treated respectfully.

I had had my weekly conversation with David just two afternoons before. We talked about his medications, we talked about pain, and we talked about his phlegm. But David had had a dream, and he was eager to share it. Working to push out his breaths and speaking with a gravelly voice, he told me the dream.

> "I was in the midst of being born.
>
> "My head was out, and I could see light and color—it was beautiful. And I really got it what love is. Love is total trust.
>
> "It felt like I knew God and God is trust. I was surrounded by love—everyone I have ever known; people I've read about, like Gandhi and Martin Luther King. And my wife Ann. It was wonderful to see her again. She was the same as before; she was 40."

David paused to breathe, then continued,

> "The ultimate lesson is that God is love and God is total trust. This has changed my life already. I am more comfortable, not afraid of dying—this revelation took away the fear. I want to live and live this [world view] many more days. I want to tell the people I trust. I told my caregivers. What a gift I could give to a 38-year-old? It all makes sense. This gift is why I'm alive."

The dream had changed David, washing away his PTSD, washing away his fears. I often wondered why David had lived through his horrific accident, why he lived through the custom karmic hell of total dependency. And now, I knew.

Rest in peace, David.

— Linda Gromko, MD

GLOSSARY FROM THE TRANSGENDER LANGUAGE PRIMER

by Greyson Simon

This glossary, which focuses on the language of the transgender and nonbinary community, was used with permission from editor Greyson Simon. For more information on the Transgender Language Primer, refer to the TLP website at translanguageprimer.com.

AGAB / DGAB / IS *(noun phrase / abbreviation)*. Assigned [Gender] At Birth or Designated [Gender] At Birth or InterSex. It is sometimes written as GAAB or GAB. This refers to what gender someone was assigned at birth. This is used when talking about a range of people who experience a set of common issues based on their birth assignment. AGAB is also used by many transgender people to talk about their gender experience without having to use narratives about "what gender they used to be," as many trans people never identified with their birth assigned gender. Sometimes seen as AGAB/IS to be inclusive of intersex people who are dealing with similar situations, but who do not identify with binary assignment labels.

Agender *(adjective)*. Agender people define their gender in a variety of ways. Some agender people define their gender as being neither a man nor a woman while others understand themselves as not having any gender at all. Agender people may or may not transition physically, legally, or socially. This is based on their understanding of their relationship with gender and their access to transitioning within their culture. Generally, agender people are considered under the nonbinary and transgender umbrellas, but they may or may not identify as transgender or nonbinary specifically.

Androgynous *(adjective | androgyny, noun | androgynously, adverb)*. This term is often used regarding outward gender expression, though it has been occasionally used as an identity term very similar to androgyne. In terms of expression, it is generally understood as having an appearance that is beyond contextually feminine or masculinity traits or specifically blending contextually gendered traits.

Asexual *(adjective | asexuality, noun)*. Sometimes shortened to "ace." A person who does not experience sexual attraction. Asexuality is a sexual orientation and is different from celibacy, in that celibacy is the choice to refrain from engaging in sexual behaviors and does not comment on one's sexual attractions. An asexual individual may choose to engage in sexual behaviors for various reasons even while not experiencing sexual attraction. Asexuality is an identity and sexual orientation; it is not a medical condition. Sexual attraction is not necessary for a person to thrive.

- ***Related Articles and Resources***
  - *AZE Journal* | Azejournal.com
  - The Asexual Visibility and Education Network (AVEN) | Asexuality.org
  - "Asexuality: The 'X' in a Sexual World" | Huffington Post

Attraction *(noun)*. There are many different types of attraction. All of these attractions are valid and may be independent from each other or interact with each other in a variety of ways. They can be present or absent in everything from friendships to life partners. Each relationship is a unique experience. This is why some people identify not only with their sexuality (heterosexual, bisexual, etc.) but also with their romantic attraction using the suffix -romantic (panromantic, homoromantic). This is especially common in the asexual community where a focus on romantic relationships or platonic relationships is more visible.

- ***Types of Attraction***
  - **Sexual attraction:** attraction that makes people desire sexual contact or shows sexual interest in another person(s). This is different from a sexual drive, which is a biological instinct distinct from someone's sexual attraction.
  - **Romantic attraction:** attraction that makes people desire romantic contact or interaction with another person(s).
  - **Aesthetic attraction:** occurs when someone appreciates the appearance or beauty of another person(s), disconnected from sexual or romantic attraction.
  - **Sensual attraction:** the desire to interact with others in a tactile, nonsexual way, such as through hugging or cuddling.
  - **Emotional attraction:** the desire to get to know someone, often as a result of their personality instead of their physicality. This type of attraction is present in most relationships including platonic friendships.
  - **Mental attraction:** the desire to engage with another in a thoughtful manner, such as having deep conversations or engaging in thought provoking activities together. This has nothing to do with western ideas of "intelligence" as something measurable, but rather an attraction to how a person thinks, how they solve problems, or how they interpret and engage with the world.

Bigender / Trigender / etc. *(adjective).* People who are two (three, etc.) genders. Some bigender people shift between genders while others are multiple genders simultaneously. Individual genders may or may not be binary. Some bigender people are both cisgender and transgender. Bigender people may or may not transition physically, legally, or socially. This is based on their understanding of their relationship with gender and their access to transitioning within their culture. Generally, bigender people are considered under the polygender, nonbinary, and transgender umbrellas but may or may not identify as polygender, nonbinary, or transgender specifically.

See also: Pangender.

- ***Related Link***
  - **"What It Means to Be Multigender: The Questions Many Have, But Are Afraid to Ask" | The Body Is Not an Apology**

Birth assignment *(noun phrase).* The gender we are assigned at birth, usually based on genitals alone. It is assumed that our identities should and will match this assignment but this isn't the case for most transgender people. It is also known as "gender assignment."

Birth stealth *(adjective phrase).* A transgender person choosing to pass universally as a cisgender person of their birth assignment. Being birth stealth can be a freely made choice, but is often due to one or multiple forms of transition being inaccessible to the individual and a need to maintain familial, employment, or housing stability. A birth stealth trans woman passes as a cisgender man; a birth stealth trans man passes as a cisgender woman, a birth stealth nonbinary person passes as whatever cisgender person shares their birth assignment. It should be noted that birth stealth (as well as stealth) can sometimes be used in derogative ways, and therefore it's best to not apply this label to others unless they self-identify with the term.

Bisexual *(adjective | bisexuality, noun).* Someone who is sexually attracted to more than one/two or more genders, but not necessarily all possible genders. Bisexuality was historically understood as people who are sexually attracted to "both men and women," but with our growing understanding of gender and its possible manifestations, the definition of bisexuality has grown to encompass not only its historical meaning, but also a wide range of experiences.

Chaser *(noun | chasers, plural).* A person who dates/hooks up with a certain "type" of person, like trans people, but who doesn't recognize their humanity beyond their "type." Chasers are usually embarrassed of their attractions and have a hard time looking past the shame that society attaches to being attracted to anyone other than white cisgender gender-conforming people.

Chosen family *(noun).* Chosen family is the concept of a family made out of those who are unaffiliated by blood. Chosen families have been around since the beginning of time, especially in marginalized communities where biological families are broken up by both external and internal bigotry.

Cisgender *(adjective).* Someone who is not transgender. Cisgender people identify with the gender they were assigned at birth. It is often shortened to cis, which comes from the Latin prefix meaning "on the same side of." Cisgender should be used instead of inaccurate terms like "bio/logical," "genetic," "natal," "real," or "born" when referring to people's genders.

Coming out *(compound verb | came out, past tense).* The act of disclosing one's gender or orientation to someone who previously did not know. Coming out can be a scary, stressful experience, but also a beautiful, transformational one.

Demigender *(adjective | demi-, prefix, e.g., demiboy, noun | demigirl, noun).* Someone who is a specific gender on some level but not completely. For example, someone who is a demigirl identifies at least partially with being a girl or woman but not completely. Demigender people may or may not transition physically, legally, or socially. This is based on their understanding of their relationship with gender and their access to transitioning within their culture. Generally, demigender people are considered under the nonbinary and transgender umbrellas but may or may not identify as transgender or nonbinary specifically.

Detransition *(verb, -s, -ed, -ing).* Detransition, sometimes called "desistance," is the process of identifying as cisgender after having already come out as transgender. While detransition/desistance does happen, the rates of it are incredibly low compared to the many trans people who transition and feel confident in their choices. Many folks who are called "detransitioners" are actually going birth stealth due to stigma and not an actual desistance of their trans identity.

- ***Related Links***
    - "Reframing 'Transgender Desistance' Debates" | Julia Serano
    - "I Detransitioned. But Not Because I Wasn't Trans" | The Atlantic
    - "The Trans People Who Are Detransitioning to Stay Safe in Trump's America" | The Establishment (through Medium.com)

Dysphoria *(noun).* Everyone experiences dysphoria differently; therefore, it can be hard to explain. Dysphoria is often described as the discomfort, pain, and unhappiness that is experienced by many transgender people in relationship to the commonly gendered parts of their body (physical dysphoria), and/or to the way people interact with them (social dysphoria), and/or to how they are legally required to fill out documentation (social dysphoria enforced by the legal system). Not all transgender people experience dysphoria. Some may not understand themselves as experiencing dysphoria but later recognize it as such. Transition is one way that folks manage their dysphoria.

See also: Gender euphoria

Eunuch *(noun)*. An AMAB person who identifies as a eunuch and has been or aims to be castrated. While many eunuchs still identify as male, others identify as third gender, nonbinary, and/or transgender. Historically, many eunuchs were castrated without their consent. Eunuch has also historically been a slur against AMAB trans people who don't identify as eunuchs, and therefore should only be used when referring to self-identified eunuchs. Eunuchs may or may not transition physically, legally, or socially. This is based on their understanding of their relationship with gender and their access to transitioning within their culture.

- ***Related Link***
    - **The Eunuch Archive** | **Eunuch.org**

Femininity / Masculinity *(noun | feminine / masculine, adjective)*. Femininity and masculinity are concepts that vary widely by culture. What is considered feminine in some places may be seen as neutral or even masculine in others. It also varies within cultures—for example, cooking in the home is seen as feminine labor in many places, but most professional chefs are men who are seen as relatively masculine. The questions of who is and is not feminine or masculine are often deeply embedded into all sorts of social and cultural activities, and many times, the ideas that our cultures have about femininity/masculinity are toxic and negative. Limiting femininity or masculinity to any one thing, or even several things would be problematic because not all "markers" of femininity or masculinity are accessible to people at various intersections of oppression and what any two people consider feminine or masculine could (and often does) vary widely.

- ***Related Links***
    - **"Who Can and Cannot be Feminine without Giving Up Their Safety?"** | **The Body Is Not an Apology**
    - **"Ain't We Femme?"** | **The Body Is Not an Apology**
    - **"Undoing the 'Manly' Myth: My 5 Steps to Finding a Healthy Masculinity"** | **The Body Is Not an Apology**

FTM / F2M / Female to male *(abbreviation / noun phrase)*. These terms are usually synonymous with trans men but is sometimes used by other AFAB people to express a generalized version of their gender experience. While widely used, it is viewed by many trans people as being too focused on binary genders and reinforcing the medicalization of transgender bodies. Many trans men have never identified with being female, so using this term generally to mean trans men is discouraged.

Gatekeeping *(verb, -s, -ed)*. The practice of limiting access to services, particularly based on a set of assumptions that there is a certain way a person should behave or present themselves in order to truly need or deserve the care they're seeking. Gatekeeping commonly occurs under the pretense of "protecting" transgender people from themselves, or requiring extra bureaucracy to prove that trans people are really sure of their own identity before providing transition treatment comparable to what a cisgender person could reasonably expect to receive. For example, a doctor who requires several letters from mental health professionals before providing hormones to a transgender person—the same hormones that any cisgender person would receive without said letters.

Gay *(adjective)*. Someone, who can be transgender or cisgender, who is generally attracted to someone of the same gender. Being gay is separate from the concept of gender identity, and so it is possible for a trans person to be both trans and gay. Also, it is generally understood that people who are trans and gay are attracted to people of the same broad category of gender, not necessarily of the same trans status. Colloquially, the term "gay" has been used as a slur to mean "stupid," and there is an ongoing effort to reclaim the word "gay" within the LGBTQ+ community. The term has also been adopted by more than just cis (or trans) men, and people of other gender identities may also use this term to describe their sexual or romantic orientation.

Gender *(noun)*. A complex combination of roles, expression, aesthetics, identities, performances, social interactions, and more that are assigned certain meanings by society. Gender is both self-defined and society-defined. How gender is embodied and defined varies from culture to culture and from person to person. Gender is often simplified—purposely, due to colonization—into a binary or a spectrum, but neither fully encapsulates the whole of gender. The model that this primer endorses is the galaxy model.

See also: Gender galaxy

Gender binary *(compound noun)*. The pervasive social system, largely a product of colonialism, that tells us there can only be presumably cisgender men and women, and that there can be no alternatives in terms of gender or expression. The binary exists in terms of the social systems that enforce it but does not actually exist in the real experience of gender, insofar as gender is much, much more than a binary. The binary is an assumption that conceals a beautiful dynamic experience of gender and life.

Gender euphoria *(compound noun)*. The opposite of dysphoria. The strong feeling of joy when one's gender is being respected and affirmed, whether through outward presentation that is being read correctly, or through inward acceptance of one's own gender. Like dysphoria, it can come in many forms, and a trans person need not feel either euphoria nor dysphoria to be trans. Cisgender people can also feel gender euphoria, but it's often overlooked as many cisgender people take their gender being affirmed for granted. Unfortunately, due to racism and colonialism, this is not accessible to all trans people equally. Black people are even more likely to be killed if they are trans, less likely to"pass" as cisgender, and less likely to have the resources and support to access the things that would enable them to experience euphoria about their gender.

Gender expression *(compound noun)*. How one expresses their gender outwardly and/or the facets of a person's expression which have gendered connotations in their culture. There is no right or wrong way to express your gender, though in imbalanced cultures masculinity and femininity are encouraged to be expressed in toxic, limited, and actively harmful ways while other expressions endanger those that are neither or other. Gendered expression has been and still is a tool that can be used to oppress people, especially Black or indigenous people.

Genderfluid / Genderflux *(adjective)*. This term can be used as a specific identity or as a way of articulating the changing nature of one's gender or expression. Genderfluid or genderflux people may have genders that shift in a pattern, shift constantly, or flip like a switch. Genderfluid people may or may not transition physically, legally, or socially. This is based on their understanding of their relationship with gender and their access to transitioning within their culture. Generally, genderfluid people are considered under the nonbinary and transgender umbrellas but may or may not identify as transgender or nonbinary specifically.

Gender galaxy *(noun phrase)*. This is a model of gender to assist in visualizing the diversity of gender identities and expression within humanity. A galaxy is a three-dimensional object in space that consists of billions of star systems, nebulae, dark matter, and other space objects, all interconnected by the force of gravity. Similarly, gender is an overarching term that consists of incredibly diverse identities that can be expressed in infinite ways. Like a galaxy, gender is an interconnected web between the relation of people's internal gender, which is unique to them, the expression of their gender, and its relation to the socialization and expectations both within their own societies and elsewhere. This model supersedes previous attempted models such as the gender binary and the gender spectrum, and we at the Primer feel it is one of the better models to begin understanding the vastness of gender.

Gender identity *(compound noun)*. An individual's internal sense of their own gender(s) or lack thereof. One's gender identity may or may not align with their birth assignment, and one's gender identity is not necessarily apparent to others.

Gender marker / Gender recognition *(noun phrase)*. Refers to any gender designation on official forms. Often seen in discussions around driver's licenses, state IDs, social security, and birth certificates.

- ***Related Link***
  - "Why Transgender People Suffer from 'ID Anxiety'" | Time

Gender-neutral pronouns *(noun phrase)*. Any pronoun can be gender-neutral, but the ones that are most commonly seen as such are those that are neither "he" nor "she." Some examples are: they, vi, sie, xe, ze, thon, it, ne, and per. There have been and will continue to be other terms, including those used by indigenous people, but many are lost to history or only locally known.

Gender-nonconforming (GNC) *(compound adjective)*. Someone who does not fully conform to the expectations around their gender that their society enforces. This may be, but is not limited to: expression, roles, or some other aspect of gender. Being GNC is distinct from being transgender, though some trans people may consider themselves gender-nonconforming. Gender nonconformity is generally apparent in people who identify as a binary gender, either cisgender or transgender. A femme trans man is just as nonconforming as a femme cis man. Some nonbinary people may also identify as gender-nonconforming for a variety of reasons.

Gender presentation *(compound noun)*. A mishmash of visual, verbal, and performative cultural signifiers that we are taught to interpret in specific ways related to gender. This largely involves the styling of one's clothing, facial adornment, hair, verbal cues, and body language, and varies across cultures and time periods. While we can control much about our presentation, there is also a significant part of presentation that relies on the perception of another person, which is why presentation isn't enough to accurately guess someone's gender.

Genderqueer *(adjective)*. This term is intentionally hard to define, much as is its sexuality counterpart queer. It can generally be understood as a gender that is neither man nor woman, possibly a mix of genders, and possibly fluid. Genderqueer people may or may not transition physically, legally, or socially. This is based on their understanding of their relationship with gender and their access to transitioning within their culture. Generally, genderqueer people are considered under the nonbinary and transgender umbrellas but may or may not identify as transgender or nonbinary specifically.

Gender spectrum *(noun phrase)*. The gender spectrum is an extension of the gender binary. The spectrum is a linear model, ranging from 100 percent man to 100 percent woman with various states in between. The gender galaxy is a further extension of this that includes space for all genders, including those left out of the gender spectrum.

Harry Benjamin Standards of Care *(noun phrase)*. An outdated set of medical transition guidelines published by the Harry Benjamin International Gender Dysphoria Association concerning the care of patients with gender identity disorders. These have been replaced by ICATH and WPATH Standards of Care. This is the origin of the now-defunct "full-time" requirement.

ICATH Standards *(abbreviation)*. *When a person gives "Informed Consent," it means that the individual possesses the cognitive ability to make an informed and independent decision about their healthcare and are choosing to do so without coercion. When giving informed consent, no therapist or letter is required, the patient is informed by the medical provider what a medication's effects (reversible, and irreversible) will be when administered. The patient, once informed, gives their consent to receive such treatment under the care of the provider. (*Credit to ICATH.info.)

Intersex *(adjective)*. A person born with any manner of supposed "ambiguity" in terms of gendered physical characteristics. This can include reproductive organs, genitals, hormones, chromosomes, or any combination thereof. Many intersex people are medically coerced as infants and children to better fit into a cisgender role and make their bodies cisnormative. Intersex people may or may not transition physically, legally, or socially. Many other folks are assumed dyadic at birth due to a lack of visible apparent intersexuality and therefore don't know their status until later, if ever. This is based on their understanding of their relationship with gender and their access to transitioning within their culture. Generally, intersex people are not immediately considered transgender, and may or may not identify as transgender and/or nonbinary specifically, despite there being significant overlap between the two communities.

- ***Related Link***
    - I'm Intersex, and It's WAY More Common Than You Think | Teen Vogue

Lesbian *(adjective)*. Someone, who can be transgender or cisgender, who generally considers themself a woman who is attracted to other women. Being a lesbian is separate from the concept of gender identity, and so it is possible for a trans person to be both trans and lesbian. Also, it is generally understood that people who are trans and lesbian are attracted to people of the same broad category of gender, not necessarily of the same trans status.

LGBTQIA+ (abbreviation). An acronym for Lesbian, Gay, Bisexual, Trans, Queer, Intersex, Agender, and others. It refers to a population of people united by having gender identities or sexual orientations that differ from the heterosexual and cisgender majority.

Medicalization *(noun | to medicalize, verb)*. Medicalization is the process by which human conditions and problems come to be defined and treated as medical conditions, and thus become the subject of medical study, diagnosis, prevention, or treatment. It also refers to the way which we refer to intrinsic things that have been medicalized as being somehow separate from ourselves.

Misgendering *(verb, -s, -ed)*. The act of attributing the wrong gender to a person, whether intentionally or not. Calling trans women "men" is misgendering. Calling someone "it" when they have asked you to use a different pronoun is misgendering. The best way to avoid misgendering people is to ask them what their gender is and what terms they prefer others to use when referring to them.

MTF / M2F / Male to female *(abbreviation / adjective phrase)*. These terms are usually synonymous with trans women but may be used by other AMAB people to express a generalized version of their gender experience. While widely used, it is viewed by many trans people as being too focused on binary genders and reinforcing the medicalization of transgender bodies. Many trans women have never identified with being male, so using this term generally to mean trans women is discouraged.

Neutrois *(adjective)*. A term very similar to agender but with a stronger emphasis on gender neutrality. Neutrois people may or may not transition physically, legally, or socially. This is based on their understanding of their relationship with gender and their access to transitioning within their culture. Generally, neutrois people are considered under the nonbinary and transgender umbrellas but may or may not identify as transgender or nonbinary specifically.

Nonbinary *(adjective)*. Nonbinary is an umbrella term for people who identify as a gender other than wo/man and/or who are not women exclusively. Well-meaning individuals sometimes write this as "gender nonbinary" but this is not correct. We don't say "gender man" or "gender woman," so "gender nonbinary" likewise makes no sense. Nonbinary is itself an adjective that modifies a noun such as "nonbinary people." Nonbinary people may or may not transition physically, legally, or socially. This is based on their understanding of their relationship with gender and their access to transitioning within their culture. Generally, nonbinary people are considered under the transgender umbrella but may or may not identify as transgender specifically. Nonbinary can also be used as an identity term by people who know they are not wo/men, but may be currently unable to find a term that fits their gender experience.

Outing *(verb | to out, verb, -ed, -ing)*. To share with others, in public, etc., an identity that was previously unknown to people, usually referring to sexual orientation or gender. You should never out someone without their consent. Outing someone without their express and prior consent is dangerous, possibly even deadly.

Pangender *(adjective)*. *Pangender, sometimes seen as "omnigender," is a nonbinary gender experience, which refers to a wide multiplicity of genders that can (or not) stretch to the infinite (meaning that this experience can go beyond the current knowledge of genders), but always within the person's own culture and life experience. This experience can be either simultaneously or over time. (*Credit to GenderWiki.)

Pronouns *(noun)*. The words by which one is referred to, whether they be "he," "she," "they," "it," "ze," "ey," or any other. It is best to always ask someone their pronouns if possible and to not make assumptions about a person's pronouns. Always be sure to respect a person's pronouns, use them, and apologize if you slip up. Everyone has preferred pronouns, not just trans people. Anyone of any gender can use any pronouns they choose, though it's important to remember that colonialism and binarism forced the abandonment of indigenous and cultural language around gender, including pronouns that are now lost.

Queer *(adjective)*. This term is intentionally hard to define, much as is its gender counterpart genderqueer. It can generally be understood as an orientation that is neither straight nor gay, but definitely LGBTQ+ and possibly fluid.

Reclamation *(noun)*. The cultural process by which a group reclaims terms that were previously used in a way disparaging of that group. This is often seen in the LGBTQ+ because of how we've been systematically deprived of the right to our own language, so we've been forced to reclaim the slurs and judgment-laden language of the cisgender people around us. This is how we've come to use words like fag/got, queer, and dyke.

- ***Related Link***
    - How—and Why—to Reclaim Your Slurs | Wear Your Voice Magazine

Sex *(noun)*. A medical term designating a certain combination of gonads, chromosomes, external organs, secondary sex characteristics, and hormonal balances. A binary system (wo/man) set by the medical establishment to reinforce white supremacy and gender oppression, usually based on genitals and sometimes chromosomes. Because this is usually divided into "male" and "female," this category ignores the existence of intersex people and natural sexual variations within the two broader recognized categories.

Sexual identity / orientation *(compound noun)*. Refers to if and to whom one is sexually attracted. Gender and sexual orientation are not the same. Sexual orientation can be flexible or rigid and may change over time. Sexual orientation can also be hard to define, given that the two primary options are based solely on binary gender people, and recognizing the true expanse of gender and sexuality throws the whole standard of classification into question.

Stealth *(adjective)*. A transgender person choosing to pass universally as a cisgender person of their gender without publicly acknowledging their transgender status or history. This often requires all forms of transition and is undertaken by binary people who are at risk of violence, or lack of job and/or home security. A stealth trans woman passes as a cisgender woman; a stealth trans man passes as a cisgender man.

See also: Birth stealth.

TERF *(acronym | adjective / noun)*. *Trans-exclusionary radical feminism (TERF) is a subgroup of radical feminism characterized by transphobia, especially transmisogyny, and hostility to the third wave of feminism. They believe that the only real women are those born with a vagina and XX chromosomes. They wish to completely enforce the classic gender binary, supporting gender essentialism. The term was likely invented by Hoyden about Town writer Viv Smythe (aka TigTog) in 2008. (*Credit to **Rational Wiki**.)

Third gender *(compound noun / adjective)*. This term is most often used as an umbrella term for indigenous genders that are beyond the gender binary that may or may not be accepted in their respective cultures. While people in western cultures may identify as third gender, it may be seen as appropriative depending on context. Third-gender people may or may not transition physically, legally, or socially. This is based on their understanding of their relationship with gender and their access to transitioning within their culture. Generally, third-gender people are considered under the nonbinary and transgender umbrellas but may or may not identify as transgender or nonbinary specifically.

Transgender *(adjective)*. Often shortened as "trans." An umbrella term for people whose gender and/or expression does not match their birth assignment. Transgender includes many of the terms in this list and may or may not include transsexuals, cross dressers, drag kings/queens, and others who defy what society tells them their gender should be. How people identify with this term depends on the individual and their relationship with their gender.

Transition *(verb | to transition, verb, -s, -ed. -ing)*. The process by which people affirm their transgender identity. This may include social, physical/medical, and/or mental/emotional transition. Specifically this may or may not include and is not limited to: changing one's name legally or socially, taking hormones, having surgery, changing legal documents to reflect one's gender, coming out to loved ones, dressing as one chooses, and accepting oneself, among many other things. Transition is an individual process. No two transitions are the same.

Transsexual *(noun)*. This term refers to (mostly binary) trans people who completely physically transition or want to do so. It can be used to be precise about a person's medical transition status and goals but is sometimes viewed as outdated and too focused on the medical aspects of transition. Transsexuals may or may not identify as transgender specifically, but categorically fall under the transgender umbrella.

Trans status *(compound noun)*. Whether someone identifies as transgender or not. Only an individual can determine their own trans status or determine when or how to disclose their status.

Two-spirit (2spirit) *(adjective)*. These are LGBTQ+ people of North American indigenous descent. Two-spirit identities are directly linked to indigenous spiritual and/or religious belief systems that vary from tribe to tribe. Two-spirit individuals do not identify with either heterosexual orientation, cisgender identity, or both. Some tribes have spiritual and religious belief systems that do not support the idea of two-spirit identities. Two-spirit people, historically, were respected spiritual leaders among their tribal nations up until the colonization of North America. Two-spirit people may or may not transition physically, legally, or socially. This is based on their understanding of their relationship with gender and their access to transitioning within their culture. Generally, people with two-spirit gender identities are considered under the nonbinary and transgender umbrellas but may or may not identify as transgender or nonbinary specifically. This term should not be used by people who are not indigenous/First Nations of Turtle Island.

- ***Related Links***
  - The Healing History of Two-Spirit, a Term That Gives LGBTQ Natives a Voice | Huffpost
  - Why Non-Natives Appropriating "Two-Spirit" Hurts | BGD
  - 8 Things You Should Know about Two-Spirit People | Indian Country Today
  - A Letter to White People Using the Term "Two Spirit" | Conspire for Change
  - Two-Spirit Resources Directory | Native Youth Sexual Health Network

WPATH Standards of Care *(noun phrase)*. A set of medical guidelines published by the World Professional Association for Transgender Health concerning the care of patients with gender dysphoria. Essentially, the transgender healthcare guidebook. You can find the WPATH SOC at wpath.org.

See also: Harry Benjamin Standards of Care, ICATH Standards.

LIST OF FIGURES AND TABLES

List of Figures

List of Tables

BIBLIOGRAPHY

ACES Too High. "What ACEs/PCEs Do You Have?" *ACES Too High News*. Accessed July 30, 2021. https://acestoohigh.com/got-your-ace-score/.

Alzahrani, Talal, Tran Nguyen, Angela Ryan, Ahmad Dwairy, James McCaffrey, Raza Yunus, Joseph Forgione et al. "Cardiovascular Disease Risk Factors and Myocardial Infarction in the Transgender Population." *Circulation: Cardiovascular Quality and Outcomes* 12, no. 4 (April 2019): 1–7. https://doi.org/10.1161/circoutcomes.119.005597.

American Psychiatric Association. *Gender Dysphoria*, DSM-5 Update (Washington DC: APA Publishing, 2013). https://www.psychiatry.org/File%20Library/Psychiatrists/Practice/DSM/APA_DSM-5-Gender-Dysphoria.pdf.

Apple. "Use Fall Detection with Apple Watch." September 17, 2020. https://support.apple.com/en-us/HT208944.

Bertoluci, Marcello Casaccia, and Viviane Zorzanelli Rocha. "Cardiovascular Risk Assessment in Patients with Diabetes." *Diabetology & Metabolic Syndrome* 9, no. 25 (April 20, 2017), https://doi.org/10.1186/s13098-017-0225-1.

Bizic, Marta, Vladimir Kojovic, Dragana Duisin, Dusan Stanojevic, Svetlana Vujovic, Aleksandar Milosevic, Gradimir Korac, and Miroslav L. Djordjevic. "An Overview of Neovaginal Reconstruction Options in Male to Female Transsexuals." *The Scientific World Journal* 2014, Article ID 638919 (May 26, 2014): 8 pages. https://doi.org/10.1155/2014/638919.

Bollinger, Alex. "A Father Slit His Son's Throat for Being Gay in an Attempt to Kill Him." *LGBTQ Nation*, November 12, 2019. https://www.lgbtqnation.com/2019/11/father-slit-sons-throat-gay-attempt-kill/.

Bonnay, Juliet. "How High ACE Scores Can Impact Adult Health." *Juliet Bonnay: Different Perspectives* (blog), November 15, 2019. https://by-julietbonnay.com/2019/11/how-high-ace-scores-can-impact-adult-health/.

Borzillo, Carrie, and Men's Health Editorial. "How Penis Rings Can Help You Have Better Sex." *Men's Health*, July 8, 2020. https://www.menshealth.com/sex-women/a19532760/cock-rings/.

Caceres, Vanessa. "9 Best Ways to Quit Smoking." *US News & World Report*. Last reviewed February 12, 2021. https://health.usnews.com/wellness/articles/best-ways-to-quit-smoking.

Capitán, Luis. "Management of Complex Revision Frontal Sinus and Forehead Cases." Lecture presented at the WPATH 26th Scientific Symposium Surgeon's Program, November 6, 2020.

Capitán, Luis, Javier Gutiérrez Santamaría, Daniel Simon, Devin Coon, Carlos Bailón, Raúl J. Bellinga, Thiago Tenório, and Fermín Capitán-Cañadas. "Facial Gender Confirmation Surgery: A Protocol for Diagnosis, Surgical Planning, and Postoperative Management." *Plastic and Reconstructive Surgery* 145, no. 4 (April 2020): 818e–28e. https://doi.org/10.1097/prs.0000000000006686.

Cardiovascular Surgery of Southern Nevada. "How Many Times Does Your Heart Beat per Day?" September 25, 2013. http://www.cvsurgnv.com/how-many-times-does-your-heart-beat-per-day/.

Cazaubon, Michèle. "Deep Vein Thrombosis and Air Travel: Risk Management in 2015." *Phlebolymphology* 22, no. 1 (January 2015): 25–32. https://www.phlebolymphology.org/deep-vein-thrombosis-and-air-travel-risk-management-in-2015/.

Centers for Disease Control and Prevention. "Heart Disease Facts." Last reviewed September 8, 2020. https://www.cdc.gov/heartdisease/facts.htm.

Centers for Disease Control and Prevention. "Leading Causes of Death." Last reviewed March 1, 2021. https://www.cdc.gov/nchs/fastats/leading-causes-of-death.htm.

Centers for Disease Control and Prevention. "Pre-Exposure Prophylaxis (PrEP)." Last reviewed June 23, 2021. https://www.cdc.gov/hiv/risk/prep/.

Centers for Disease Control and Prevention. "Preventing Adverse Childhood Experiences." Last reviewed April 6, 2021. https://www.cdc.gov/violenceprevention/aces/fastfact.html.

Centers for Disease Control and Prevention. "Preventing Adverse Childhood Experiences (ACEs) to Improve US Health." Last reviewed April 6, 2021. https://www.cdc.gov/media/releases/2019/p1105-prevent-aces.html.

Cirillo, Dominic J., Robert B. Wallace, Rebecca J. Rodabough, Philip Greenland, Andrea Z. LaCroix, Marian C. Limacher, and Joseph C. Larson. "Effect of Estrogen Therapy on Gallbladder Disease." *The Journal of the American Medical Association* 293, no. 3 (January 19, 2005): 330–39. https://doi.org/10.1001/jama.293.3.330.

City of Seattle. "CPR Training (Medic II)." Accessed July 28, 2021. http://www.seattle.gov/fire/safety-and-community/medic-ii-cpr-training.

Colby, Christine. "Dying Trans: Preserving Identity in Death." *The Order of the Good Death*, January 10, 2017. http://www.orderofthegooddeath.com/dying-trans-preserving-identity-death.

Connor, Kathryn M., and Jonathan R. T. Davidson. "Development of a New Resilience Scale: The Connor-Davidson Resilience Scale (CD-RISC)." *Depression and Anxiety* 18, no. 2 (September 2003): 76–82. http://dx.doi.org/10.1002/da.10113.

Craft, Lynette L., and Frank M. Perna. "The Benefits of Exercise for the Clinically Depressed." *The Primary Care Companion to the Journal of Clinical Psychiatry* 6, no. 3 (February 2004): 104–11, doi: 10.4088/pcc.v06n0301.

De Luca, Maurizio, Luigi Angrisani, Jacques Himpens, Luca Busetto, Nicola Scopinaro, Rudolf Weiner, Alberto Sartori et al. "Indications for Surgery for Obesity and Weight-Related Diseases: Position Statements from the International Federation for the Surgery of Obesity and Metabolic Disorders (IFSO)." *Obesity Surgery* 26, no. 8 (July 2016): 1659–96. https://doi.org/10.1007/s11695-016-2271-4.

Deschamps-Braly, Jordan C., Caitlin L. Sacher, Jennifer Fick, and Douglas K. Ousterhout. "First Female-to-Male Facial Confirmation Surgery with Description of a New Procedure for Masculinization of the Thyroid Cartilage (Adam's Apple)." *Plastic & Reconstructive Surgery* 139, no. 4 (April 2017): 883e–87e. https://doi.org/10.1097/prs.0000000000003185.

Deutsch, Madeline B. "Overview of Feminizing Hormone Therapy." Transgender Care, University of California-San Francisco. June 17, 2016. https://transcare.ucsf.edu/guidelines/feminizing-hormone-therapy.

Deutsch, Madeline B. "Screening for Breast Cancer in Transgender Women." Transgender Care, University of California-San Francisco. June 17, 2016. https://transcare.ucsf.edu/guidelines/breast-cancer-women.

Doughton, Sandi. "UW Psychologist Kristina Olson Thought the MacArthur Foundation Had the Wrong 'Genius.'" *Pacific NW Magazine, Seattle Times*, September 1, 2019. https://www.seattletimes.com/pacific-nw-magazine/uw-psychologist-kristina-olson-thought-the-macarthur-foundation-had-the-wrong-genius/.

Dowden, Richard V. "Transumbilical Breast Augmentation Is Safe and Effective." *Seminars in Plastic Surgery* 22, no. 1 (February 2008): 51–9. https://doi.org/10.1055/s-2007-1019143.

Drugs.com. "Varencline." Last updated on September 8, 2020. https://www.drugs.com/ppa/varenicline.html.

Elkin, Irene, M. Tracie Shea, John T. Watkins, Stanley D. Imber, Stuart M. Sotsky, Joseph F. Collins, David R. Glass, Paul A. Pilkonis, William R. Leber, John P. Docherty et al. "National Institute of Mental Health Treatment of Depression Collaborative Research Program: General Effectiveness of Treatments." *Archives of General Psychiatry* 46, no. 11 (December 1989): 971–82. https://doi.org/10.1001/archpsyc.1989.01810110013002.

Ellen, Jane. "The Adverse Childhood Experiences Study—the Largest, Most Important Public Health Study You Never Heard of—Began in an Obesity Clinic." *ACES Too High News*. October 3, 2012. https://acestoohigh.com/2012/10/03/the-adverse-childhood-experiences-study-the-largest-most-important-public-health-study-you-never-heard-of-began-in-an-obesity-clinic/.

Family and Youth Services Bureau, US Department of Health and Human Services. "Asking: 'What's Happened to You?' A Focus on Trauma-Informed Care." *NCFY Reports, Summer 2011*, July 27, 2012. https://www.acf.hhs.gov/archive/fysb/newsletter/fysbnewsletter/asking-whats-happened-you-focus-trauma-informed-care.

Felitti, Vincent J. "The Relation between Adverse Childhood Experiences and Adult Health: Turning Gold into Lead." *The Permanente Journal* 6, no. 1 (Winter 2002): 44–7. https://www.ncbi.nlm.nih.gov/pubmed/30313011.

Felitti, Vincent J., Robert F. Anda, Dale Nordenberg, David F. Williamson, Alison M. Spitz, Valerie Edwards, Mary P. Koss, and James S. Marks. "Relationship of Childhood Abuse and Household Dysfunction to Many of the Leading Causes of Death in Adults: The Adverse Childhood Experiences (ACE) Study." *American Journal of Preventive Medicine* 14, no. 4 (May 1998): 245–58. https://doi.org/10.1016/s0749-3797(98)00017-8.

Fookes, C. "Drug Half-life Explained." *Drugs.com*, March 8, 2019. https://www.drugs.com/article/drug-half-life.html.

FSA Store. "Transgender Counseling or Surgery: FSA Eligibility." Accessed July 28, 2021. https://fsastore.com/FSA-Eligibility-List/T/Transgender-Counseling-or-Surgery-E717.aspx.

Games, Finlay. "Phalloplasty Final Stage | AMS Implant Review." *Finn the InFinncible*, May 25, 2019. http://finlaygames.com/phalloplasty-final-stage-ams-implant-review.

Gillis, Chelsia, and Paul E. Wischmeyer. "Preoperative Nutrition and the Elective Surgical Patient: Why, How and What?" *Anaesthesia* 74, Supplement 1 (January 2019): 27–35. https://doi.org/10.1111/anae.14506.

Gorner, Peter. "Work That Led to Viagra Wins Americans a Nobel." *Chicago Tribune*, October 13, 1998. https://www.chicagotribune.com/news/ct-xpm-1998-10-13-9810130307-story.html.

Grant, Jaime M., Lisa A. Mottet, and Justin Tanis. *National Transgender Discrimination Survey Report on Health and Health Care*. Washington DC: National Center for Transgender Equality, 2010. https://cancer-network.org/wp-content/uploads/2017/02/National_Transgender_Discrimination_Survey_Report_on_health_and_health_care.pdf.

Grant, Jaime M., Lisa A. Mottet, Justin Tanis, Jack Harrison, Jody L. Herman, and Mara Keisling. *Injustice at Every Turn: A Report of the National Transgender Discrimination Survey*. Washington DC: National Center for Transgender Equality and National Gay and Lesbian Task Force, 2011. https://transequality.org/sites/default/files/docs/resources/NTDS_Report.pdf.

Gromko, Linda. *Where's MY Book?: A Guide for Transgender and Gender-Nonconforming Youth, Their Parents, & Everyone Else*. Seattle: Bainbridge Books, 2015.

Harvard Health Publishing. "Can Relationships Boost Longevity and Well-Being?" *Harvard Medical School*, June 1, 2017. https://www.health.harvard.edu/mental-health/can-relationships-boost-longevity-and-well-being.

Hassan, Adeel. "Hate-Crime Violence Hits 16-Year High, F.B.I. Reports." *New York Times*, December 11, 2019. https://www.nytimes.com/2019/11/12/us/hate-crimes-fbi-report.html.

Hattenstone, Simon. "The Dad Who Gave Birth: 'Being Pregnant Doesn't Change Me Being a Trans Man.'" *Guardian*, April 20, 2019. https://www.theguardian.com/society/2019/apr/20/the-dad-who-gave-birth-pregnant-trans-freddy-mcconnell.

Heightman, A. J. "Early Citizen Response/CPR/AEDs; Uninterrupted Compressions and Dispatcher-Assisted CPR Emphasized by EMS Experts at CPR Summit." *Journal of Emergency Medical Services*, special report from the Cardiac Arrest Survivors Summit. December 12, 2019. https://www.jems.com/patient-care/cardiac-resuscitation/early-citizen-response/.

Herman, Jody L., Ann P. Haas, and Philip L. Rodgers. *Suicide Attempts among Transgender and Gender Non-Conforming Adults*. Los Angeles: The Williams Institute, UCLA. 2014. https://escholarship.org/uc/item/8xg8061f.

Hess, Jochen, A. Henkel, J. Bohr, Christian Rehme, Andrej Panic, L. Panic, R. Rossi Neto, B. Hadaschik, and Y. Hess. "Sexuality after Male-to-Female Gender Affirmation Surgery." *BioMed Research International* 2018, no. 36 (May 2018): 1–7. http://dx.doi.org/10.1155/2018/9037979.

Hillis, Susan D., Robert F. Anda, Shanta R. Dube, Vincent J. Felitti, Polly A. Marchbanks, and James S. Marks. "The Association between Adverse Childhood Experiences and Adolescent Pregnancy, Long-Term Psychosocial Consequences, and Fetal Death." *Pediatrics* 113, no. 2 (February 2004): 320–27. doi: 10.1542/peds.113.2.320.

Hillis, Susan D., Robert F. Anda, Vincent J. Felitti, and Polly A. Marchbanks. "Adverse Childhood Experiences and Sexual Risk Behaviors in Women: A Retrospective Cohort Study." *Family Planning Perspectives* 33, no. 5 (September 2001): 206–11. doi: 10.2307/2673783.

Hochman, Gloria. "When One Spouse Changes Gender, Can the Marriage Be Saved?" *The Philadelphia Inquirer*, December 29, 2016. https://www.inquirer.com/philly/health/When-one-spouse-changes-gender-can-the-marriage-be-saved.html.

Howard, Jacqueline. "Covid-19 Likely Ranks as the Third Leading Cause of Death in the US in 2020, CDC Statisticians Say." *CNN*, January 5, 2021. https://www.cnn.com/2021/01/05/health/covid-third-leading-cause-of-death-cdc-wellness/index.html.

Huang, Catherine K., and Neal Handel. "Effects of Singulair (Montelukast) Treatment for Capsular Contracture." *Aesthetic Surgery Journal* 30, no. 3 (July 2010): 404–8. https://doi.org/10.1177/1090820x10374724.

Jackowich, Robyn A., Rachel Vale, Kayla Vale, Richard J. Wassersug, and Thomas W. Johnson. "Voluntary Genital Ablations: Contrasting the Cutters and Their Clients." *Sexual Medicine* 2, no. 3 (August 2014): 121–32. https://doi.org/10.1002/sm2.33.

James, Sandy E., Carter Brown, and Isaiah Wilson. *2015 U.S. Transgender Survey: Report on the Experiences of Black Respondents*. Washington, DC and Dallas, TX: National Center for Transgender Equality, Black Trans Advocacy, and National Black Justice Coalition, 2017. https://transequality.org/sites/default/files/docs/usts/USTS-Black-Respondents-Report.pdf.

James, Sandy E., Jody L. Herman, Susan Rankin, Mara Keisling, Lisa Mottet, and Ma'ayan Anafi. *The Report of the 2015 U.S. Transgender Survey*. Washington, DC: National Center for Transgender Equality, 2016. https://transequality.org/sites/default/files/docs/usts/USTS-Full-Report-Dec17.pdf.

Jarrett, Brooke A., Alexandra L. Corbet, Ivy H. Gardner, Jamie D. Weinand, and Sarah M. Peitzmeier. "Chest Binding and Care Seeking among Transmasculine Adults: A Cross-Sectional Study." *Transgender Health* 3, no. 1 (December 2018): 170–78. https://doi.org/10.1089/trgh.2018.0017.

Judd, Lewis L., Hagop Akiskal, Pamela J. Schettler, Jean Endicott, Jack Maser, David A. Solomon, Andrew C. Leon, John A. Rice, and Martin B. Keller. "The Long-term Natural History of the Weekly Symptomatic Status of Bipolar 1 Disorder." *Archives of General Psychiatry* 59, no. 6 (July 2002): 530–37. https://doi.org/10.1001/archpsyc.59.6.530.

Kanhai, Robert C. J. "Sensate Vagina Pedicled-Spot for Male-to-Female Transsexuals: The Experience in the First 50 Patients." *Aesthetic Plastic Surgery* 40, no. 2 (February 18, 2016): 284–7. https://doi.org/10.1007/s00266-016-0620-2.

Kenney, William Larry, and Percy Chiu. "Influence of Age on Thirst and Fluid Intake." *Medicine and Science in Sports and Exercise* 33, no. 9 (October 2001): 1524–32. https://doi.org/10.1097/00005768-200109000-00016.

Kiprop, Victor. "Average Height of American Men." *World Atlas*, March 25, 2019. https://www.worldatlas.com/articles/what-is-the-average-height-of-american-men.html.

Kornfield, Meryl. "VA Plans to Offer Gender-Confirmation Surgery to Transgender Veterans, Reversing Ban." *The Washington Post*, June 19, 2021. https://www.washingtonpost.com/national-security/2021/06/19/veterans-gender-affirmation-surgery/.

Kuhar, David T., David K. Henderson, Kimberly A. Struble, Walid Heneine, Vasavi Thomas, Laura W. Cheever, Ahmed Gomaa, Adelisa L. Panlilio, and the US Public Health Service Working Group. "Updated US Public Health Service Guidelines for the Management of Occupational Exposures to Human Immunodeficiency Virus and Recommendations for Postexposure Prophylaxis." *Infection Control and Hospital Epidemiology* 34, no. 9 (September 2013): 875–92. https://doi.org/10.1086/672271.

Law, Anica C., Gary E. Weissman, and Theodore J. Iwashyna. "A Dangerous Myth: Does Speaking Imply Breathing?" *Annals of Internal Medicine* 173 (2020): 754–55. https://doi.org/10.7326/M20-4186.

Lee, Jasmine, Ian T. Nolan, Marco Swanson, Cameron J. Kneib, Christopher S. Crowe, Erik M. Wolfswinkel, Shane D. Morrison et al. "A Review of Hand Feminization and Masculinization Techniques in Gender Affirming Therapy." *Aesthetic Plastic Surgery* 45, no. 2 (April 2021): 589–601. https://doi.org/10.1007/s00266-020-01963-0.

March of Dimes. "Miscarriage." Last reviewed November 2017. https://www.marchofdimes.org/complications/miscarriage.aspx.

Martin, Paul. "CPR to Stayin' Alive Beat Helps Keep Proper Rate." *ProTrainings*. Last updated October 25, 2018. https://www.procpr.org/blog/training/cpr-stayin-alive-song.

Masic, Izet, Milan Miokovic, and Belma Muhamedagić. "Evidence-Based Medicine—New Approaches and Challenges." *Acta Informatica Medica* 16, no. 4 (November 2008): 219–25. https://doi.org/10.5455/aim.2008.16.219-225.

Mayo Clinic. "Antidepressants: Selecting One That's Right for You." *Mayo Clinic*, December 31, 2019. https://www.mayoclinic.org/diseases-conditions/depression/in-depth/antidepressants/art-20046273.

Mayo Clinic. "Heart Attack: Symptoms and Causes." *Mayo Clinic*, June 16, 2020. https://www.mayoclinic.org/diseases-conditions/heart-attack/symptoms-causes/syc-20373106.

Merriam-Webster. S.v. "orgasm." Accessed July 14, 2021. https://www.merriam-webster.com/dictionary/orgasm.

Morche, Johannes, Tim Mathes, and Dawid Pieper. "Relationship Between Surgeon Volume and Outcomes: A Systematic Review of Systematic Reviews." *Systematic Reviews* 5, no. 1 (November 2016): 1–15. https://doi.org/10.1186/s13643-016-0376-4.

Movement Advancement Project. *Conversion Therapy Laws*. Updated July 16, 2021. https://www.lgbtmap.org/img/maps/citations-conversion-therapy.pdf.

Movement Advancement Project. "Equality Maps: Conversion 'Therapy' Laws." Accessed July 28, 2021. https://www.lgbtmap.org/equality-maps/conversion_therapy.

Nagoski, Emily. *Come as You Are: The Surprising New Science That Will Transform Your Sex Life*. New York: Simon & Schuster, 2015.

National Center for PTSD, US Department of Veterans Affairs. "Complex PTSD." Updated January 31, 2020. https://www.ptsd.va.gov/professional/treat/essentials/complex_ptsd.asp.

National Center for Transgender Equality. "Understanding Non-Binary People: How to Be Respectful and Supportive." *Issues and Resources*, October 5, 2018. https://transequality.org/issues/resources/understanding-non-binary-people-how-to-be-respectful-and-supportive.

National Institute on Aging. "What Is a Heart Attack?" Reviewed June 1, 2018. https://www.nia.nih.gov/health/what-heart-attack.

Nolan, Ian T., Christopher J. Kuhner, and Geolani W. Dy. "Demographic and Temporal Trends in Transgender Identities and Gender Confirming Surgery." *Translational Andrology and Urology* 8, no. 3 (June 2019): 184–90. doi: 10.21037/tau.2019.04.09.

Olson-Kennedy, Johanna. "The Medical Needs of Transgender Youth: Puberty Delay and Cross Hormones." Lecture at the Gender Odyssey International Conference, Seattle, WA, August 20, 2015.

O'Reilly, Richard L., Lisa Bogue, and Shiva M. Singh. "Pharmacogenetic Response to Antidepressants in a Multicase Family with Affective Disorder." *Biological Psychiatry* 36, no. 7 (October 1994): 467–71. https://doi.org/10.1016/0006-3223(94)90642-4.

Our Bodies, Ourselves contributors. "Models of Sexual Response." *Our Bodies, Ourselves*, October 15, 2011. https://www.ourbodiesourselves.org/book-excerpts/health-article/models-sexual-response/.

Peitzmeier, Sarah, Ivy Gardner, Jamie Weinand, Alexandra Corbet, and Kimberlynn Acevedo. "Health Impact of Chest Binding among Transgender Adults: A Community-Engaged, Cross-Sectional Study." *Culture, Health & Sexuality* 19, no. 1 (June 2016): 1–12. https://doi.org/10.1080/13691058.2016.1191675.

Petrucelli, Nancie, Mary B. Daly, and Tuya Pal. "BRCA1- and BRCA2-Associated Hereditary Breast and Ovarian Cancer." In *GeneReviews*, edited by Margaret P. Adam et al. Seattle: University of Washington, 1993–2020, September 4, 1998, updated December 15, 2016. https://www.ncbi.nlm.nih.gov/books/NBK1247/.

Radix, Asa, and Madeline B. Deutsch. "Cardiovascular Disease." Transgender Care, University of California-San Francisco. June 17, 2016. https://transcare.ucsf.edu/guidelines/cardiovascular.

Rodriguez, Alvaro H. "Male-to-Female Gender Affirming Surgery Using Nile Tilapia Fish Skin as a Biocompatible Graft." Presentation at the WPATH 26th Scientific Symposium Surgeon's Program, November 7, 2020.

Ruiz, Don Miguel. *The Four Agreements: A Practical Guide to Personal Freedom*. San Francisco: Amber-Allen, 2018.

Runyowa, Simba. "Microaggressions Matter." *Atlantic*, September 18, 2015. https://www.theatlantic.com/politics/archive/2015/09/microaggressions-matter/406090/.

Sanders, Linley. "What Is Gender X? New Identity Is Accepted in These States, and Washington and Vermont Could Be Next." *Newsweek*, January 19, 2018. https://www.newsweek.com/gender-x-new-identity-states-washington-vermont-775221.

Scutti, Susan. "First Baby Born to Woman with Uterus Transplanted from Deceased Donor." *CNN*, December 5, 2018. https://www.cnn.com/2018/12/04/health/uterus-transplant-deceased-donor-study/index.html.

Shaeer, Osama Kamal Zaki. "Shaeer's Technique: A Minimally Invasive Procedure for Monsplasty and Revealing the Concealed Penis," *PRS Global Open* 4, no. 8 (August 29, 2016): e1019. https://dx.doi.org/10.1097%2FGOX.0000000000001019.

Shepherd, Brittany. "Biden Tells Transgender Americans, 'Your President Has Your Back.'" *Yahoo News*, April 28, 2021. https://news.yahoo.com/biden-tells-transgender-americans-your-president-has-your-back-023259977.html?guccounter=1&guce_.

Shupe, Jamie. "I Was America's First 'Nonbinary' Person. It Was All a Sham." *The Daily Signal*, March 10, 2019. https://www.dailysignal.com/2019/03/10/I-was-Americas-first-non-binary-person-it-was-all-a-sham.

Siegel, Fabian P., and Petro E. Petrides. "Congenital and Acquired Polycythemias." *Deutsches Ärzteblatt International* 105, no. 4 (January 2008): 62–8. DOI: 10.3238/arztebl.2008.0062.

Sosin, Kate. "U.S. to Add 'X' Gender Marker on Passports." *The 19th*, June 30, 2021. https://19thnews.org/2021/06/u-s-to-add-x-gender-marker-on-passports/.

Tello, Monique. "Trauma-Informed Care: What It Is, and Why It's Important." *Harvard Health Blog*, Harvard Health Publishing, October 16, 2018. https://www.health.harvard.edu/blog/trauma-informed-care-what-it-is-and-why-its-important-2018101613562.

Toomey, Russell B., Amy K. Syvertsen, and Maura Shramko. "Transgender Adolescent Suicide Behavior." *Pediatrics* 142, no. 4 (October 1, 2018): 2017–4218. https://doi.org/10.1542/peds.2017-4218.

Transgender Legal Defense and Education Fund. *Medical Necessity of Facial Gender Reassignment Surgery for Transgender Women: Literature Review*. Washington, DC: Transgender Legal Defense and Education Fund, September 10, 2020. https://transhealthproject.org/documents/34/Facial_surgery_medical_necessity_literature_review.pdf.

Traumadissociation.com. "Complex Posttraumatic Stress Disorder." Accessed June 24, 2021. http://traumadissociation.com/complexptsd.

Truth Initiative. "Tobacco Use in LGBT Communities." *Fact Sheet*, February 18, 2018. https://truthinitiative.org/sites/default/files/media/files/2019/03/Truth_LGBT%20FactSheet_FINAL.pdf.

Under Armour. *Myfitnesspal*. V. 20.7.0.29453. 2020.

Unilever. "Dove Evolution." October 6, 2006. YouTube video, https://www.youtube.com/watch?v=iYhCn0jf46U.

US Food and Drug Administration. "FDA Warns about Illegal Use of Injectable Silicone for Body Contouring and Associated Health Risks." November 13, 2017. https://www.fda.gov/news-events/press-announcements/fda-warns-about-illegal-use-injectable-silicone-body-contouring-and-associated-health-risks.

US Food and Drug Administration. "Questions and Answers about Breast Implant-Associated Anaplastic Large Cell Lymphoma (BIA-ALCL)." Updated October 23, 2019. https://www.fda.gov/medical-devices/breast-implants/questions-and-answers-about-breast-implant-associated-anaplastic-large-cell-lymphoma-bia-alcl.

US Food and Drug Administration. "Risks and Complications of Breast Implants." Updated September 28, 2020. https://www.fda.gov/medical-devices/breast-implants/risks-and-complications-breast-implants#Capsular_Contracture.

US Food and Drug Administration. "Tobacco Use in the LGBT Community: A Public Health Issue." Updated June 2, 2021. https://www.fda.gov/tobacco-products/health-information/tobacco-use-lgbt-community-public-health-issue.

Van der Kolk, Bessel. *The Body Keeps the Score*. New York: Penguin Books, 2014.

Venken, K., F. Callewaert, S. Boonen, and D. Vanderschueren. "Sex Hormones, Their Receptors and Bone Health." *Osteoporosis International* 19, no. 11 (November 2008): 1517–25. https://doi.org/10.1007/s00198-008-0609-z.

Virupaksha, H. G., Daliboyina Muralidhar, and Jayashree Ramakrishna. "Suicide and Suicidal Behavior among Transgender Persons." *Indian Journal of Psychological Medicine* 38, no. 6 (November–December 2016): 505–09. http://dx.doi.org/10.4103/0253-7176.194908.

Wassersug, Richard J., and Thomas W. Johnson. "Modern-Day Eunuchs: Motivations for and Consequences of Contemporary Castration." *Perspectives in Biology and Medicine* 50, no. 4 (Autumn 2007): 544–56. http://doi.org/10.1353/pbm.2007.0058.

White, Christine Cissy. "Putting Resilience and Resilience Surveys under the Microscope." *ACES Too High News*. February 5, 2017. https://acestoohigh.com/2017/02/05/__trashed-4/.

Yoon, Hahna. "How to Respond to Microaggressions." *New York Times*, March 3, 2020. https://www.nytimes.com/2020/03/03/smarter-living/how-to-respond-to-microaggressions.html.

PHOTO AND ILLUSTRATION CREDITS

Title Page
Holding the World, Jacqui Beck

Foreword
Tree House, Jacqui Beck

Introduction
In the Trees, Jacqui Beck

Section 1 | Gender, Sexual Orientation, Puberty, and Gender Dysphoria
Avian Gossip, Jacqui Beck

Chapter 1 | The Critical 911 Message
In the Very Middle, Jacqui Beck

Chapter 2 | Defining Gender
Chicken Connection, Jacqui Beck
Ultrasound fetal head, ultrasound labia, and ultrasound penis; anonymous contributor
Human Karyotype, iStock, somersault18:24
X for the Third Gender Category, iStock, nito100

Chapter 3 | Sexual Orientation
Sister Dance, Jacqui Beck

Chapter 4 | Deciding What You Want and Need
Plenty, Jacqui Beck

Chapter 5 | A Review of Puberty and Reproduction
Watching Over, Jacqui Beck
Homologues of External Genitalia, Frank Netter, MD, Netterimages.com
Sperm (Close Up), iStock, ktsimage
Female Reproductive System, iStock, 7activestudio
Menstrual Cycle, Endometrium, and Hormone, iStock, ttsz
Male Reproductive System, iStock, pixologicstudio
The Tanner Stages, used with permission from New England Journal of Medicine; Jean-Claude Carel and Juliane Léger, "Clinical Practice. Precocious Puberty," *New England Journal of Medicine* no. 358 (May 29, 2008): 2366–77, https://doi.org/10.1056/nejmcp0800459

Chapter 6 | Gender Dysphoria
Housework, Jacqui Beck
Sheep Conversion Therapy, NakedPastor.com
Confident Teenager Gives Important Message about Being Happy with Your Own Gender Identity, iStock, RS-photography
EPPY-EGG, Cynthia Radthorne

Section 2 | Hormones
To Fill, Jacqui Beck

Chapter 7 | Starting Hormones
Finding Our Way, Jacqui Beck
Odor in the Elevator, iStock, diane39
Vector Skeletal Formula of Spironolactone, Adobe Stock, Maxim Grebeshkov
Structural Formulas of Testosterone Molecule, Adobe Stock, logos2012
Pulmonary Embolism (2), iStock, JFalcetti
The Part of Internal Human Digestive System, iStock, rendixalextian
Human Heart Anatomy [Internal], iStock, melazerg
Human Heart Anatomy [External], iStock, melazerg

Anatomy of a Heart Attack, iStock, elenabs
Stent Angioplasty Procedure, iStock, blueringmedia
Heart Bypass Surgery, iStock, Graphic_BKK1979
5-Step CPR Guidelines, iStock, spkphotostock
Blood Plasma and Formed Elements in Test Tube, iStock, ttsz

Section 3 | Presentation: The Nonsurgical Things We Do to Show Who We Are
In a Bee Loud Glade, Jacqui Beck

Chapter 8 | Nonsurgical Ways to Appear More Feminine
What My Reflection Shows, Jacqui Beck
Hair Growth Cycle, iStock, neyro2008
The Alaskan Malamute, Adobe Stock, ekim
Floral Boots, Adobe Stock, I-Wei Huang
Erica Sciarretta portrait, Jenna Karwoski, jfkstudios.com
Image makeovers of Rachel and Jenny Robinson, Erica Sciarretta, Sorella Photos, sorellaphotos.com
Carla Petrulli portrait, Erica Sciarretta, Sorella Photos, sorellaphotos.com
Fashion Hipster Clothes Accessories Set, Adobe Stock, evgenij918
Capsule Clothes, iStock, Elizaveta Shishlyannikova

Chapter 9 | Nonsurgical Ways to Appear More Masculine
Perched, Jacqui Beck
Lancer Forney portrait, courtesy of Lancer Forney, Emerson Salon, emersonsalon.com
Juan Cardenas portrait, courtesy of Juan Cardenas, Prodigy Hair Studio, prodigyhairstudio.com
Vintage Smart Casual Outfit, Adobe Stock, ClaudiK
TransTape, courtesy of Kaiyote Jackson, TransTape, transtape.life
pStyle STP device, courtesy of Scout Rose, TransGuy Supply, transguysupply.com

Section 4 | Gender-Affirming Surgeries
Nature Reflecting, Jacqui Beck

Chapter 10 | Planning for Your Surgery
Many Socks, Jacqui Beck
Break Down Cigarette, Adobe Stock, Nopphon

Chapter 11 | The Surgeries Themselves
Conversation, Jacqui Beck
Feminizing Surgeries
Business Is Good! [stereotypically male and female faces], iStock, Yuri_Arcurs
Male and Female Skulls, used with permission from Addicus Books; Douglas K. Ousterhout, Facial Feminization Surgery; *A Guide for the Transgendered Woman*, Omaha: Addicus Books, 2010
Facial Feminization Surgery, Hillary Wilson, hwilsonillustration.com
Breast Implant Over and Under, Bob Bost
Homologues of External Genitalia, Frank Netter, MD, Netterimages.com
Male-to-Female Vaginoplasty [four illustrations], Hillary Wilson, hwilsonillustration.com
Perineum Anatomy Engraving 1886, iStock, THEPALMER
Scheme of the Course of the Peritoneum in Women, iStock, ilbusca
Peritoneum (Male), iStock, ilbusca
Large Intestine, Colon Sections Labeled in Male Abdominal Anatomy, iStock, Hank Grebe
Masculinizing Surgeries
Birdhouse, Jacqui Beck
Tracheal Augmentation, Chris Gralapp, chrisgralapp.com
Top-Surgery Scars, Bob Bost
Female Reproductive System, iStock, 7activestudio
Structure of the Skin, iStock, Paladjai
Forearm Flap Phalloplasty [three illustrations], Hillary Wilson, hwilsonillustration.com
Pedicle Flap Phalloplasty Steps, Bob Bost
Penis-Preserving Peritoneal Pull-Through Vaginoplasty, Bob Bost

Chapter 12 | Taking Care of Yourself after Surgery
Feels Like Home, Jacqui Beck
Resting on Your Side with Pillows, Bob Bost
Elevation of the Legs, Bob Bost
The Great Wall of Vagina, Panel 4, Jamie McCartney, jamiemccartney.com
Tyrannosaurus rex, iStock, Warpaintcobra
Pink Pockets, courtesy of Pink Pockets, pink-pockets.com
3D nipple tattoo, courtesy of the Vinnie Myers Team, vinniemyersteam.com
Saline Solution, iStock, kckate16
Phalloplasty tattoos, courtesy of FTM Tattoo, ftmtattoo.com/phalloplasty

Section 5 | Surviving and Thriving
Sueño de Milagros, Jacqui Beck

Chapter 13 | Coming Out
Not the Same, Jacqui Beck
Caring Mother Supporting Teen Boy, iStock, Motortion
Mature Woman with Man Relaxing, Adobe Stock, contrastwerkstatt
Little School Girl, iStock, fizkes
Two Women Sitting Together, Cynthia Radthorne

Chapter 14 | Finding Gender-Friendly Healthcare and Counseling
Earth Flying, Jacqui Beck
Medical Alert Bracelet, iStock, duckycards
Washington State POLST form, courtesy of Washington State Hospital Association, washington-state-hospital-association.myshopify.com

Chapter 15 | Education and Career Planning
Time Enough, Jacqui Beck
Businesswoman Analyzing Graph on Laptop, Adobe Stock, Andrey Popov

Chapter 16 | Microaggressions, Personal Safety, and Bullying
Catwatch, Jacqui Beck
Suffering Cyber Bullying, iStock, Marcos Calvo
The Upstander Pledge, courtesy of the Tyler Clementi Foundation, tylerclementi.org
Mac Scotty McGregor portrait, courtesy of Mac Scotty McGregor

Chapter 17 | Recognizing and Treating Depression
Comfort Found, Jacqui Beck
Woman Hand Holding Yellow Sponge, Adobe Stock, Ljiljana
Neuron, iStock, wetcake
Teenager Girl with Depression, Adobe Stock, Stanislaw Mikulski
Happy Woman with Mirror, Unsplash, Caroline Veronez
Reflection of Mystery Man, Adobe Stock, zephyr_p

Chapter 18 | Trauma-Informed Care and Resilience: Adverse Childhood Experiences and PTSD
Hidden Underneath, Jacqui Beck
Drawing Shows Young Girl's Inner Feelings about Being Abused, iStock, chameleonseye
Finding Your ACES Score, adapted from acestoohigh.com/got-your-ace-score/

Chapter 19 | Changing Your Documents
Inattention to Detail, Jacqui Beck
People Holding Passports, Adobe Stock, photobyphotoboy

Chapter 20 | Traveling
Tree in Cat, Jacqui Beck
Stealth Brothers HRT travel kit, courtesy of Stealth Bros & Co., stealthbrosco.com

Chapter 21 | Pregnancy Planning—and Avoidance—for Transgender Folks
Who I Listen To, Jacqui Beck
Breastfeeding, iStock, szeyuen
Slender Seahorse (Hippocampus reidi), iStock, wrangel
Jack Shephard and daughter photos, courtesy of Jack Shephard

Chapter 22 | Sex and Relationships
I Belong, Jacqui Beck
Online Dating by Phone, iStock, AnnaStills
Female Hand Pulling White Sheets in Ecstasy, Orgasm, Adobe Stock, Stavros
The Lost Keychain, Adobe Stock, Евгений Медведев
Buck Angel's T-Lube and Buck-Off, courtesy of Buck Angel, buckangel.com
Fascination Sleeves, courtesy of Joseph Mudge, GenderCat, gendercat.com
OK, Adobe Stock, リンドウ
Close Male and Female Friends Walking Down City Street Together, Adobe Stock, Mangostar
Prescription Drugs, Adobe Stock, JJAVA

Chapter 23 | How Transgender and Gender-Nonconforming Individuals Can Live Long, Healthy Lives
The Birthday Cat and the Giraffe Piñata, Jacqui Beck
All photos of Ginger Chien, Alison Peacock
Stephanie Dykes Sings with Seattle Men's Chorus, John Pai, courtesy of Seattle Men's Chorus
Christmas Eve in Las Cruces, Katherine Johnson

Conclusion
Still Forest, Jacqui Beck

About the Author
Linda Gromko portrait, Erica Sciarretta, Sorella Photos, sorellaphotos.com
Jacqui Beck portrait, Akasha Schutz

ACKNOWLEDGMENTS

A Practical Reference for Transgender and Gender-Nonconforming Adults brought together a committed group of professionals and an email reunion of the folks who contributed their talents to create *Where's MY Book? A Guide for Transgender and Gender Non-Conforming Youth, Their Parents, & Everyone Else.*

This project evolved over time into something much larger and more complex than I had originally envisioned. For this reason, we had two phases. I am eternally grateful to book designer Kathryn Campbell for getting this project off the ground. I learned that she truly embraced the transgender and gender-nonconforming community with great honor and care. I saw this especially in our last, somewhat revolutionary chapter—the one about living long and living well.

The bulk of the copyediting and secondary phase of design was completed by editor Mi Ae Lipe. Mi Ae also executed the important task of fact-checking and further elevated the graphic design and subject matter integration to a level I'd only envisioned. This book combined the best medical illustrations I could find, plus photographs, graphs, complex medical content, and a hodgepodge of personal stories—beautifully drawn together by Mi Ae into a credible whole. I am further grateful for Mi Ae's gentle midwifery in the enormous tasks of locating the proper ebook integrator and printers who made all the difference in getting this book out to the world. Thank you for your patience, Mi Ae.

I am grateful to my long-time friend Bob Bost. Bob's line drawings offer more medical clarity, helping me to explain tough concepts more effectively. Our butterfly logo, also Bob's design, is the registered trademark representing our practice. Combining the medical caduceus and the butterfly for transformation, Bob captured the essence of what we do.

Jacqui Beck's art is liberally sprinkled through this book, giving it more dimension and passion. What a joy to have her paintings in a book yet again. Read more about Jacqui's work on page 507. Thanks also to Richard Nicol, who photographed these paintings.

I recognize all my coworkers at Queen Anne Medical Associates and Transformative Aesthetics for weathering another book project. Most especially, I recognize and thank office manager Barbara Boni and Suzi Spinner, the director of Queen Anne Medical Electrolysis and Laser. Thanks to Carol Keenholts, ARNP, and Rachel Arnold, ARNP, our outstanding nurse practitioners—and to all of our staff.

I am grateful to Marsha Botzer, the founder of Seattle's internationally known Ingersoll Gender Center, for her mentorship, her foreword, and a friendship that spans decades.

As in the first book, I called on a village of professionals in trans medicine and related fields. These folks took their time to review my chapters and make additions and corrections. One of the surgeons, when asked to review this work, said, "It's a pandemic. I have some time on my hands!" These folks made their contributions with no expectation of remuneration—it was simply to add to the collective knowledge and to serve people, and they are listed here. And there must be people who have been inadvertently omitted; I thank them and ask their forgiveness.

I am supremely grateful to the following professionals who served as volunteer consultants and contributors for this book. In most cases, they reviewed specific chapters dealing with areas of expertise for accuracy. They often added comments, which are generally noted as quotations in the text. They are listed here in the approximate order of their appearance in the book. Contact and credential information may be found on their respective websites. Certain individuals are listed for other informational contributions.

Marsha Botzer	ingersollgendercenter.org
Aidan Key	genderdiversity.org
E. Antonio Mangubat, MD	labelleviecosmetic.com
Jennifer Hastings, MD	
Johanna Olson-Kennedy, MD	Dr. Olson-Kennedy's profile at Children's Hospital Los Angeles
Cynthia Radthorne	cynthiaradthorne.com
Toby R. Meltzer, MD	themeltzerclinic.com
Madeline Deutsch, MD, MPH	Dr. Deutsch's profile at the University of California-San Francisco Transgender Care
Ryan Tennant, DDS	2thstudio.com
Greyson Simon	translanguageprimer.com
J. Samuel Tolman, MD	Dr. Tolman's profile at Peace Health
Joseph Mudge	gendercat.com
Matthew D. Davies, MD, PhD	Dr. Davies's profile at Swedish Medical Center
Sandy Hirsch, MS CCC-SLP	givevoice.com
Robert Niedbalski, DO	hairreplacementsurgeon.com
William Collier	williamcollierdesign.com
Carla Petrulli	seattlemakeupartist.com
Erica Sciaretti	sorellaphotos.com
Amy E. White	linkedin.com/in/amyewhite44
Joanna Watson	linkedin.com/in/joanna-watson-0a1549163
Lancer Forney	emersonsalon.com
Juan Cardenas	prodigyhairstudio.com
Kaiyote Jackson	transtape.life
Scout Rose	transguysupply.com
Richard Santucci, MD	cranects.com
Curtis Crane, MD	cranects.com
Noah E. Lewis, Esq.	linkedin.com/in/noahelewis
Christine McGinn, DO	drchristinemcginn.com
M. Dru Lavasseur, Esq.	linkedin.com/in/mdlevasseur
Marci L. Bowers, MD	marcibowers.com
Jordan Deschamps-Braly, MD	deschamps-braly.com
Fermín Capitán, PhD	facialteam.eu
Scott Mosser, MD	genderconfirmation.com
Douglas K. Ousterhout, MD	deschamps-braly.com/dr-ousterhout-facial-feminization-surgeon-ffs

Thomas Satterwhite, MD	alignsurgical.com
Heidi Wittenberg, MD	mozaiccare.net
Geoffrey Stiller, MD	stilleraesthetics.com
Alvaro H. Rodriguez, MD	cecmcolombia.com
Harlowe Rayne Thunderword-Cohen	linkedin.com/in/harlowerayne-thunderword-cohen-4aba0b11a
Dev Gurjala, MD	alignsurgical.com
Finlay Games	finlaygames.com
Jamie McCartney	jamiemccartney.com
Vinnie Myers	vinniemyersteam.com
Shane Wallin	garnettattoo.com
Meiko Xavier	questhouseservices.wordpress.com
Stacey Prince, PhD	livingroomseattle.com/stacey-prince-phd.html
Jana Ekdahl, MA	transunfolds.homestead.com
Jane Clementi	tylerclementi.org
Mac Scotty McGregor	goodmenproject.com
Steven R. Mitchell, MD PhD	Dr. Mitchell's profile at Swedish Medical Center
Elaine Duncan, MA LMHC	counselinginbothell.com
Jack Shephard, RN	linkedin.com/in/jack-shephard-559318b1
Emily Nagoski, PhD	emilynagoski.com
Tina Schermer Sellers, PhD LMFT	tinaschermersellers.com
Ellie Zara Ley, MD	themeltzerclinic.com
Buck Angel	buckangel.com
NadjaDee	Contact Linda Gromko, MD, to reach NadjaDee
Andy Duran and Lisa Finn	www.babeland.com
Carol Queen, PhD	www.goodvibrations.com
Andrew M. Faulk, MD	smashwords.com/profile/view/Culbertson
Rachel Drake	www.consent.academy
Paulette de Coriolis, MA, LMHCA	paulettecounseling.com
Ginger Chien	linkedin.com/in/gingerchien
Stephanie Dykes, PhD	linkedin.com/in/stephanie-dykes-9828a2b
Katherine Johnson	unavocesola.wordpress.com
Barbara Sehr	barbarasehr.com

Gratitude to Our Financial Contributors

Finally, many thanks to the individuals who donated to my GoFundMe campaign—guardian angels do exist! While I did not include names of individuals out of respect for privacy, I must recognize Dr. Bob Niedbalski, Dr. Andrew Faulk, and David Hamilton for their extraordinary contributions!

I invite anyone wishing to contribute to cover book printing expenses and promotion to go to GoFundMe.com and search "Linda Gromko transgender book." (And thank you.)

INDEX

Page numbers with an *f* refer to a figure or a caption; *t* refers to a table; and *n* indicates a footnote.

D

F

G

H

I

N

O

P

Q

R

S

T

X

Y

Z

ABOUT THE AUTHOR

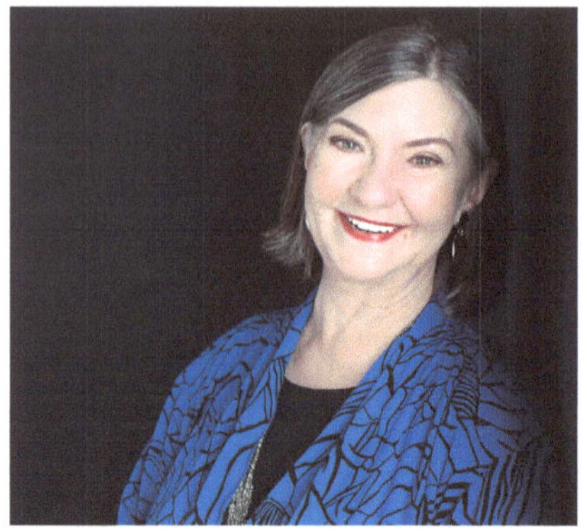

Linda Gromko, MD is a board-certified family practice physician who has worked with the transgender community since 1998, when a caller asked, "Does Dr. Gromko treat transgender women?" Dr. Gromko replied, "Not yet."

Thus began a decades-long commitment to transgender healthcare and education. Early experiences are discussed in the preface of this book, *A Practical Reference for Transgender and Gender-Nonconforming Adults*. Today, she is one of the few Seattle physicians who treats transgender folk of all ages, along with the rest of her broad-ranging family practice.

Dr. Gromko's interest in healthcare goes back to the age of 14 when she volunteered as a candy striper. She earned both her bachelor's and master's degrees in nursing from the University of Washington. While working as a nurse practitioner at Planned Parenthood in Seattle, Dr. Gromko began her premed classes and enrolled in the University of Washington School of Medicine when her son Tim was only 4 years old.

After graduation from the University of Washington Family Medicine Residency program, Dr. Gromko worked in a large emergency room and a number of women's clinics while setting up her own practice, which opened in 1989. Initially, the practice focused on women's healthcare and obstetrics. Dr. Gromko stopped delivering babies in 2005.

In mid-life, Dr. Gromko found the love of her life in Steve Williams. When Steve's health plummeted as a result of diabetic kidney failure, Dr. Gromko quickly learned to perform home kidney dialysis, which the couple did for more than 3 years before Steve's death in 2011. The experience of providing home care to a critically ill spouse made Dr. Gromko a bit of a zealot in promoting home kidney dialysis, as well as in preventing diabetes and kidney failure. Her two memoirs about this period won several awards, as did the award-winning guide, *Arranging Your Life When Dialysis Comes Home: The Underwear Factor,* written with interior designer Jane C. McClure.

Dr. Gromko loves to speak about transgender health and welcomes speaking invitations.

She makes her home in Seattle and spends free time kayaking, riding a "bike that goes nowhere," and writing.

Linda@LindaGromkoMD.com
LindaGromkoMD.com (Website and blog)
QueenAnneMedicalAssociates.com (Office)

ABOUT ARTIST JACQUI BECK

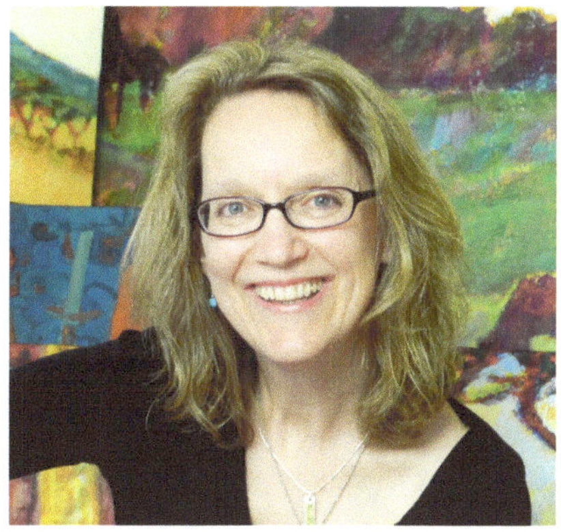

Jacqui Beck is an artist, art educator, and creativity coach living in Seattle, Washington. She has been teaching students of all ages for more than 15 years and is an adjunct professor of art at Seattle Pacific University. Her award-winning expressive acrylic paintings are collected and exhibited in the United States, Canada, Europe, and New Zealand. She has a master's degree in counseling psychology from the University of Victoria and is a trained life coach and creativity coach. She has studied at the Gage Academy of Art and with many nationally known artists.

In Jacqui Beck's words,

> "I create paintings using acrylics and mixed media. My artwork is colorful, personal, and expressive, and I keep in mind both the depth and whimsy of life. I often paint animal totem protectors representing the fierce strength of ourselves and those who love us. This strength, ideally, is tempered by a sense of paradox, irony, and humor. We can't always recognize our protectors by their appearance (notice chickens, birds, cats, and various strange or imaginary animals). The most powerful beings have an understanding of, and compassion for, our uniqueness and fallibility.
>
> "Like life, painting is an unfolding process of intention and accident. I notice what shows up and decide what to keep or enhance, and what to prune. The subject matter and meaning of my paintings are an exploration of what being a person means to me. I paint to explore my questions about life, about strength, fear, confusion, curiosity, and joy."

Jacqui Beck's project, Gender Personal, explores and celebrates gender variance through art, poetry, and recorded interviews. Its vision is to lead to social change and acceptance and to foster understanding by increasing awareness of the natural experience of gender variance. As the mother of a transgender son, Jacqui has a personal connection with this work. Many of the paintings in this book and in Gromko's earlier *Where's MY Book?* were done as part of the Gender Personal Project (**genderpersonal.org**). For more information on Jacqui Beck's more recent work, visit her website at **jacquibeck.com**.

www.ingramcontent.com/pod-product-compliance
Lightning Source LLC
LaVergne TN
LVHW070943210926
848482LV00002B/77
9780982514344